Morphea and Related Disorders

Edited by

Tasleem Arif

*Department of Dermatology, STDs, Leprosy and Aesthetics
Dar As Sihha Medical Center, Dammam, Saudi Arabia*

Ellahi Medicare Clinic, Srinagar, Kashmir, India

Morphea and Related Disorders

Editor: Tasleem Arif

ISBN (Online): 978-981-5080-98-8

ISBN (Print): 978-981-5080-99-5

ISBN (Paperback): 978-981-5123-00-5

First published in 2024.

need for a court order if at any point you breach any terms of this License Agreement. In no event will any delay or failure by Bentham Science Publishers in enforcing your compliance with this License Agreement constitute a waiver of any of its rights.

3. You acknowledge that you have read this License Agreement, and agree to be bound by its terms and conditions. To the extent that any other terms and conditions presented on any website of Bentham Science Publishers conflict with, or are inconsistent with, the terms and conditions set out in this License Agreement, you acknowledge that the terms and conditions set out in this License Agreement shall prevail.

Bentham Science Publishers Pte. Ltd.
80 Robinson Road #02-00
Singapore 068898
Singapore
Email: subscriptions@benthamscience.net

BENTHAM SCIENCE

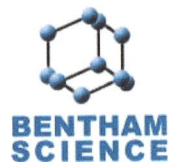

CONTENTS

FOREWORD

I feel privileged to write this foreword for the book titled "Morphea and Related Disorders", edited by Dr. Tasleem Arif unquestionably one of my most exceptionally brilliant students. Dr. Tasleem did his postgraduation in dermatology under my supervision as the head of the Postgraduate Department of Dermatology, Venereology, and Leprosy at Government Medical College Srinagar, Jammu and Kashmir, India. Throughout his post-graduation, Dr. Tasleem manifested a profound interest in Morphea and related disorders, leading him to select these disorders as the focal point of his thesis.

This remarkably comprehensive book efficaciously addresses the missing gaps in our understanding of the range of these disorders.

Focus on the classification of Morphea, a comprehensive account of topics like linear atrophoderma of Moulin, Idiopathic Atrophoderma of Pasini and Pierini, Parry-Romberg syndrome, and Extragenital Lichen sclerosus makes it interesting for the readers thereby transforming it into an invaluable resource book for dermatologists as well as rheumatologists

I congratulate Dr. Tasleem for coming forth with a book on a spectrum of disorders that are still an enigma for the practicing dermatologist.

Iffat Hassan
Government Medical College Srinagar, Jammu and Kashmir, India

PREFACE

The aim of this book titled "Morphea and related disorders" is to give a comprehensive and detailed description of morphea and some of the disorders related to it. Morphea as a subject, has not been addressed adequately as other topics in dermatology like pigmentary dermatoses, bullous disorders, psoriasis, atopic dermatitis, etc. Patients of morphea are mainly managed by dermatologists and rheumatologists though other specialties like pediatrics, internal medicine, gynecology and obstetrics, and orthopedics are also involved in managing such patients. There have been several debates regarding various aspects of morphea especially its terminology, classification, etc. Unfortunately, I couldn't come across a single book, which has exclusively addressed morphea in total. Moreover, there has been plenty of confusion regarding certain conditions like Linear atrophoderma of Moulin, Parry Romberg syndrome, Idiopathic atrophoderma of Pasini and Pierini, Eosinophilic fasciitis and Lichen sclerosus; whether they constitute subtypes of morphea or they are separate disease entities. Thus, there existed an unmet need for a book giving an in-depth understanding of morphea and to give a compendious account of such bewildering conditions. Through this book, I have tried to address such issues.

The inspiration for writing the book on this subject came in 2012 during my dermatology residency programme when I was assigned thesis related to scleroderma. My research was based on both localized (morphea) as well as systemic (systemic sclerosis) forms of scleroderma. Since, the enrollment of my first patient for thesis research, I have been collecting data, figures, etc. as a preparation for this unique book project. So in other words, the drafting for book has been for the last 2-3 years but the actual preparation has been there for a decade. One of the major boosts to my confidence to write on this subject came from New England Journal of medicine (NEJM). Every physician is well aware of the impact and reputation which NEJM has in medical science. My basic research on morphea and systemic sclerosis was published in 2015 in BMC Gastroenterology Journal. That research was reviewed by NEJM in their journal watch and they concluded their journal watch based on findings of our research. That gave me an impetus to write on scleroderma. Since then, I have consistently made research on scleroderma and published around 25 research articles related to it. With such numbers and expertise in scleroderma, I felt probably I can attempt to edit and author a book on morphea. The everlasting prayers of my parents for my success have been a pillar in shaping my career.

Being the solo editor as well as author/co-author of 12 chapters (out of 20 chapters) of this book, the journey of this book for the past 2-3 years has seen lots of ups and downs. One of the major reasons was Covid-19. Apart from that, this era has been full of trials to me and my family. We have faced practically some calamities. At one stage, the circumstances became so difficult that I felt I will not be able to edit or author this book. But massive credit goes to my wife, Dr Marwa Sami, who knew what this book means to me. Despite our strenuous and back-breaking conditions, she kept me motivating and giving me timely reminders to complete this book. I don't feel this book could have been accomplished without her continuous motivation.

There are several features which add uniqueness to this book. Probably, the first book which has been written exclusively on morphea describing it's all parameters ranging from etiology to treatment. There are individual chapters' on topics like linear atrophoderma of Moulin, Parry Romberg syndrome, Idiopathic atrophoderma of Pasini and Pierini, Eosinophilic fasciitis, Lichen sclerosus and Pediatric morphea. Even in the most advanced textbooks of dermatology, we can hardly find any substantial account on such topics. Every chapter begins with a table having the main substance summarized in the form of chapter synopsis. Learning points in the form of a table are provided at the end of each chapter so that readers can conclude what they have learnt from the chapter. The text of each chapter is enriched with ample number of boxes and tables to enhance the readability. Boxes are provided to summarize the content of a particular section for quick revision. This book will serve as reference book to dermatologists, rheumatologists and physicians ranging from resident to professor as well as practicing physicians. Ultimately, I am hopeful that readers will unveil several horizons related to morphea and its related disorders while reading this book.

Tasleem Arif
Department of Dermatology, STDs, Leprosy and Aesthetics
Dar As Sihha Medical Center, Dammam, Saudi Arabia

Ellahi Medicare Clinic, Srinagar, Kashmir, India

DEDICATION

This book is dedicated to:

............If anyone killed an innocent human, it would be as if he killed all mankind; And if anyone saved a life, it would be as if he saved the life of entire mankind.........

(The Glorious Quran; Chapter 5: Verse 32.)

As an editor and author/co-author (of 12 chapters out of 20) of this book, if only one human gets correctly diagnosed and treated as a result of this book, I will feel that I have done my job.

List of Contributors

Adriana Polańska
Department of Dermatology and Venereology, University of Medical Sciences, Poznan, Poland

Aleksandra Dańczak-Pazdrowska
Department of Dermatology, University of Medical Sciences, Poznan, Poland

Anju George
Department of Dermatology, Christian Medical College, Vellore, Tamil Nadu, India

Abid Keen
Dermatology Clinic, Esthetica Skin, Hair and Dental Institute. Nai Basti, Anantnag, Kashmir, India

Dorota Krasowska
Department of Dermatology, Venereology and Pediatric Dermatology, Medical University of Lublin, Lublin, Poland

Defne Ozkoca
Department of Dermatology and Venereology, Cerrahpasa Medical Faculty, Istanbul University-Cerrahpasa, Istanbul, Turkey

Katarzyna Wolska-Gawron
Department of Dermatology, Venereology and Pediatric Dermatology, Medical University of Lublin, Lublin, Poland

Marwa Sami
Department of Dermatology, Venereology and Andrology, Ministry of Health, Algharbeya, Egypt

Mohammad Adil
Department of Dermatology, Jawaharlal Nehru Medical College (JNMC), Aligarh Muslim University (AMU), Aligarh, India

Muazzez Cigdem Oba
Department of Dermatology and Venereology, Sancaktepe Sehit Prof. Dr. Ilhan Varank Research and Training Hospital, Istanbul, Turkey

Marcia Ramos-e-Silva
Sector of Dermatology and Post-Graduation Course in Dermatology, University Hospital and School of Medicine, Federal University of Rio de Janeiro, Rio de Janeiro, Brazil

Ovgu Aydin Ulgen
Department of Pathology, Cerrahpaşa Medical Faculty, Istanbul University-Cerrahpasa, Istanbul, Turkey

Ömer Kutlu
Department of Dermatology and Venereology, Tokat Gaziosmanpasa University, School of Medicine, Tokat, Turkey

Özge Aşkin
Department of Dermatology, Cerrahpasa Medicine Faculty İstanbul University-Cerrahpaşa, İstanbul, Turkey

Ola Ahmed Bakry
Department of Dermatology, Andrology and STDs, Faculty of Medicine, Menoufiya University, Menoufiya Governorate, Egypt

Parvaiz Anwar Rather
Department of Dermatology, Venereology & Leprosy, Government Medical College, Baramulla, Jammu and Kashmir, India

Ryszard Żaba
Department of Dermatology and Venereology, University of Medical Sciences, Poznan, Poland

Renata Cavalcante
Sector of Dermatology and Post-Graduation Course in Dermatology, University Hospital and School of Medicine, Federal University of Rio de Janeiro, Rio de Janeiro, Brazil

Sueli Carneiro   Sector of Dermatology and Post-Graduation Course in Dermatology, University Hospital and School of Medicine, Federal University of Rio de Janeiro, Rio de Janeiro, Brazil

Sabha Mushtaq   Department of Dermatology, Venereology and Leprosy, Government Medical College, Jammu, Jammu and Kashmir, India

Safia Bashir   Medical officer, Jammu & Kashmir Health Services, Kashmir. Jammu & Kashmir, India

Shazia Jeelani   Department of Dermatology, STDs and Leprosy, Government Medical College, Srinagar, Kashmir, India

Tasleem Arif   Department of Dermatology, STDs, Leprosy and Aesthetics, Dar As Sihha Medical Center, Dammam, Saudi Arabia
Ellahi Medicare Clinic, Srinagar, Kashmir, India

Tugba Kevser Uzuncakmak   Memorial Health Group, Sisli Hospital, Istanbul, Turkey

Yasmeen Jabeen Bhat   Department of Dermatology, Venereology and Leprosy, Government Medical College Srinagar, University of Kashmir, Jammu & Kashmir, India

Zygmunt Adamski   Department of Dermatology, University of Medical Sciences, Poznan, Poland

Introduction and History

Tasleem Arif[1,2,*]

[1] *Department of Dermatology, STD's, Leprosy and Aesthetics, Dar As Sihha Medical center, Dammam, Saudi Arabia*

[2] *Ellahi Medicare Clinic, Srinagar, Kashmir, India*

Chapter Synopsis.
• Scleroderma is a spectrum of disorders characterized by thickening and/ or hardening of the skin and fibrosis of the involved tissues. It is divided into localized and systemic forms. The localized form is called morphea and the systemic form is the systemic sclerosis.
• The terms 'Localized scleroderma' and 'morphea' are not synonymous though they have been frequently used interchangeably.
• Morphea is differentiated from systemic sclerosis by the absence of sclerodactyly, vascular symptoms in the form of Raynaud's phenomenon, abnormalities of the nail fold capillaries, and specific internal organ system involvement like gastrointestinal tract, lung, and kidneys.
• Clinically, morphea is characterised by round or oval, irregular or linear plaques that are initially dull red or violaceous or brownish, smooth and indurated/sclerosed but later turn atrophic.
• Previously, morphea was considered a self-limiting disease. Currently, there is ample evidence to suggest that it can have a protracted, relapsing–remitting course. Certain types of morphea if left untreated, can cause significant cosmetic and functional disability.
• Several treatment options are available for morphea which include topicals, phototherapy, and systemic agents.

Keywords: Anti-nuclear antibody, Diffuse cutaneous systemic sclerosis, Fibrosis, Flexion contractures, Generalized localized scleroderma, Idiopathic atrophoderma of Pasini and Pierini, Keloid of Alibert, Lichen sclerosus, Limited cutaneous systemic sclerosis, Linear atrophoderma of Moulin, Localized scleroderma, Methotrexate, Morphea, Parry Romberg syndrome, Raynaud's phenomenon, Sclerosis, Scleroderma, Sclerodactyly, Systemic sclerosis, Systemic scleroderma.

* **Corresponding author Tasleem Arif:** Department of Dermatology, STD's, Leprosy and Aesthetics, Dar As Sihha Medical center, Dammam, Saudi Arabia and Ellahi Medicare Clinic, Srinagar, Kashmir, India; E-mail: dr_tasleem_arif@yahoo.com

INTRODUCTION

Morphea is a group of chronic inflammatory diseases which is characterized by sclerosis of the skin as a result of excessive collagen deposition in the dermis and subcutaneous tissue [1]. The word scleroderma has been widely used to account for any condition where there are skin lesions associated with sclerosis of the skin. However, to be precise, the term scleroderma is used to connote a spectrum of disorders, which are characterized by sclerotic skin lesions as their primary disease process and presentation. These include a localized and a systemic form. The localized type which has been inappropriately termed as *'localized scleroderma'*, denotes a group of related disorders characterized by varying degrees of sclerosis, fibrosis and atrophy in the skin and subcutaneous tissues, that can occasionally extend deep into the fascia, muscle, bone and brain. However, the term *localized scleroderma* is not appropriate and a more apt term "Morphea" has been introduced in the literature to account for the confusion created by the term localized scleroderma'. Firstly, under the umbrella term of *localized scleroderma*, other disorders can be incorporated into it whose primary manifestation is not scleroderma; scleroderma is one of their secondary manifestations. There is a long list of such diseases which can have lesions similar to *localized scleroderma,* notable among them are chronic graft-versus-host disease, lipodermatosclerosis, porphyria cutanea tarda, *etc.* Secondly, among the types of morphea, there is an entity called generalized morphea which can be read as *'generalized localized scleroderma'* if we use the term *localized scleroderma* instead of morphea. The term *"generalized localized scleroderma"* will be a source of confusion to the authors as well as to the readers. Hence, this term *localized scleroderma* is discouraged and that is the reason throughout this book the term morphea will be preferred instead of *localized scleroderma.* On the other hand, the systemic form of scleroderma is systemic sclerosis (SSC), which, in addition to sclerotic skin lesions, is characterized by the presence of sclerodactyly, vascular symptoms in the form of Raynaud phenomenon, abnormalities of the nail fold capillaries, and specific internal organ system involvement like gastrointestinal tract, lung, kidneys, *etc.* Though the process of development of sclerosis in the skin may follow similar mechanisms in the two diseases (morphea and systemic sclerosis); these are considered as two distinct entities with different antibody profiles, prognosis and treatment.

SSC has been further classified into two subtypes: limited cutaneous systemic sclerosis (LcSSC) and diffuse cutaneous systemic sclerosis (DcSSC). The former affects the distal extremities leading to sclerodactyly. It is associated with a long preceding history of Raynaud phenomenon, telangiectasias, and gastrointestinal involvement, and conveys a risk of isolated pulmonary artery hypertension. On the contrary, DcSSC is differentiated from LcSSC by proximal (above the knee and elbow and trunk) involvement of the skin. Though patients with DcSSC also suffer from sclerodactyly, they have a shorter history of onset of the Raynaud phenomenon, telangiectasias, and gastrointestinal involvement. These patients are at increased risk of interstitial lung fibrosis and renal crisis. These two subsets also have contrasting specific antibody profiles [2 - 5].

Morphea is an uncommon, autoimmune disease though relatively benign, characterized by round or oval, irregular or linear plaques that are initially dull red or violaceous or brownish (Fig. **1.1**), smooth and indurated/sclerosed but later turn atrophic. They are histologically characterized by sclerosis of the dermis and/or subcutaneous tissue (Fig. **1.2**) [1]. They are commonly confined to the skin and subcutaneous tissues; less commonly they can extend deeper and involve fat, fascia, muscle, bone and joints and rarely involve the eyes and brain. Like most of the other autoimmune diseases, morphea has been reported as more common in females. Though autoantibodies such as antinuclear antibody (ANA), antihistone, and anti-ssDNA can be found in the patients of morphea; however the SSC-specific autoantibodies such as anticentromere, anti-topoisomerase, and anti-RNA polymerase antibodies are rarely found in these patients. In addition, the organ system involvement that is typical of SSC, viz., gastrointestinal tract involvement, lung involvement and scleroderma renal disease does not occur in morphea. Though, nearly one-fifth to one-quarter of patients with morphea have been reported to experience extracutaneous manifestations but the SSC-specific organ system involvement doesn't occur in morphea. Previously, morphea was considered a self-limiting disease. However in the last decade, many reviews have been published on morphea and there is ample evidence to suggest that a protracted, relapsing–remitting course may be common in morphea. Certain types of morphea if left untreated, can cause significant cosmetic and functional morbidity. Though the disease itself doesn't seem to increase the chance of mortality; however, the disease can lead to significant morbidity as a result of flexion contractures, limb and facial asymmetry, extracutaneous manifestations, eye and CNS involvement; and psychological disability [6 - 9].

The treatment of morphea has been updated. Currently, there are several treatment options available for morphea which include topicals, phototherapy, systemic drugs, and recently biologicals. The choice of agent for treatment will depend upon several factors like the type of the morphea, the extent of the disease, the activity of the disease, the presence of deformities, *etc*. In the treatment of severe morphea, methotrexate in combination with systemic steroids and ultraviolet A1 light phototherapy has been the most effective treatment option [7].

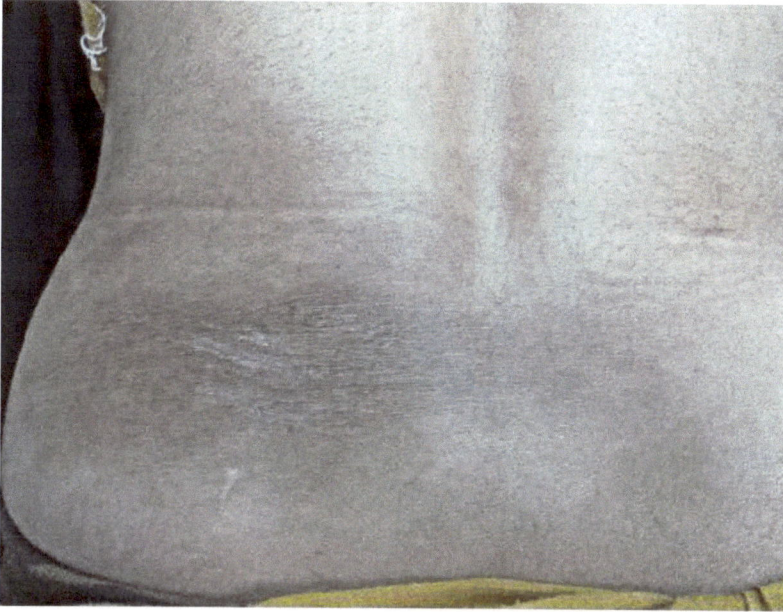

Fig. (1.1). Morphea: Ill-defined brownish hyperpigmented indurated plaque over lower back. [Copyright: Arif T, Hassan I, Nisa N. Morphea and vitiligo-A very uncommon association. Our Dermatol Online. 2015;6(2):232-234].

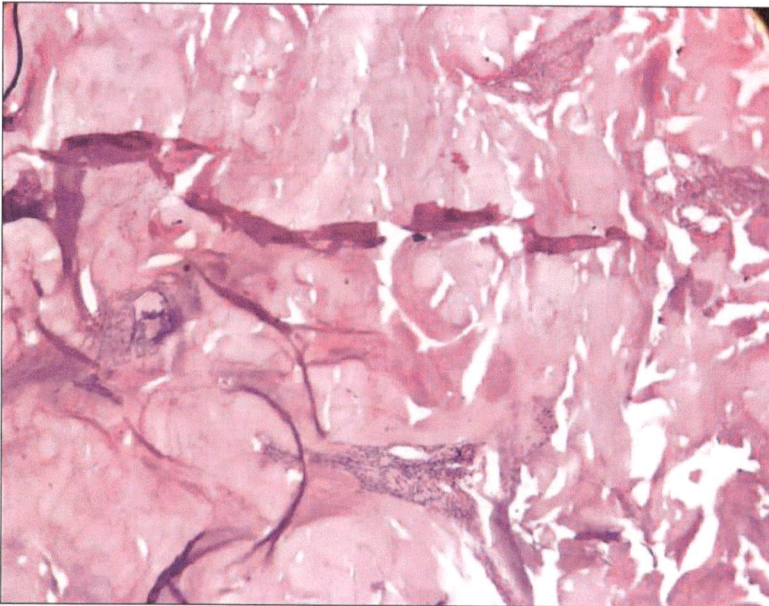

Fig. (1.2). Histopathology of morphea showing dense homogenized bundles of collagen in the dermis (H and E, 100x).

There are several other dermatoses which have been described in close relation with morphea. They can cause great diagnostic confusion as they may be seen occurring in association with morphea. They can possess similar clinical and histopathological findings. These include *idiopathic atrophoderma of Pasini and Pierini* (IAPP), *linear atrophoderma of Moulin* (LAM), *Parry Romberg syndrome* (PRS), *Eosinophilic fasciitis* (EF) and *lichen sclerosus (LS)*. These have been discussed separately and in appropriate chapters in the book.

HISTORY

The history of morphea dates back to some 400 BC (Table **1.1**) when Hippocrates mentioned a condition of thickened skin. Literally, the word "scleroderma" has been derived from the Greek words '*skleros*' meaning 'hard or indurated' and '*derma*' referring to skin. Curzio of Naples described the first case of generalized "hardness" of the skin in a young woman in 1752.

Table 1.1. History of Scleroderma.

400 B.C	Hippocrates mentioned a condition of thickened skin
1752	Curzio of Naples described a case of generalized "hardness" of the skin in a young woman
1847	Gintrac coined the term "sclérodermie"
1854	Thomas Addison introduced the concept "Keloid of Alibert" and tried to differentiate it from true keloid.
1924	Matsui described the typical histopathologic changes of scleroderma
1930	O'Leary and Nomland elaborated on the differentiating features of morphea and systemic sclerosis.

The term *"sclérodermie"* was coined by the French physician Gintrac in 1847. The first detailed description of morphea was given by Thomas Addison. He described a few cases with keloidal lesions and referred to them as *"Keloid of Alibert"* in 1854. He tried to differentiate it from the true keloid. He used the term *"Keloid of Alibert"* as he believed that Alibert was the first to discriminate and accurately describe this condition [10]. The typical histopathologic changes of scleroderma, including the increase in collagen and thickening of vessel walls in the involved skin were described by Matsui in 1924. The differentiating features of morphea and systemic sclerosis were described by O'Leary and Nomland in 1930 [11].

Box 1.1: Learning points.
• Morphea is a type of scleroderma characterized predominantly by the involvement of the skin, commonly confined to the skin and subcutaneous tissues; less commonly can extend deeper and involve fat, fascia, muscle, bone and joints and rarely involve the eyes and the brain.
• About one-fifth to one-quarter of patients with morphea experience extracutaneous manifestations. However, the organ system involvement that is typical of SSC doesn't occur in it.
• Once considered a self-limiting disease, it can follow a protracted, relapsing-remitting course. Some types of morphea if left untreated, can lead to significant functional and cosmetic disability but the overall prognosis is better than systemic sclerosis.

REFERENCES

[1]   Arif T, Adil M, Amin SS, *et al.* Clinico-epidemiological Study of Morphea from a Tertiary Care Hospital. Curr Rheumatol Rev 2018; 14: 201-204.
         [PMID: 29637865]

[2]   Arif T, Adil M, Sodhi JS. Upper gastrointestinal endoscopy in systemic sclerosis: A cross sectional study. J Pak Assoc Dermatol 2019;29 (4):374-383.

[3]   Arif T, Hassan I. Raynauds phenomenon in systemic sclerosis: Its prevalence and its relationship with the disease onset and subset-An experience from the Kashmir valley, India. West Indian Med journal 2018; 67 (1): 52-56.

[4]   Arif T, Adil M, Singh Sodhi J, Hassan I. Assessment of modified Rodnan skin score and esophageal manometry in systemic sclerosis: a study correlating severity of skin and esophageal involvement by objective measures. Acta Dermatovenerol Alp Pannonica Adriat. 2018; 27: 169-173.
         [PMID: 30564828]

[5]   Arif T, Adil M, Hassan I. Antibody profile in systemic sclerosis patients: A cross sectional study from Kashmir Valley of India. J Pak Assoc Derm 2018; 28(1): 45-50.

[6]   Fett N, Werth VP. Update on morphea: part I. Epidemiology, clinical presentation, and pathogenesis. J Am Acad Dermatol 2011; 64(2): 217–28.
         [http://dx.doi.org/10.1016/j.jaad.2010.05.045] [PMID: 21238823]

[7]   Fett N, Werth VP. Update on morphea: part II. Outcome measures and treatment. J Am Acad Dermatol 2011; 64(2): 231–42.
         [http://dx.doi.org/10.1016/j.jaad.2010.05.046] [PMID: 21238824]

[8]   Fett N. Scleroderma: nomenclature, etiology, pathogenesis, prognosis, and treatments: facts and controversies. Clin Dermatol 2013; 31(4): 432–7.
         [http://dx.doi.org/10.1016/j.clindermatol.2013.01.010] [PMID: 23806160]

[9]   Arif T, Majid I, Haji MLI. Late onset 'en coup de sabre' following trauma: Rare presentation of a rare disease. Our Dermatol Online 2015; 6(1): 49-51.
         [http://dx.doi.org/10.7241/ourd.20151.12]

[10]   Addison T. On the keloid of Alibert, and on true keloid. Med Chirurg Trans. 1854; 37: 27.
         [http://dx.doi.org/10.1177/095952875403700106] [PMID: 20896031]

[11]   O'Leary PA, Nomland R. A clinical study of one hundred and three cases of scleroderma. Am J Med Sci. 1930; 180: 95.
         [http://dx.doi.org/10.1097/00000441-193007000-00013]

CHAPTER 2

Classification

Tasleem Arif[1,2,*] and **Marwa Sami**[3]

[1] *Department of Dermatology, STDs, Leprosy and Aesthetics, Dar As Sihha Medical Center, Dammam, Saudi Arabia*

[2] *Ellahi Medicare Clinic, Srinagar, Kashmir, India*

[3] *Department of Dermatology, Venereology and Andrology, Ministry of Health, Algharbeya, Egypt*

Chapter Synopsis.
• Morphea comprises a group of distinct conditions that primarily involve the skin and subcutaneous tissues.
• Involvement of internal organ systems like lungs, gastrointestinal tract, kidneys and heart is usually absent in morphea.
• There are several types of morphea. Each type has a different clinical presentation and level of tissue involvement. However, the common denominator among the types of morphea is the presence of skin thickening (induration) with an increased amount of collagen in the lesion.
• Due to the broad clinical spectrum, several attempts have been made to classify morphea. However, to date no universally accepted classification system has been proposed which can account for all the heterogeneity seen in the clinical spectrum of this disease.
• Conditions like linear atrophoderma of Moulin (LAM), Idiopathic Atrophoderma of Pasini and Pierini (IAPP), Lichen sclerosus (LS), Eosinophilic fasciitis (EF) and Parry-Romberg syndrome (PRS) are related to morphea. Their relation with the morphea has been a topic of debate. These conditions need to be discussed thoroughly.

Keywords: Bullous morphea, Circumscribed morphea, Deep morphea, Disabling pansclerotic morphea, En coup de sabre, Eosinophilic fasciitis, Guttate morphea, Generalized morphea, Idiopathic atrophoderma of Pasini and Pierini, Keloidal morphea, Lichen sclerosus, Limited plaque morphea, Linear morphea, Mixed morphea, Morphea en plaque, Nodular morphea, Parry-Romberg syndrome, Plaque morphea, Progressive hemifacial atrophy, Subcutaneous morphea.

INTRODUCTION

Morphea, inappropriately also called as, localized scleroderma, comprises a group of distinct conditions that primarily involve the skin and subcutaneous tissues.

---

[*] **Corresponding author Tasleem Arif:** Department of Dermatology, STDs, Leprosy and Aesthetics, Dar As Sihha Medical center, Dammam, Saudi Arabia and Ellahi Medicare Clinic, Srinagar, Kashmir, India;
E-mail: dr_tasleem_arif@yahoo.com

Lesions clinically range from very small plaques limited to the skin only, to diseases that have the potential to cause significant physiological and aesthetic deformities, with a wide range of extracutaneous manifestations. Based on the specific subtype and localization, structures near the skin that include fascia, muscles, fat, bones and joints can also get affected. Involvement of internal organ systems like the lungs, gastrointestinal tract, kidneys and the heart is usually absent in morphea. Morphea should be viewed as a distinct entity from systemic sclerosis because of its almost exclusive cutaneous involvement and absence of visceral organ involvement except in rare instances. The differences between morphea and systemic sclerosis have already been discussed in chapter 1.

There are several types of morphea. Each type has a different clinical presentation and level of tissue involvement. However, the common denominator among the types of morphea is the presence of skin thickening (Induration) with an increased amount of collagen in the indurated lesion at any stage of disease evolution [1, 2]. Due to its broad clinical spectrum, several different attempts have been made to classify morphea. However, to date, no universally accepted classification system has been proposed which can account for all the heterogeneity seen in the clinical spectrum of morphea. Despite several classification systems which have categorized the disease, there are still controversies among authors as to which conditions should be included within the spectrum of morphea. This is particularly relevant with the three related atrophic variants *viz.*, linear atrophoderma of Moulin (LAM), Idiopathic Atrophoderma of Pasini and Pierini (IAPP) and Parry-Romberg syndrome (PRS). A similar fate is faced by Eosinophilic fasciitis and Lichen sclerosus (LS). There has been controversy regarding bullous morphea and deep morphea. Whether the two should be kept as separate subtypes or not. Another headache to the system of classification is what constitutes generalized morphea as it has been defined in different ways by different authors. In this chapter, the authors will describe the various classification systems that have been suggested for morphea. However, in view of the lack of a single universally accepted classification system of morphea, the author has suggested a simple classification which can avoid most of the controversies by taking some suggestions from the already published classification systems. That classification system will be followed throughout this book.

CLASSIFICATION BY O' LEARY *ET AL.*

The earliest attempt to classify scleroderma was made by O'Leary and Nomland. They published their clinical study of 103 cases of scleroderma in 1930. They broadly classified scleroderma into two types: 1) Generalized forms of scleroderma (associated with a varying degree of systemic involvement), 2) Localized forms of scleroderma, usually without systemic manifestations. Localized scleroderma is further divided into two types Table (**2.1**). A) Morphea and B) Other types [3, 4]. The classification of localized scleroderma is described as follows:

Table 2.1. Classification of localized scleroderma by O' leary *et al.*

Localized Scleroderma	
I. Morphea	**II. Other types**
Localized	Linear
Generalized	Localized forms associated with hemiatrophy including en coup de sabre

Morphea

Localized

According to them, a localized variant of morphea comprised of cutaneous patches having a variable size of 2 to 20 cm. These patches were having varied clinical presentations ranging from the classically sclerosed, carnauba wax-colored plaque to hyperpigmented atrophic areas present over the trunk and extremities. These lesions have signs of inflammation and later involute of their own.

Generalized

In generalized morphea, numerous plaques are present which at times may involve the entire trunk, though they didn't give the definite criteria to diagnose generalized morphea. These plaques have pigmentation, atrophy and sclerosis depending upon the stage of evolution of the disease. The prognosis of this type was considered good.

Other Types

Linear

In this type, there are linear bands or streaks of waxy/sclerosed skin involving a limb. It may or may not be associated with plaque morphea.

Localized Forms Associated with Hemiatrophy

This subtype may present with a small indurated plaque on the forehead or scalp and can include linear morphea en coup de sabre. There can be atrophy of bone or muscle of the face in collaboration with the involvement of upper or lower limbs or both. Though there is hardly any risk of mortality, there is variable morbidity depending upon the magnitude of hemiatrophy and any associated congenital defects.

This classification though kick-started the process of classifying morphea, however, there were many limitations in the classification system. Some of them are mentioned as follows. Firstly, there was no clear-cut definition of generalized morphea with regard to the number of lesions or the size of lesions or the number of anatomic areas affected by the disease. Secondly, the most severe form of morphea, the pansclerotic type was not mentioned in the classification. Thirdly, the classification broadly divided scleroderma into localized and systemic forms, however, the intermediate forms like linear atrophoderma of Moulin (LAM), Idiopathic Atrophoderma of Pasini and Pierini (IAPP), Lichen sclerosus (LS), *etc.* were left out. Finally, a mixed type of morphea where different types can be present in the same patient was lacking in the system.

CLASSIFICATION OF LOCALIZED SCLERODERMA BY RODNAN ET AL (1979)

Rodnan, Jablonska and Medsger in 1979 divided localized scleroderma into two broad types: 1) Morphea and 2) Linear scleroderma [5, 6]. Their classification is mentioned in Table **2.2**.

Table 2.2. Classification of localized scleroderma by Rodnan *et al.*

Localized Scleroderma	
I. Morphea	**II. Linear scleroderma**
Plaque	Scleroderma en coup de sabre with or without associated facial hemiatrophy
Generalized	
Guttate	
Subcutaneous	
Bullous	
Keloidal	
Superficial primary atrophic morphea (atrophoderma of Pasini and Pierini)	

Morphea

Morphea was further divided into plaque type, generalized, guttate, subcutaneous type, keloidal, bullous type and superficial primary atrophic morphea (atrophoderma of Pasini and Pierini)

Linear Scleroderma

Scleroderma en coup de sabre with or without associated facial hemiatrophy. This classification system was a refined one over the previous classification. Some new terms were introduced in the classification like guttate morphea, bullous type, keloidal form, *etc.* However, it had similar limitations as the previous one. Generalized morphea was not defined with respect to the number or size of plaques. Similarly, intermediate scleroderma entities like LAM, LS, *etc.* were not mentioned in the classification, though they tried to accommodate the atrophoderma of Pasini and Pierini in the morphea classification system [6].

MODIFIED AMERICAN RHEUMATISM ASSOCIATION (ARA) CLASSIFICATION FOR LOCALIZED SCLERODERMA

The classification of localized scleroderma by ARA has been mentioned in Table **2.3**. They broadly divided localized scleroderma into two types: morphea and linear scleroderma both having subtypes.

Table 2.3. Modified ARA Classification of localized scleroderma.

S. No.	Type
1.	**Morphea**
	Limited
	Plaque
	Guttate
	Generalized
	Others (deep)
	Nodular
	Subcutaneous
	Profunda
2.	**Linear scleroderma**
	Linear
	En coup de sabre

According to them, plaque-type morphea can occur at any part of the body rarely involving the face and extremities. The size of the plaque may vary from 1cm to the palm of the hand. As a rule of thumb, skin is moveable over the underlying tissues. The plaque may start as an erythematous and edematous area or as an ivory white plaque with the lilac ring. The disease is usually self-limiting in 3-5 years but rarely may persist for as long as 25 years.

Guttate morphea usually presents with multiple superficial white papules of varying sizes (2-10 mm). The sites of predilection include the shoulders and chest. The lesions lack follicular plugging, a feature differentiating them from LS. The lesions are arranged in a linear band.

Generalized morphea presents with lesions similar to plaque-type morphea but in widespread distribution and the lesions show a tendency to coalesce with one another and extend peripherally. Generalized morphea is usually bilateral and lesions may show secondary changes like pigmentation, development of bullae, calcinosis and purpura. Such patients may develop complications like ulcers, contracture and disability. Long-standing ulcers may develop malignant change. These patients usually suffer from morbidity and disability for years.

Linear scleroderma usually involves the pediatric population although it can persist till adulthood. It usually involves the upper and lower limbs. Atrophy, sclerosis, contractures and limitations of limb movement can occur. When linear scleroderma involves the forehead and scalp causing atrophy, and sclerosis and can extend to the underlying bone, it is termed as en coup de sabre [7].

This classification considered three subtypes for the deep morphea *viz.*, nodular, subcutaneous and profunda. This classification too had several drawbacks like what constitutes the generalized morphea. Objective criteria to define generalized morphea was lacking. They did not include the Idiopathic Atrophoderma of Pasini and Pierini (IAPP) in the classification system owing to the controversial relationship between morphea and IAPP. A good percentage of patients have two or more than two types of morphea called mixed morphea. That was also missing in the classification. Similar was the case with LAM, PRS and Pansclerotic morphea.

CLASSIFICATION OF MORPHEA BY PETERSON *ET AL.*

In view of the limitations of ARA classification of localized scleroderma, *Peterson et al.* in 1995 came up with a better classification scheme [8]. They classified morphea into five general types: plaque morphea, generalized morphea, bullous morphea, linear morphea, and deep morphea Table **2.4**. This classification has been widely used by dermatologists throughout the globe though it was also having some limitations. This classification tried to give a holistic approach to classifying morphea. An account of this classification is as follows:

Table 2.4. Classification of morphea by *Peterson et al.*

S. No.	Type
1.	**Plaque morphea** • Morphea en plaque • Guttate morphea • Atrophoderma of Pasini and Pierini • Keloid morphea (nodular morphea) • Lichen sclerosus
2.	**Generalized morphea**
3.	**Bullous morphea**
4.	**Linear morphea** • Linear morphea (linear scleroderma) • En coup de sabre • Progressive hemifacial atrophy
5.	**Deep morphea** • Subcutaneous morphea • Eosinophilic fasciitis • Morphea profunda • Disabling pansclerotic morphea of children

Plaque Morphea

This type represents the superficial type of morphea which is usually restricted to the dermis and rarely involves the subcutaneous tissue. It has been further divided into several subtypes:

Morphea en Plaque

This is the most common variant of plaque-type morphea. It usually involves only one or two anatomic sites. The trunk is the most common site affected followed by extremities. The face is rarely involved. Plaques have well-defined borders which separate them from the surrounding normal skin. It usually starts with one or more round or oval indurated plaques which are larger than 1 cm in size. An erythematous halo or a violaceous ring (lilac ring) if present is characteristic of the plaque. As the disease progresses, the skin overlying the lesion becomes sclerotic while the inflammation subsides. After a variable disease course which may span from months to years, the disease burns out, there is softening of the plaque and atrophy ensues. There can be areas of hyperpigmentation or hypopigmentation in the plaque.

Guttate Morphea

This type of morphea presents with multiple oval lesions of varying size (2 to 10 mm) in diameter. The upper part of the trunk is the most common affected site. There is mild erythema surrounding these lesions. As the disease progresses, lesions develop mild induration with dyspigmentation (hyperpigmentation or hypopigmentation).

Atrophoderma of Pasini and Pierini

Peterson et al. grouped IAPP as a subtype of plaque morphea which later faced criticism. It is characterized by hyperpigmented atrophic plaques with characteristic "cliff-drop borders". The plaques are asymptomatic and usually involve the trunk. Such plaques usually fail to develop induration. Hence, due to the absence of overt inflammation and sclerosis in the lesions, it was considered as a "burnt-out morphea." It can present alone or occur with other morphea subtypes.

Keloid Morphea

It is characterized by nodular lesions that look similar to keloids in the presence of typical lesions of morphea. These nodules can be solitary or confluent.

Lichen Sclerosus (LS)

LS is characterized by shiny atrophic white plaques. Such plaques are usually preceded by violaceous skin lesions. The ano-genital area is the most commonly affected site, however, extragenital LS affecting the trunk and extremities also occur. Peterson *et al.* classified LS as a subtype of plaque morphea which was a controversial aspect of the classification.

Generalized Morphea

The onset of this type of morphea is usually insidious. Generalized morphea is considered when individual plaques enlarge to become confluent or plaques disseminate and involve more than two anatomic sites.

Bullous Morphea

In this type of morphea, there are tense sub-epidermal bullae in the presence of typical lesions of morphea. The lesions usually involve the limbs, trunk, face, or neck. Lesions can be superficial or extend deep into the dermis. A plausible explanation for Bulla formation was attributed to the lymphatic obstruction caused by the sclerodermatous process or due to the localized trauma.

Linear Morphea

This type is characterized by one or more linear indurated streaks that can involve extremities and face or scalp or all three areas in the pediatric population. In this morphea, the disease can extend to the dermis, subcutaneous tissue, fascia, muscle, and even the underlying bone.

Linear Morphea (Linear Scleroderma)

This type of morphea usually manifests as a discrete linear induration mainly involving the limbs. It may or may occur in a zosteriform distribution. In 95% of the cases, the disease is unilateral. It may lead to several complications like limb atrophy, joint contractures and consequent deformities. The disease can extend beyond the subcutaneous tissue of the limbs to affect the growth and development of bony structures. In a study of patients having linear morphea, 20% of the patients had atrophy of underlying muscle and bone affecting lower limbs, having a leg length discrepancy of 1.5- to 7-cm. Contractures usually develop when linear morphea involves a joint. This type of morphea can result in severe flexural deformity which may need amputation [9].

En Coup de Sabre

When linear morphea involves the face or scalp, the lesions often resemble a stroke from a sword (sabre), hence the name 'en coup de sabre'. The usual site of affection is the paramedian forehead. The disease is mostly unilateral, however, bilateral cases rarely occur. It can lead to several complications like ptosis, loss of eyelashes or eyebrows, uveitis, pseudo-oculomotor palsy, lingual atrophy and dental problems [10 - 13].

Progressive Hemifacial Atrophy

Progressive hemifacial atrophy (Parry-Romberg syndrome) causes hemifacial atrophy. The primary disease site is the subcutaneous tissue, muscle or bone. Most often skin remains mobile lacking sclerosis as the affliction of the dermis is a secondary change. However, in linear morphea, the dermis and subcutaneous tissues are the primary affected sites, and later the deep tissues are involved [14]. The relationship between Parry-Romberg syndrome and morphea en coup de sabre is a topic of debate and has been discussed in detail in chapter 17.

Deep Morphea

Deep morphea involves the deeper dermis, subcutaneous tissue, fascia, or superficial muscle. The lesions of deep morphea are usually more diffuse and are not present in a linear pattern, a feature that differentiates it from linear morphea. Though the level of depth of involvement may vary, the histopathological changes of different types of deep morphea are similar. They divided deep morphea into 4 types

Subcutaneous Morphea

As the name suggests, subcutaneous tissue is the primary site of involvement of subcutaneous morphea. Contrary to the lesions of 'morphea en plaque', the plaques of subcutaneous morphea are deeper and bound down. It was termed subcutaneous morphea by Jablonska [6]. A clinical study of 16 patients with subcutaneous morphea was described by Person and Su. According to them, the plaques were ill-defined, hyperpigmented and symmetrically distributed. The inflammation was more pronounced than that associated with other types of morphea. The rapid onset of sclerosis and pronounced inflammation were the characteristic features of this type [15].

Eosinophilic Fasciitis

It is a deep fibrotic condition involving fascia affecting the extremities proximal to the hands and feet. The fascia is the primary site of disease. There have been two schools of thought regarding the placement of this disease. Several authors have described it as a separate entity and kept it distinct from the typical morphea. However, histopathology may share features with deep morphea subtypes. In addition, eosinophilic fasciitis has been reported in patients having morphea and systemic sclerosis [16, 17]. Based on such features, *Peterson et al* classified eosinophilic fasciitis as a subtype of morphea and placed it in the deep morphea group. Eosinophilic fasciitis has been described in detail in chapter 20.

Morphea Profunda

This entity was introduced by Su and Person in 1981 based on a histopathological study of 23 cases. In this type of morphea, the entire skin feels taut, thickened and bound down. For diagnosing morphea profunda, they suggested a triad of criteria based on clinical, histopathological and therapeutic aspects of the disease: (1) Diffuse, bound-down, taut and deep cutaneous sclerosis; (2) Significant thickening and hyalinization of collagen bundles of both the subcutaneous tissue and the fascia along with a dense inflammatory cell infiltrate; and (3) Response to systemic corticosteroids, antimalarial agents, or other anti-inflammatory drugs [18]. Whittaker *et al.* in 1989 described patients with solitary indurated plaques having features of morphea profunda [19].

Disabling Pansclerotic Morphea of Children

This type of morphea was first reported by Diaz-Perez *et al.* in 1980 [20]. It is a mutilating variant of morphea with an aggressive disease course having significant disease morbidity. Clinically, patients present with generalized disease involving the trunk, extremities, scalp and face. The toes and fingertips are spared. The disease usually affects patients before the age of 14 years. The sclerotic plaques that develop in this disease extend deep into the subcutaneous tissue, fascia, muscle, and even bone, hence the name "Pansclerotic". This type of morphea is considered to have the worst prognosis [8].

The classification system proposed by *Peterson et al.* was widely used by authors throughout the world. However, this classification had several drawbacks. Firstly, they classified the Atrophoderma of Pasini and Pierini and Lichen sclerosus as sub-types of morphea. Though both of them bear some relationship with morphea. However, there is still controversy about it and to date it has not been solved. Hence keeping them with morphea was not justified. Similarly, Eosinophilic fasciitis which primarily involves fascia and skin involvement is a secondary phenomenon in it; has been kept under morphea. Though morphea and EF have been reported to be present in the same patient but that doesn't justify it being a subtype of morphea. Secondly, generalized morphea has not been defined completely. Thirdly, a good percentage of patients have more than one type of morphea, described as mixed type, and was missing in the classification. Additionally, regarding deep morphea, any type of morphea can extend beneath the dermis and involve subjacent tissues. Finally, terms like subcutaneous morphea and morphea profunda are similar. It looked very difficult to differentiate them. Some of these deficiencies were later discussed by Laxer/Zulian and Kreuter *et al.* in their classifications coming ahead.

CLASSIFICATION OF MORPHEA BY EUROPEAN PEDIATRIC RHEUMATOLOGY SOCIETY

To address certain deficiencies in the classification system proposed by *Peterson et al.*, the Pediatric Rheumatology European Society in 2006 proposed a new classification system of juvenile localized scleroderma Table **2.5**. Their classification, also known as Laxer and Zulian classification, included five subtypes: circumscribed morphea, generalized morphea, linear scleroderma, pansclerotic morphea and the new subtype "mixed" when two or more subtypes are present in the same patient [21]. This classification excluded Lichen sclerosus, atrophoderma of Pasini and Pierini, and eosinophilic fasciitis, however, they retained Parry Romberg syndrome. Certain modifications were introduced in the existing subtypes. Salient features of their classification are discussed below:

Table 2.5. Classification of morphea by Pediatric Rheumatology European Society.

S. No.	Types
1.	**Circumscribed morphea** Superficial Deep
2.	**Linear morphea** Trunk/limbs Head
3.	**Generalized morphea**
4.	**Pansclerotic morphea**
5.	**Mixed morphea**

Circumscribed Morphea

It has been divided into two types-superficial and deep variants. In the superficial variant, there are round or oval circumscribed areas of induration that are limited to the epidermis and dermis. Such plaques can be single or multiple and most often have altered pigmentation and possess a violaceous, erythematous halo (lilac ring) which is more obvious in fair skin. In the deep variant, they have put the morphea profunda and subcutaneous morphea subtypes of *Peterson et al.* Oval or round circumscribed areas of deep skin induration extend to the subcutaneous tissue or fascia or underlying muscle (morphea profunda subtype of *Peterson et al*). The lesions can be single or multiple. Occasionally, the primary site of involvement is in the subcutaneous tissue without the involvement of the skin (subcutaneous type of *Peterson et al*).

Generalized Morphea

For generalized morphea, they proposed some discrete criteria which were missing in the previous classifications. Generalized morphea was considered when individual plaques are four or more in number and each plaque is larger than 3cm and becomes confluent involving at least two out of seven anatomic sites (right upper extremity, left upper extremity, right lower extremity, left lower extremity, head/neck, anterior trunk and posterior trunk). They also suggested that unilateral generalized morphea (usually having onset in childhood) should be regarded as an extreme variant.

Linear Morphea

Linear morphea can involve either the limbs/trunk or head/neck. It is considered as the most common subtype in pediatric population. It is characterized by one or more linear areas of induration that can involve the dermis, panniculus, muscle or even the underlying bone. It can lead to significant deformities. Not only upper and lower extremities can get involved but also the head and neck can get affected. Accordingly, linear morphea in the form of en coup de sabre variety (ECDS) (as the lesions resemble a stroke from the sword) and Parry Romberg syndrome characterize the linear morphea affecting the face/scalp. ECDS is considered a milder variant characterized by linear induration that affects the face and the scalp and sometimes involves muscle and underlying bone. On the other hand, PRS is considered a severe form of the disease that is characterized by hemifacial atrophy of the skin and tissue of the lower face (below the forehead) with only mild or absent involvement of the superficial skin [22, 23]. There is enough evidence to consider PRS as the severe end of the spectrum of ECDS. This could be the reason that they have classified it in the linear morphea affecting the head/neck. The presence of similar associated conditions like CNS, ocular and dental abnormalities has been reported in both conditions with similar prevalence [24 - 26]. In addition, the author and colleagues have carried out a recent review of literature in which they have shown enough evidence to suggest that PRS and ECDS lie on the same spectrum with ECDS being a milder variant while PRS lies on the severe end of the spectrum [23]. The relationship between ECDS and PRS has been discussed in detail also in chapter 17.

Pansclerotic Morphea

Pansclerotic morphea is the most severe type of morphea, fortunately very rarely encountered in the clinical set-up. There is generalized full-thickness involvement of the skin of the extremities, trunk, scalp and face. However, there is sparing of the toes and fingertips. Though the entire body can be affected by it but internal organ involvement is rarely seen. This feature differentiates it from systemic sclerosis. Chronic ulcers in pansclerotic morphea can evolve into squamous cell carcinoma which is a life-threatening complication [27 - 29]

Mixed Morphea

When two or more of the previous subtypes of morphea are present, the term mixed morphea is applied. This subtype has been missing in the previous classifications. According to a multicenter study comprising 750 children, it was found to constitute about 15% of the whole group [30].

Laxer and Zulian's classification has been widely used by researchers. It was a refined classification in comparison to Peterson *et al.* The addition of mixed subtypes made it more comprehensive. However, certain questions remain to be answered. Generalized morphea has been defined as 4 or more plaques each more than 3 cm involving at least two anatomic regions. However, if there is a large plaque (or less than 4 plaques) covering the entire trunk or one complete limb, how it will be labelled. Is the area of involvement the only parameter needed or the deeper extension of disease is also important? In addition, disease entities like IAPP, EF, LS, and LAM which are somehow related to morphea have not been discussed in the classification.

CLASSIFICATION OF MORPHEA BY GERMAN DER-MATOLOGICAL SOCIETY

The German Dermatological Society in 2009 proposed S1 guidelines for the diagnosis and treatment of localized scleroderma that included a new classification which divided morphea broadly into 4 types: limited, linear, generalized, and deep types Table **2.6**. This classification included idiopathic atrophoderma of Pasini and Pierini and eosinophilic fasciitis. However, it excluded Lichen sclerosus and mixed sub-type. This classification has claimed some advantages over the previous classifications. Firstly, the classification is a simplified one. This simple classification was based on clinico-therapeutic outcome meaning that there was a therapeutic algorithm correlating with a specific subtype of morphea. Secondly, this classification also predicts the prognosis of the disease [31]. For instance, in the limited type, resolution of the disease occurs in about 2.5 years in approximately 50% of patients [32, 33]. On the contrary, the mean duration of disease in linear, deep and generalized subtypes has been reported to be longer (around 5.5 years) [30]. These guidelines also had recommendations for serological, histopathological and biometric diagnostic procedures for morphea subtypes. Salient features of this classification are discussed briefly below:

Table 2.6. Classification of morphea by German Dermatological Society (2009).

S. No.	Types
1.	**Limited type** • Morphea (plaque type) • Guttate morphea • Idiopathic atrophoderma of Pasini and Pierini

(Table 2.6) cont.....

S. No.	Types
2.	**Generalized type** • Generalized localized scleroderma (involvement of 3 or more anatomic sites) • Disabling pansclerotic morphea • Eosinophilic fasciitis
3.	**Linear type** • Linear localized scleroderma (usually with the involvement of the extremities) • Linear localized scleroderma, "en coup de sabre" type. • Parry Romberg syndrome.
4.	**Deep type**

Limited Type of Localized Scleroderma

The commonest type of morphea is the plaque type. It is characterized by lesions having a size of more than 1 cm, affecting one or two anatomic areas of the body. Trunk is the most frequently affected site. In the beginning stage, round to oval-shaped lesions present with an erythematous appearance that is more apparent in fair skin. Later the lesion becomes indurated and may acquire an ivory-white color. An active lesion is characterized by a violaceous rim/halo (called as "lilac ring") surrounding the hardened area. Sometimes long standing sclerotic lesions burnt out and become softer again over the course of many years of the disease. Such lesions can develop atrophy, or develop dyspigmentation (hyper-hypopigmentation). The fibrosis associated with the disease can cause loss of hair as well as loss of cutaneous appendages.

The guttate subtype is also called "morphea guttata". This type presents clinically with multiple small sclerotic lesions, yellowish-white in color and having a glistening surface. The size of the lesions is usually less than 1 cm having a similar "lilac ring" in active lesions. Similar to plaque morphea, guttate morphea is frequently seen to affect the trunk. This type of morphea can simply present as erythematous macules at the onset of the disease.

IAPP is possibly an early abortive type of guttate morphea. It is frequently seen to affect during childhood. Clinically, it is characterized by lesions usually less than 1cm in size placed symmetrically over the trunk. Occasionally, lesions are erythematous. Due to the loss of connective tissue such lesions can become wedge-shaped depressions lying below the level of the skin surface. Histopathological findings are similar to the late atrophic stage of morphea [34].

Generalized Type of Localized Scleroderma

Generalized localized scleroderma is defined when lesions involve three or more anatomic sites. The trunk, thighs, and lumbosacral area are the most frequently involved sites. Usually, indurated plaques are present in a symmetrical distribution and have the tendency to coalesce to form larger plaques. Lesions may be present in their different stages of evolution.

Disabling pansclerotic morphea is an extremely rare subtype of the generalized type of morphea. This is considered the severe form of the disease. It can lead to complications like contractures, ulcerations, *etc.* It may show little tendency to reverse fibrotic changes involved in this disease.

Eosinophilic fasciitis (EF), also known as Shulman's syndrome has been related to morphea by several researchers. According to this classification, EF is a type of morphea and has been placed as a subtype of generalized morphea.

Linear Type of Localized Scleroderma

According to this classification, linear localized scleroderma can involve extremities or frontoparietal area in the form of en coup de sabre or cause progressive hemifacial atrophy (Parry Romberg syndrome).

Linear localized morphea involving extremities is clinically characterized by linear band-like streaks which are arranged longitudinally. The lesions may resolve leaving hyperpigmentation in mild disease. In certain cases, healing of lesions may result in the formation of sclerotic bands crossing joints and leading to restriction of limb movement. It may be associated with the atrophy of underlying bone or muscle.

En coup de sabre is a special type of linear localized scleroderma in which the lesions pass over the frontoparietal area. Frequently, lesions are present in a paramedian location extending from the eyebrows upwards into the hairy scalp where the lesions culminate into the cicatricial alopecia. CNS involvement has been frequently reported.

Progressive facial hemiatrophy (Parry Romberg syndrome) is related to linear localized scleroderma. There is atrophy of the affected subcutaneous tissue which frequently extends deep to the muscles and osteocartilaginous tissues. Cutaneous fibrosis is rarely reported. Disease onset usually occurs during childhood or adolescence. Severe facial atrophy causing asymmetry is not uncommon. En coup de sabre type of linear localized scleroderma and Parry Romberg syndrome are frequently seen together in the same patient in about 40% of the cases [35]. Central nervous system involvement is usually encountered in PRS. In 50% of the cases, antinuclear antibodies have been reported.

Deep Type of Localized Scleroderma

This classification considered the deep type as the rarest variant seen in less than 5% of cases. The deep type is defined when the cutaneous fibrosis extends to the deeper layers like subcutaneous fat tissue, fascia, and subjacent muscles. Lesions are usually present on the extremities in a symmetrical distribution. Less often deep morphea can present without a preceding inflammatory phase.

Though this classification provided some good advantages but it has certain limitations and shortcomings. The mixed subtype of morphea as introduced by laxer-Zulian was dropped from the classification which doesn't seem to be justified. Secondly, some bizarre terms were introduced. It doesn't sound good to write generalized localized scleroderma which is really confusing to the reader. It should have been better written as generalized morphea. Thirdly, classifying EF as a subtype of morphea can't be justified at present. Though there exists some relationship between EF and morphea but there is enough evidence to set EF apart from morphea and the relationship between the two is still debatable and it has not been agreed globally that EF is a subtype of morphea. The relationship between the two has been discussed in chapter 20. Additionally, the definition of generalized morphea seems to be incomplete. Just the mere involvement of three or more anatomic areas doesn't seem to be sufficient. If a person has three plaques each 1cm and present in three anatomic areas. Would that qualify for generalized morphea? Questions like that needed to be clarified.

UPDATED CLASSIFICATION OF MORPHEA BY GERMAN DERMATOLOGICAL SOCIETY

In 2016, a group of German dermatology association presented updated guidelines regarding diagnosis and therapy of localized scleroderma. These guidelines provided a refined perspective of different aspects of localized scleroderma like definition, classification, epidemiology, pathogenesis, histopathology, and laboratory workup. These guidelines also included scoring for localized scleroderma and imaging and other device-assisted workup. Treatment protocols were presented in an algorithm corresponding to the clinical subtype. Their updated classification of morphea is mentioned in Table **2.7**.

Table 2.7. Updated Classification of morphea by German dermatological society (2016).

S. No.	Types
1.	**Limited form** • Morphea (plaque type) • Guttate morphea (a special form of morphea) • Idiopathic atrophoderma of Pasini and Pierini (a special form of morphea)

(*Table 2.7) cont.....*

S. No.	Types
2.	**Generalized form** • Generalized localized scleroderma (affecting at least three anatomic sites) • Disabling pansclerotic morphea (severe special form) • Eosinophilic fasciitis (a special form predominantly affecting the fasciae)
3.	**Linear form** • Linear localized scleroderma (usually affecting the extremities) • Linear localized scleroderma en coup de sabre • Progressive facial hemiatrophy (synonym: Parry-Romberg syndrome)
4.	**Deep form**
5.	**Mixed form**

This classification included mixed form which was dropped in the previous version (2009). In addition, it considered guttate morphea, IAPP and EF as special forms of morphea [36]. Excluding mixed morphea, the criticism to this classification remains the same as that of the previous version.

HOLISTIC CLASSIFICATION OF MORPHEA AND RELATED DISORDERS

From the proceeding discussion it is clear that to date, no single classification has covered all the aspects of morphea or is without any disagreements. In order to describe the morphea and its variants in a lucid and detailed way, the author has suggested a holistic classification (Box **2.1**) for morphea and certain disorders which are related to morphea. This classification will be followed throughout the book. This classification has been framed by taking inputs from most of the classification systems of morphea discussed already in the chapter.

The five disorders namely, IAPP, LS, PRS, EF and LAM have been put in a separate category named as "Morphea Related disorders". These are the disorders which share several features with morphea and are related to morphea having a variable strength of relationship with it. But at the same time, there are several recognizable differences between them and morphea which set them apart from morphea. There have been plenty of publications which have debated over the relationship between them and morphea and the controversy has not been solved to date. In order to simplify the situation and avoid confusion among the readers, a simple and holistic way of classifying morphea and disorders related to it has been followed throughout this book.

Box 2.1: Holistic classification of morphea and related disorders.
I. Morphea

Circumscribed Morphea
   • Superficial variant
   • Deep variant
Linear Morphea
   • Linear morphea involving trunk/ limbs
   • En coup de sabre
Generalized morphea
Pansclerotic morphea
Mixed morphea
Other types:
   • Guttate
   • bullous
   • Keloidal/nodular

II. Morphea-Related disorders
Idiopathic atrophoderma of Pasini and Pierini **Lichen sclerosus** **Parry Romberg Syndrome** **Eosinophilic fasciitis** **Linear atrophoderma of Moulin**

One of the aims of this classification to keep these 5 entities in a separate group is that, since this book is exclusively on morphea and related disorders, so there was an obvious need to give a detailed and comprehensive account of morphea as well as these 5 disease entities. If we look at the best and most comprehensive textbooks of dermatology, we can hardly find a paragraph or couple on topics like LAM, PRS, IAPP, *etc.* As a result, there was an unmet need for a detailed account of these entities. Keeping them separate, it gives the authors of this book an open opportunity to discuss them at detail comprising all the disease parameters ranging from epidemiology to treatment in a lucid way. Had these entities been amalgamated with morphea, it would have been difficult to give such a comprehensive account of each of these entities in the form of separate chapters.

Additionally, in all five chapters based on IAPP, LS, PRS, EF and LAM, authors have discussed the relationship between morphea and these entities in a detailed manner.

Among these five, PRS seems to have the strongest relationship with the morphea and is very closely related to the linear morphea en coup de sabre with which sometimes it becomes difficult to differentiate. The author has given a detailed account of the relation between the two in chapter 17 and has proposed a classification for the spectrum of diseases having PRS and linear morphea en coup de sabre at the two ends.

Regarding deep morphea/morphea profunda, any type of morphea can extend beyond the dermis to be logically called as Deep morphea. This can occur in plaque/circumscribed, linear, generalized types of morphea. So it is not necessary to form a separate category for deep morphea. A good way to designate deep morphea is to put the word "deep" following the name of the morphea subtype, once histopathology has confirmed deep involvement. The author has come across several cases of en coup de sabre morphea where there was no deeper involvement and few of them have been published. Similarly, a generalized case of morphea has been reported by the author where the disease was restricted to the dermis. Thus the deeper extension of disease is not present in every case of linear or generalized morphea. Thus, the correct diagnosis of a subtype of morphea should give information on whether the disease has deeper involvement or not irrespective of the morphea subtype. *e.g.*, if a patient has linear morphea involving one of the limbs with histopathology ruling out deeper involvement, his diagnosis will be simply "linear morphea". However, if skin biopsy confirms deeper involvement, the diagnosis should be "linear morphea-deep". This will certainly have therapeutic implications. The treatment of the two forms will be different. Remember skin biopsy is not mandatory to confirm the deeper involvement. A simple clinical examination involving palpation of involved skin will give you clue whether the disease is superficial or has deeper involvement. However, in case one is not sure, histopathology can confirm it.

In case of generalized morphea, we have followed Laxer and Zulian classification system. However, there is a scope for improvement in defining it in a better way. A couple of deep infiltrating plaques on the neck can be more problematic to a patient than involving a superficially large surface area of the back. Thus, a mere number of plaques and their surface area is not sufficient for defining generalized morphea. There should be a scoring system for defining generalized morphea encompassing features like surface area, deeper extension, complications, *etc.*

Box 2.2: Learning points.
• There exist various classification systems that have been suggested for morphea. However, till date not a single classification has covered all the aspects of heterogeneity of this disease.
• Five related conditions namely linear atrophoderma of Moulin (LAM), Idiopathic Atrophoderma of Pasini and Pierini (IAPP), Lichen sclerosus (LS), Eosinophilic fasciitis (EF) and Parry-Romberg syndrome (PRS) are related to morphea with a variable strength of relationship which has been a topic of controversy. A plausible way to give a detailed account of them is to classify them as "morphea-related disorders" to simplify the debate.
• Despite having several clinical types, the common denominator among all the types of morphea is the presence of induration at any stage of disease evolution which is considered the hallmark of morphea lesions.

REFERENCES

[1]   Su WPD, Powel Fe. Morphea and morphea profunda. In: Arndt KA, Leboit PE, Robinson JK, Sintroub BU, Eds. Cutaneous Medicine and Surgery. Philadelphia: Saunders 1995; pp. 895-900.

[2]   Buckingham RB, Prince RK, Rodnan GP, Barnes EL. Collagen accumulation by dermal fibroblast cultures of patients with linear localized scleroderma. J Rheumatol 1980; 7(2): 130-42.
[PMID: 7373615]

[3]   O'Leary PA, Nomland R. A Clinical Study of 103 Cases of Scleroderma. Am J Med Sci 1930; 180: 95-112.
[http://dx.doi.org/10.1097/00000441-193007000-00013]

[4]   O'Leary PA, O'Leary PA, Ragsdale WE Jr. Dermatohistopathology of various types of scleroderma. Arch Dermatol 1957; 75(1): 78-87.
[http://dx.doi.org/10.1001/archderm.1957.01550130080008] [PMID: 13381197]

[5]   Rodnan GP, Jablonska S, Medsger TA Jr. Classification and nomenclature of progressive systemic sclerosis (scleroderma). Clin Rheum Dis 1979; 5(1): 5-13.
[http://dx.doi.org/10.1016/S0307-742X(21)00050-3]

[6]   Jablonska S, Rodnan GP. Localized forms of scleroderma. Clin Rheum Dis 1979; 5(1): 215-41.
[http://dx.doi.org/10.1016/S0307-742X(21)00062-X]

[7]   Schachter RK. Localized scleroderma. Curr Opin Rheumatol 1989; 1(4): 505-11.
[http://dx.doi.org/10.1097/00002281-198901040-00015] [PMID: 2702053]

[8]   Peterson LS, Nelson AM, Su WPD. Classification of morphea (localized scleroderma). Mayo Clin Proc 1995; 70(11): 1068-76.
[http://dx.doi.org/10.4065/70.11.1068] [PMID: 7475336]

[9]   Kornreich HK, King KK, Bernstein BH, Singsen BH, Hanson V. Scleroderma in childhood. Arthritis Rheum 1977; 20(2 Suppl.): 343-50.
[PMID: 263911]

[10]   Dilley JJ, Perry HO. Bilateral linear scleroderma en coup de sabre. Arch Dermatol 1968; 97(6): 688-9.
[http://dx.doi.org/10.1001/archderm.1968.01610120078012] [PMID: 5652974]

[11]   Goldenstein-Schainberg C, Pereira RMR, Gusukuma MC, Messina WC, Cossermell W. Childhood linear scleroderma? en coup de sabre? with uveitis. J Pediatr 1990; 117(4): 581-4.
[http://dx.doi.org/10.1016/S0022-3476(05)80693-6]

[12]   Tang RA, Mewis-Christmann L, Wolf J, Wilkins RB. Pseudo oculomotor palsy as the presenting sign of linear scleroderma. J Pediatr Ophthalmol Strabismus 1986; 23(5): 236-8.
[http://dx.doi.org/10.3928/0191-3913-19860901-09] [PMID: 3772692]

[13]   Suttorp-Schulten MS, Koornneef L. Linear scleroderma associated with ptosis and motility disorders. Br J Ophthalmol 1990; 74(11): 694-5.
[http://dx.doi.org/10.1136/bjo.74.11.694] [PMID: 2223709]

[14]   Lehman TJ. The Parry Romberg syndrome of progressive facial hemiatrophy and linear scleroderma en coup de sabre. Mistaken diagnosis or overlapping conditions? J Rheumatol 1992; 19(6): 844-5.
[PMID: 1404118]

[15]   Person JR, Su WPD. Subcutaneous morphoea: a clinical study of sixteen cases. Br J Dermatol 1979; 100(4): 371-80.
[http://dx.doi.org/10.1111/j.1365-2133.1979.tb01636.x] [PMID: 454564]

[16]   Michet CJ Jr, Doyle JA, Ginsburg WW. Eosinophilic fasciitis: report of 15 cases. Mayo Clin Proc 1981; 56(1): 27-34.
[PMID: 7453247]

[17]   Coyle HE, Chapman RS. Eosinophilic fasciitis (Shulman syndrome) in association with morphoea and systemic sclerosis. Acta Derm Venereol 1980; 60(2): 181-2.

[http://dx.doi.org/10.2340/0001555560181182] [PMID: 6154917]

[18] Su DWP, Person JR. Morphea profunda. Am J Dermatopathol 1981; 3(3): 251-60.
[http://dx.doi.org/10.1097/00000372-198110000-00003] [PMID: 6172992]

[19] Whittaker SJ, Smith NP, Jones RR. Solitary morphoea profunda. Br J Dermatol 1989; 120(3): 431-40.
[http://dx.doi.org/10.1111/j.1365-2133.1989.tb04171.x] [PMID: 2785401]

[20] Diaz-Perez JL, Connolly SM, Winkelmann RK. Disabling pansclerotic morphea of children. Arch Dermatol 1980; 116(2): 169-73.
[http://dx.doi.org/10.1001/archderm.1980.01640260045011] [PMID: 7356347]

[21] Laxer RM, Zulian F. Localized scleroderma. Curr Opin Rheumatol 2006; 18(6): 606-13.
[http://dx.doi.org/10.1097/01.bor.0000245727.40630.c3] [PMID: 17053506]

[22] Jablonska S, Blaszczyk M. Long-lasting follow-up favours a close relationship between progressive facial hemiatrophy and scleroderma en coup de sabre. J Eur Acad Dermatol Venereol 2005; 19(4): 403-4.
[http://dx.doi.org/10.1111/j.1468-3083.2005.00979.x] [PMID: 15987282]

[23] Arif T, Fatima R, Sami M. Parry-Romberg syndrome: a mini review. Acta Dermatovenerol Alp Panonica Adriat 2020; 29(4): 193-9.
[PMID: 33348939]

[24] Menni S, Marzano AV, Passoni E. Neurologic abnormalities in two patients with facial hemiatrophy and sclerosis coexisting with morphea. Pediatr Dermatol 1997; 14(2): 113-6.
[http://dx.doi.org/10.1111/j.1525-1470.1997.tb00216.x] [PMID: 9144696]

[25] Blaszczyk M, Jablonska S. Linear scleroderma en Coup de Sabre. Relationship with progressive facial hemiatrophy (PFH). Adv Exp Med Biol 1999; 455: 101-4.
[http://dx.doi.org/10.1007/978-1-4615-4857-7_14] [PMID: 10599329]

[26] Sommer A, Gambichler T, Bacharach-Buhles M, von Rothenburg T, Altmeyer P, Kreuter A. Clinical and serological characteristics of progressive facial hemiatrophy: A case series of 12 patients. J Am Acad Dermatol 2006; 54(2): 227-33.
[http://dx.doi.org/10.1016/j.jaad.2005.10.020] [PMID: 16443052]

[27] Wollina U, Buslau M, Weyers W. Squamous cell carcinoma in pansclerotic morphea of childhood. Pediatr Dermatol 2002; 19(2): 151-4.
[http://dx.doi.org/10.1046/j.1525-1470.2002.00033.x] [PMID: 11994182]

[28] Parodi PC, Riberti C, Draganic Stinco D, Patrone P, Stinco G. Squamous cell carcinoma arising in a patient with long-standing pansclerotic morphea. Br J Dermatol 2001; 144(2): 417-9.
[http://dx.doi.org/10.1046/j.1365-2133.2001.04041.x] [PMID: 11251587]

[29] Maragh SH, Davis MDP, Bruce AJ, Nelson AM. Disabling pansclerotic morphea: Clinical presentation in two adults. J Am Acad Dermatol 2005; 53(2 Suppl. 1): S115-9.
[http://dx.doi.org/10.1016/j.jaad.2004.10.881] [PMID: 16021158]

[30] Zulian F, Athreya BH, Laxer R, *et al.* Juvenile Scleroderma Working Group of the Pediatric Rheumatology European Society (PRES). Juvenile localized scleroderma: clinical and epidemiological features in 750 children. An international study. Rheumatology 2006; 45(5): 614-20.
[http://dx.doi.org/10.1093/rheumatology/kei251] [PMID: 16368732]

[31] Kreuter A, Krieg T, Worm M, *et al.* Diagnosis and therapy of localized scleroderma. J Deut Dermatol Gesell 2009; 7 (Suppl. 6): S1-S14.

[32] Christianson HB, Dorsey CS, Kierland RR, O'Leary PA. Localized Scleroderma. AMA Arch Derm 1956; 74(6): 629-39.
[http://dx.doi.org/10.1001/archderm.1956.01550120049012] [PMID: 13371921]

[33] Peterson LS, Nelson AM, Su WP, Mason T, O'Fallon WM, Gabriel SE. The epidemiology of morphea (localized scleroderma) in Olmsted County 1960-1993. J Rheumatol 1997; 24(1): 73-80.

[PMID: 9002014]

[34]   Kencka D, Blaszczyk M, Jabłońska S. Atrophoderma Pasini-Pierini is a primary atrophic abortive morphea. Dermatology 1995; 190(3): 203-6.
[http://dx.doi.org/10.1159/000246685] [PMID: 7599381]

[35]   Jablonska S. Facial hemiatrophy and it's relation to localized scleroderma. In: Jablonska S, Ed. Scleroderma and pseudoscleroderma. Warsaw: PZWL 1975a; pp. 537-48.

[36]   Kreuter A, Krieg T, Worm M, *et al.* German guidelines for the diagnosis and therapy of localized scleroderma. J Dtsch Dermatol Ges 2016; 14(2): 199-216.
[http://dx.doi.org/10.1111/ddg.12724] [PMID: 26819124]

CHAPTER 3

Epidemiology

Parvaiz Anwar Rather[1,*] and Tasleem Arif[2,3]

[1] *Department of Dermatology, Venereology & Leprosy, Government Medical College, Baramulla, Jammu and Kashmir, India*

[2] *Department of Dermatology, STDs, Leprosy and Aesthetics, Dar As Sihha Medical Center, Dammam, Saudi Arabia*

[3] *Ellahi Medicare Clinic, Srinagar, Kashmir, India*

Chapter Synopsis.
• Knowledge of the epidemiological aspects of any disease is of paramount importance in order to acquire a better understanding of the concerned disease condition.
• There is limited knowledge available in the literature on the detailed epidemiology of morphea, despite continuous research efforts.
• Rarity of morphea can be understood by its very low incidence rate reported in the literature, ranging from 0.3 to 3 cases per 100,000 population.
• Morphea can present at any age. However, it has been reported to have bimodal age of onset, with two peaks.
• The mean age of onset of morphea in the pediatric population is between 6-9 years. On the contrary, the mean age of occurrence in adult population has been reported to be between 20 and 40 years of age.
• There is a need to undertake large-scale population studies in order to get a detailed understanding of the epidemiology of morphea.

Keywords: Adult morphea, Autoimmune, Bimodal age, Caucasian race, Circumscribed morphea, Collagen vascular disease, Co-morbidity, Congenital morphea, Epidemiology, Female preponderance, Generalized morphea, Incidence and prevalence, Linear morphea, Localized scleroderma, Morbidity, Morphea, Morphea profunda, Pansclerotic morphea, Pediatric morphea, Plaque morphea, Psychological and physical disability.

INTRODUCTION

Morphea is a rare localized connective tissue (collagen vascular) disease presenting with different clinical forms. A detailed description of this disease,

---

* **Corresponding author Parvaiz Anwar Rather:** Department of Dermatology, Venereology & Leprosy, Government Medical College, Baramulla, Jammu and Kashmir, India; E-mail: parvaizanwar@gmail.com

especially its epidemiology, is missing in the literature, mainly because of the rarity of this dermatoses. So far, very few studies have been dedicated to exclusively describe various epidemiological aspects of this rare skin condition. In this chapter, an attempt has been made to give a brief overview of the epidemiology of morphea, after a thorough review of the related literature. There is an absolute need to conduct large-scale population-based studies, in order to further understand the details of the epidemiological aspects of this rare dermatological condition.

MAGNITUDE OF MORPHEA AS PUBLIC HEALTH PROBLEM

Being a rare skin condition, morphea is expected to have less incidence. But at the same time, owing to chronicity, it has a relatively higher prevalence. Just to refresh the existing knowledge, it is appropriate to mention here that the incidence is the number of new cases occurring in a population over a period of time and the prevalence is the number of old and new cases present in the population at a point of time.

The rarity of morphea is reflected by its very less incidence rate reported in the literature, ranging from 0.3 to 3 cases per 100,000 population, with a slight variation between different studies [1 - 6].

In one of the best analytical studies on this topic to date from Olmsted County, Minnesota, wherein an attempt was made to register all patients with morphea from 1960 to 1993, the annual incidence rate of 27 per million (2.7 per 100,000) population was reported [7].

A general look at the literature shows that the overall incidence of morphea appears to have been increasing over time, most likely, because of better awareness among the patients who report it earlier and also better/ advanced diagnostic tools available now, than it was previously [8]. These aspects are summarized in Table **3.1**.

AGE OF INVOLVEMENT

Although morphea can present at any age, it has been reported to have a bimodal age of onset, with two peaks. The peak age for onset in the pediatric population is 6-11 years [4, 9 - 11], and that for adults, it is 44-47 years [4, 10, 11].

Although morphea has been described in infants and even neonates, the mean age of onset of the disease in the pediatric population is between 6-9 years [9, 12 - 15]. In children, morphea occurs at least 10 times more often than systemic sclerosis [16].

Table 3.1. Magnitude of morphea as a public health problem [1-8].

Incidence and Prevalence	The incidence of morphea is very less owing to the rarity of the disease condition, but because of its chronic nature, it has a considerable prevalence rate.
Average incidence rate	The average incidence rate ranges from 0.3-3 per 100,000 population, with some inter-study variations.
Annual incidence rate	One of the best analytical studies on this topic to date from Olmsted County, Minnesota, reported an annual incidence rate of 2.7 per 100,000 population.
Overall incidence	The overall incidence of morphea has increased with time, attributable to better patient awareness who report it earlier and due to the availability of advanced diagnostic tools now.

The mean age of occurrence in the adult population is between 20 and 40 years of age, with a slight variation between different studies [17 - 19]. Similarly, the age group of 20-29 years was most commonly affected in a study from India [5, 20].

Congenital forms, with a presentation at birth, have also been reported in the literature [15, 21, 22].

As a general statement, it can be stated that the prevalence of morphea increases with age [8]. The age-related aspects of morphea have been mentioned in (Box 3.1).

Box 3.1: Age of involvement in morphea [4, 8, 10, 11, 15, 16, 21, 22].
• Morphea has bimodal age of onset. The peak age for onset in the pediatric population is 6-11 years while in adults, it is 44-47 years.
• In children, morphea occurs at least 10 times more often than systemic sclerosis.
• Cases of congenital morphea have also been reported.
• As a general rule, the prevalence of morphea increases with age.

CLINICAL ASPECTS OF MORPHEA VERSUS AGE GROUP

Although no specific age group is more susceptible or immune to the development of a particular clinical subtype of morphea, there is enough evidence in the literature that some clinical subtypes of morphea are more common in adults than in the pediatric age group and vice versa [23].

Circumscribed (plaque) morphea, which is the most common subtype of morphea, has been found to usually affect adults between 40 and 50 years of age [4, 6, 24]. In the Olmsted County study, 56% of patients had plaque-type of morphea [7].

Linear morphea has more frequent occurrence in children aged 2–14 years [6, 24], and there is enough evidence in the literature that patients with morphea in the pediatric age group are less likely to have the generalized subtype, plaque subtype, and other subtypes of morphea [10].

In a study involving 750 children with pediatric morphea, it was found that the linear subtype of morphea was the most common type, found in 65% of patients, and plaque lesions, generalized involvement, and deep lesions were respectively found in 26%, 12% and 2% patients [9].

Linear pattern with unilateral occurrence in most cases and presentation in the pediatric population, has led to a hypothesis that these affected patients have genetically susceptible cells in this distribution, with a subsequent development of disease triggered by environmental exposure.

In general, patients with pediatric-onset morphea are less likely to have other comorbid medical conditions, as compared to that with adult-onset morphea [10].

However, there seems to be no difference between pediatric and adult morphea with respect to anti-nuclear antibody (ANA) positivity, and personal and family history of other associated autoimmune diseases [10].

As expected, the duration of the disease has been found to be higher in the pediatric population than in the adult population [10].

GENDER CONSIDERATIONS OF MORPHEA

It is a universal and established fact that morphea, like that of most other autoimmune and connective tissue diseases, has more of a female preponderance.

On average, the female-to-male ratio varies from 2.4-5 to 1 [4, 9, 11, 12, 15, 25]. In some studies, a ratio of 2.6-6 to 1 has been described [6, 24, 26].

In Olmsted County, the female-to-male ratio was 2.6 to 1 [7], and in a study from India, it was reported to be 3.7 females for every male [5]. The exception to this general rule is the pansclerotic subtype of morphea, which has been reported in some studies to be found more commonly in males as compared to females. Also in the linear morphea subtype, no gender preference has been described [27]. The epidemiological aspects of gender in morphea are summarized in (Box **3.2**).

Box 3.2: Gender aspects of morphea. [4, 6, 7, 9, 11, 12, 15, 24-27].
• There is a definite female preponderance, with female to male ratio reported as 2.4-6 females to 1 male, depending on some inter-study variations.
• In the Olmsted County study, the female to male ratio was 2.6 to 1.
• Pansclerotic and linear subtypes of morphea are an exception to this general rule of female preponderance, with former reported to be more common in males and no gender preference described in the latter.

RACIAL PREDISPOSITION

Morphea has been found to be more common in Caucasians [7, 15]. In another study, among the adult-onset group of morphea patients, a higher proportion of white and African-American patients were found, and a higher proportion of Hispanic patients were found in the pediatric-onset group of morphea patients [10]. Morphea has been reported to be less common in the black race and Asians [20, 28].

MORBIDITY

Morphea is generally considered having a benign nature and not posing life-threatening risk to the patients. In the Olmsted County study, the survival rate of patients with morphea was generally found to be somewhat similar to that of the general population [7]. Although there is a low mortality rate specific to morphea, but it has substantial morbidity in terms of psychological and physical disability.

Disability can occur in morphea depending on the depth of skin involvement, clinical subtype of morphea, age of onset, site of involvement, and body surface area involved. Correspondingly, some of the predisposing factors for physical and psychological disability in morphea are deeper forms of morphea (for example morphea profunda), linear morphea, early age of onset, lesions on the face and over joints, and a larger area of the body surface involved.

Lesions on the face can result in more psychological disability, whereas lesions on the joints and larger body area involvement can cause more physical disability.

In the Olmsted County study, 11% of the patients had a substantial disability, occurring primarily with a linear form of morphea with onset less than 18 years of age in almost two-thirds of patients [7].

Box 3.3: Learning points.
• Morphea is a very rare dermatoses, with a very low incidence rate, but exists in the community with a considerable prevalence and there is limited literature available to describe its epidemiology.
• Morphea has a bimodal age of onset and can occur in both pediatric and adult populations. Circumscribed (plaque) type of morphea is the most common form in the adult age group, whereas the linear form is the most common type seen in pediatric population.
• Like most of the other autoimmune diseases, morphea has a female preponderance.
• Caucasians are the most commonly involved racial group. The involvement of Asians and black race is less commonly reported in the literature.
• Although disease-specific mortality due to morphea is very rare, it causes significant morbidity in the form of psychological and physical disability.

REFERENCES

[1]   Silman A, Jannini S, Symmons D, Bacon P. An epidemiological study of scleroderma in the West Midlands. Rheumatology 1988; 27(4): 286-90.
        [http://dx.doi.org/10.1093/rheumatology/27.4.286] [PMID: 3261609]

[2]   Herrick AL, Ennis H, Bhushan M, Silman AJ, Baildam EM. Incidence of childhood linear scleroderma and systemic sclerosis in the UK and Ireland. Arthritis Care Res 2010; 62(2): 213-8.
        [http://dx.doi.org/10.1002/acr.20070] [PMID: 20191520]

[3]   Knobler R, Moinzadeh P, Hunzelmann N, *et al.* European Dermatology Forum S1-guideline on the diagnosis and treatment of sclerosing diseases of the skin, Part 1: localized scleroderma, systemic sclerosis and overlap syndromes. J Eur Acad Dermatol Venereol 2017; 31(9): 1401-24.
        [http://dx.doi.org/10.1111/jdv.14458] [PMID: 28792092]

[4]   Mertens JS, Seyger MMB, Thurlings RM, Radstake TRDJ, de Jong EMGJ. Morphea and Eosinophilic Fasciitis: An Update. Am J Clin Dermatol 2017; 18(4): 491-512.
        [http://dx.doi.org/10.1007/s40257-017-0269-x] [PMID: 28303481]

[5]   Arif T, Adil M, Amin SS, *et al.* Clinico-epidemiological Study of Morphea from a Tertiary Care Hospital. Curr Rheumatol Rev 2018; 14(3): 251-4.
        [http://dx.doi.org/10.2174/1573397114666180410115553] [PMID: 29637865]

[6]   Wolska-Gawron K, Bartosińska J, Krasowska D. MicroRNA in localized scleroderma: A review of literature. Arch Dermatol Res 2020; 312(5): 317-24.
        [http://dx.doi.org/10.1007/s00403-019-01991-0] [PMID: 31637470]

[7]   Peterson LS, Nelson AM, Su WP, Mason T, O'Fallon WM, Gabriel SE. The epidemiology of morphea (localized scleroderma) in Olmsted County 1960-1993. J Rheumatol 1997; 24(1): 73-80.
        [PMID: 9002014]

[8]   Mayes MD. Classification and epidemiology of scleroderma. Semin Cutan Med Surg 1998; 17(1): 22-6.
        [http://dx.doi.org/10.1016/S1085-5629(98)80058-8] [PMID: 9512103]

[9]   Zulian F, Athreya BH, Laxer R, *et al.* Juvenile Scleroderma Working Group of the Pediatric Rheumatology European Society (PRES). Juvenile localized scleroderma: clinical and epidemiological features in 750 children. An international study. Rheumatology 2006; 45(5): 614-20.
        [http://dx.doi.org/10.1093/rheumatology/kei251] [PMID: 16368732]

[10]   Condie D, Grabell D, Jacobe H. Comparison of outcomes in adults with pediatric-onset morphea and those with adult-onset morphea: A cross-sectional study from the morphea in adults and children cohort. Arthritis Rheumatol 2014; 66(12): 3496-504.

[http://dx.doi.org/10.1002/art.38853] [PMID: 25156342]

[11]   Mertens JS, Seyger MMB, Kievit W, *et al.* Disease recurrence in localized scleroderma: A retrospective analysis of 344 patients with paediatric- or adult-onset disease. Br J Dermatol 2015; 172(3): 722-8.
[http://dx.doi.org/10.1111/bjd.13514] [PMID: 25381928]

[12]   Christen-Zaech S, Hakim MD, Afsar FS, Paller AS. Pediatric morphea (localized scleroderma): Review of 136 patients. J Am Acad Dermatol 2008; 59(3): 385-96.
[http://dx.doi.org/10.1016/j.jaad.2008.05.005] [PMID: 18571769]

[13]   Weibel L, Laguda B, Atherton D, Harper JI. Misdiagnosis and delay in referral of children with localized scleroderma. Br J Dermatol 2011; 165(6): 1308-13.
[http://dx.doi.org/10.1111/j.1365-2133.2011.10600.x] [PMID: 21895625]

[14]   Li SC. Scleroderma in children and adolescents: Localized scleroderma and systemic sclerosis. Pediatr Clin North Am 2018; 65(4): 757-81.
[http://dx.doi.org/10.1016/j.pcl.2018.04.002] [PMID: 30031497]

[15]   George R, George A, Kumar TS. Update on management of morphea (Localized Scleroderma) in children. Indian Dermatol Online J 2020; 11(2): 135-45.
[http://dx.doi.org/10.4103/idoj.IDOJ_284_19] [PMID: 32477969]

[16]   Murray KJ, Laxer RM. Scleroderma in children and adolescents. Rheum Dis Clin North Am 2002; 28(3): 603-24.
[http://dx.doi.org/10.1016/S0889-857X(02)00010-8] [PMID: 12380372]

[17]   Heite HJ. Ergebnisse häufi gkeitanalytischer Untersuchungen bei der Sklerodermie. Arch Derm Syphilol 1955; 200: 426-33.

[18]   Christianson HB, Dorsey CS, O'Leary PA, *et al.* Localized Scleroderma. AMA Arch Derm 1956; 74(6): 629-39.
[http://dx.doi.org/10.1001/archderm.1956.01550120049012]

[19]   Sehgal VN, Srivastava G, Aggarwal AK, Behl PN, Choudhary M, Bajaj P. Localized scleroderma/morphea. Int J Dermatol 2002; 41(8): 467-75.
[http://dx.doi.org/10.1046/j.1365-4362.2002.01469.x] [PMID: 12207760]

[20]   Arif T, Masood Q, Singh J, Hassan I. Assessment of esophageal involvement in systemic sclerosis and morphea (localized scleroderma) by clinical, endoscopic, manometric and pH metric features: A prospective comparative hospital based study. BMC Gastroenterol 2015; 15(1): 24.
[http://dx.doi.org/10.1186/s12876-015-0241-2] [PMID: 25888470]

[21]   Mansour M, Liy Wong C, Zulian F, *et al.* Natural history and extracutaneous involvement of congenital morphea: Multicenter retrospective cohort study and literature review. Pediatr Dermatol 2018; 35(6): 761-8.
[http://dx.doi.org/10.1111/pde.13605] [PMID: 30187959]

[22]   Zulian F, Vallongo C, de Oliveira SKF, *et al.* Congenital localized scleroderma. J Pediatr 2006; 149(2): 248-51.
[http://dx.doi.org/10.1016/j.jpeds.2006.04.052] [PMID: 16887444]

[23]   Johnson W, Jacobe H. Morphea in adults and children cohort II: Patients with morphea experience delay in diagnosis and large variation in treatment. J Am Acad Dermatol 2012; 67(5): 881-9.
[http://dx.doi.org/10.1016/j.jaad.2012.01.011] [PMID: 22382198]

[24]   Kreuter A, Krieg T, Worm M, *et al.* German guidelines for the diagnosis and therapy of localized scleroderma. J Dtsch Dermatol Ges 2016; 14(2): 199-216.
[http://dx.doi.org/10.1111/ddg.12724] [PMID: 26819124]

[25]   Kreuter A, Wischnewski J, Terras S, Altmeyer P, Stücker M, Gambichler T. Coexistence of lichen sclerosus and morphea: A retrospective analysis of 472 patients with localized scleroderma from a German tertiary referral center. J Am Acad Dermatol 2012; 67(6): 1157-62.

[http://dx.doi.org/10.1016/j.jaad.2012.04.003] [PMID: 22533994]

[26]   Leitenberger JJ, Cayce RL, Haley RW, Adams-Huet B, Bergstresser PR, Jacobe HT. Distinct autoimmune syndromes in morphea: A review of 245 adult and pediatric cases. Arch Dermatol 2009; 145(5): 545-50.
[http://dx.doi.org/10.1001/archdermatol.2009.79] [PMID: 19451498]

[27]   Kim A, Marinkovich N, Vasquez R, Jacobe HT. Clinical features of patients with morphea and the pansclerotic subtype: A cross-sectional study from the morphea in adults and children cohort. J Rheumatol 2014; 41(1): 106-12.
[http://dx.doi.org/10.3899/jrheum.130029] [PMID: 24293577]

[28]   Warner Dharamsi J, Victor S, Aguwa N, *et al.* Morphea in adults and children cohort III: nested case-control study. The clinical significance of autoantibodies in morphea. JAMA Dermatol 2013; 149(10): 1159-65.
[http://dx.doi.org/10.1001/jamadermatol.2013.4207] [PMID: 23925398]

CHAPTER 4

Predisposing Factors

Sabha Mushtaq[1,*] and Tasleem Arif[2,3]

[1] *Department of Dermatology, Venereology and Leprosy, Government Medical College, Jammu, Jammu and Kashmir, India*

[2] *Department of Dermatology, STDs, Leprosy and Aesthetics, Dar As Sihha Medical Center, Dammam, Saudi Arabia*

[3] *Ellahi Medicare Clinic, Srinagar, Kashmir, India*

Chapter Synopsis.
• Morphea is a chronic inflammatory and fibrotic skin condition that classically presents as hyperpigmented sclerotic plaque with lilac-colored borders.
• The exact etiology of morphea is not known but many factors have been proposed to initiate the fibrotic cascade.
• Both genetic and environmental factors like infection, trauma, radiation, drugs and chemicals, vaccination, *etc.* underlie the pathogenesis of morphea.
• Several types of trauma have been implicated in the causation of morphea like blunt trauma, mechanical compression, and friction, penetrating trauma, trauma due to radiation, *etc.*
• The presence of autoantibodies and a high prevalence of personal and familial autoimmune diseases point to the autoimmune nature of the disease.

Keywords: ANA, Autoimmunity, Chemicals, Drugs, Endocrine dysfunction, Etiology, Fibrosis, HLA, Infection, Localized scleroderma, Microchimerism, Morphea, Predisposing factors, Pregnancy, Radiation, Risk factors, Thyroid disorder, Trauma, Triggers, Vaccination.

INTRODUCTION

Morphea, often inappropriately referred to as localized scleroderma, is an inflammatory skin condition affecting the dermis and subcutaneous tissue leading to varying degrees of sclerosis and atrophy. Unlike systemic sclerosis, internal organ fibrosis is not seen in morphea but cutaneous sclerosis, joint contractures, and restricted mobility have a substantial impact on the quality of life of affected

* **Corresponding author Sabha Mushtaq:** Department of Dermatology, Venereology and Leprosy, Government Medical College, Jammu, Jammu and Kashmir, India; E-mail: smqazi.gmc@gmail.com

patients. The pathophysiology of morphea involves increased collagen deposition and vascular changes in a background of autoimmunity [1]. A wide range of factors (Fig. **4.1**) may act as triggering events in the causation of morphea (Box **4.1**, **4.2**). This chapter will discuss these predisposing factors in detail.

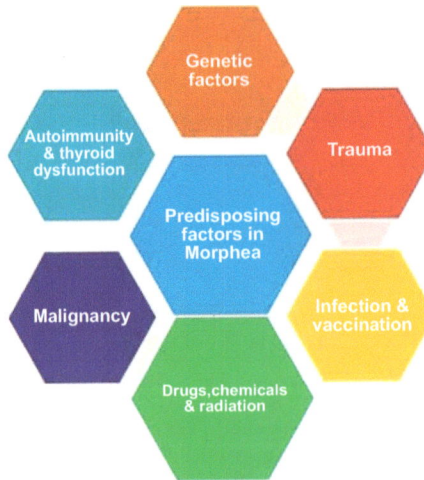

Fig. (4.1). Various predisposing factors implicated in the development of morphea.

GENETIC FACTORS

The role of genetics in morphea is suggested by HLA predisposition and familial occurrence in many cases [2 - 4] (Box **4.1**). Jacob *et al.* reported that certain HLA class I alleles like HLA DRB1*04:04 and HLA-B*37 confer increased susceptibility, particularly in linear and generalised subtypes [2]. X-chromosome inactivation has also been demonstrated in the pathogenesis of morphea [5]. The blaschkoid involvement in linear morphea indicates regional genetic susceptibility which can be attributed to cutaneous mosaicism [6, 7]. The role of micro RNAs (miRNAs) in the pathogenesis of morphea is emerging. Skin and serum of patients with morphea have been found to have downregulated antifibrotic miRNA-7 and miRNa-196a, which contributes to the overexpression of type I collagen [8, 9].

Box 4.1: Genetic factors involved in morphea.
HLA class I alleles HLA DRB1*04:04 and HLA-B*37
Downregulation of antifibrotic miRNA-7 and miRNa-196a
X-chromosome inactivation
Cutaneous mosaicism in linear morphea

EXTERNAL FACTORS

A variety of external factors and stimuli act as triggering factors in patients genetically predisposed to the development of morphea (Box **4.2**).

Box 4.2: Predisposing factors causing morphea.
Trauma
Infection
Vaccination
Drugs
Chemicals
Malignancy
Thyroid disorders
Autoimmunity
Radiation
Pregnancy

Trauma

Morphea has been reported following an array of traumatic events including physical injury, mechanical compression and friction, *etc.*, (Box **4.3**).

Box 4.3: Types of trauma implicated in the development of morphea.
Blunt trauma
Penetrating trauma
Mechanical compression (slim belt, *etc.*)
Chronic friction due to clothing (brassiere, waist band, *etc.*)
Injection site trauma
Trauma due to waxing of hair
Surgical trauma
Radiation trauma

Blunt trauma, injection site trauma, following waxing for excessive hair, and use of slim belt have been reported as triggering factors in different reports [1, 10 - 17]. A survey of the Morphea in Adults and Children (MAC) cohort studied the role of skin trauma in morphea. In this survey, morphea was reported to occur as an isomorphic phenomenon and also as an isotopic response following surgery, penetrating trauma, injection, herpes zoster, radiation and extreme exercise.

Isomorphic morphea was defined as morphea occurring at the site of repeated trauma and included patients with lesions distributed in areas of chronic friction like that caused by brassiere and waistband. Isotopic morphea was defined as morphea appearing at the site of past trauma within 6 months of the onset of lesions. The proportion of patients in which trauma was the inciting event was up to 16% and this was predominantly observed in adults with generalised morphea. Patients with the isotopic distribution of morphea lesions were reported to have greater clinical severity with a higher modified Rodnan skin score (mRSS) as compared to those with isomorphic lesions [11]. Trauma-induced morphea is believed to be related to the up-regulation of Toll- like receptor ligands which activate the innate immune system leading to enhanced fibrogenesis [18].

Infection

Many viral and bacterial infections have been proposed to be associated with the causation of morphea (Box **4.4**). These include *Borrelia*, cytomegalovirus, Epstein-Barr virus, hepatitis C, varicella zoster and HIV [19 - 28].

Box 4.4: Various infectious agents involved in morphea.
Borrelia burgdorferi
Borrelia afzellii
Borrelia garinii
Cytomegalovirus
Epstein-barr virus
Hepatitis C virus
Human immunodeficiency virus
Varicella

Of these, infection with *Borrelia burgdorferi* is the most extensively studied and researched with reports of *Borrelia* DNA detected within morphea lesions [25 - 28]. In the USA, *Borrelia burgdorferi* is the predominant type whereas, in European and Japanese patients, *Borrelia afzellii* and *Borrelia garinii* have also been detected [29]. *"Borrelia* –associated early onset morphea" is a distinct clinical entity described as a combination of onset of disease at a young age, infection with *Borrelia* and autoimmune phenomenon evident as high-titre antinuclear antibodies [30]. However, the association is still controversial as many studies have not found a definitive evidence of *Borrelia* infection in morphea, based on PCR and serologic assays [31 - 33].

Vaccination

Apart from viral and bacterial infection, some vaccines are also known to induce morphea. There are reports of morphea profunda triggered by vaccination against hepatitis B, tetanus, diphtheria-pertussis-tetanus (DPT) vaccine and pneumococcal vaccine [34 - 36]. Measles mumps rubella (MMR) vaccination has also been reported to induce morphea (Box **4.5**) [37].

Box 4.5: Vaccines implicated in the development of morphea.
Measles mumps rubella (MMR)
Diphtheria pertussis tetanus (DPT)
Hepatitis B
Tetanus
Pneumococcal vaccines

The mechanism underlying vaccination-induced morphea is not clearly elucidated. It can be due to the trauma of the injection or the adjuvant vaccine constituents [10].

Drugs & Chemicals

Drug-induced morphea is a rare phenomenon and has been reported with balicatib, pembrolizumab, ustekinumab and interferon β-1b [38 - 41]. Balicatib, a cathepsin K inhibitor was found to be associated with the development of morphea lesions over the trunk in a patient after 9 months of therapy [38]. Cheng *et al.* reported a case of generalised morphea with the use of pembrolizumab in a patient with choroidal melanoma [39]. Ustekinumab administered for the management of ulcerative colitis resulted in sclerotic plaques suggestive of morphea in an 84-year old female [40]. Several other drugs have been implicated in the development of morphea which include pentazocine, bleomycin, cocaine, uracil-tegafur, gemcitabine, bromocryptine, bisoprolol, 1-5-hydroxytryptophan with carbidopa, ibuprofen, mitomycin C, melphalan limb perfusion, valproate, docetaxel, *etc* [42 - 45] Table **4.1**.

Inflammatory lymphocytic response and autoantibody production specific to the drug result in vascular injury, oxidative stress and production of cytokines (IL-1, TGF-β, TNF-α) leading to morphea [10]. Morphea-like scleroderma has also been described due to occupational exposure to organic solvents like perchloroethylene [46, 47].

Table 4.1. Drugs implicated in the development of morphea.

Balicatib	Ustekinumab
Interferon β-1b	Pembrolizumab,
l-5-hydroxytryptophan with carbidopa	Peplomycin
Cocaine	Pentazocine
Progestin	Vitamin K
Vitamin B12	Docetaxel
D-penicillamine	Methysergide
Bisoprolol	Uracil-tegafur combination
Paclitaxel	Mitomycin C
Gemcitabine	Valproate
Bleomycin	Bromocryptine
Melphalan limb perfusion	Ibuprofen

Radiation

Radiation-induced morphea also known as post-irradiation morphea (PIM) or radiation port morphea is distinct from the late irreversible effects of radiation therapy like telangiectasias, fibrosis, and liponecrosis. PIM is a chronic progressive radiation-induced inflammatory condition that results in sclerodermoid skin change [48]. It has largely been reported in cases of breast cancer and is mostly confined to the irradiated site. In about 25% of the cases, it can affect sites distant from the irradiated skin zone [10, 48 - 51]. The interval between radiotherapy and the onset of RIM can vary from 1 month to as long as 32 years [52]. PIM is believed to be caused due to increased levels of IL-4, IL-5, and TGF-β [53].

Malignancy

Morphea can sometimes occur as a paraneoplastic phenomenon. It has been reported in association with malignancies like endometrial cancer, breast cancer, prostate cancer, cholangiogenic cancer and adrenal adenoma (Box **4.6**).

Sclerodermatous plaques may be seen before the underlying malignancy is detected or they can present simultaneously with the tumor. It can present as localized plaques or generalized morphea. Patients with paraneoplastic morphea are often older with a sudden onset of localized morpheaform plaques [54, 55]. Cytokines released from the tumor cells may be responsible for the induction of sclerotic skin changes [54].

Box 4.6: Malignancies reported in association with morphea.
Endometrial carcinoma
Carcinoma breast
Carcinoma prostate
Cholangiogenic cancer
Adrenal adenoma

Thyroid Dysfunction

In a study by Hassan *et al.*, abnormal thyroid function test in the form of elevated Thyroid stimulating hormone was demonstrated in 7 out of 17 (41.2%) patients with morphea. Of these, six patients had plaque-type morphea and one had generalized morphea. The authors concluded that abnormal thyroid function tests observed in their patients should be considered as a preliminary finding and further larger studies should be carried out to support or refute a definite association [56]. Another study by Dańczak-Pazdrowska *et al.* evaluated 42 patients of morphea for the presence of anti-thyroid antibodies [anti-peroxidase antibodies (TPO-Ab), and anti-thyroglobulin antibodies] and found increased levels of anti-thyroid antibodies in only 10 patients. The study did not find any significant difference in the levels of anti-thyroid antibodies between localized and generalized forms of morphea. The association of morphea with autoimmune thyroid disorders was therefore refuted and it was concluded that routine screening of patients with thyroid disorders is not mandatory [57].

Pregnancy

Morphea can be triggered by pregnancy in some cases. There can be de novo development of morphea during pregnancy or worsening of the pre-existing disease [58]. In one case report, a 22- year old primigravida developed skin thickening over the breast which was confirmed on histopathology to be morphea. A complete resolution was observed in the post-partum period [58]. In another case, linear morphea developed during the first trimester in a patient with Grave's disease and CMV IgM positivity [59]. Cases of worsening of morphea (en coup de sabre) have also been reported during pregnancy [60]. Several mechanisms have been proposed for pregnancy-triggered morphea. These include microchimerism, alteration in the immune system during pregnancy and the role of mechanical injury caused by breast swelling and subsequent trauma caused by bra straps [60].

Autoimmunity

The role of autoimmunity in the pathogenesis of morphea is suggested by personal or family history of autoimmune and rheumatological diseases in about 9-46% of cases [10]. Morphea can occur concomitantly with other autoimmune diseases like vitiligo, autoimmune hepatitis, systemic lupus erythematosus, primary biliary cirrhosis, and myasthenia gravis. The generalized type of morphea has a greater prevalence of autoimmune associations when compared to other types [61]. Furthermore, a variety of autoantibodies can be detected in patients with morphea. Anti-nuclear antibody (ANA) levels are found to be elevated in 18-68% of cases. ANA positivity is associated with deeper tissue involvement and with a more widespread disease extent [10, 62]. Anti-histone antibodies (AHA) positivity was found in 47% of a Japanese cohort of morphea patients [63]. Antibodies against extractable nuclear antigens like anti-ds DNA, Smith/RNP, SSA/B, anti-centromere Abs and anti-Scl-70 are less commonly detected in morphea with 1-15% positivity reported in various studies [62]. The role of autoimmunity and of different auto-antibodies in the pathogenesis of morphea has been discussed in detail in chapter 5.

Box 4.7: Learning points.
• Both genetic and external factors can act as predisposing factors for the development of morphea.
• Genetic factors like HLA association, downregulation of anti-fibrotic mi-RNAs, microchimerism and mosaicism increase the susceptibility to develop morphea.
• Among the external factors, the role of infection with *Borrelia* has been most extensively researched followed by trauma and other agents like drugs and chemicals, radiation, vaccination and malignancy.
• The autoimmune nature of morphea is supported by its association with other autoimmune disorders like vitiligo, SLE, autoimmune hepatitis, *etc.* and also by the presence of autoantibodies (anti-nuclear antibodies, anti-histone antibodies *etc.*)
• The role of thyroid disorders in morphea is still a matter of debate.

REFERENCES

[1]　Arif T, Adil M, Amin SS, *et al.* Clinico-epidemiological study of morphea from a tertiary care hospital. Curr Rheumatol Rev 2018; 14(3): 251-4.
[http://dx.doi.org/10.2174/1573397114666180410115553] [PMID: 29637865]

[2]　Jacobe H, Ahn C, Arnett FC, Reveille JD. Major histocompatibility complex class I and class II alleles may confer susceptibility to or protection against morphea: findings from the Morphea in Adults and Children cohort. Arthritis Rheumatol 2014; 66(11): 3170-7.
[http://dx.doi.org/10.1002/art.38814] [PMID: 25223600]

[3]　Pham CM, Browning JC. Morphea affecting a father and son. Pediatr Dermatol 2010; 27(5): 536-7.
[http://dx.doi.org/10.1111/j.1525-1470.2010.01277.x] [PMID: 21182646]

[4]　Brownell I, Soter NA, Jr AGF. Familial linear scleroderma (en coup de sabre) responsive to antimalarials and narrowband ultraviolet B therapy. Dermatol Online J 2007; 13(1): 11.
[http://dx.doi.org/10.5070/D383K6X3TB] [PMID: 17511944]

[5]   Karaca NE, Aksu G, Karaca E, *et al.* Progressive morphea of early childhood tracing Blaschko's lines on the face: involvement of X chromosome monosomy in pathogenesis and clinical prognosis. Int J Dermatol 2011; 50(11): 1406-10.
[http://dx.doi.org/10.1111/j.1365-4632.2011.04900.x] [PMID: 22004499]

[6]   Soma Y, Kawakami T, Yamasaki E, Sasaki R, Mizoguchi M. Linear scleroderma along Blaschko's lines in a patient with systematized morphea. Acta Derm Venereol 2003; 83(5): 362-4.
[http://dx.doi.org/10.1080/00015550310013088] [PMID: 14609105]

[7]   McKenna DB, Benton EC. A tri-linear pattern of scleroderma 'en coup de sabre' following Blaschko's lines. Clin Exp Dermatol 1999; 24(6): 467-8.
[http://dx.doi.org/10.1046/j.1365-2230.1999.00535.x] [PMID: 10606951]

[8]   Etoh M, Jinnin M, Makino K, *et al.* MicroRNA-7 down-regulation mediates excessive collagen expression in localized scleroderma. Arch Dermatol Res 2013; 305(1): 9-15.
[http://dx.doi.org/10.1007/s00403-012-1287-4] [PMID: 22965811]

[9]   Makino T, Jinnin M, Etoh M, *et al.* Down-regulation of microRNA-196a in the sera and involved skin of localized scleroderma patients. Eur J Dermatol 2014; 24(4): 470-6.
[http://dx.doi.org/10.1684/ejd.2014.2384] [PMID: 25152444]

[10] Saracino AM, Denton CP, Orteu CH. The molecular pathogenesis of morphoea: from genetics to future treatment targets. Br J Dermatol 2017; 177(1): 34-46.
[http://dx.doi.org/10.1111/bjd.15001] [PMID: 27553363]

[11] Grabell D, Hsieh C, Andrew R, *et al.* The role of skin trauma in the distribution of morphea lesions: A cross-sectional survey of the Morphea in Adults and Children cohort IV. J Am Acad Dermatol 2014; 71(3): 493-8.
[http://dx.doi.org/10.1016/j.jaad.2014.04.009] [PMID: 24880663]

[12] Ahn JG, Kim YT, Lee CW. Trauma-induced isomorphic lesions in morphea: A brief case report. J Korean Med Sci 1995; 10(2): 152-4.
[http://dx.doi.org/10.3346/jkms.1995.10.2.152] [PMID: 7576296]

[13] Arif T, Majid I, Ishtiyaq Haji ML. Late onset 'en coup de sabre' following trauma: Rare presentation of a rare disease. Nasza Dermatol Online 2015; 6(1): 49-51.
[http://dx.doi.org/10.7241/ourd.20151.12]

[14] Arif T, Adil M, Amin SS, Sami M, Raj D. Concomitant en coup de sabre and plaque type morphea in the same patient: A rare occurrence. Przegl Dermatol 2017; 5(5): 570-4.
[http://dx.doi.org/10.5114/dr.2017.71222]

[15] Arif T, Majid I. Can lesions of 'en coup de sabre' progress after being quiescent for a decade? Indian J Dermatol 2016; 2(18): 77-9.

[16] Arif T, Hassan I, Anwar P, Suhail Amin S. Slim belt induced morphea-Price paid for a slimmer look. Nasza Dermatol Online 2015; 6(3): 347-9.
[http://dx.doi.org/10.7241/ourd.20153.93]

[17] Arif T, Fatima R, Sami M. Morphea due to waxing at a salon: The first case report. J Turk Acad Dermatol 2022; 16(1): 31-32.

[18] Ciechomska M, Cant R, Finnigan J, van Laar JM, O'Reilly S. Role of toll-like receptors in systemic sclerosis. Expert Rev Mol Med 2013; 15: e9.
[http://dx.doi.org/10.1017/erm.2013.10] [PMID: 23985302]

[19] Goulabchand R, Khellaf L, Forestier A, *et al.* Acute and regressive scleroderma concomitant to an acute CMV primary infection. J Clin Virol 2014; 61(4): 604-7.
[http://dx.doi.org/10.1016/j.jcv.2014.10.003] [PMID: 25453335]

[20] Longo F, Saletta S, Lepore L, Pennesi M. Localized scleroderma after infection with Epstein-Barr virus. Clin Exp Rheumatol 1993; 11(6): 681-3.

[PMID: 8299265]

[21]   de Oliveira FL, de Barros Silveira LK, Rambaldi ML, Barbosa FC. Localized scleroderma associated with chronic hepatitis C. Case Rep Dermatol Med 2012; 2012

[22]   Noh TW, Park SH, Kang YS, Lee UH, Park HS, Jang SJ. Morphea developing at the site of healed herpes zoster. Ann Dermatol 2011; 23(2): 242-5.
[http://dx.doi.org/10.5021/ad.2011.23.2.242] [PMID: 21747631]

[23]   Qu T, Fang K. Bullous morphea arising at the site of a healed herpes zoster. J Dermatol 2014; 41(6): 553-4.
[http://dx.doi.org/10.1111/1346-8138.12427] [PMID: 24750285]

[24]   Mosquera JA, Ojea R, Navarro C. HIV infection associated with scleroderma: report of two new cases. J Clin Pathol 2010; 63(9): 852-3.
[http://dx.doi.org/10.1136/jcp.2010.080044] [PMID: 20819885]

[25]   Espinoza-León F, Arocha F, Hassanhi M, Arévalo J. Using the polymerase chain reaction to Borrelia burgdorferi infection in localized scleroderma injure (morphea), in Venezuelan patients. Invest Clin 2010; 51(3): 381-90.
[PMID: 21305774]

[26]   Santos M, Ribeiro-Rodrigues R, Talhari C, Ferreira LCL, Zelger B, Talhari S. Presence *of Borrelia burgdorferi Sensu Lato* in patients with morphea from the Amazonic region in Brazil. Int J Dermatol 2011; 50(11): 1373-8.
[http://dx.doi.org/10.1111/j.1365-4632.2011.05081.x] [PMID: 22004491]

[27]   Moniuszko A, Gińdzieńska-Sieśkiewicz E, Pancewicz SA, Czupryna P, Zajkowska J, Sierakowski S. Evaluation of skin thickness lesions in patients with Lyme disease measured by modified Rodnan total skin score. Rheumatol Int 2012; 32(10): 3189-91.
[http://dx.doi.org/10.1007/s00296-011-2157-7] [PMID: 21960047]

[28]   Miglino B, Zavattaro E, Valente G, Viana M, Bonin S, Colombo E. Localized scleroderma unius lateri and Borrelia burgdoferi infection. Ind J Dermatol Venereol Leprol 2012; 78(3): 383-5.
[http://dx.doi.org/10.4103/0378-6323.95460] [PMID: 22565449]

[29]   Fujiwara H, Fujiwara K, Hashimoto K, *et al.* Detection of Borrelia burgdorferi DNA (B garinii or B afzelii) in morphea and lichen sclerosus et atrophicus tissues of German and Japanese but not of US patients. Arch Dermatol 1997; 133(1): 41-4.
[http://dx.doi.org/10.1001/archderm.1997.03890370047008] [PMID: 9006371]

[30]   Prinz JC, Kutasi Z, Weisenseel P, Pótó L, Battyáni Z, Ruzicka T. Borrelia-associated early-onset morphea: A particular type of scleroderma in childhood and adolescence with high titer antinuclear antibodies? J Am Acad Dermatol 2009; 60(2): 248-55.
[http://dx.doi.org/10.1016/j.jaad.2008.09.023] [PMID: 19022534]

[31]   Zollinger T, Mertz KD, Schmid M, Schmitt A, Pfaltz M, Kempf W. *Borrelia* in granuloma annulare, morphea and lichen sclerosus: A PCR-based study and review of the literature. J Cutan Pathol 2010; 37(5): 571-7.
[http://dx.doi.org/10.1111/j.1600-0560.2009.01493.x] [PMID: 20015188]

[32]   Gutiérrez-Gómez C, Godínez-Hana AL, García-Hernández M, *et al.* Lack of IgG antibody seropositivity to *Borrelia burgdorferi* in patients with Parry-Romberg syndrome and linear morphea *en coup de sabre* in Mexico. Int J Dermatol 2014; 53(8): 947-51.
[http://dx.doi.org/10.1111/ijd.12105] [PMID: 24527729]

[33]   Weide B, Schittek B, Klyscz T, *et al.* Morphoea is neither associated with features of Borrelia burgdorferi infection, nor is this agent detectable in lesional skin by polymerase chain reaction. Br J Dermatol 2000; 143(4): 780-5.
[http://dx.doi.org/10.1046/j.1365-2133.2000.03775.x] [PMID: 11069456]

[34]   Mlika RB, Kenani N, Badri T, *et al.* Morphea profunda in a young infant after hepatitis B vaccination.

J Am Acad Dermatol 2010; 63(6): 1111-2.
[http://dx.doi.org/10.1016/j.jaad.2009.02.047] [PMID: 21093674]

[35]   Khaled A, Kharfi M, Zaouek A, *et al.* Postvaccination morphea profunda in a child. Pediatr Dermatol 2012; 29(4): 525-7.
[http://dx.doi.org/10.1111/j.1525-1470.2011.01548.x] [PMID: 21854420]

[36]   Viladomiu EA, Valls A, Zabaleta B, Pérez NO, Moreno AJ. Deep morphea in a child after pneumococcal vaccination. Indian J Dermatol Venereol Leprol 2014; 80(3): 259-60.
[http://dx.doi.org/10.4103/0378-6323.132259] [PMID: 24823409]

[37]   Weibel L. Localized scleroderma (morphea) in childhood. Hautarzt 2012; 63(2): 89-96.
[http://dx.doi.org/10.1007/s00105-011-2199-5] [PMID: 22290277]

[38]   Peroni A, Zini A, Braga V, Colato C, Adami S, Girolomoni G. Drug-induced morphea: Report of a case induced by balicatib and review of the literature. J Am Acad Dermatol 2008; 59(1): 125-9.
[http://dx.doi.org/10.1016/j.jaad.2008.03.009] [PMID: 18410981]

[39]   Cheng MW, Hisaw LD, Bernet L. Generalized morphea in the setting of pembrolizumab. Int J Dermatol 2019; 58(6): 736-8.
[http://dx.doi.org/10.1111/ijd.14097] [PMID: 29931792]

[40]   Steuer AB, Peterson E, Lo Sicco K, Franks AG Jr. Morphea in a patient undergoing treatment with ustekinumab. JAAD Case Rep 2019; 5(7): 590-2.
[http://dx.doi.org/10.1016/j.jdcr.2019.05.008] [PMID: 31312709]

[41]   Gupta M, Yamauchi PS, Bagot M, *et al.* Uncommon presentation of morphea related to interferon beta in a patient with concomitant multiple sclerosis and chronic hepatitis C: A case report. Clin Case Rep 2020; 8(9): 1647-50.
[http://dx.doi.org/10.1002/ccr3.2971] [PMID: 32983469]

[42]   Orteu CH. Morphea and allied scarring and sclerosing inflammatory dermatoses.Rook's Textbook of Dermatology. 9th Ed.. West Sussex: Wiley-Blackwell 2016; p. 22.

[43]   Goihman-Yahr M, Leal G, Essenfeld-Yahr E. Generalized morphea: A side effect of valproate sodium? Arch Dermatol 1980; 116(6): 621.
[http://dx.doi.org/10.1001/archderm.1980.01640300009007] [PMID: 6769395]

[44]   Bouchard SM, Mohr MR, Pariser RJ. Taxane-induced morphea in a patient with CREST syndrome. Dermatol Reports 2010; 2(1): e9.
[http://dx.doi.org/10.4081/dr.2010.e9]

[45]   Landau M, Brenner S, Gat A, Klausner JM, Gutman M. Reticulate scleroderma after isolated limb perfusion with melphalan. J Am Acad Dermatol 1998; 39(6): 1011-2.
[http://dx.doi.org/10.1016/S0190-9622(98)70279-8] [PMID: 9843018]

[46]   Hinnen U, Schmid-Grendelmeier P, Müller E, Elsner P. [Exposure to solvents in scleroderma: disseminated circumscribed scleroderma (morphea) in a painter exposed to perchloroethylene]. Schweiz Med Wochenschr 1995; 125(50): 2433-7.
[PMID: 8553031]

[47]   Yamakage A, Ishikawa H. Generalized morphea-like scleroderma occurring in people exposed to organic solvents. Dermatology 1982; 165(3): 186-93.
[http://dx.doi.org/10.1159/000249939] [PMID: 6215270]

[48]   Partl R, Regitnig P, Tauber G, Pötscher M, Bjelic-Radisic V, Kapp KS. Radiation-induced morphea: A rare but severe late effect of adjuvant breast irradiation : Case report and review of the literature. Strahlenther Onkol 2018; 194(11): 1060-5.
[http://dx.doi.org/10.1007/s00066-018-1336-9] [PMID: 30014236]

[49]   Akay BN, Sanli H, Heper AO. Postirradiation linear morphoea. Clin Exp Dermatol 2010; 35(4): e106-8.
[http://dx.doi.org/10.1111/j.1365-2230.2009.03717.x] [PMID: 19874351]

[50]   Bleasel NR, Stapleton KM, Commens C, Ahern VA. Radiation-induced localized scleroderma in breast cancer patients. Australas J Dermatol 1999; 40(2): 99-102.
[http://dx.doi.org/10.1046/j.1440-0960.1999.00330.x] [PMID: 10333622]

[51]   Khamaganova I. Localized Scleroderma: Predisposing and Triggering Factors. The Open Dermatol J 2017; 11(1): 1-11.

[52]   Schaffer JV, Carroll C, Dvoretsky I, Huether MJ, Girardi M. Postirradiation morphea of the breast presentation of two cases and review of the literature. Dermatology 2000; 200(1): 67-71.
[http://dx.doi.org/10.1159/000018322] [PMID: 10681621]

[53]   Kumar S, Kolozsvary A, Kohl R, Lu M, Brown S, Kim JH. Radiation-induced skin injury in the animal model of scleroderma: implications for post-radiotherapy fibrosis. Radiat Oncol 2008; 3(1): 40.
[http://dx.doi.org/10.1186/1748-717X-3-40] [PMID: 19025617]

[54]   Jedlickova H, Durčanská V, Vašků V. Paraneoplastic scleroderma: Are there any clues? Acta Dermatovenerol Croat 2016; 24(1): 78-80.
[PMID: 27149136]

[55]   Desmond BL, Blattner CM, Young J III. Generalized morphea as the first sign of breast carcinoma: A case report. Dermatol Online J 2016; 22(2): 13030/qt2tr4496q.
[http://dx.doi.org/10.5070/D3222030094] [PMID: 27267193]

[56]   Hassan I, Arif T, Anwar P. Thyroid dysfunctions in morphoea: A preliminary report. Indian J Dermatol Venereol Leprol 2014; 80(6): 579.
[http://dx.doi.org/10.4103/0378-6323.144230] [PMID: 25382535]

[57]   Dańczak-Pazdrowska A, Polańska A, Synakiewicz J, *et al.* Morphea and antithyroid antibodies. Postepy Dermatol Alergol 2018; 35(5): 470-3.
[http://dx.doi.org/10.5114/ada.2018.75839] [PMID: 30429703]

[58]   Pham AK, Srivastava B, Deng A. Pregnancy-associated morphea: A case report and literature review. Dermatol Online J 2017; 23(1): 13030/qt5qv9f9h3.
[http://dx.doi.org/10.5070/D3231033691] [PMID: 28329476]

[59]   Wong B, Piliouras P, Mortimore R, Zonta M, Tucker S. Lower limb linear morphoea in a pregnant woman with known Graves' disease and cytomegalovirus immunoglobulin M positivity. Australas J Dermatol 2015; 56(4): e96-8.
[http://dx.doi.org/10.1111/ajd.12173] [PMID: 24712973]

[60]   Noda S, Asano Y, Ashida R, Tomita M, Kawashima T, Sato S. Localized scleroderma en coup de sabre exacerbated during pregnancy followed by postpartum development of rheumatoid arthritis. Eur J Dermatol 2011; 21(3): 441-2.
[http://dx.doi.org/10.1684/ejd.2011.1342] [PMID: 21524983]

[61]   Leitenberger JJ, Cayce RL, Haley RW, Adams-Huet B, Bergstresser PR, Jacobe HT. Distinct autoimmune syndromes in morphea: A review of 245 adult and pediatric cases. Arch Dermatol 2009; 145(5): 545-50.
[http://dx.doi.org/10.1001/archdermatol.2009.79] [PMID: 19451498]

[62]   Khatri S, Torok KS, Mirizio E, Liu C, Astakhova K. Autoantibodies in Morphea: An Update. Front Immunol 2019; 10: 1487.
[http://dx.doi.org/10.3389/fimmu.2019.01487] [PMID: 31354701]

[63]   Sato S, Ihn H, Soma Y, *et al.* Antihistone antibodies in patients with localized scleroderma. Arthritis Rheum 1993; 36(8): 1137-41.
[http://dx.doi.org/10.1002/art.1780360815] [PMID: 8343189]

CHAPTER 5

Pathogenesis

Mohammad Adil[1,*] and Tasleem Arif[2,3]

[1] *Department of Dermatology, Jawaharlal Nehru Medical College (JNMC), Aligarh Muslim University (AMU), Aligarh, India*

[2] *Department of Dermatology, STDs, Leprosy and Aesthetics, Dar As Sihha Medical Center, Dammam, Saudi Arabia*

[3] *Ellahi Medicare Clinic, Srinagar, Kashmir, India*

Chapter Synopsis.
• Morphea is a disease of variable clinical presentation characterized by an increase in collagen deposition and extracellular matrix production.
• It is believed to be an autoimmune disease triggered by an extraneous agent in genetically susceptible individuals.
• Patients of morphea have an increased susceptibility to other autoimmune and rheumatological diseases. HLA-B*37 and HLA-DRB1*04:04 have been linked to increased susceptibility to morphea.
• The likely role of mosaicism is proposed in linear morphea which follows the lines of Blaschko.
• Epigenetic factors such as DNA methylation and histone acetylation may act as a link between genetic and extraneous factors in disease pathogenesis.
• Morphea is associated with several autoantibodies, but their role in pathogenesis and disease activity is not as specific as in SSC.
• Trauma, radiation, infections, and drugs may trigger morphea in susceptible individuals.
• Vascular endothelial injury is one of the earliest and most important steps in the pathogenesis of morphea.
• Keratinocytes produce several factors that lead to dermal fibrosis. Epidermal-dermal signalling pathways assist in the same.
• The early phase of inflammation is mediated by Th1 cytokines followed by the phase of induction of fibrosis characterized by Th17 cytokines. The final phase of sclerosis is mediated by Th2 cytokines.
• Myofibroblasts are the cells primarily responsible for fibrosis. The process of fibrosis goes on unchecked in morphea under the influence of several growth factors and activating signals.
• Morphea and SSC share common pathogenic features. However, there are differences in the triggering factors, genetic susceptibility, autoantibodies and cytokine levels.

* **Corresponding author Mohammad Adil:** Department of Dermatology, Jawaharlal Nehru Medical College (JNMC), Aligarh Muslim University (AMU), Aligarh, India; E-mail: dr.mohd.adil@gmail.com

Keywords: Autoantibodies, Autoimmune disease, Borrelia, Chemokines, Chimerism, Cytokines, Cytomegalovirus, Dendritic cell, Endothelial injury, Epigenetics, Extracellular matrix, Fibroblasts, Genetic susceptibility, Human leucocyte antigen, Insulin-like growth factor, Interleukins, Matrix metalloproteinase, Mesenchyme, Micro-RNA, Mosaicism, Positional identity, Radiation, Sclerosis, T-helper cell, Transforming growth factor-β, Trauma, Tumor necrosis factor-α.

INTRODUCTION

Morphea is a disease that shows wide variation in clinical presentation. The exact etiopathogenesis of the disease is still uncertain and is largely extrapolated from systemic sclerosis (SSC) as both diseases show increased collagen deposition and an increase in extracellular matrix production. The etiological and susceptibility factors of morphea have been discussed in the previous chapter. The discussion in this chapter shall be focussed on the pathogenesis of morphea. It is believed that the occurrence of morphea requires an external environmental insult in a genetically predisposed individual [1]. This insult leads to vascular changes and the release of several pro-inflammatory and pro-fibrotic cytokines involving epidermal signalling and mesenchymal drivers which ultimately produce skin sclerosis [2]. While the clinical features may show variability, the various subsets of morphea probably share inflammatory and fibrotic molecular pathogenetic mechanisms [2]. A greater understanding of disease pathogenesis and its subsets is important for insights into clinical features and targeted therapeutic solutions.

The pathogenesis of morphea involves the role of genetic factors, epigenetic factors, vascular factors, autoantibodies, and inflammatory cytokines. The role of both innate and adaptive immunity has been postulated. Environmental factors such as trauma, radiation, infections (*e.g.* Borrelia, Cytomegalovirus, *etc.*), and drugs are possible triggers for the occurrence of the disease. All these factors are discussed individually in the upcoming sections of this chapter. Fig. (**5.1**) describes the basic steps in the pathogenesis of morphea in the form of a flowchart.

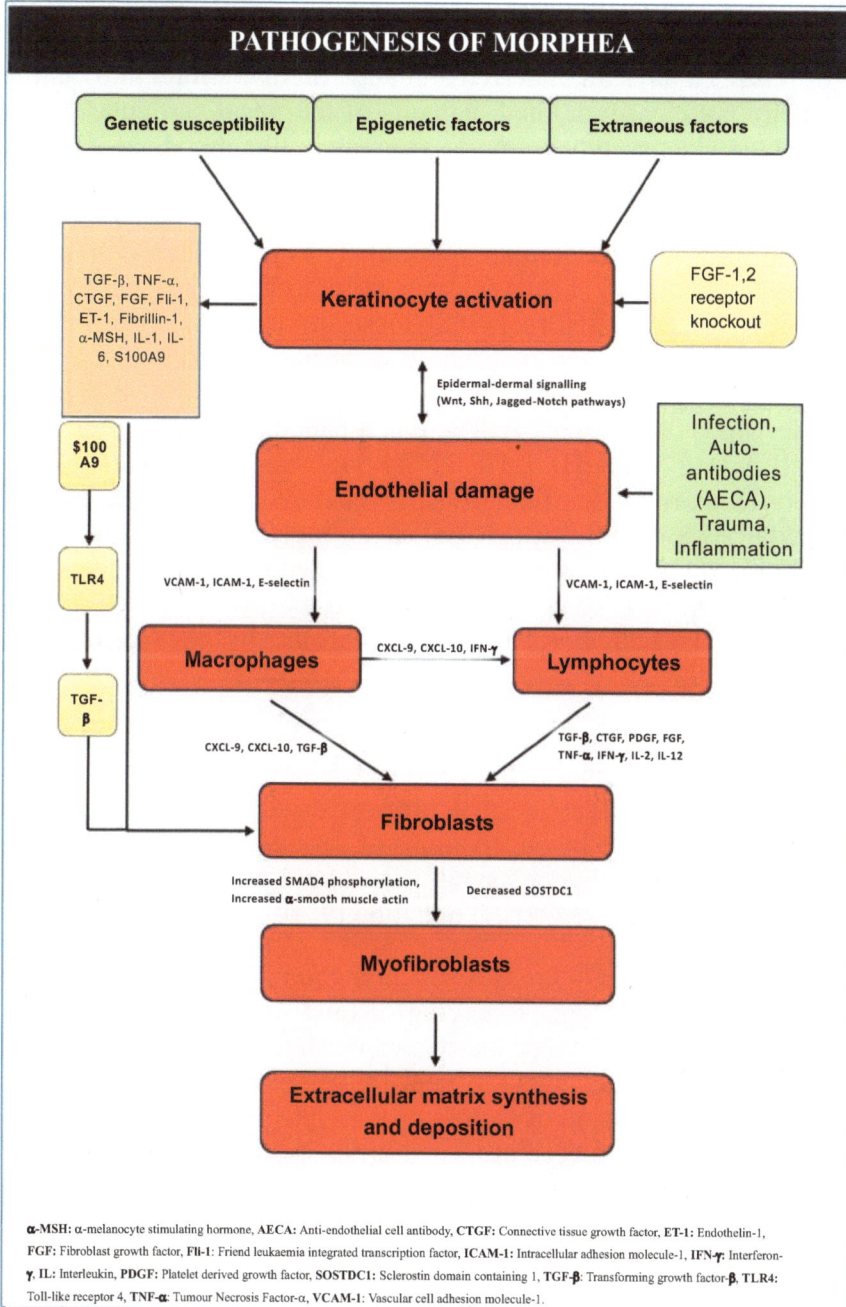

PATHOGENESIS OF MORPHEA

Genetic susceptibility | Epigenetic factors | Extraneous factors

TGF-β, TNF-α, CTGF, FGF, Fli-1, ET-1, Fibrillin-1, α-MSH, IL-1, IL-6, S100A9

Keratinocyte activation

FGF-1,2 receptor knockout

Epidermal-dermal signalling (Wnt, Shh, Jagged-Notch pathways)

S100 A9

Endothelial damage

Infection, Auto-antibodies (AECA), Trauma, Inflammation

TLR4

VCAM-1, ICAM-1, E-selectin   VCAM-1, ICAM-1, E-selectin

TGF-β

Macrophages   CXCL-9, CXCL-10, IFN-γ   **Lymphocytes**

CXCL-9, CXCL-10, TGF-β   TGF-β, CTGF, PDGF, FGF, TNF-α, IFN-γ, IL-2, IL-12

Fibroblasts

Increased SMAD4 phosphorylation, Increased α-smooth muscle actin   Decreased SOSTDC1

Myofibroblasts

Extracellular matrix synthesis and deposition

α-MSH: α-melanocyte stimulating hormone, **AECA**: Anti-endothelial cell antibody, **CTGF**: Connective tissue growth factor, **ET-1**: Endothelin-1, **FGF**: Fibroblast growth factor, **Fli-1**: Friend leukaemia integrated transcription factor, **ICAM-1**: Intracellular adhesion molecule-1, **IFN-γ**: Interferon-γ. **IL**: Interleukin, **PDGF**: Platelet derived growth factor, **SOSTDC1**: Sclerostin domain containing 1, **TGF-β**: Transforming growth factor-β, **TLR4**: Toll-like receptor 4, **TNF-α**: Tumour Necrosis Factor-α, **VCAM-1**: Vascular cell adhesion molecule-1.

Fig. (5.1). The basic outline of the pathogenesis of morphea.

GENETIC FACTORS

Patients of morphea have an underlying genetic predisposition, though the genes responsible are not clearly defined. Patients of morphea, particularly those with generalized and linear types, have a greater likelihood of having other autoimmune diseases, which may be up to 46% in generalized morphea. Chances of a concomitant autoimmune disease or rheumatic disease are more common in adults [3]. Significantly, children are more likely to present with a family history of morphea than adults [3]. These findings point to the fact that morphea shares certain genetic susceptibility foci with these autoimmune and rheumatologic diseases. The gene expression in genome-wide patterns with the help of DNA microarrays from a skin biopsy of 3 morphea patients linked them to an inflammatory signature cluster [4]. There is a paucity of studies linking HLA to morphea. HLA-B*37 and HLA-DRB1*04:04 have been linked to increased susceptibility to morphea, particularly the generalized and linear subtypes [5]. Since HLA-DRB1*04:04 has been linked strongly to rheumatoid arthritis, a common genetic susceptibility to morphea and rheumatoid arthritis is, therefore, implied [6]. The role of CD8 or natural killer cells is proposed by the association of HLA class I alleles with morphea and indicates loss of tolerance to an unknown antigen [5].

The likely role of mosaicism for mutations that predispose to morphea is proposed based on the observation that linear morphea is strongly related to the lines of Blaschko [7, 8]. A primarily dermal process driven by fibroblasts following Blaschko lines is supported by observations of dermal diseases such as granuloma annulare and focal dermal hypoplasia in Blaschkoid distribution, which is due to porcupine homologue gene (*PORCN*) mutation [9, 10].

Positional identity refers to the phenomenon of immunologically and phenotypically similar fibroblasts having distinct gene expressions at different locations. The *HOX* genes are primarily responsible for this positional identity. The site-specific gene signatures are vital for region-specific mesenchymal cell differentiation and expression of factors such as TGF-β and ultimately determine fibrosis [11]. Their role has been proposed in SSC-related skin and internal organ involvement but studies regarding their role in morphea, though relevant, are lacking [12]. (Box **5.1**) summarises the genetic susceptibility mechanisms in morphea.

Box 5.1: Factors supporting genetic susceptibility mechanisms in morphea.
Family history of morphea
Personal history of other autoimmune diseases
Shared genetic loci with other autoimmune or rheumatologic diseases
HLA subtype
Mosaicism
Positional identity of mesenchymal cell differentiation

MICROCHIMERISM

The clinical and histopathological similarities between morphea and graft versus host disease point to the possible role of chimeric cells in the pathogenesis of morphea. These cells are transferred during pregnancy from the mother to the foetus or vice-versa. This theory is supported by the observation that children and parous women in their reproductive years are most commonly affected by morphea [13]. Chimeric cells have been found to be present in morphea patients using the polymerase chain reaction (PCR) technique, but their number is similar to healthy controls. However, lesional skin has chimeric cells of epithelial origin while non-lesional skin has chimeric cells with markers of T cells and macrophages [14, 15]. The significance of this observation is still to be explored.

EPIGENETIC FACTORS

Epigenetic factors (Box **5.2**) act as a bridge between genetic susceptibility and extraneous susceptibility factors. Patients of SSC demonstrate altered patterns of DNA methylation and histone acetylation at several genetic loci. Of great significance is the transcriptional silencing of repressive genes in fibroblasts, which leads to increased expression of pro-fibrotic genes and transforming growth factor (TGF-β) genes [16]. Altered methylation of genes on X-chromosomes, which are responsible for apoptosis, inflammation and oxidative stress on SSC-identified sites may provide an explanation for the higher prevalence of SSC and morphea in women [17].

Box 5.2: Epigenetic factors in morphea.
Altered DNA methylation of genes involved in apoptosis and inflammation
Histone acetylation of genes involved in fibrosis
Transcriptional silencing of repressive genes of fibroblasts
Increased expression of micro RNA (miRNA-483 5p, miRNA-30b, miRNA-21, miRNA-155)
Decreased expression of miRNA (miRNA-30b, miRNA-7, miRNA-196a, miRNA-let7a)

Several micro RNAs (miRNAs) have been found to be dysregulated in the skin of patients with scleroderma. miRNA-21 and miR-155 are expressed in greater than normal amounts in SSC and are pro-fibrotic in nature [18]. miRNA-483 5p is a specific marker of skin fibrosis and is also upregulated in SSC and morphea [19]. Its overexpression in endothelial cells leads to myofibroblast differentiation [20]. miRNA-30b is related to increased expression of platelet-derived growth factor (PDGF) on the dermal fibroblasts and its expression correlates inversely with the extent of skin involvement in SSC (as measured by the modified Rodnan skin score) [21]. Levels of miRNA-7 in tissue and serum are significantly decreased in morphea and lead to higher expression of α2 type-1 collagen. In fact, serum levels of miRNA-7 may be used as a disease marker for morphea [22]. Similarly, serum and tissue levels of miRNA-196a and miRNA-let7a have been shown to be decreased in morphea with consequent overexpression of collagen type 1 [23].

AUTOANTIBODIES

SSC is not only characterized by the presence of autoantibodies, but these autoantibodies are also important for disease classification and internal organ involvement. The role of autoantibodies and their clinical implications in morphea is, however, not clearly defined.

Antinuclear antibodies (ANA) in morphea have been shown in 20-80% of patients with the speckled pattern being most common [24 - 27]. The positivity of ANA is associated with deeper tissue involvement and involvement of extracutaneous sites [28, 29]. The severity of skin disease, assessed by the body surface area involved, modified Rodnan skin score (mRSS), and the number of lesions, and the number of sites involved was found to be significantly associated with positivity to ANA in the morphea in adults and children (MAC) cohort and the National registry of childhood onset scleroderma (NRCOS) studies [30, 31]. Positive ANA also predisposes to relapse of morphea after remission by an odds ratio of 4.8 [32]. SSC-related autoantibodies such as anti-centromere, anti-topoisomerase, anti-U3 ribonucleoprotein (anti-U3RNP), *etc.* are seen in a small subset of morphea patients and correlate with skin symptoms, skin thickness, joint contractures and musculoskeletal system involvement [33]. Rheumatoid factor has been found to be positive in 3-16% of all morphea patients and correlated with musculoskeletal and joint manifestations [34].

Anti-histone antibodies may be seen in up to half of all morphea patients and correlate with the number of skin lesions, their distribution, linear subtype, and deep tissue involvement in the form of joint contractures [35]. Anti-single-stranded DNA antibodies (anti-ssDNA) are also seen in around half of all patients and show correlation with joint contractures and active disease of more than two years' duration and with inflammatory cytokines [31, 36, 37]. Positivity to anti-histone as well as anti-ssDNA indicates severe disease, larger body surface involvement, severe skin damage and functional limitation in the linear type of morphea [30].

Antibodies to dense fine speckled 70 kDa antigen (anti-DFS70) are seen in juvenile morphea. Anti-DFS70 are more commonly seen in those who do not have antinuclear antibody-associated rheumatic disease [38].

Anti-DNA topoisomerase II α (anti topo-IIα) of IgG and IgM type were found to be relatively specific for morphea and showed positivity in 76% of patients with localized morphea and 85% patients with the generalized form of morphea. This is in contrast to low positivity of 14% in SSC, 8% in systemic lupus erythematosus (SLE) and 10% in dermatomyositis. These antibodies correlated with a greater number of sclerotic lesions and the number of plaque lesions of localized morphea [39].

Anti-U1-RNP and anti-U3-RNP have been reported in morphea patients [40]. Anti-endothelial cell antibodies (AECA) are elevated in 22-86% of SSC patients and are likely elevated in morphea as well [41]. The AECA is a cause of vascular injury by inducing apoptosis of endothelial cells, generating free radicals and expression of adhesion molecules on endothelial cells [42]. Vascular endothelial injury is proposed as one of the earliest events in the pathogenesis of morphea [43]. The various antibodies seen in morphea and their clinical significance have been summarized in Table **5.1**.

Table 5.1. Autoantibodies in morphea and their clinical correlation.

Autoantibody	Positivity (%)	Clinical Correlation
Anti-nuclear antibody (ANA) [24, 32]	20-80%	• Deeper tissue involvement • Extracutaneous involvement • Number of lesions • Number of sites involved • Modified Rodnan skin score • Generalized and linear subtypes • Probability of flare after remission (Odds ratio=4.8)
Anti-topoisomerase (anti-Scl-70), Anti-centromere (ACA), Anti-U3 ribonucleoprotein (anti-U3RNP) [33]	6-16%	• Joint contractures • Musculoskeletal involvement • Skin thickness • Skin symptoms (tingling, pain)

(Table 5.1) cont.....

Autoantibody	Positivity (%)	Clinical Correlation
Anti-histone antibody (AHA) [35]	47%	• Number of lesions • Distribution of lesions • Depth of lesions • Muscle & joint involvement • Linear subtype > generalized subtype • No correlation with relapse
Anti-single-stranded DNA antibody (anti-ssDNA) [31, 36, 37]	50%	• Deep tissue involvement • Joint contractures • Longer duration of disease activity • Extensive skin involvement • No correlation with relapse
AHA & anti-ssDNA [30]	23%	• Deep tissue involvement • Joint contracture • Extensive skin involvement • Functional limitation in linear subtype
Rheumatoid factor (RF) [34]	3-16%	• Musculoskeletal & joint involvement
Anti-dense fine speckled 70 kDa antigen (anti-DFS70) [38]	4.5-13.8%	• Joint involvement (in ANA-negative children)
Anti-DNA topoisomerase II α (anti topo-IIα) [39]	76-85%	• Relatively specific for morphea • Number of sclerotic lesions • Number of plaque lesions • Seen in generalized > localized disease
Anti-endothelial cell antibody (AECA) [1]	22-86%	• Details not available
Anti- Sjogren syndrome related antigen A and B (anti-SSA and anti-SSB) [33]	2%	• Skin tightness & hypopigmentation • Neurological manifestations
Anti-Smith ribonucleoproteins [33]	2-12%	• Shiny skin • Hypo- and hyper-pigmentation
Anti-U1 ribonucleoprotein (anti-U1RNP) [40]	3%	• Possibly with linear morphea • No extracutaneous involvement

EXTRINSIC FACTORS

As already discussed, morphea occurs when a genetically susceptible individual is exposed to a 'second hit', which can be environmental insults such as trauma, radiation, surgery, infection, or drugs or can occur due to the presence of autoantibodies.

Trauma

Preceding history of mechanical trauma has been seen in approximately 13% of children in two retrospective studies involving nearly 900 patients [24, 34].

Reports of morphea developing after vaccination have also been ascribed to the trauma from injection or to preservatives used in vaccines [44]. There have been reports of morphea developing at compression sites [45, 46]. Trauma may induce an unchecked healing process leading to excessive fibrosis. However, what causes delayed induction of morphea following trauma several years back is not known [47].

Radiation

Post-radiation morphea is common and is seen in one out of every 500 patients [48]. It usually develops within a year of radiotherapy, though reports of morphea after several years of having received radiotherapy are described [49]. Breast cancer patients on adjuvant radiotherapy are at the greatest risk [50]. A quarter of all patients develop morphea beyond the boundaries of the radiation field and even at a remote areas [51, 52]. It is believed that radiation may trigger an isomorphic response, may selectively activate fibroblasts, or may produce self-antigens as a result of radiation-induced tissue damage [1].

Infections

The role of *Borrelia* in the causation of morphea is controversial. Several studies have refuted its role in disease pathogenesis [53 - 55]. Eidendle *et al.* reported that half of all patients with morphea showed positivity for *Borrelia* [56]. A retrospective review by Prinz *et al.* in 90 patients of morphea found a highly significant association between high titres of ANA and *Borrelia* serology in patients with early onset of morphea in childhood or adolescence [57]. Further, it is interesting to note that reports associating the disease with *Borrelia* are mostly from Europe [1], which is caused by *Borrelia afzelii* or *Borrelia garinii*, unlike American *Borrelia* infection which is caused by *Borrelia burgdorferi* (*sensu stricto*). The organism can adhere to and penetrate human fibroblasts, which may somehow lead to their activation or lipoprotein expression, which may invite inflammatory cells and mediators [58].

Cytomegalovirus (CMV) may also be one of the etiologic agents and case reports of morphea developing secondary to CMV infection have been reported [59]. Antibodies to CMV have been found in patients of SSC [60], though no such study is available for morphea. However, the propensity of CMV to infect and damage vascular endothelium, induction of B-cells leading to immune dysregulation and its ability for recruitment of macrophages makes it a potential etiologic agent in morphea as well [61]. Molecular mimicry between CMV late protein UL-94 and NAG-2 and surface protein of endothelial cells may lead to endothelial damage [62].

Antibodies to *Toxoplasma gondii*, *Epstein Barr* virus and hepatitis B virus were found to be higher in patients of SSC than healthy controls [60]. However, no such study has been undertaken in patients of morphea so far.

Drugs

Drug-induced morphea is extremely uncommon. Cases have been described after the intake of bisoprolol, bleomycin, peplomycin, d-penicillamine, bromocriptine, 5-hydroxytryptophane and carbidopa, pentazocine, vitamin B_{12}, vitamin K and balicatib (also see chapter 4, Table **4.1**, for more drugs reported to cause morphea). The latency period from the start of the drug to the onset of lesions ranged from a few days to 3 years [63]. Bleomycin, peplomycin, beta blockers, and dopaminergic drugs may produce morphea by inducing fibroblast growth and collagen synthesis [63]. Penicillamine interferes with collagen and elastin maturation [64]. Ergot derivatives and pentazocine may induce morphea by producing ischemic damage [63]. The induction of morphea due to vitamin K and vitamin B_{12} has been attributed to the toxic effects of the oil-based vehicle used or to benzyl alcohol used as a preservative [65, 66]. The common extraneous causes of morphea and the proposed mechanism of the disease are summarised in Table **5.2**.

Table 5.2. Mechanism of morphea caused by extraneous agents.

Category	Name of Agent	Proposed Pathogenesis of morphea
TRAUMA		Induction of the healing process that goes on unchecked and leads to excessive fibrosis [47].
RADIATION		Triggering of isomorphic response, production of self-antigens and selective activation of fibroblasts [1].
INFECTIONS	Borrelia	Penetration and activation of human fibroblasts and lipoprotein expression, which cause an influx of inflammatory cells and mediators [58].
	Cytomegalovirus	Infection and damage to vascular endothelium by molecular mimicry between CMV late proteins and surface proteins of the endothelium, immune dysregulation by induction of B cells and recruitment of macrophages [61, 62]
	Parvovirus B19	Infects endothelial cells and fibroblasts and leads to production of tumour necrosis factor-alpha

(Table 5.2) cont.....

Category	Name of Agent	Proposed Pathogenesis of morphea
DRUGS	Bleomycin, Peplomycin, Beta blockers, Dopaminergic drugs	Induction of fibroblast growth and collagen synthesis [63].
	Penicillamine	Interference with collagen and elastin maturation and synthesis, decreased regulatory T cells [64]
	Ergot derivatives, Pentazocine	Production of ischemic damage leading to endothelial injury and influx of profibrotic cytokines [63]
	Vitamin K, Vitamin B$_{12}$	Toxic effects of oil-based vehicle or benzyl alcohol used as a preservative or due to hypersensitivity [65, 66]
	Balicatib	Deposition of excessive extracellular matrix proteins deposition [63]

VASCULAR FACTORS

Vascular injury has been proposed to be one of the earliest and most important steps in the pathogenesis of SSC. This is probably mediated by external triggers such as drugs, infections or by AECA. Fresch *et al.* demonstrated interstitial edema, fibrosis, endothelial cell swelling and lamellation of the basal layer in patients of SSC [67]. Further, early morphea lesions show decreased capillary density, perivascular inflammation and perivascular activation of fibroblasts on histopathology and endothelial cell destruction along with the duplication of capillary endothelial cells on electron microscopy [68].

Endothelial cell injury is mediated by interleukin-6 (IL-6) released from neutrophils and Fas-mediated apoptotic pathway with the help of antibody-dependant cell-mediated toxicity [69, 70]. Higher plasma levels of microparticles, small membrane-bound vesicles that participate in intercellular signalling, have been detected in SSC patients [71]. Phagocytosis of these microparticles and acid sphingomyelinase activity may lead to apoptosis of circulating angiogenic cells [72]. Dermal fibroblasts have high expression of anti-apoptotic proteins such as cFLIP and cIAP. They are also deficient in acid sphingomyelinase enzyme. This makes the dermal fibroblasts partially resistant to apoptosis and provides an explanation for their increased survival and resultant increased extracellular matrix deposition [73, 74].

It is believed that endothelial cell injury upregulates the expression of cytokines such as Vascular cell adhesion molecule-1(VCAM-1), intercellular adhesion molecule-1 (ICAM-1) and E-selectin [75]. This leads to the influx of inflammatory cells such as T-cells, macrophages and eosinophils, which increases the production of profibrotic cytokines, such as IL-4, IL-6 and transforming growth factor-β (TGF-β), leading to tissue fibrosis [76, 77].

ROLE OF EPIDERMIS

Keratinocytes

The epidermal cells presumably play an important role in the pathogenesis of morphea, though most evidence is from SSC or animal-based studies. Experimental studies have shown that connective tissue growth factors (CTGF), fibronectin and collagen type 1 are altered by keratinocytes, which influences extracellular matrix genes [78]. Keratinocytes produce several factors causing dermal fibrosis, such as TGF-β, tumor necrosis factor-α (TNF-α), IL-1, IL-6, endothelin-1, fibrillin-1, fibroblast growth factor (FGF), chemokine (c-c motif) ligand 2 (CCL2), friend leukaemia integrated transcription factor-1 (Fli-1), S100A9, α-melanocyte stimulating factor (α-MSH), *etc* [79]. Keratinocytes primarily via IL-1, mediate fibrosis by inducing keratinocyte growth factor (KGF) and metalloproteinases in fibroblasts [80]. Skin involved in SSC has an increased proliferation of keratinocytes [81]. Keratinocytes also promote the activation of myofibroblasts, even without the stimulation of TGF- β, and have an imbalance between NFκB1 and peroxisome proliferator-activated receptor gamma (PPAR-γ), which produces cytokines and upregulates CCL5 [82].

CTGF has been demonstrated in dermal fibroblasts in morphea lesions [83]. Keratinocytes produce S100A9 in times of stress, which in conjunction with toll-like receptor-4 (TLR-4) increases CTGF expression and stimulates fibroblasts [84]. TLR-4 itself has a profibrotic effect via TGF-β. The role of fibroblast growth factor (FGF) has been linked to fibrosis in animal studies. FGF receptor knockout mice show increased trans-epidermal water loss, prompting keratinocytes to produce IL-1, S100A8 and S100A9, leading to fibrosis [85]. α-MSH mediates fibrosis and cytokine production by keratinocytes and fibroblasts and is important for homeostasis of fibrosis. Mice lacking its receptor, the melanocortin-1 receptor (MC1R) have shown susceptibility to fibrosis [86]. Fibrillin-1, a major component of the extracellular matrix mediates binding to integrin and has been linked to skin sclerosis. Antibodies to fibrillin-1 have been demonstrated in morphea [87]. Fibrillin-1 mutation leads to stiff skin syndrome, a morphea-like clinical picture [88]. Similarly, keratinocyte Fli-1 knockout mice demonstrate increased skin fibrosis apart from the expression of cytokines like IL-1, IL-6 and IL-8 [2, 89]. Further, Fli-1 downregulation produces an SSC-like picture in vessels, fibroblasts and macrophages [2, 90].

Epidermal-dermal Signalling

Several epidermal-dermal signalling pathways are being explored as potential mechanisms leading to dermal fibrosis. Of particular interest are the sonic hedgehog pathway (Shh) and the Jagged-Notch pathway. These have been demonstrated to be involved in SSC and may be relevant in patterns and morphological variations seen in morphea [91, 92]. Wnt signalling pathway begins in the epidermis and stimulates fibroblasts leading to the expression of β-catenin mediated collagen, other matrix proteins, CTGF, increased proliferation of fibroblasts and differentiation of myofibroblasts [93]. Wnt ligands and receptors are overexpressed while Wnt antagonists are decreased in SSC. PPAR-γ is an antagonist of Wnt-β-catenin pathway and has been shown to be decreased in SSC [93]. Wnt also decreases the epidermal response to FGF. Keratinocyte-derived Wnt-5a, which is β-catenin independent, is expressed in greater amounts in dermal fibroblasts in SSC. Wnt-5a knockout mice are relatively resistant to skin sclerosis induced by bleomycin [94]. The Jagged-Notch pathways and Shh pathways are both elevated in fibroblasts in SSC [95, 96]. There is, however, scarce literature supporting the role of these pathways in morphea. Table **5.3** discusses the major mediators of pathogenesis in the epidermis.

Table 5.3. Pathogenic mediators of morphea in the epidermis.

Keratinocyte Growth Factor (KGF)	Produced by Keratinocytes *via* Interleukin-1, mediates fibrosis [80]
S100A9	In conjunction with Toll-like receptor-4 (TLR-4), increases CTGF expression and stimulates fibroblasts [84].
Toll-like receptor 4 (TLR4)	Profibrotic action via TGF-β increases CTGF expression and stimulates fibroblasts under influence of S100A9 [84].
Fibroblast growth factor (FGF)	Keratinocyte FGF receptor knockout leads to increased trans-epidermal water loss, prompting keratinocytes to produce Interleukin-1, S100A8, and S100A9, leading to fibrosis [85].
α-melanocyte stimulating factor (α-MSH)	Mediates homeostasis in fibrosis and cytokine production by keratinocytes and fibroblasts [86].
Fibrillin-1	A major component of the extracellular matrix that mediates the binding to integrin, antibodies against it are seen in morphea [87], and mutation produces stiff skin syndrome [88].
Friend leukaemia integrated transcription factor-1 (Fli-1)	Downregulation produces skin fibrosis and expression of interleukins 1, 6, 8, producing an SSC like the picture in vessels, macrophages and fibroblasts [89, 90].
Wingless and int homologue (Wnt) pathway	Stimulates fibroblasts and enhances the expression of collagen, other matrix proteins, connective tissue growth factor (CTGF), increases fibroblast proliferation and myofibroblast differentiation decreases epidermal response to fibroblast growth factor [2, 93].

(Table 5.3) cont.....

Jagged-Notch pathway & Sonic Hedgehog (Shh) pathway	Found to be elevated in fibroblasts of SSC [95, 96], proposed to be relevant in patterns and morphological variation seen in morphea [91, 92]

THE IMMUNE RESPONSE

Innate Immunity

The role of innate immune response in triggering the pro-inflammatory cascade is under investigation. Type 1 interferon (IFN-1) is supposedly the key mediator in fibrosis, which via TLR signalling increases the responsiveness of fibroblasts to TGF-β and increases other pro-inflammatory and pro-fibrotic cytokines and chemokines [97]. Studies on mice have demonstrated that TLR3 ligand induces the expression of several extracellular matrix genes in fibroblasts and dermal fibrosis [98]. Activation of interferon genes is controlled by interferon regulatory factor 5 (IRF-5). The role of IRF-5 in pulmonary fibrosis has been established and it has been coined a susceptibility factor for SSC [99]. The signal transducer and activator of transcription 4 (STAT4) is also one of the inducers of IFN-1 and mice deficient in STAT4 develop less fibrosis compared to controls when exposed to bleomycin [99]. STAT4 also produces several pro-inflammatory cytokines such as IL-2, IL-6 and TNF-α. This is particularly relevant as fibrosis in morphea is a result of inflammation.

The levels of IL-1β and NACHT-LLR-PYD-containing protein-3 (NLRP-3) inflammasome correlate with the severity of skin involvement, assessed by modified Rodnan skin score in SSC and can be seen in the epidermis of SSC skin on immunohistochemistry [100]. Nuclear factor kappa B (NFkB) is the chief mediator of innate immunity. One of its five subunits, the c-Rel, has been shown to play a profibrotic role in experimental mice and its link to SSC is suggested [101].

Acquired Immunity

The cytokine profile-based model of the immunopathogenesis of morphea shows three disease phases (Fig. **5.2**).

The early phase of the disease shows active inflammation and is mediated by Th1 cytokines such as IL-2, IL-6 and TNF-α. The second stage shows ongoing inflammation and the onset of fibrosis. This stage is guided by the Th17 cytokines such as IL-17, IL-22, IL-1 and by TGF-β. The Th2 cytokines produce the final stage of sclerosis and atrophy. This stage is mediated by IL-4 and IL-13 [102].

CYTOKINE PROFILE IN VARIOUS STAGES OF MORPHEA

EARLY STAGE OF ACTIVE INFLAMMATION

Th1 cytokines (IL-2, IL-6, TNF-α)

STAGE OF ONGOING INFLAMMATION & ONSET OF FIBROSIS

Th17 cytokines (IL-17, IL22, IL-1) & TGF-β

FINAL STAGE OF SCLEROSIS & ATROPHY

Th2 cytokines (IL-4, IL-13)

IL: Interleukin, **TNF-α:** Tumour Necrosis Factor-α, **TGF-β:** Transforming Growth Factor-β

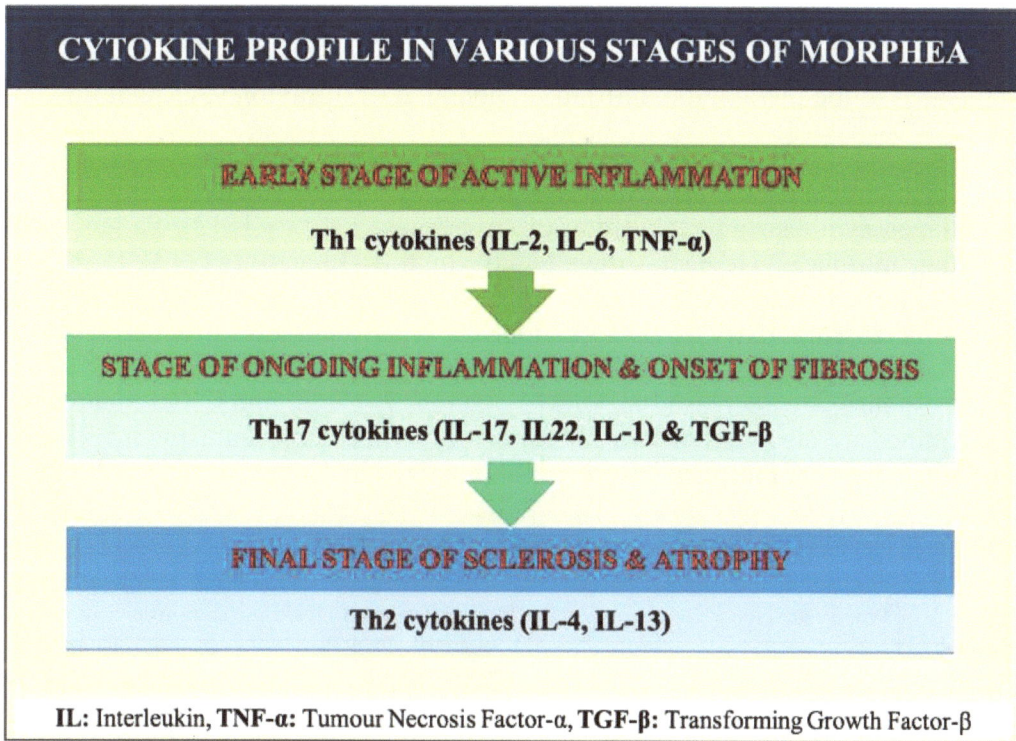

Fig. (5.2). Cytokine profile in various stages of morphea.

The serum levels of TNF-α, IL-2, IL-1, IL-6 and their receptors are found to be raised in the early lesions of morphea and correlate with the severity of skin involvement and antibody titres [102, 103]. IL-1 and IL-6 levels are raised during the first few months of disease onset [104]. Collagen transcription, CTGF expression and fibroblast activation is triggered by IL-1, via its action on IL-6 and platelet derived growth factor (PDGF) [105].

IL-1 and IL-6 are Th17 inducers and IL-17F and IL-22, which are chief effectors of the Th17 pathway, are elevated after 1-2 years of disease onset. IL-22 and TNF-activated keratinocytes produce a profibrotic response [106]. The levels of IL-17A correlate inversely with IL-22 and TGF-β in the setting of polymerised collagen treatment and normalization of dermal architecture in morphea skin [107].

TGF-β is the principal regulator involved in wound healing and is responsible primarily for pathological fibrosis. Skin biopsy and serum levels of TGF-β and its receptors are increased in morphea [108]. TGF-β also promotes the extracellular matrix and inhibits its degradation by the regulation of matrix metalloproteinases

(MMP) [109]. MMP-12 has an increased expression in SSC and corresponds to the extent of skin involvement and disease duration [110]. MMP-12 has been implicated in the therapeutic antifibrotic potential of ultraviolet A1 phototherapy [111].

The Th2 cytokine profile related to IL-4 and IL-13 is involved in the upregulation of collagen synthesis and inhibition of collagenase activity [112]. Patients with late-stage morphea have been shown to have high IL-13 activity [113]. IL-13 also is linked to TGF-β and CCL2. Gene expression profiling of morphea patients has shown increased activity of IL-13 and CCL2 [4]. B cells also produce IL-6 and TGF-β and a profibrotic Th2 response. Regulatory B cells, which inhibit Th1 and Th17 response, are decreased in SSC [2]. CCL5, 7, 17, 22 and CXCL8 and other chemokines are also responsible for fibrosis [114]. The mechanisms involved in the pathogenesis of morphea have been summarized in Table **5.4**.

Table 5.4. Inflammatory mediators in the pathogenesis of morphea.

Innate immunity	Type 1 interferon	Key mediator of fibrosis, increases responsiveness of fibroblasts to transforming growth factor-β and increases pro-inflammatory and pro-fibrotic cytokines and chemokines [97].
	Toll-like receptor 3 ligand (TLR3)	Increases responsiveness of fibroblasts to transforming growth factor-β, increases other pro-inflammatory and pro-fibrotic cytokines in conjunction with interferon type 1 [98].
	Interferon regulatory factor-5 (IRF-5)	Regulates the expression of interferon genes [99].
	Signal transducer and activator of transcription 4 (STAT4)	Induces interferon type 1, produces pro-inflammatory cytokines interleukin-2, interleukin-6, tumour necrosis factor-α [99].
	NACHT, LLR and PYD-domain--containing protein-2 (NLR-3) inflammasome	Levels correlate with modified Rodnan skin score [100].
	Nuclear factor kappa B (NFkB)	c-Rel subunit has a pro-fibrotic role [101].
Acquired immunity	Th1 cytokines (Interleukin 2,6 & Tumour necrosis factor-α)	Raised in the early phase of the disease (within 2 years), interleukin-6 increases collagen and promotes fibroblast activation [105].
	Th17 cytokines (Interleukin 1, 17, 22)	Raised later (2-4 years after disease onset), interleukin-1 increases the expression of connective tissue growth factor (CTGF), collagen transcription and fibroblast activation [105].

(Table 5.4) cont.....

	Transforming growth factor-β	Principal regulator of pathological fibrosis, promotes extracellular matrix deposition and increases matrix metalloproteinase [109].
	Th2 cytokines (interleukin 4, 13)	Upregulate collagen synthesis and inhibit collagenase activity [112].

ROLE OF MESENCHYME & FIBROBLASTS

Myofibroblasts are the chief cells responsible for fibrosis. Fibroblasts migrate at the site of an epithelial defect and change to secretory myofibroblasts producing healing. In morphea, this process of fibrosis goes on unchecked under the influence of TGF-β, CTGF, FGF and other activating signals [96]. Fibrotic skin diseases also show trans-differentiation of fibroblasts from differentiated cells of other cell lineages. Epithelial to myofibroblast trans-differentiation is mediated by Bone morphogenetic protein 2 (BMP-2) induced TNF-α, TGF-β, CTGF, FGF, Smad signalling, Wnt, Shh and Jagged-Notch pathways [115 - 117]. Apart from trans-differentiation, aberrant differentiation of bone marrow related fibrocytes into fibroblasts also takes place in SSC [118]. The small molecule GTPase Rac1, which helps cell trafficking and migration may play an important role in the persistence of myofibroblasts in morphea [119]. As discussed previously, dermal fibroblasts are resistant to Fas-mediated apoptosis due to a deficiency of acid sphingomyelinase and the increased levels of cFLIP and cIAP.

ROLE OF DENDRITIC CELLS

Dendritic cells have been proposed to play an important role in the pathogenesis of morphea. The plasmacytoid dendritic cells, in response to an unknown ligand, produce IFN-α and IFN-γ. The myeloid dendritic cells are activated which in turn produce autoreactive B and T cells via MHC molecules [120]. This produces skin autoimmunity by T cell activation and then morphea (Fig. **5.3**).

CD8-bearing apoptotic bodies activating CD205 of dendritic cells have been demonstrated in *In-vivo* T cell subtyping studies. CD205 present on myeloid dendritic cells has the ability to induce tolerance to autoantigens released during apoptosis or necrosis of tissue by recognizing and trapping them [121]. High numbers of plasmacytoid dendritic cells have been demonstrated in the lesional skin of morphea in the deep dermis, around blood vessels and in collagen bundles [122].

ROLE OF INSULIN-LIKE GROWTH FACTOR-1 (IGF-1)

The potential role of IGF-1 was indicated by its increased expression in morphea lesional and non-lesional skin and serum compared to controls. IGF-1 in lesional skin was significantly higher than that present in non-lesional skin. The levels of IGF-1 in the lesional skin correlated with the Rodnan skin score [123]. IGF-1 is a profibrotic compound expressed on all connective tissue. It increases the production of collagen and the deposition of extracellular matrix and recruits fibroblasts. It activates pre-B cells to produce immunoglobulins and causes T-cell expansion [123].

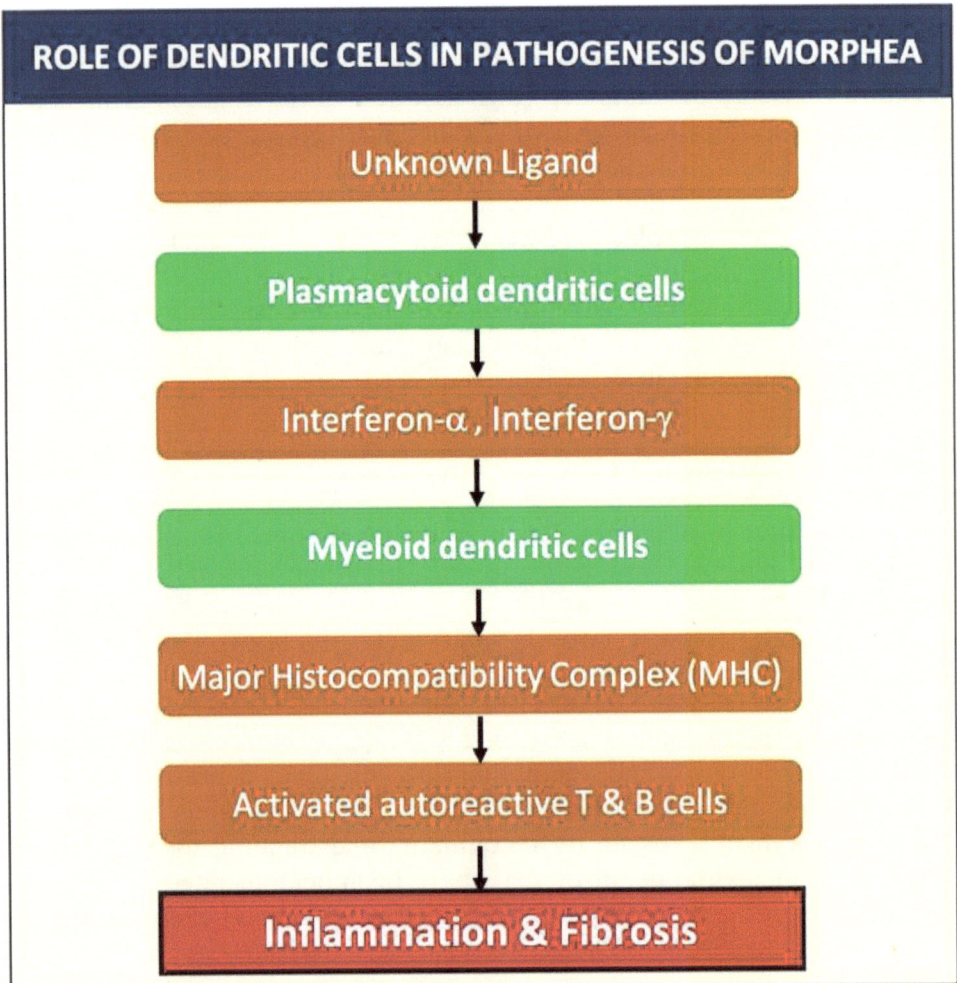

Fig. (5.3). Role of dendritic cells in the pathogenesis of morphea.

MORPHEA SUBTYPES AND PATHOGENESIS

Morphea presents with a wide variety of anatomic and morphologic variability. This may be the result of local susceptibility factors which include regional genetic and epigenetic disturbances or distinct pathogenic mechanisms. The stepwise pathogenic pathway of inflammation followed by sclerosis and atrophy shows inter-individual and intra-individual variability. Epigenetic factors, positional identity, Wnt signalling or α-MSH may be responsible for the same [2]. As already discussed, the pathogenesis of blaschkoid morphea can be explained on the basis of PORCN mutations seen in focal dermal hypoplasia [9]. Friction and radiation may also act as location-specific triggers while positional identity, site specific expression of TGF and FGF, epidermal signalling, epidermal-mesenchymal trans-differentiation, positional identity and innate pathways may lead to regional susceptibility to morphea [2].

DISTINCTIVENESS OF PATHOGENESIS OF MORPHEA IN CHILDREN

Apart from the age of onset, morphea in children shows distinct features (Box **5.3**). There is a higher chance of extracutaneous involvement and deep tissue involvement in children. Children also have a longer mean duration of disease. They have a higher frequency of linear, mixed and pan-sclerotic subtypes of morphea compared to adults [124]. These factors are responsible for the higher frequency of morbidity in children [124]. The age-related differences in immune response may be the cause. Chapter 19 has been exclusively dedicated to pediatric morphea. Readers are referred to chapter 19 for a detailed account of pediatric morphea.

Box 5.3: Distinctive features of childhood morphea.
Greater extracutaneous involvement
Greater chance of deeper tissue involvement
Longer mean duration of disease
Higher risk of linear, pan-sclerotic and mixed morphea
Greater morbidity
Reduced number of regulatory T-cells
Higher activation of innate immunity
Increased number of Th1, Th17 and Th2 cells
Accelerated immune system development to adult form

Normally, children show a higher number of T-regulatory cells, monocytes and natural killer cells but lower levels of CD4 and CD8 cells than adults. Childhood is also the time of generation of immune repertoire for lymphocytes. Diseased children show a reduced number of T-regulatory cells, higher activation of innate immune cells and an increased number of Th1, Th17 and Th2 cells compared to healthy children. This immune pattern resembles that of healthy adults. While autoreactivity may be a contributor to disease pathogenesis, it has been speculated that the above-mentioned immune cell distribution and activity may be due to an accelerated immune system development to a more permissive form [6]. This is distinct from the ageing of the immune system where senescent inflammatory cells are seen.

DIFFERENCES IN THE PATHOGENESIS OF MORPHEA AND SSC

Morphea and SSC broadly share similar pathogenesis, though the two conditions are clinically quite distinct. In both these conditions, the twin hit (genetic and environmental) results in vascular endothelial injury. This results in the recruitment of inflammatory cells by the release of cell adhesion molecules and chemokines. These inflammatory cells are of Th1, Th17 and Th2 types. Inflammation ensues, fibroblasts are activated, and fibrosis occurs. However, there are some differences in the pathogenesis of morphea and SSC Table **5.5**.

Table 5.5. Differences in the pathogenesis of morphea and SSC.

Parameter	Morphea	SSC
Genetic factors	Specific genes not identified, linked to HLA class I	Specific genes such as *IRF5*, *BANK1*, *STAT4*, *CD247*, *BLK* and *TNFSF4*.
External agents	Radiation, trauma, Borrelia and viral infections and certain drugs (carbidopa, Vitamin K. Vitamin B1, pentazocine, bleomycin)	Infections (CMV, Parvovirus B19), medications (bleomycin, pentazocine) and chemicals (silica, vinyl chloride and organic solvents)
Autoantibodies	Anti-nuclear, anti-histone, anti-single-stranded and anti-topoisomerase IIα	Anti-nuclear, anti-centromere, anti-topoisomerase I and anti-RNA polymerase III antibodies.
Interleukin-2, 6	Higher levels	Lower levels
Interleukin-13	Lower levels	Higher levels
Matrix metalloproteinase	Higher levels in peripheral blood mononuclear cells	Lower levels in peripheral blood mononuclear cells.
Epidermal growth factor, Platelet derived growth factor	Lower levels	Higher levels
Tumour Necrosis Factor-α	Lower levels	Higher levels

(Table 5.5) cont.....

Parameter	Morphea	SSC
Inflammatory cells	CD3, CD4, CD8 positive T cells	CD8 positive T cells
Role of Dendritic cells	Stronger evidence	Less evidence

Genetic studies have revealed definite association of SSC with genetic loci such as *IRF5, BANK1, STAT4, CD247, BLK* and *TNFSF4* genes [125]. Such strong genetic association is yet to be established for morphea, though HLA class I alleles have been linked to it [5, 6]. While SSC has been linked to external agents such as infections (CMV, Parvovirus B19), medications (bleomycin, pentazocine) and chemicals (silica, vinyl chloride and organic solvents), morphea is known to be triggered by radiation, trauma, Borrelia and viral infections and certain drugs (carbidopa, Vitamin K. Vitamin B1, pentazocine, bleomycin) [1, 126]. The levels of IL-2 and IL-6 are higher in morphea than that of SSC patients [103]. Peripheral blood mononuclear cells of patients of SSC have a lower level of matrix metalloproteinase-1 and a higher level of epidermal growth factor, platelet-derived growth factor, TNF-α and IL-13 [127]. The autoantibody profile of the two conditions is quite different. Patients of SSC mostly show antinuclear antibodies and almost exclusively show anti-centromere, anti-topoisomerase I and anti-RNA polymerase III antibodies. Morphea, on the other hand, shows anti-histone, anti-single-stranded and anti-topoisomerase IIα antibodies. Gene array analysis has demonstrated that gene signatures in morphea and SSC are different [4]. SSC is initiated and maintained by CD8 + T cells while morphea shows a greater number of cells with CD3+, CD4+ and CD8+ T cells and strong evidence of the role of dendritic cells as well [120].

Box 5.4: Learning points.
• Adults with morphea are more likely to have another concomitant autoimmune disease while children are more likely to have a family history of morphea.
• Altered methylation of genes on X chromosome which are responsible for apoptosis, inflammation and oxidative stress on SSC-identified sites may provide an explanation for the higher prevalence of SSC and morphea in women.
• Several microRNAs hava e greater expression in morphea, whleadslead to fibrosis. Serum levels of miRNA-7 may be used as a disease marker for morphea.
• Antinuclear antibody positivity in morphea is associated with deeper tissue and extracutaneous involvement, number of lesions, number of sites involved and modified Rodnan skin scores.
• Anti-histone and anti-single stranded DNA antibodies are seen in more than half of all morphea patients. Positivity to both indicates larger surface area involvement, severe skin disease and functional limitation in linear morphea.
• Anti-DNA topoisomerase II α antibodies are relatively specific for morphea and are seen in 85%of patients of generalised morphea and 76% patients with localized disease.

(Box 5.4) cont.....

Box 5.4: Learning points.
• Radiation may lead to morphea by selective activation of fibroblasts, triggering of isomorphic response or production of self-antigens.
• Disease caused by *Borrelia afzelii* or *Borrelia garinii* has been associated with morphea but not *Borrelia burgdorferi*.
• Dermal fibroblasts have high expression of anti-apoptotic proteins and have deficient acid sphingomyelinase activity. This makes them resistant to apoptosis, increasing their survival and leading to excessive extracellular matrix deposition.
• Morphea in children is attributed to an accelerated immune system development to an adult permissive form with higher activation of Th1, Th17 and Th2 inflammatory cells.

REFERENCES

[1]   Fett N, Werth VP. Update on morphea. J Am Acad Dermatol 2011; 64(2): 217-28.
        [http://dx.doi.org/10.1016/j.jaad.2010.05.045] [PMID: 21238823]

[2]   Saracino AM, Denton CP, Orteu CH. The molecular pathogenesis of morphoea: from genetics to future treatment targets. Br J Dermatol 2017; 177(1): 34-46.
        [http://dx.doi.org/10.1111/bjd.15001] [PMID: 27553363]

[3]   Leitenberger JJ, Cayce RL, Haley RW, Adams-Huet B, Bergstresser PR, Jacobe HT. Distinct autoimmune syndromes in morphea: A review of 245 adult and pediatric cases. Arch Dermatol 2009; 145(5): 545-50.
        [http://dx.doi.org/10.1001/archdermatol.2009.79] [PMID: 19451498]

[4]   Milano A, Pendergrass SA, Sargent JL, *et al.* Molecular subsets in the gene expression signatures of scleroderma skin. PLoS One 2008; 3(7): e2696.
        [http://dx.doi.org/10.1371/journal.pone.0002696] [PMID: 18648520]

[5]   Jacobe H, Ahn C, Arnett FC, Reveille JD. Major histocompatibility complex class I and class II alleles may confer susceptibility to or protection against morphea: findings from the Morphea in Adults and Children cohort. Arthritis Rheumatol 2014; 66(11): 3170-7.
        [http://dx.doi.org/10.1002/art.38814] [PMID: 25223600]

[6]   Torok KS, Li SC, Jacobe HM, *et al.* Immunopathogenesis of pediatric localized scleroderma. Front Immunol 2019; 10: 908.
        [http://dx.doi.org/10.3389/fimmu.2019.00908] [PMID: 31114575]

[7]   Weibel L, Harper JI. Linear morphoea follows Blaschko's lines. Br J Dermatol 2008; 159(1): 175-81.
        [http://dx.doi.org/10.1111/j.1365-2133.2008.08647.x] [PMID: 18503590]

[8]   Jue MS, Kim MH, Ko JY, Lee CW. Digital image processing for the acquisition of graphic similarity of the distributional patterns between cutaneous lesions of linear scleroderma and Blaschko's lines. J Dermatol 2011; 38(8): 778-83.
        [http://dx.doi.org/10.1111/j.1346-8138.2010.01162.x] [PMID: 21366680]

[9]   Paller AS. Wnt signaling in focal dermal hypoplasia. Nat Genet 2007; 39(7): 820-1.
        [http://dx.doi.org/10.1038/ng0707-820] [PMID: 17597772]

[10]   Morice-Picard F, Boralevi F, Lepreux S, Labrèze C, Lacombe D, Taïeb A. Severe linear form of granuloma annulare along Blaschko's lines preceding the onset of a classical form of granuloma annulare in a child. Br J Dermatol 2007; 157(5): 1056-8.
        [http://dx.doi.org/10.1111/j.1365-2133.2007.08141.x] [PMID: 17725676]

[11]   Chang HY, Chi JT, Dudoit S, *et al.* Diversity, topographic differentiation, and positional memory in human fibroblasts. Proc Natl Acad Sci 2002; 99(20): 12877-82.
        [http://dx.doi.org/10.1073/pnas.162488599] [PMID: 12297622]

[12]   Bhattacharyya S, Wei J, Varga J. Understanding fibrosis in systemic sclerosis: Shifting paradigms, emerging opportunities. Nat Rev Rheumatol 2012; 8(1): 42-54.
[http://dx.doi.org/10.1038/nrrheum.2011.149] [PMID: 22025123]

[13]   McNallan KT, Aponte C, el-Azhary R, *et al.* Immunophenotyping of chimeric cells in localized scleroderma. Rheumatology 2007; 46(3): 398-402.
[http://dx.doi.org/10.1093/rheumatology/kel297] [PMID: 17085771]

[14]   Lambert NC, Pang JM, Yan Z, *et al.* Male microchimerism in women with systemic sclerosis and healthy women who have never given birth to a son. Ann Rheum Dis 2005; 64(6): 845-8.
[http://dx.doi.org/10.1136/ard.2004.029314] [PMID: 15550532]

[15]   Rak JM, Pagni PP, Tiev K, *et al.* Male microchimerism and HLA compatibility in French women with sclerodema: A different profile in limited and diffuse subset. Rheumatology 2009; 48(4): 363-6.
[http://dx.doi.org/10.1093/rheumatology/ken505] [PMID: 19208687]

[16]   Wang Y, Fan PS, Kahaleh B. Association between enhanced type I collagen expression and epigenetic repression of theFLI1 gene in scleroderma fibroblasts. Arthri Rheum 2006; 54(7): 2271-9.
[http://dx.doi.org/10.1002/art.21948] [PMID: 16802366]

[17]   Selmi C, Feghali-Bostwick CA, Lleo A, *et al.* X chromosome gene methylation in peripheral lymphocytes from monozygotic twins discordant for scleroderma. Clin Exp Immunol 2012; 169(3): 253-62.
[http://dx.doi.org/10.1111/j.1365-2249.2012.04621.x] [PMID: 22861365]

[18]   Yan Q, Chen J, Li W, Bao C, Fu Q. Targeting miR-155 to treat experimental scleroderma. Sci Rep 2016; 6(1): 20314.
[http://dx.doi.org/10.1038/srep20314] [PMID: 26828700]

[19]   Chouri E, Servaas NH, Bekker CPJ, *et al.* Serum microRNA screening and functional studies reveal miR-483-5p as a potential driver of fibrosis in systemic sclerosis. J Autoimmun 2018; 89: 162-70.
[http://dx.doi.org/10.1016/j.jaut.2017.12.015] [PMID: 29371048]

[20]   Wolska-Gawron K, Bartosińska J, Krasowska D. MicroRNA in localized scleroderma: A review of literature. Arch Dermatol Res 2020; 312(5): 317-24.
[http://dx.doi.org/10.1007/s00403-019-01991-0] [PMID: 31637470]

[21]   Tanaka S, Suto A, Ikeda K, *et al.* Alteration of circulating miRNAs in SSc: miR-30b regulates the expression of PDGF receptor β. Rheumatology 2013; 52(11): 1963-72.
[http://dx.doi.org/10.1093/rheumatology/ket254] [PMID: 23893664]

[22]   Etoh M, Jinnin M, Makino K, *et al.* MicroRNA-7 down-regulation mediates excessive collagen expression in localized scleroderma. Arch Dermatol Res 2013; 305(1): 9-15.
[http://dx.doi.org/10.1007/s00403-012-1287-4] [PMID: 22965811]

[23]   Makino T, Jinnin M, Etoh M, *et al.* Down-regulation of microRNA-196a in the sera and involved skin of localized scleroderma patients. Eur J Dermatol 2014; 24(4): 470-6.
[http://dx.doi.org/10.1684/ejd.2014.2384] [PMID: 25152444]

[24]   Christen-Zaech S, Hakim MD, Afsar FS, Paller AS. Pediatric morphea (localized scleroderma): Review of 136 patients. J Am Acad Dermatol 2008; 59(3): 385-96.
[http://dx.doi.org/10.1016/j.jaad.2008.05.005] [PMID: 18571769]

[25]   Khan Mohammad Beigi P. The Immunogenetics of Morphea and Lichen Sclerosus. Adv Exp Med Biol 2022; 1367: 155-72.
[http://dx.doi.org/10.1007/978-3-030-92616-8_7] [PMID: 35286696]

[26]   Arkachaisri T, Fertig N, Pino S, Medsger TA Jr. Serum autoantibodies and their clinical associations in patients with childhood- and adult-onset linear scleroderma. A single-center study. J Rheumatol 2008; 35(12): 2439-44.
[http://dx.doi.org/10.3899/jrheum.080098] [PMID: 19004036]

[27]   Takehara K, Sato S. Localized scleroderma is an autoimmune disorder. Br J Rheumatol 2005; 44(3): 274-9.
[http://dx.doi.org/10.1093/rheumatology/keh487] [PMID: 15561734]

[28]   Zulian F, Vallongo C, Woo P, *et al.* Juvenile Scleroderma Working Group of the Pediatric Rheumatology European Society (PRES). Localized scleroderma in childhood is not just a skin disease. Arthritis Rheum 2005; 52(9): 2873-81.
[http://dx.doi.org/10.1002/art.21264] [PMID: 16142730]

[29]   Wu EY, Li SC, Torok KS, *et al.* Childhood Arthritis and Rheumatology Research Alliance (CARRA) Legacy Registry Investigators. Baseline description of the juvenile localized scleroderma subgroup from the childhood arthritis and rheumatology research alliance legacy registry. ACR Open Rheumatol 2019; 1(2): 119-24.
[http://dx.doi.org/10.1002/acr2.1019] [PMID: 31777788]

[30]   Warner Dharamsi J, Victor S, Aguwa N, *et al.* Morphea in adults and children cohort III: nested case-control study--the clinical significance of autoantibodies in morphea. JAMA Dermatol 2013; 149(10): 1159-65.
[http://dx.doi.org/10.1001/jamadermatol.2013.4207] [PMID: 23925398]

[31]   Falanga V, Medsger TA Jr, Reichlin M, Rodnan GP. Linear Scleroderma. Ann Intern Med 1986; 104(6): 849-57.
[http://dx.doi.org/10.7326/0003-4819-104-6-849] [PMID: 3486617]

[32]   Kurzinski KL, Zigler CK, Torok KS. Prediction of disease relapse in a cohort of paediatric patients with localized scleroderma. Br J Dermatol 2019; 180(5): 1183-9.
[http://dx.doi.org/10.1111/bjd.17312] [PMID: 30315656]

[33]   Khatri S, Torok KS, Mirizio E, Liu C, Astakhova K. Autoantibodies in morphea: An update. Front Immunol 2019; 10: 1487.
[http://dx.doi.org/10.3389/fimmu.2019.01487] [PMID: 31354701]

[34]   Zulian F, Athreya BH, Laxer R, *et al.* Juvenile Scleroderma Working Group of the Pediatric Rheumatology European Society (PRES). Juvenile localized scleroderma: clinical and epidemiological features in 750 children. An international study. Rheumatology 2006; 45(5): 614-20.
[http://dx.doi.org/10.1093/rheumatology/kei251] [PMID: 16368732]

[35]   Sato S, Ihn H, Soma Y, *et al.* Antihistone antibodies in patients with localized scleroderma. Arthritis Rheum 1993; 36(8): 1137-41.
[http://dx.doi.org/10.1002/art.1780360815] [PMID: 8343189]

[36]   el-Azhary RA, Aponte CC, Nelson AM, Weaver AL, Homburger HA. Antihistone antibodies in linear scleroderma variants. Int J Dermatol 2006; 45(11): 1296-9.
[http://dx.doi.org/10.1111/j.1365-4632.2006.02891.x] [PMID: 17076709]

[37]   Zhu JL, Paniagua RT, Chen HW, *et al.* Autoantigen microarrays reveal myelin basic protein autoantibodies in morphea. J Transl Med 2022; 20(1): 41.
[http://dx.doi.org/10.1186/s12967-022-03246-5] [PMID: 35073943]

[38]   Schmeling H, Mahler M, Levy DM, *et al.* Autoantibodies to dense fine speckles in pediatric diseases and controls. J Rheumatol 2015; 42(12): 2419-26.
[http://dx.doi.org/10.3899/jrheum.150567] [PMID: 26472409]

[39]   Hayakawa I, Hasegawa M, Takehara K, Sato S. Anti-DNA topoisomerase II? autoantibodies in localized scleroderma. Arthritis Rheum 2004; 50(1): 227-32.
[http://dx.doi.org/10.1002/art.11432] [PMID: 14730620]

[40]   Yamane K, Ihn H, Kubo M, Asano Y, Yazawa N, Tamaki K. Anti-U3 snRNP antibodies in localised scleroderma. Ann Rheum Dis 2001; 60(12): 1157-8.
[http://dx.doi.org/10.1136/ard.60.12.1157] [PMID: 11760725]

[41]   Mihai C, Tervaert JWC. Anti-endothelial cell antibodies in systemic sclerosis. Ann Rheum Dis 2010;

69(2): 319-24.
[http://dx.doi.org/10.1136/ard.2008.102400] [PMID: 20107031]

[42] Sartori-Valinotti JC, Tollefson MM, Reed AM. Updates on morphea: role of vascular injury and advances in treatment. Autoimmune Dis 2013; 2013: 1-8.
[http://dx.doi.org/10.1155/2013/467808] [PMID: 24319593]

[43] Sgonc R, Gruschwitz MS, Dietrich H, Recheis H, Gershwin ME, Wick G. Endothelial cell apoptosis is a primary pathogenetic event underlying skin lesions in avian and human scleroderma. J Clin Invest 1996; 98(3): 785-92.
[http://dx.doi.org/10.1172/JCI118851] [PMID: 8698871]

[44] Torrelo A, Suárez J, Colmenero I, Azorín D, Perera A, Zambrano A. Deep morphea after vaccination in two young children. Pediatr Dermatol 2006; 23(5): 484-7.
[http://dx.doi.org/10.1111/j.1525-1470.2006.00289.x] [PMID: 17014648]

[45] Ehara M, Oono T, Yamasaki O, Matsuura H, Iwatsuki K. Generalized morphea-like lesions arising in mechanically-compressed areas by underclothes. Eur J Dermatol 2006; 16(3): 307-9.
[PMID: 16709501]

[46] Arif T, Hassan I, Anwar P, Suhail Amin S. Slim belt induced morphea-Price paid for a slimmer look. Nasza Dermatol Online 2015; 6(3): 347-9.
[http://dx.doi.org/10.7241/ourd.20153.93]

[47] Arif T, Majid I, Ishtiyaq Haji ML. Late onset 'en coup de sabre' following trauma: Rare presentation of a rare disease. Nasza Dermatol Online 2015; 6(1): 49-51.
[http://dx.doi.org/10.7241/ourd.20151.12]

[48] Bleasel NR, Stapleton KM, Commens C, Ahern VA. Radiation-induced localized scleroderma in breast cancer patients. Australas J Dermatol 1999; 40(2): 99-102.
[http://dx.doi.org/10.1046/j.1440-0960.1999.00330.x] [PMID: 10333622]

[49] Schaffer JV, Carroll C, Dvoretsky I, Huether MJ, Girardi M. Postirradiation morphea of the breast presentation of two cases and review of the literature. Dermatology 2000; 200(1): 67-71.
[http://dx.doi.org/10.1159/000018322] [PMID: 10681621]

[50] Partl R, Regitnig P, Tauber G, Pötscher M, Bjelic-Radisic V, Kapp KS. Radiation-induced morphea: A rare but severe late effect of adjuvant breast irradiation : Case report and review of the literature. Strahlenther Onkol 2018; 194(11): 1060-5.
[http://dx.doi.org/10.1007/s00066-018-1336-9] [PMID: 30014236]

[51] Spalek M, Jonska-Gmyrek J, Gałecki J. Radiation□induced morphea: A literature review. J Eur Acad Dermatol Venereol 2015; 29(2): 197-202.
[http://dx.doi.org/10.1111/jdv.12704] [PMID: 25174551]

[52] Kushi J, Csuka ME. Generalized morphea after breast cancer radiation therapy. Case Rep Rheumatol 2011; 2011: 1-4.
[http://dx.doi.org/10.1155/2011/951948] [PMID: 22937449]

[53] Espinoza-León F, Hassanhi-Hassanhi M, Arocha-Sandoval F, Urbina-López M. Absence of Borrelia burgdorferi antibodies in the sera of Venezuelan patients with localized scleroderma (morphea). Invest Clin 2006; 47(3): 283-8.
[PMID: 17672287]

[54] Weide B, Schittek B, Klyscz T, *et al.* Morphoea is neither associated with features of Borrelia burgdorferi infection, nor is this agent detectable in lesional skin by polymerase chain reaction. Br J Dermatol 2000; 143(4): 780-5.
[http://dx.doi.org/10.1046/j.1365-2133.2000.03775.x] [PMID: 11069456]

[55] Dillon WI, Saed GM, Fivenson DP. Borrelia burgdorferi DNA is undetectable by polymerase chain reaction in skin lesions of morphea, scleroderma, or lichen sclerosus et atrophicus of patients from North America. J Am Acad Dermatol 1995; 33(4): 617-20.

[http://dx.doi.org/10.1016/0190-9622(95)91281-9] [PMID: 7673495]

[56]   Eisendle K, Grabner T, Zelger B. Morphoea: A manifestation of infection with Borrelia species? Br J Dermatol 2007; 157(6): 1189-98.
[http://dx.doi.org/10.1111/j.1365-2133.2007.08235.x] [PMID: 17941947]

[57]   Prinz JC, Kutasi Z, Weisenseel P, Pótó L, Battyáni Z, Ruzicka T. "Borrelia-associated early-onset morphea": A particular type of scleroderma in childhood and adolescence with high titer antinuclear antibodies? J Am Acad Dermatol 2009; 60(2): 248-55.
[http://dx.doi.org/10.1016/j.jaad.2008.09.023] [PMID: 19022534]

[58]   Vasudevan B, Chatterjee M. Lyme borreliosis and skin. Indian J Dermatol 2013; 58(3): 167-74.
[http://dx.doi.org/10.4103/0019-5154.110822] [PMID: 23723463]

[59]   Bernstein S, Meskey T, Helm K, Miller J, Foulke G, Chung C. Localized cutaneous sclerodermoid changes secondary to human cytomegalovirus infection: An uncommon presentation in an immunocompetent host. JAAD Case Rep 2016; 2(2): 119-21.
[http://dx.doi.org/10.1016/j.jdcr.2016.01.002] [PMID: 27051849]

[60]   Arnson Y, Amital H, Guiducci S, *et al.* The role of infections in the immunopathogensis of systemic sclerosis--evidence from serological studies. Ann N Y Acad Sci 2009; 1173(1): 627-32.
[http://dx.doi.org/10.1111/j.1749-6632.2009.04808.x] [PMID: 19758208]

[61]   Pandey JP, LeRoy EC. Current Comment: Human cytomegalovirus and the vasculopathies of autoimmune diseases (especially scleroderma), allograft rejection, and coronary restenosis. Arthritis Rheum 1998; 41(1): 10-5.
[http://dx.doi.org/10.1002/1529-0131(199801)41:1<10::AID-ART2>3.0.CO;2-P] [PMID: 9433864]

[62]   Pastano R, Dell'Agnola C, Bason C, *et al.* Antibodies against human cytomegalovirus late protein UL94 in the pathogenesis of scleroderma-like skin lesions in chronic graft-versus-host disease. Int Immunol 2012; 24(9): 583-91.
[http://dx.doi.org/10.1093/intimm/dxs061] [PMID: 22773152]

[63]   Peroni A, Zini A, Braga V, Colato C, Adami S, Girolomoni G. Drug-induced morphea: Report of a case induced by balicatib and review of the literature. J Am Acad Dermatol 2008; 59(1): 125-9.
[http://dx.doi.org/10.1016/j.jaad.2008.03.009] [PMID: 18410981]

[64]   Liddle BJ. Development of morphoea in rheumatoid arthritis treated with penicillamine. Ann Rheum Dis 1989; 48(11): 963-4.
[http://dx.doi.org/10.1136/ard.48.11.963] [PMID: 2596888]

[65]   Morell A, Betlloch I, Sevila A, Bañuls J, Botella R. Morphea-like reaction from vitamin K1. Int J Dermatol 1995; 34(3): 201-2.
[http://dx.doi.org/10.1111/j.1365-4362.1995.tb01569.x] [PMID: 7751098]

[66]   Ho J, Rothchild YH, Sengelmann R. Vitamin B12-associated localized scleroderma and its treatment. Dermatol Surg 2004; 30(9): 1252-5.
[PMID: 15355372]

[67]   Frech TM, Revelo MP, Drakos SG, *et al.* Vascular leak is a central feature in the pathogenesis of systemic sclerosis. J Rheumatol 2012; 39(7): 1385-91.
[http://dx.doi.org/10.3899/jrheum.111380] [PMID: 22660809]

[68]   Helmbold P, Fiedler E, Fischer M, Marsch WC. Hyperplasia of dermal microvascular pericytes in scleroderma. J Cutan Pathol 2004; 31(6): 431-40.
[http://dx.doi.org/10.1111/j.0303-6987.2004.00203.x] [PMID: 15186431]

[69]   Barnes TC, Spiller DG, Anderson ME, Edwards SW, Moots RJ. Endothelial activation and apoptosis mediated by neutrophil-dependent interleukin 6 trans-signalling: A novel target for systemic sclerosis? Ann Rheum Dis 2011; 70(2): 366-72.
[http://dx.doi.org/10.1136/ard.2010.133587] [PMID: 21068092]

[70]   Sgonc R, Gruschwitz MS, Boeck G, Sepp N, Gruber J, Wick G. Endothelial cell apoptosis in systemic

sclerosis is induced by antibody-dependent cell-mediated cytotoxicity via CD95. Arthritis Rheum 2000; 43(11): 2550-62.
[http://dx.doi.org/10.1002/1529-0131(200011)43:11<2550::AID-ANR24>3.0.CO;2-H]   [PMID: 11083280]

[71]   Guiducci S, Distler JHW, Jungel A, *et al*. The relationship between plasma microparticles and disease manifestations in SSC. Arthritis Rheum 2008; 58: 2845-53.
[http://dx.doi.org/10.1002/art.23735] [PMID: 18759303]

[72]   Distler JHW, Akhmetshina A, Dees C, *et al*. Induction of apoptosis in circulating angiogenic cells by microparticles. Arthritis Rheum 2011; 63(7): 2067-77.
[http://dx.doi.org/10.1002/art.30361] [PMID: 21437873]

[73]   Chabaud S, Corriveau MP, Grodzicky T, *et al*. Decreased secretion of MMP by non-lesional late-stage scleroderma fibroblasts after selection via activation of the apoptotic fas-pathway. J Cell Physiol 2011; 226(7): 1907-14.
[http://dx.doi.org/10.1002/jcp.22520] [PMID: 21506121]

[74]   Samuel GH, Lenna S, Bujor AM, Lafyatis R, Trojanowska M. Acid sphingomyelinase deficiency contributes to resistance of scleroderma fibroblasts to Fas-mediated apoptosis. J Dermatol Sci 2012; 67(3): 166-72.
[http://dx.doi.org/10.1016/j.jdermsci.2012.06.001] [PMID: 22771321]

[75]   Yamane K, Ihn H, Kubo M, *et al*. Increased serum levels of soluble vascular cell adhesion molecule 1 and E-selectin in patients with localized scleroderma. J Am Acad Dermatol 2000; 42(1): 64-9.
[http://dx.doi.org/10.1016/S0190-9622(00)90010-0] [PMID: 10607321]

[76]   Dańczak-Pazdrowska A, Kowalczyk MJ, Szramka-Pawlak B, *et al*. Transforming growth factor-β1 in plaque morphea. Postepy Dermatol Alergol 2013; 6(6): 337-42.
[http://dx.doi.org/10.5114/pdia.2013.39431] [PMID: 24493995]

[77]   Higashi-Kuwata N, Makino T, Inoue Y, Takeya M, Ihn H. Alternatively activated macrophages (M2 macrophages) in the skin of patient with localized scleroderma. Exp Dermatol 2009; 18(8): 727-9.
[http://dx.doi.org/10.1111/j.1600-0625.2008.00828.x] [PMID: 19320738]

[78]   Ghaffari A, Kilani RT, Ghahary A. Keratinocyte-conditioned media regulate collagen expression in dermal fibroblasts. J Invest Dermatol 2009; 129(2): 340-7.
[http://dx.doi.org/10.1038/jid.2008.253] [PMID: 18787532]

[79]   Kondo S. The roles of keratinocyte-derived cytokines in the epidermis and their possible responses to UVA-irradiation. J Investig Dermatol Symp Proc 1999; 4(2): 177-83.
[http://dx.doi.org/10.1038/sj.jidsp.5640205] [PMID: 10536996]

[80]   Russo B, Brembilla NC, Chizzolini C. Interplay between keratinocytes and fibroblasts: A systematic review providing a new angle for understanding skin fibrosing disorders. Front Immunol 2020; 11: 648.
[http://dx.doi.org/10.3389/fimmu.2020.00648] [PMID: 32477322]

[81]   Aden N, Shiwen X, Aden D, *et al*. Proteomic analysis of scleroderma lesional skin reveals activated wound healing phenotype of epidermal cell layer. Rheumatology 2008; 47(12): 1754-60.
[http://dx.doi.org/10.1093/rheumatology/ken370] [PMID: 18829709]

[82]   McCoy SS, Reed TJ, Berthier CC, *et al*. Scleroderma keratinocytes promote fibroblast activation independent of transforming growth factor beta. Rheumatology 2017; 56(11): 1970-81.
[http://dx.doi.org/10.1093/rheumatology/kex280] [PMID: 28968684]

[83]   Igarashi A, Nashiro K, Kikuchi K, *et al*. Connective tissue growth factor gene expression in tissue sections from localized scleroderma, keloid, and other fibrotic skin disorders. J Invest Dermatol 1996; 106(4): 729-33.
[http://dx.doi.org/10.1111/1523-1747.ep12345771] [PMID: 8618012]

[84]   Nikitorowicz-Buniak J, Shiwen X, Denton CP, Abraham D, Stratton R. Abnormally differentiating

keratinocytes in the epidermis of systemic sclerosis patients show enhanced secretion of CCN2 and S100A9. J Invest Dermatol 2014; 134(11): 2693-702.
[http://dx.doi.org/10.1038/jid.2014.253] [PMID: 24933320]

[85] Meyer M, Müller AK, Yang J, Šulcová J, Werner S. The role of chronic inflammation in cutaneous fibrosis: fibroblast growth factor receptor deficiency in keratinocytes as an example. J Investig Dermatol Symp Proc 2011; 15(1): 48-52.
[http://dx.doi.org/10.1038/jidsymp.2011.1] [PMID: 22076327]

[86] García-Borrón JC, Olivares C. Melanocortin 1 receptor and skin pathophysiology: beyond colour, much more than meets the eye. Exp Dermatol 2014; 23(6): 387-8.
[http://dx.doi.org/10.1111/exd.12310] [PMID: 24372738]

[87] Arnett FC, Tan FK, Uziel Y, *et al.* Autoantibodies to the extracellular matrix microfibrillar protein, fibrillin 1, in patients with localized scleroderma. Arthritis Rheum 1999; 42(12): 2656-9.
[http://dx.doi.org/10.1002/1529-0131(199912)42:12<2656::AID-ANR22>3.0.CO;2-N] [PMID: 10616014]

[88] Loeys BL, Gerber EE, Riegert-Johnson D, *et al.* Mutations in fibrillin-1 cause congenital scleroderma: stiff skin syndrome. Sci Transl Med 2010; 2(23): 23ra20.
[http://dx.doi.org/10.1126/scitranslmed.3000488] [PMID: 20375004]

[89] Maier CSG, Distler J, Beyer C. Inhibition of phosphodiesterase 4 (PDE4) reduces dermal fibrosis by interfering with the release of profibrotic cytokines from M2-macrophages. J Scleroderma Relat Disord 2016; 1: 28.

[90] Bujor AM, El Adili F, Parvez A, Marden G, Trojanowska M. Fli1 downregulation in scleroderma myeloid cells has profibrotic and proinflammatory effects. Front Immunol 2020; 11: 800.
[http://dx.doi.org/10.3389/fimmu.2020.00800] [PMID: 32508810]

[91] Horn A, Kireva T, Palumbo-Zerr K, *et al.* Inhibition of hedgehog signalling prevents experimental fibrosis and induces regression of established fibrosis. Ann Rheum Dis 2012; 71(5): 785-9.
[http://dx.doi.org/10.1136/annrheumdis-2011-200883] [PMID: 22402139]

[92] Aoyagi-Ikeda K, Maeno T, Matsui H, *et al.* Notch induces myofibroblast differentiation of alveolar epithelial cells via transforming growth factor-beta-Smad3 pathway. Am J Respir Cell Mol Biol 2011; 45(1): 136-44.
[PMID: 21749980]

[93] Hamburg-Shields E, DiNuoscio GJ, Mullin NK, Lafyatis R, Atit RP. Sustained β-catenin activity in dermal fibroblasts promotes fibrosis by up-regulating expression of extracellular matrix protein-coding genes. J Pathol 2015; 235(5): 686-97.
[http://dx.doi.org/10.1002/path.4481] [PMID: 25385294]

[94] Shi J, Chi S, Xue J, Yang J, Li F, Liu X. Emerging role and therapeutic role of Wnt signalling pathways in autoimmune diseases. J Immunol Res 2016; 2016: 1-18.
[http://dx.doi.org/10.1155/2016/9392132] [PMID: 27110577]

[95] Dees C, Zerr P, Tomcik M, *et al.* Inhibition of Notch signaling prevents experimental fibrosis and induces regression of established fibrosis. Arthritis Rheum 2011; 63(5): 1396-404.
[http://dx.doi.org/10.1002/art.30254] [PMID: 21312186]

[96] Gilbane AJ, Denton CP, Holmes AM. Scleroderma pathogenesis: A pivotal role for fibroblasts as effector cells. Arthritis Res Ther 2013; 15(3): 215.
[http://dx.doi.org/10.1186/ar4230] [PMID: 23796020]

[97] Wu M, Assassi S. The role of type 1 interferon in systemic sclerosis. Front Immunol 2013; 4: 266.
[http://dx.doi.org/10.3389/fimmu.2013.00266] [PMID: 24046769]

[98] Dumoitier N, Lofek S, Mouthon L. Pathophysiology of systemic sclerosis: State of the art in 2014. Presse Med 2014; 43(10): e267-78.
[http://dx.doi.org/10.1016/j.lpm.2014.08.001] [PMID: 25179277]

[99]   Martínez-Godínez MA, Cruz-Domínguez MP, Jara LJ, *et al.* Expression of NLRP3 inflammasome, cytokines and vascular mediators in the skin of systemic sclerosis patients. Isr Med Assoc J 2015; 17(1): 5-10.
        [PMID: 25739168]

[100]   Fullard N, Moles A, O'Reilly S, *et al.* The c-Rel subunit of NF-κB regulates epidermal homeostasis and promotes skin fibrosis in mice. Am J Pathol 2013; 182(6): 2109-20.
        [http://dx.doi.org/10.1016/j.ajpath.2013.02.016] [PMID: 23562440]

[101]   Kurzinski K, Torok KS. Cytokine profiles in localized scleroderma and relationship to clinical features. Cytokine 2011; 55(2): 157-64.
        [http://dx.doi.org/10.1016/j.cyto.2011.04.001] [PMID: 21536453]

[102]   Ihn H, Sato S, Fujimoto M, Kikuchi K, Takehara K. Demonstration of interleukin-2, interleukin-4 and interleukin-6 in sera from patients with localized scleroderma. Arch Dermatol Res 1995; 287(2): 193-7.
        [http://dx.doi.org/10.1007/BF01262331] [PMID: 7763091]

[103]   Torok KS, Kurzinski K, Kelsey C, *et al.* Peripheral blood cytokine and chemokine profiles in juvenile localized scleroderma: T-helper cell-associated cytokine profiles. Semin Arthritis Rheum 2015; 45(3): 284-93.
        [http://dx.doi.org/10.1016/j.semarthrit.2015.06.006] [PMID: 26254121]

[104]   Aden N, Nuttall A, Shiwen X, *et al.* Epithelial cells promote fibroblast activation via IL-1alpha in systemic sclerosis. J Invest Dermatol 2010; 130(9): 2191-200.
        [http://dx.doi.org/10.1038/jid.2010.120] [PMID: 20445556]

[105]   Lonati PA, Brembilla NC, Montanari E, *et al.* High IL-17E and low IL-17C dermal expression identifies a fibrosis-specific motif common to morphea and systemic sclerosis. PLoS One 2014; 9(8): e105008.
        [http://dx.doi.org/10.1371/journal.pone.0105008] [PMID: 25136988]

[106]   Furuzawa-Carballeda J, Ortíz-Ávalos M, Lima G, Jurado-Santa Cruz F, Llorente L. Subcutaneous administration of polymerized type I collagen downregulates interleukin (IL)-17A, IL-22 and transforming growth factor-β1 expression, and increases Foxp3-expressing cells in localized scleroderma. Clin Exp Dermatol 2012; 37(6): 599-609.
        [http://dx.doi.org/10.1111/j.1365-2230.2012.04385.x] [PMID: 22731679]

[107]   Higley H, Persichitte K, Chu S, Waegell W, Vancheeswaran R, Black C. Immunocytochemical localization and serologic detection of transforming growth factor beta 1. Association with type I procollagen and inflammatory cell markers in diffuse and limited systemic sclerosis, morphea, and Raynaud's phenomenon. Arthritis Rheum 1994; 37(2): 278-88.
        [http://dx.doi.org/10.1002/art.1780370218] [PMID: 7510487]

[108]   Denton CP, Abraham DJ. Transforming growth factor-β and connective tissue growth factor: key cytokines in scleroderma pathogenesis. Curr Opin Rheumatol 2001; 13(6): 505-11.
        [http://dx.doi.org/10.1097/00002281-200111000-00010] [PMID: 11698729]

[109]   Manetti M, Guiducci S, Romano E, *et al.* Increased serum levels and tissue expression of matrix metalloproteinase-12 in patients with systemic sclerosis: correlation with severity of skin and pulmonary fibrosis and vascular damage. Ann Rheum Dis 2012; 71(6): 1064-72.
        [http://dx.doi.org/10.1136/annrheumdis-2011-200837] [PMID: 22258486]

[110]   Tewari A, Grys K, Kollet J, Sarkany R, Young AR. Upregulation of MMP12 and its activity by UVA1 in human skin: potential implications for photoaging. J Invest Dermatol 2014; 134(10): 2598-609.
        [http://dx.doi.org/10.1038/jid.2014.173] [PMID: 24714202]

[111]   Oriente A, Fedarko NS, Pacocha SE, Huang SK, Lichtenstein LM, Essayan DM. Interleukin-13 modulates collagen homeostasis in human skin and keloid fibroblasts. J Pharmacol Exp Ther 2000; 292(3): 988-94.
        [PMID: 10688614]

[112] Hasegawa M, Sato S, Nagaoka T, Fujimoto M, Takehara K. Serum levels of tumor necrosis factor and interleukin-13 are elevated in patients with localized scleroderma. Dermatology 2003; 207(2): 141-7.
[http://dx.doi.org/10.1159/000071783] [PMID: 12920362]

[113] Yamamoto T. Chemokines and chemokine receptors in scleroderma. Int Arch Allergy Immunol 2006; 140(4): 345-56.
[http://dx.doi.org/10.1159/000094242] [PMID: 16804319]

[114] Yan C, Grimm WA, Garner WL, *et al.* Epithelial to mesenchymal transition in human skin wound healing is induced by tumor necrosis factor-alpha through bone morphogenic protein-2. Am J Pathol 2010; 176(5): 2247-58.
[http://dx.doi.org/10.2353/ajpath.2010.090048] [PMID: 20304956]

[115] O'Kane D, Jackson MV, Kissenpfennig A, *et al.* SMAD inhibition attenuates epithelial to mesenchymal transition by primary keratinocytes *in vitro*. Exp Dermatol 2014; 23(7): 497-503.
[http://dx.doi.org/10.1111/exd.12452] [PMID: 24848428]

[116] Takahashi M, Akamatsu H, Yagami A, *et al.* Epithelial-mesenchymal transition of the eccrine glands is involved in skin fibrosis in morphea. J Dermatol 2013; 40(9): 720-5.
[http://dx.doi.org/10.1111/1346-8138.12235] [PMID: 23855882]

[117] Gomer RH. Circulating progenitor cells and scleroderma. Curr Rheumatol Rep 2008; 10(3): 183-8.
[http://dx.doi.org/10.1007/s11926-008-0031-8] [PMID: 18638425]

[118] Liu S, Kapoor M, Shi-Wen X, *et al.* Role of Rac1 in a bleomycin☐induced scleroderma model using fibroblast☐specific Rac1☐knockout mice. Arthritis Rheum 2008; 58(7): 2189-95.
[http://dx.doi.org/10.1002/art.23595] [PMID: 18576327]

[119] Osmola-Mańkowska A, Teresiak-Mikołajczak E, Dańczak-Pazdrowska A, Kowalczyk M, Żaba R, Adamski Z. The role of dendritic cells and regulatory T cells in the pathogenesis of morphea. Cent Eur J Immunol 2015; 1(1): 103-8.
[http://dx.doi.org/10.5114/ceji.2015.50841] [PMID: 26155191]

[120] Shrimpton RE, Butler M, Morel AS, Eren E, Hue SS, Ritter MA. CD205 (DEC-205): A recognition receptor for apoptotic and necrotic self. Mol Immunol 2009; 46(6): 1229-39.
[http://dx.doi.org/10.1016/j.molimm.2008.11.016] [PMID: 19135256]

[121] Ghoreishi M, Vera Kellet C, Dutz JP. Type 1 IFN-induced protein MxA and plasmacytoid dendritic cells in lesions of morphea. Exp Dermatol 2012; 21(6): 417-9.
[http://dx.doi.org/10.1111/j.1600-0625.2012.01475.x] [PMID: 22507598]

[122] Fawzi MMT, Tawfik SO, Eissa AM, El-Komy MHM, Abdel-Halim MRE, Shaker OG. Expression of insulin-like growth factor-I in lesional and non-lesional skin of patients with morphoea. Br J Dermatol 2008; 159(1): 86-90.
[http://dx.doi.org/10.1111/j.1365-2133.2008.08592.x] [PMID: 18489607]

[123] Li SC. Scleroderma in children and adolescents: localized scleroderma and SSC. Pediatr Clin North Am 2018; 65(4): 757-81.
[http://dx.doi.org/10.1016/j.pcl.2018.04.002] [PMID: 30031497]

[124] Romano E, Manetti M, Guiducci S, Ceccarelli C, Allanore Y, Matucci-Cerinic M. The genetics of systemic sclerosis: An update. Clin Exp Rheumatol 2011; 29(2) (Suppl. 65): S75-86.
[PMID: 21586222]

[125] Katsumoto TR, Whitfield ML, Connolly MK. The pathogenesis of systemic sclerosis. Annu Rev Pathol 2011; 6(1): 509-37.
[http://dx.doi.org/10.1146/annurev-pathol-011110-130312] [PMID: 21090968]

[126] Brown M, Postlethwaite AE, Myers LK, Hasty KA. Supernatants from culture of type I collagen-stimulated PBMC from patients with cutaneous systemic sclerosis versus localized scleroderma demonstrate suppression of MMP-1 by fibroblasts. Clin Rheumatol 2012; 31(6): 973-81.
[http://dx.doi.org/10.1007/s10067-012-1962-z] [PMID: 22367096]

[127] Fett N. Scleroderma: Nomenclature, etiology, pathogenesis, prognosis, and treatments: Facts and controversies. Clin Dermatol 2013; 31(4): 432-7.
[http://dx.doi.org/10.1016/j.clindermatol.2013.01.010] [PMID: 23806160]

CHAPTER 6

Histopathology

Muazzez Çigdem Oba[1,*] and **Ovgu Aydin Ulgen[2]**

[1] *Department of Dermatology and Venereology, Sancaktepe Sehit Prof. Dr. Ilhan Varank Research and Training Hospital, Istanbul, Turkey*

[2] *Department of Pathology, Cerrahpaşa Medical Faculty, Istanbul University-Cerrahpasa, Istanbul, Turkey*

Chapter Synopsis.
• This chapter presents the best available knowledge on histopathological features of morphea that was retrieved from the earliest to the latest literature.
• The chapter begins with a brief introduction about the rationale for obtaining histopathological sample in morphea as well as the correct techniques for tissue sampling.
• It then presents histopathological findings that should be assessed and noted on the histopathological report.
• Individual features of different histologic variants of morphea and clinical variants of morphea that have special histopathological features are discussed.
• The chapter concludes with a detailed list of differential diagnoses that may resemble morphea histopathologically.

Keywords: Collagen, Collagen anomalies, Dermatopathology, Diagnosis, En coup de sabre, Fibrosis, Inflammation, Linear morphea, Line sign, Nodular morphea, Morphea, Morphea profunda, Mucin, Panniculitis, Pathology, Scleroderma, Sclerosing panniculitis, Sclerosis, Square sign, Superficial morphea.

INTRODUCTION

Morphea, or localized scleroderma, is a primary sclerosing skin disease, which may occasionally involve fat tissue, muscle, and fascia [1]. Skin biopsy is an adjunct to clinical examination in the work-up of morphea. Histopathological examination reveals depth of involvement and severity of inflammation [2]. These findings may assist clinicians in the choice of treatment modality [3]. In the light of the recent scientific reports, a low threshold for histopathological confirmation is recommended to better identify various clinicopathologic variants of morphea and related disorders [3].

---

[*] **Corresponding author Muazzez Çigdem Oba:** Department of Dermatology and Venereology, Sancaktepe Sehit Prof. Dr. Ilhan Varank Research and Training Hospital, Istanbul, Turkey; E-mail: muazzez.oba@istanbul.edu.tr

Tasleem Arif (Ed.)

In clinical practice, four millimeter punch biopsy is the most commonly performed biopsy technique [2]. However, as several subtypes of morphea involve primarily subcutis or fascia, incisional or excisional biopsies of sufficient depth are indicated [4, 5].

In inflammatory lesions, specimens should be obtained at the erythematous rim; while in lesions without clinically overt inflammation, biopsy should be performed at the center of the lesion. The biopsy site should be noted for better clinicopathologic correlation [2].

REPORTING OF THE HISTOPATHOLOGICAL FINDINGS

Hematoxylin and Eosin Stain (H&E)

Hematoxylin and eosin (H&E) stained specimens are assessed for severity and histologic location of sclerosis and inflammation [2].

Severity of fibrosis is graded as mild (grade 1), moderate (grade 2) and severe (grade 3). To determine the histological grade of fibrosis, each of the four dermal layers (papillary dermis, and the superficial, median and deep reticular dermis) are assessed semi-quantitatively (none, light, moderate, and extensive) for fibrosis. Specimens with no fibrosis in papillary dermis and light fibrosis in superficial, or median or deep reticular dermis are reported as grade 1. Grade 3 fibrosis has two definitions: either severe fibrosis in deep and median reticular dermis irrespective of the extent of fibrosis involving papillary and superficial reticular dermis, or severe fibrosis in deep reticular layer along with moderate fibrosis in the remaining three dermal layers. Finally, grade 2 fibrosis is attributed to all cases, which do not have features of grade 1 or 3 fibrosis [6]. Histological grades of fibrosis are summarized in Table **6.1**.

Table 6.1. Histological grades of fibrosis.

Grade of Fibrosis	Papillary Dermis	Superficial Reticular Dermis	Median Reticular Dermis	Deep Reticular Dermis
Mild (grade 1)	None	None/light	None/ light	None/light
Moderate (grade 2)	Others	Others	Others	Others
Severe (grade 3)	Any	Any	Severe	Severe
	Moderate	Moderate	Moderate	Severe

Histologic location of sclerosis is assessed to determine the pattern of sclerosis. Fibrosis limited to papillary and superficial reticular dermis is defined as a top-heavy pattern, while fibrosis involving exclusively deep reticular dermis and subcutis corresponds to the bottom-heavy pattern. The full thickness pattern is characterized by sclerosis throughout the dermis [2].

Localization of inflammatory infiltrate is defined as perivascular and periadnexal if aggregates of more than 10 cells are observed around capillaries and adnexal structures, respectively. Other localizations include interstitial, dermal subcutaneous junction, septal or lobular parts of subcutaneous tissue. Severity of inflammation is graded as mild, moderate and severe. Mild and moderate inflammation is defined as the presence of a mild perivascular infiltrate and dense perivascular infiltrate, respectively. Severe inflammation is noted when the inflammatory infiltrate is as extensive as to form round, nodular collections located in perivascular, periadnexal, and/or interstitial space or at the dermal subcutaneous junction. Table **6.2** summarizes degrees of inflammation.

Table 6.2. Severity of inflammation.

Mild	Mild Perivascular Infiltrate
Moderate	Dense perivascular infiltrate
Severe	Dense infiltrate forming round, nodular collections located in perivascular, periadnexal, and/or interstitial space or at the dermal subcutaneous junction

Cell types (lymphocytes, plasma cells, and eosinophils *etc.*) observed in the inflammatory infiltrate should be reported. Of note, a cell type is documented only if more than 5 cells are observed at low power examination [2].

Special Stains

Mucin deposition is not considered as a typical feature of morphea, however it may be present. Results of the scientific studies are conflicting. On H&E stained sections, Jindal *et al.* reported the presence of interstitial mucin in 31 of 40 cases of morphea, while Yang *et al.* reported a sensitivity of 1% [7, 8]. Alcian blue stain and colloidal iron are special stains that are employed to detect the presence of mucin that is not readily seen in routine stains [9, 10]. Deposition of fair or slight amounts of mucin in deep dermis and interlobular septa was reported as a consistent finding in specimens of morphea and systemic scleroderma by Rongioletti *et al.* [10]. Mucin deposition in lower dermis and subcutis was described in cases of morphea profunda [9, 11]. Exceptionally, abundant mucin deposition in reticular dermis was reported in cases of nodular morphea [12, 13].

Calcium deposition, which is rarely seen in morphea, may be better detected using von Kossa stain [9].

Immunohistochemistry

CD34 (human progenitor cell antigen) staining targets dermal dendrocytes and endothelium [14]. CD34 staining is normally observed in interstitial, perivascular and periadnexal areas of the dermis [15]. Immunohistochemical studies showed a loss of CD34 expressing cells in lesional skin of morphea [16].

Factor XIIIa is another useful immunostain that targets dermal dendrocytes [17]. Lesional skin of morphea displays an increased staining of factor XIIIa in the dermis [16, 17]. Rabbit monoclonal antibody is preferred over mouse monoclonal antibody, as the latter may stain keratinocytes [18].

Cutaneous perineural inflammation, which is a common finding in morphea, is better detected by the immunohistochemical staining than by the routine staining. The Schwann cell marker S-100 or the axonal marker protein gene product (PGP) 9.5 can be used. Pattern of perineural inflammation may either be concentric, involving 75% or more of the nerve circumference, or marginal, involving less than 75% of the nerve circumference. Infiltration of mononuclear inflammatory cells within the nerve is termed as intraneural inflammation [19].

However, none of these immunohistochemical stains are mandatory for diagnosis.

Direct Immunofluorescence

Direct immunofluorescence (DIF) has no substantial role in the diagnosis of morphea and it is usually negative [1].

Fontan *et al.* first described positive DIF findings in four of six pediatric cases of linear morphea. Three patients had deposits of IgM on dermoepidermal junction, and one patient had IgG epidermal nuclear staining [20]. Vincent *et al.* reported a case of linear scleroderma where immunofluorescence studies showed IgG deposits around dermal vessels and C1q deposits at the basement membrane [21].

Kulthanan *et al.* reported positive DIF findings in six of eleven patients with morphea. The most common pattern was IgM and C3 deposition at the dermoepidermal junction. Less frequent sites of deposits were at colloid bodies, appendage area, blood vessel wall and epidermal nuclear staining [22]. Positive DIF findings were also reported in two cases of localized morphea that developed secondary to the injection of vitamin K_1 [23, 24]. Sanders and Winkelmann reported C3 and fibrinogen deposition in blood vessels, whereas Alonso-Llamazares and Ahmed described an unusual continuous linear deposition of IgA along basement membrane [23, 24]. The latter was considered as an epiphenomenon due to cutaneous injury by the authors [24].

Lesional skin DIF test showed immunoreactants deposited on basement membrane zone and fibrinogen deposition in dermal collagen, in 10 and 7 specimens of bullous morphea, respectively [25].

Lastly, in a case of pansclerotic morphea of childhood positive DIF findings consisting of IgG, IgA and IgM deposition was seen on the hair shaft [26].

Specific Histopathological Signs

Several histopathological signs that can be assessed at scanning magnification have been described as useful clues for the diagnosis of morphea. These features include the line sign, square biopsy sign, cookie cutter sign and high eccrine glands sign [7, 8]. However, interobserver discordance is a disadvantage of the named signs and none of them is specific for morphea [7, 8].

Line sign is defined as a prominent straight or linear interface that is present between the subcutis and adjacent sclerotic collagen of the reticular dermis and or subcutaneous septa [27]. Thus, line sign can only be assessed if subcutis is present and is of a sufficient depth [7]. Reported rates of sensitivity and specificity of the line sign differ among studies (45% to 82% for sensitivity, and 27% to 87% for specificity) [7, 8, 27]. This difference is mostly attributable to difference in the number of included case and control biopsies with adequate depth [7]. Line sign can also be observed in lipodermatosclerosis, eosinophilic fasciitis, and sclerodermoid porphyria cutanea tarda [27].

Square biopsy sign (SBS) refers to the square shape of the biopsy, such that four corners of the tissue specimen are placed at approximately 90-degree angles with each other [7]. **Cookie cutter sign (CCS)** is defined as the straight and parallel lateral edges of the punch biopsy specimen [7]. Square biopsy sign and cookie cutter sign are mostly dependent on biopsy technique, being less useful in incisional or excisional biopsies [7]. Yang *et al.* reported the sensitivity of square biopsy sign and cookie cutter sign as 13% and 20% respectively. However, Jindal *et al.* reported higher rates of sensitivity for SBS and CCS, which are 62.5% and 70% respectively. The latter study reported a specificity of 70% for both signs, while Yang *et al.* noted 82% and 85% specificity of SBS and CCS, respectively [7, 8].

High eccrine glands sign is defined as the presence of eccrine glands on the upper two thirds of the biopsy specimen [7] (Fig. **6.1**). Eccrine gland displacement seems to be the most sensitive diagnostic sign [7, 8].

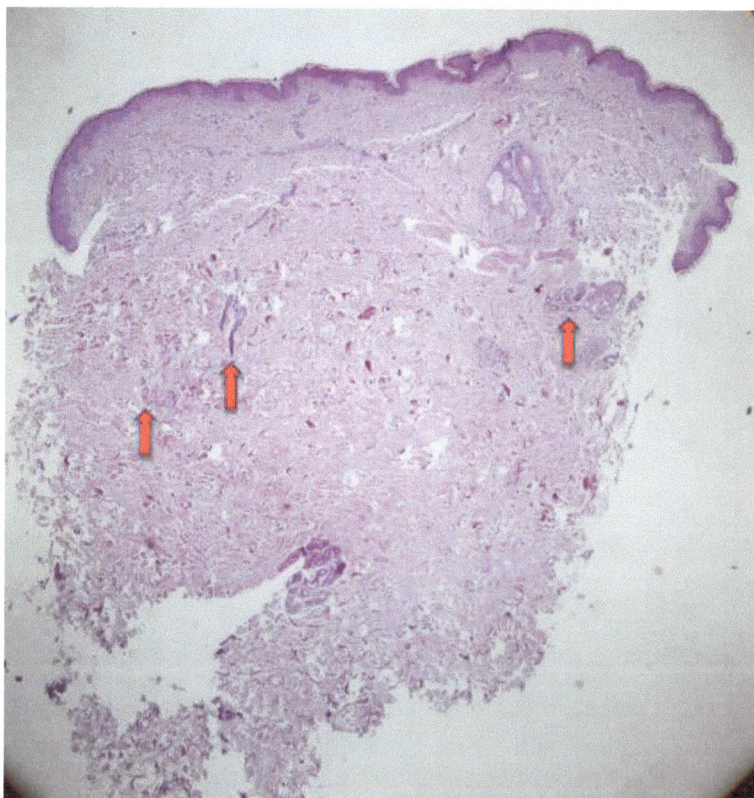

Fig. (6.1). The eccrine glands (red arrows) are located in mid dermis. HEx40

Lastly, Perez-Chua *et al.* reported the **"floating sign"** in 2 cases of circumscribed morphea. Floating sign, a finding previously described in interstitial granulomatous dermatitis, is the presence of histiocytes that form pseudorosettes around individual collagen fibers [28].

HISTOLOGIC VARIANTS OF MORPHEA

Classical Morphea, Early Stage

Biopsies from early stage lesions of morphea are often nonspecific and tend to display subtle changes as dermal sclerosis may be minimal [5, 29]. Early stage lesions of morphea are characterized by the presence of a moderately dense inflammatory infiltrate at the dermal subcutaneous junction, perivascularly, between collagen bundles and around eccrine glands (Figs. **6.2-6.3**).

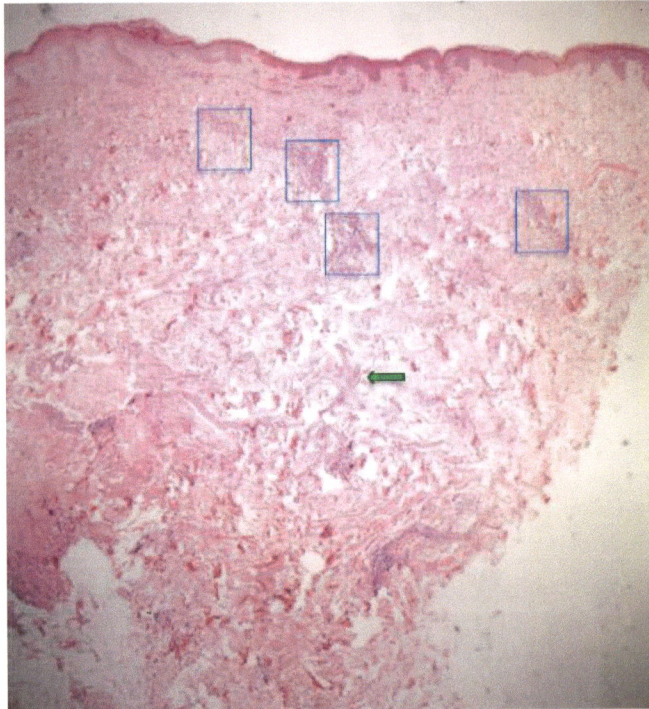

Fig. (6.2). Early inflammatory stage of Morphea. Moderate perivascular inflammatory infiltrate (blue squares), thickening of collagen bundles in lower third of dermis (green arrow). HEx40.

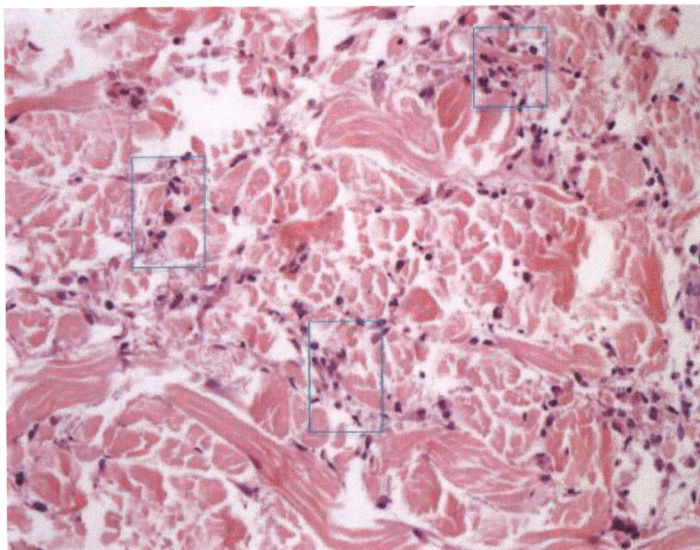

Fig. (6.3). Early inflammatory stage of Morphea. Interstitial inflammatory infiltrate (blue squares) can be seen. HEx400

This inflammatory cell infiltration is more marked in early lesions than in late lesions [1, 4, 28]. Inflammatory infiltrate is predominantly composed of lymphocytes in vast majority of the specimens. Plasma cells are documented as the second most commonly seen cell type. Eosinophils and histiocytes may also be present [2, 4]. The papillary dermis is either unaffected or appear homogenized [5]. Papillary dermal edema fluid similar to lichen sclerosus may be present in early lesions [1]. Prominent findings may be seen in reticular dermis, which displays thick and eosinophilic bundles of collagen with few fibroblasts between them, also known as *"the red desert of the dermis"* [30]. Bundles of collagen typically run parallel to the skin surface [4]. Edema of blood vessel walls and mild endothelial swelling may be observed [28]. Overlying epidermis may be normal or atrophic [4]. Perineural inflammation, which has been demonstrated in all pathological stages of morphea, is most striking at inflammatory stage. Concentric perineural inflammation rich of plasma cells is typically observed [19]. Histologic findings of early stage classic morphea are summarized in (Box **6.1**).

Box 6.1. Histologic findings of early stage classic morphea.
• Dense inflammatory infiltrates of lymphocytes, plasma cells at dermal subcutaneous junction, perivascularly, between collagen bundles and around eccrine glands (main feature)
• Dermal sclerosis may be minimal; if present involves reticular dermis
• Normal or atrophic epidermis
• Superficial dermal edema
• Edema of vessel walls, endothelial swelling
• Perineural inflammation

Classical Morphea, Late Stage

Late stage lesions of classical morphea characteristically contain closely packed, highly eosinophilic, thickened collagen bundles (Figs. **6.4-6.5**) [4, 28]. Square sign, described above, is better appreciated in late stage lesions due to loss of elasticity in sclerotic skin [28, 29]. Lesions display little or no inflammation; foci of inflammatory infiltrates may be present in advancing border [28]. There is a decrease in adnexal structures. Eccrine glands are atrophic and entrapped by sclerotic collagen (Fig. **6.6**).

As the subcutaneous fat tissue is replaced by collagen, the location of eccrine glands is higher in dermis [31]. There may be thickening of the blood vessel walls and narrowing of their lumen [28]. Dystrophic calcification is an infrequently reported finding in longstanding lesions of morphea [9, 32, 33]. Histologic findings of late stage classic morphea are summarized in (Box **6.2**).

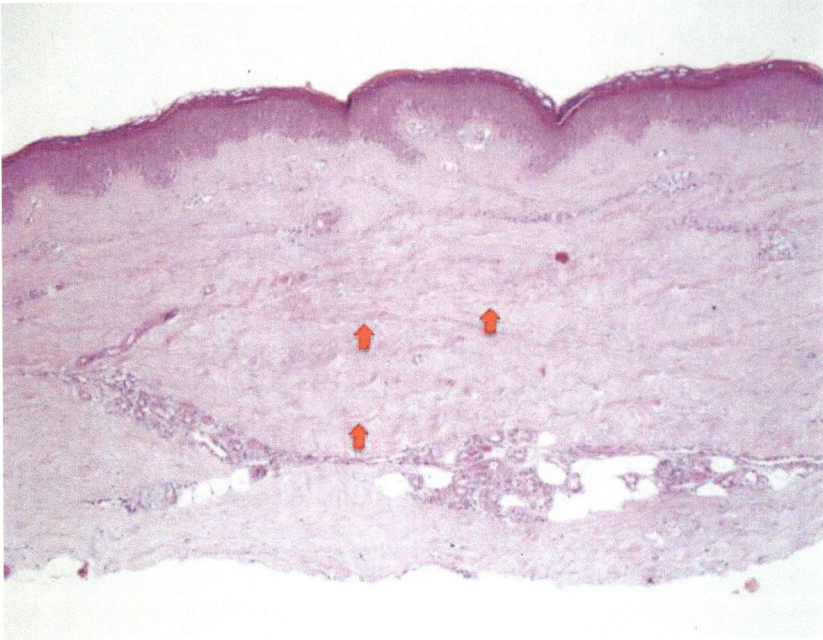

Fig. (6.4). The collagen fibers (red arrows) are sclerotic and parallel to the epidermis. HEx100

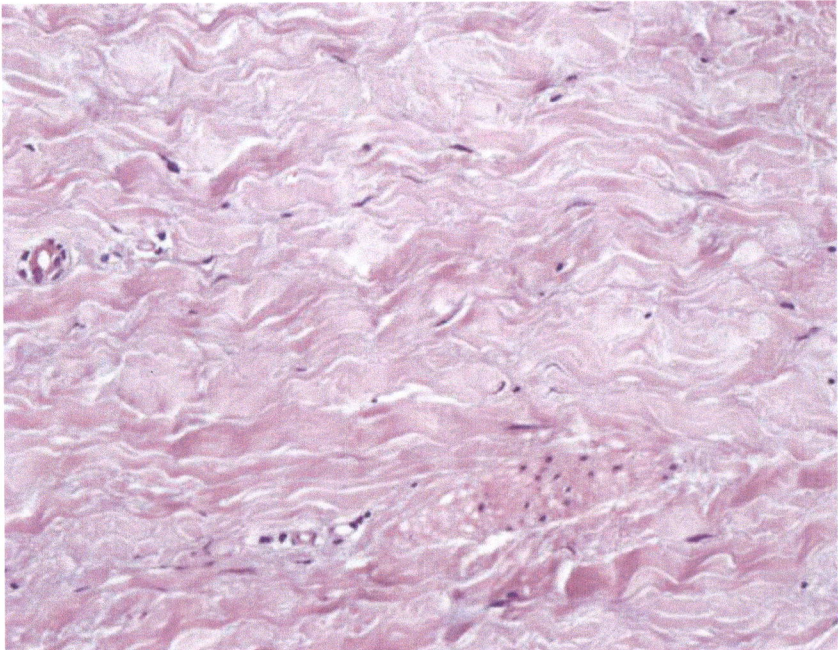

Fig. (6.5). Close view of dense collagen fibers in morphea. HEx400.

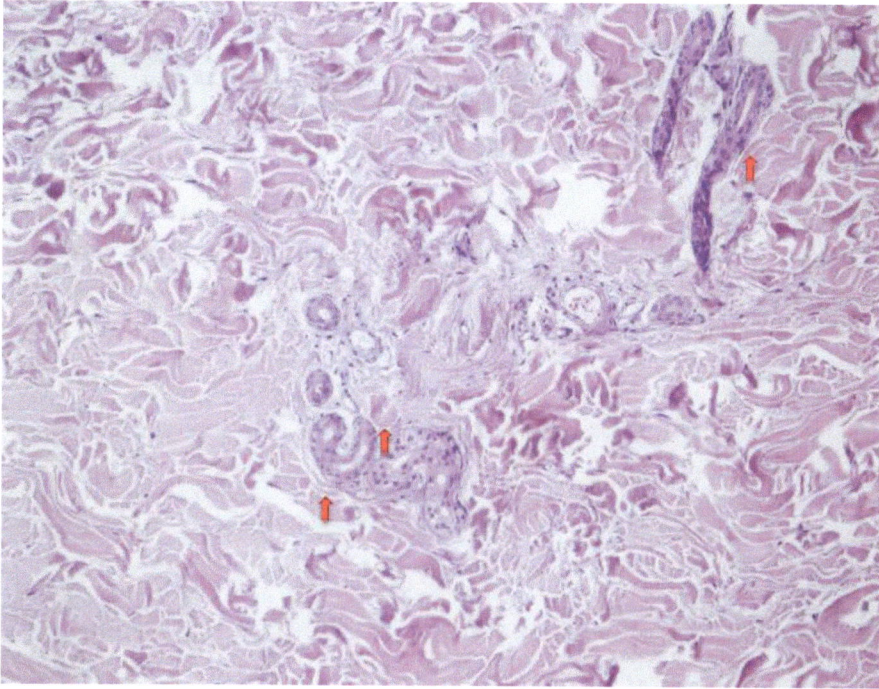

Fig. (6.6). Perieccrine fat tissue is lost. Collagen (red arrows) replaces small fat lobules around the eccrine glands in late stage. HEx200

Box 6.2. Histologic findings of late stage classic morphea.
• Marked dermal sclerosis (Main feature)
• Little or no inflammation
• Atrophy of adnexa
• High eccrine gland sign
• Thickening of the blood vessel walls and narrowing of their lumen
• Dystrophic calcification (rare)

Superficial Morphea

Superficial morphea was first described by McNiff *et al.* Authors reported six cases of morphea that exhibited thickened collagen fibers restricted to superficial reticular dermis and that did not show features of Lichen sclerosus (LS) [34]. This pattern of sclerosis sparing the deep dermis was termed as "top-heavy" sclerosis pattern by Walker *et al.* [2]. In a recent study involving 28 patients with superficial morphea, two patterns of sclerosis were reported. In 38.9% of specimens, thickened collagen fibers involved papillary dermis only, whereas in remaining 61.1% both papillary and upper reticular dermis were involved [35].

Other findings of superficial morphea include decreased number of skin appendages, a relatively decreased density of fibroblast nuclei and the presence of perivascular, periadnexal and/or interstitial inflammatory infiltrate exclusively in the superficial reticular dermis [15, 36]. Basal melanin hyperpigmentation was frequently observed, especially in focal localization [35]. Diminished CD34 staining in the superficial dermis with sparing of the deep dermis is reported in superficial morphea [15]. Specimens of superficial morphea display a unique pattern in elastic fiber staining, which consists of parallel arrangement of elastic fibers in superficial dermis, whereas LS is characterized by loss of elastic fibers in the superficial dermis [34, 36, 37]. In addition, follicular plugging, hyperkeratosis, interface dermatitis and dermal pallor, which are findings suggestive of LS, are not expected in superficial morphea [15, 36]. (Box **6.3**) summarizes histologic findings of superficial morphea.

Box 6.3. Histologic findings of superficial morphea.
• Sclerosis confined to upper dermis ("top-heavy" sclerosis)
• Inflammatory infiltrate confined to superficial reticular dermis
• Decreased appendageal structures in upper dermis
• Relatively decreased density of fibroblast nuclei in upper dermis
• Basal melanin hyperpigmentation
• Diminished CD34 staining in superficial dermis
• Parallel arrangement of elastic fibers in superficial dermis
• Lack of epidermal changes such as follicular plugging, hyperkeratosis, interface dermatitis

Bullous Morphea

Bullous morphea is a rare variant of morphea, histopathologically characterized by subepidermal blistering [25, 38 - 40]. Rencic *et al.* grouped bullous morphea cases under three histopathological patterns, namely lymphangiectatic blisters, Lichen sclerosus (LS) like blisters, and autoimmune blisters [40]. Lymphangiectatic blister pattern is the most common pattern reported [40]. In a study including 13 cases of bullous morphea, dilated lymphatics were reported in 10 specimens [25]. Lymphangioma-like pattern is characterized by dilated lymphatics located in the superficial dermis with the thinning of the epidermis and hyperkeratosis [40]. Histologic examination of the Lichen sclerosus (LS) like blisters shows hyperkeratosis, thinned epidermis, subepidermal bulla along with dermal sclerosis and perivascular and interstitial inflammation [25, 38 - 40]. Hemorrhagic bulla content is commonly reported [25, 39]. Lastly, autoimmune blister pattern occurs due to autoimmune blistering diseases such as bullous pemphigoid that develops on lesions of morphea [40, 41]. Immunofluorescence studies are mandatory to rule out autoimmune blistering disorders [39]. Table **6.3** summarizes distinctive features of three histologic patterns of bullous morphea.

Table 6.3. Histopathological patterns of bullous morphea and their distinctive features.

Lymphangiectatic blister pattern	• Dilated lymphatics located in superficial dermis
Lichen sclerosus (LS) like blister pattern	• Hyperkeratosis • Dermal sclerosis • Perivascular and interstitial inflammation
Autoimmune blister pattern	• Coexisting autoimmune blistering disease

CLINICAL VARIANTS OF MORPHEA WITH SPECIAL HISTOPATHOLOGICAL FEATURES

Morphea Profunda

Morphea profunda was first described by Su and Person in 1981 [42]. Also termed subcutaneous morphea, morphea profunda is classified under predominantly-septal panniculitides [43]. Typical histopathological findings of morphea profunda are sclerosis of deep dermis, prominent fibrosis and thickening of subcutaneous septae with hyalinized and sclerotic collagen bundles and fascial fibrosis [42 - 45]. Moreover, there is loss of hair follicles, sebaceous glands and periadnexal fat tissue [46, 47]. Active lesions demonstrate inflammatory infiltrate of lymphocyte and plasma cells at the periphery of fat lobules and underlying fascia [42, 45]. Plasma cells and multinucleated giant cells may be seen between collagen bundles [45, 48]. Mucin deposition may be seen in deep dermis [47]. Eosinophils were detected in subcutis in 25% of patients with morphea profunda [49]. Lipomembranous changes, which are degenerative changes in fat tissue characterized by cysts lined by lipomembranes, have been reported [50]. Areas of muscle inflammation have been described [46]. There have been rare reports of osteoma cutis arising in morphea profunda [51, 52]. Histopathologicalal features of morphea profunda are listed in (Box **6.4**).

Box 6.4. Histopathological features of morphea profunda.
• Thickened, hyalinized collagen in deep dermis, subcutaneous septae and fascia (main finding)
• Inflammatory infiltrate of lymphocytes and plasma cells in subcutis, fascia and interstitially
• Loss of adnexa
• Mucin deposition in deep dermis
• Eosinophils in subcutis
• Lipomembranous changes

Plasma cell panniculitis is a rare histopathological subtype of morphea profunda, characterized by the presence of predominant plasma cell infiltrate [53 - 55].

Although morphea profunda is considered a morphea subtype, other morphea subtypes, namely linear, plaque and generalized subtypes may also show histological features of morphea profunda [2]. Plasma cell panniculitis was also reported in a case of linear scleroderma [21].

Nodular Morphea

Nodular morphea is a rare variant of morphea characterized by fibrotic lesions arising on sclerotic plaques of localized or systemic scleroderma [56]. Nodular morphea and keloidal morphea are used synonymously in the literature [57]. Histopathological findings reported in cases of nodular morphea range from features of a normal scar tissue, hypertrophic scar, keloid, morphea or the combination of features of hypertrophic scar and morphea [12, 13, 56, 58 - 61]. Nodular morphea cases that show histopathological features of hypertrophic scars are characterized by bundles of collagen that are oriented parallel to the skin surface accompanied by increased number of fibroblasts and perpendicularly oriented capillaries [56, 61]. In contrast, nodular morphea cases with histopathological changes of keloid typically display haphazardly distributed, thick and brightly eosinophilic collagen bundles along with reduced vascularity [57]. Of note, some authors stress that the terms nodular and keloidal should not be used interchangeably [13, 57]. Ohata *et al.* proposed that the diagnosis of nodular morphea should be reserved for cases with histologic evidence of scleroderma [57]. Table **6.4** shows the comparison of histopathological features of nodular morphea subtypes with classical morphea. Abundant mucin deposition in reticular dermis has been reported in cases of nodular morphea [12, 13].

Table **6.4.** Comparison of histopathological features of nodular morphea subtypes with classical morphea.

Morphea subtypes	Collagen	Fibroblasts	Vascularity
Classical morphea	Thick Parallel to skin surface	Decreased	No characteristic change
Nodular morphea (hypertrophic scar type)	Thin Parallel to skin surface	Increased	Perpendicularly oriented
Nodular morphea (keloidal type)	Thick Haphazard distribution	Decreased	Reduced

En Coup De Sabre Morphea

Histopathologicalal analysis of 16 cases of en coup de sabre morphea revealed the presence of interface dermatitis in all cases, which is an unexpected finding in morphea [34, 62]. All of the specimens displayed spongiosis, epidermal lymphocytic infiltrates and vacuolar changes of dermoepidermal junction. Perivascular and/or periadnexal lymphocytic infiltrate and vacuolar degeneration of the follicular epithelium are typically observed in early lesions of en coup de sabre morphea [62].

Typical findings in histopathology of alopecia in en coup de sabre morphea are the decreased number of hair follicles and the presence of sclerosis [63]. Observation of perineural lymphoplasmacytic infiltration on scalp biopsies was reported to be a clue to the diagnosis of alopecia due to morphea [64, 65]. A case of early en coup de sabre morphea revealed perineural inflammation extending to subcutis and fascia on histopathological examination of alopecic scalp [64]. In addition, perineural lymphocytic inflammation was observed in the histopathological examination of a rare case of long-standing plaque type solitary morphea affecting the scalp [65].

Upon histopathological examination of a case of en coup de sabre morphea alopecia, Pierre-Louis *et al.* reported the presence of columnar, atrophic epithelial structures that represent non-viable follicular remnants [63]. These structures resembled telogen follicles but lacked terminal hair differentiation on horizontal section of the scalp biopsy [63]. Similar findings were previously described in permanent alopecia related to chemotherapy, thus they are not considered specific to morphea [63, 66]. Histopathological features of en coup de sabre alopecia are summarized in Box **6.5**.

Box 6.5. Histopathologicalal features of en coup de sabre alopecia.
• Sclerosis and decreased number of hair follicles (main finding)
• Loss of adnexal structures
• Perivascular, perifollicular lymphocytic inflammatory infiltrate
• Perineural lymphoplasmacytic infiltration
• Basaloid structures (case report)

Oral mucosa may be involved in patients with en coup de sabre morphea and even without concomitant cutaneous sclerosis [67 - 69]. Histopathological examination reveals thickened and hyalinized collagen and perivascular lymphocytic infiltrate [68, 69].

Idiopathic Atrophoderma of Pasini-Pierini

Some authors consider superficial morphea and idiopathic atrophoderma Pasini-Pierini (IAPP) as same diseases [70]. However, other authors stress clinical and histopathological differences between two entities [71]. Clinically, the presence of a cliff-drop border of the lesions and a younger age of onset are in favor of IAPP. Histopathologically, lesions of IAPP lack evident sclerosis [72, 73]. Elastic tissue stains are usually normal in IAPP [71, 74]. Reduction and fragmentation of elastic fibers have also been reported [74]. The detailed histopathological features of IAPP have been described in chapter 15.

The histopathological findings of Linear atrophoderma of Moulin (LAM), Parry-Romberg syndrome (PRS), Lichen sclerosus (LS) and Eosinophilic fasciitis (EF) have been described in detail in chapters 16, 17, 18 and 20 respectively.

DIFFERENTIAL DIAGNOSIS

Various histopathological mimickers of morphea that are discussed below are summarized in Table **6.5**.

Table 6.5. Histopathological differential diagnosis of morphea.

Mimicker	Clues to Differential Diagnosis
Normal thick skin	• Check biopsy site. • Search for histopathological findings of morphea other than thickened collagen.
Scar tissue	• Elastic fiber staining decreased in scar *vs.* preserved in morphea.
Lichen sclerosus (LS)	• Hyperkeratosis, follicular plugging, basal cell vacuolar degeneration and band-like infiltrate in mid dermis favor LS. • Elastic fiber staining decreased in LS *vs.* preserved in morphea.
Systemic scleroderma (SSc)	• Differentiation is sometimes impossible. • Thickened and hyalinized vessel walls and narrowing of the vessel lumina and absence of sclerosis in papillary dermis favor SSc.
Chronic graft-versus-host (GVHD) disease, sclerodermoid type	• Differentiation is sometimes impossible. • Interface dermatitis favors GVHD
Nephrogenic systemic fibrosis (NSF)	• Increased dermal cellularity in NFS *vs.* acellular dermis in morphea • Dermal CD34 staining increased in NSF *vs.* lost in morphea
Post-irradiation panniculitis	• Mixed lobular and septal panniculitis in post-irradiation panniculitis *vs.* predominant septal panniculitis in morphea profunda.
Lupus panniculitis	• Vacuolar changes at dermoepidermal junction, follicular plugs, predominant lobular panniculitis and positive direct immunofluorescence findings favor lupus panniculitis.

(Table 6.5) cont.....

Mimicker	Clues to Differential Diagnosis
Foreign material injections	• Polarized light microscopy helps in identifying foreign material.
Eosinophilic fasciitis (EF)	• Presence of eosinophils in fascia and loss of CD34 staining in fascia favor EF
Interstitial mycosis fungoides (MF)	• Interstitial plasma cells and inflammatory infiltrates at dermal subcutaneous junction are more typical of morphea. • CD7 expression is lost in MF *vs.* preserved in morphea.
Patch-type granuloma annulare	• Interstitial pattern of granulomatous inflammation and mucin deposition in dermis favor patch-type granuloma annulare.
Necrobiosis lipoidica (NL)	• Palisading necrobiotic granulomas centered in lower dermis in NL.
Paucibacillar leprosy	• Search associated clinical findings and follow-up.
Acquired port-wine stain	• May be indistinguishable from early morphea. • Close clinical follow-up is recommended.
Vitiligo	• Decreased CD34 and increased factor XIIIa staining favor morphea.

Normal thick skin, such as the skin of the back, displays thickened collagen and may be mistaken for morphea [14, 75]. Thus, biopsy site should be taken in consideration and other findings including inflammation and eccrine gland entrapment *etc.* should be evaluated [75].

Scar tissue and morphea can be difficult to differentiate, as both conditions display dermal sclerotic collagen and loss of CD34 staining [37]. Elastic fiber staining is helpful to differentiate the two conditions. While elastic fibers are diminished, thinned or lost in scar tissue; they are preserved in morphea [37, 76].

It may be difficult to differentiate morphea and Lichen sclerosus (LS), especially when there is intense papillary dermal edema and in cases of superficial morphea as discussed above [75]. Succaria *et al.* reported the presence of lichen sclerosus-like changes, defined as edematous homogenized hyalinized collagen, in the papillary dermis in 9 of 73 cases of morphea. All of the cases had associated epidermal atrophy [77]. The presence of papillary dermal sclerosis and the clinical association of lichen sclerosus and morphea has led some authors to regard lichen sclerosus and morphea as belonging to the same disease spectrum [28, 78, 79]. However, hyperkeratosis, follicular plugging, basal cell vacuolar degeneration and band-like infiltrate in mid dermis are findings that are prototypical of lichen sclerosus [75]. Whereas sclerosis of reticular dermis and subcutis and loss of adnexal structures are features of morphea [5]. In addition, elastic fibers are decreased or lost in lichen sclerosus, while they are preserved in morphea [30]. Occasionally, cases of LS with deep dermal and subcutaneous sclerosis occur and are termed as lichen sclerosus/morphea overlap [29]. A case of coexistent morphea profunda and LS was reported [11].

Systemic sclerosis (SSc) and morphea have similar histopathological findings and are better differentiated by clinical examination and serologic findings [1]. Histopathology of both conditions display inflammation, thickened and homogenized collagen fibers in dermis and subcutis and vascular changes. However, specimens of morphea exhibit higher degrees of inflammation as compared to SSc [77, 80]. In addition, observation of thickened and hyalinized vessel walls and narrowing of the vessel lumina and absence of sclerosis in papillary dermis are suggestive of the diagnosis of SSc [1, 80]. Presence of perineural inflammation is also reported as a clue to the diagnosis of morphea rather than SSc [77].

Chronic graft-versus-host (GVHD) disease, sclerodermoid type, displays deep dermal sclerosis, which is also a typical histopathological feature of morphea [1, 7]. Clinical information is of importance to differentiate two entities [1]. Accompanying interface dermatitis favors the diagnosis of GVHD [29].

Nephrogenic systemic fibrosis (NSF) manifests dermal and subcutaneous sclerosis. Interstitial mucin, which is often present in NFS, can also be observed in morphea. Differentiating the two conditions, dermal cellularity is increased in NFS due to the presence of abundant fibroblasts, whereas dermis is acellular in morphea [29, 30]. In addition, dermal CD34 staining is increased in nephrogenic systemic fibrosis in contrast to loss of CD34 staining observed in morphea [30, 75].

Morphea profunda is very similar to post-irradiation panniculitis both clinically and histologically [43]. However, in contrast to a predominant septal panniculitis in idiopathic morphea profunda, post-irradiation panniculitis shows a mixed lobular and septal panniculitis [81].

Another histologic differential diagnosis of morphea profunda is lupus panniculitis [9, 29]. Sclerotic and hyalinized collagen bundles in subcutis favor the diagnosis of morphea profunda but they can also be observed in lupus panniculitis. Mucin deposition in the dermis and the presence of focal lymphoid follicles in subcutis are typically observed in lupus panniculitis, but these findings may also be seen in morphea profunda [9, 82]. Epidermal changes such as vacuolar changes at dermoepidermal junction and follicular plugs, observation of a mostly lobular panniculitis and positive direct immunofluorescence findings help in histopathological diagnosis of lupus panniculitis [9, 82].

Subcutaneous sclerosis and lymphoplasmacytic inflammatory infiltration mimicking morphea profunda may occur following foreign material injections, especially vitamin K [82, 83]. A foreign body reaction may be suspected in rare cases of deep morphea that develop following various types of vaccination. Polarized light microscopy may be applied to identify foreign material [46].

Morphea profunda also shows overlapping histopathological findings with eosinophilic fasciitis (EF) [84]. While eosinophilic fasciitis is considered by some authors to be a variant of morphea [85], others describe EF as a separate entity due to clinical differences [47]. In a recent comparative study involving 16 patients with EF and 11 patients with morphea profunda, the presence of eosinophils in fascia and loss of CD34 staining in fascia were reported as histologic findings predictive of eosinophilic fasciitis. However, absence of eosinophils does not exclude the diagnosis of EF [84].

Early morphea and mycosis fungoides (MF) may closely resemble each other both clinically and histologically [86, 87]. As pointed out above; early stage morphea is characterized most frequently by a dermal perivascular lymphoplasmacytic infiltrate, a nonspecific finding that may also be present in mycosis fungoides. Cases of early morphea showing lymphocytic epidermotropism were misdiagnosed as mycosis fungoides [86, 87]. Interstitial mycosis fungoides, a rare histologic variant of MF, histologically simulates inflammatory morphea [88]. Both entities are characterized by the presence of interstitial lymphoid cells, however, interstitial plasma cells are more commonly seen in morphea than in interstitial MF. Inflammatory infiltrates at the dermal subcutaneous junction is also typically observed in morphea. In addition, squamatization of the basal layer, attenuation of rete ridges, and slight vacuolar interphase changes are suggestive of morphea [89]. CD7 immunoreactivity may be helpful in differentiating two diseases [87]. Tumoral cells of MF frequently lack CD7 expression, while it is preserved in morphea. In equivocal cases, molecular tests can be performed in order to search for monoclonal populations of T-cells. However, T lymphocyte monoclonality is not always a reliable indicator of malignancy. In fact, monoclonality has been demonstrated in many inflammatory dermatoses and pseudoclonality is a pitfall in specimens with few lymphocytes. Close clinical follow-up and repeat biopsies are necessary for a correct diagnosis [86].

Patch-type granuloma annulare, also known as interstitial granuloma annulare, is a rare variant of granuloma annulare that may mimic inflammatory morphea clinically and histopathologically. Perivascular lymphocytic infiltration is seen in both conditions. Although presence of plasma cells is a typical finding of morphea, Khanna and North reported that one-third of interstitial granuloma annulare cases also display plasma cells. Patch type granuloma annulare is characterized by interstitial pattern of granulomatous inflammation and mucin deposition in dermis. Thus, CD68 staining of histiocytes along with increased dermal mucin helps establish the diagnosis of patch-type granuloma annulare [90].

Necrobiosis lipoidica also displays deep dermal sclerosis and lymphoplasmacytic inflammatory infiltrate [7, 91]. Presence of typical palisading necrobiotic granulomas centered in lower dermis establishes the diagnosis of necrobiosis lipoidica [91].

Paucibacillary leprosy shares similar clinical and histopathological findings with morphea. Perivascular and perineural lymphocytic inflammation of morphea may be misdiagnosed as leprosy, especially in countries where this infectious disease is frequently encountered [92].

Acquired port-wine stain may mimic early inflammatory morphea both clinically and histologically [93]. Histopathologically, port-wine stain is characterized by multiple ectatic capillaries located in papillary and reticular dermis [94]. Biopsies obtained from early stage morphea that display telangiectatic dermal vessels and lack inflammatory infiltrate may be misdiagnosed as port-wine stain [28]. Patients with a diagnosis of acquired port-wine stain should be closely followed-up to check for progression to localized morphea [93].

Early hypopigmented lesions of morphea without overt fibrosis may resemble vitiligo clinically. Moreover, in histopathological examination, decreased number of melanocytes at dermoepidermal junction can be observed in both conditions. CD34 and factor XIIIa immunohistochemistry helps in the differential diagnosis. Decreased CD34 and increased factor XIIIa staining points to the diagnosis of morphea [95].

Box 6.6. Learning points.
• Morphea has many clinicopathologic variants and a vast clinical and histological differential diagnosis. Thus, a low threshold for histopathological confirmation is recommended.
• Early stage lesions of classic morphea are characterized by the presence of a moderately dense inflammatory infiltrate at dermal subcutaneous junction, perivascularly, between collagen bundles and around eccrine glands. Whereas, late stage lesions have little or no inflammation and contain closely packed, highly eosinophilic collagen bundles.
• Superficial morphea is characterized by thickened collagen fibers restricted to superficial reticular dermis without features of lichen sclerosus.
• Bullous morphea is a rare variant of morphea, characterized by subepidermal blistering.
• Differential diagnosis of morphea includes conditions exhibiting dermal perivascular lymphoplasmacytic infiltrate for early morphea and sclerosing conditions in late morphea.

REFERENCES

[1]   Rongioletti F, Ferreli C, Atzori L, Bottoni U, Soda G. Scleroderma with an update about clinico-pathological correlation. G Ital Dermatol Venereol 2018; 153(2): 208-15.
[PMID: 29368844]

[2]   Walker D, Susa JS, Currimbhoy S, Jacobe H. Histopathological changes in morphea and their clinical correlates: Results from the Morphea in Adults and Children Cohort V. J Am Acad Dermatol 2017; 76(6): 1124-30.
[http://dx.doi.org/10.1016/j.jaad.2016.12.020] [PMID: 28285783]

[3]   Nouri S, Jacobe H. Recent developments in diagnosis and assessment of morphea. Curr Rheumatol Rep 2013; 15(2): 308.
[http://dx.doi.org/10.1007/s11926-012-0308-9] [PMID: 23307579]

[4]   Kreuter A. Localized scleroderma. Dermatol Ther 2012; 25(2): 135-47.
[http://dx.doi.org/10.1111/j.1529-8019.2012.01479.x] [PMID: 22741933]

[5]   Luzar B, Calonje E. Idiopathic connective tissue disorders. McKee's Pathology of the Skin 2020.

[6]   Verrecchia F, Laboureau J, Verola O, et al. Skin involvement in scleroderma--where histological and clinical scores meet. Rheumatology 2007; 46(5): 833-41.
[http://dx.doi.org/10.1093/rheumatology/kel451] [PMID: 17255134]

[7]   Yang S, Draznin M, Fung MA. The Line Sign Is a Rapid and Efficient Diagnostic "Test" for Morphea: Clinicopathological Study of 73 Cases. Am J Dermatopathol 2018; 40(12): 873-8.
[http://dx.doi.org/10.1097/DAD.0000000000001177] [PMID: 30475273]

[8]   Jindal R, Shirazi N, Chauhan P. Histopathology of morphea: Sensitivity of various named signs, a retrospective study. Indian J Pathol Microbiol 2020; 63(4): 600-3.
[http://dx.doi.org/10.4103/IJPM.IJPM_67_20] [PMID: 33154313]

[9]   Ito T, Mori T, Miura T, Yamamoto T. Pediatric-onset solitary morphea profunda. Int J Dermatol 2021; 60(3): e116-7.
[http://dx.doi.org/10.1111/ijd.15078] [PMID: 32955115]

[10]   Rongioletti F, Gambini C, Micalizzi C, Pastorino A, Rebora A. Mucin deposits in morphea and systemic scleroderma. Dermatology 1994; 189(2): 157-8.
[http://dx.doi.org/10.1159/000246821] [PMID: 8075444]

[11]   Fujisawa A, Morita K, Yonezawa MM, Miyachi Y, Utani A. Solitary morphea profunda with a prominent mucinous deposit. Pediatr Dermatol 2007; 24(2): 201-2.
[http://dx.doi.org/10.1111/j.1525-1470.2007.00380.x] [PMID: 17461829]

[12]   Jain K, Dayal S, Jain VK, Aggarwal K, Bansal A. Blaschko linear nodular morphea with dermal mucinosis. Arch Dermatol 2007; 143(7): 945.
[http://dx.doi.org/10.1001/archderm.143.7.953] [PMID: 17638753]

[13]   Hsu S, Lee MWC, Carlton S, Kramer EM. Nodular morphea in a linear pattern. Int J Dermatol 1999; 38(7): 529-30.
[http://dx.doi.org/10.1046/j.1365-4362.1999.00728.x] [PMID: 10440283]

[14]   Rapini RP. Alterations of Connective Tissue.Practical Dermatopathology. Edinburgh: Elsevier-Saunders 2012; pp. 139-49.
[http://dx.doi.org/10.1016/B978-0-323-06658-7.00009-9]

[15]   Jacobson L, Palazij R, Jaworsky C. Superficial morphea. J Am Acad Dermatol 2003; 49(2): 323-5.
[http://dx.doi.org/10.1067/S0190-9622(03)00429-8] [PMID: 12894089]

[16]   Skobieranda K, Helm KF. Decreased expression of the human progenitor cell antigen (CD34) in morphea. Am J Dermatopathol 1995; 17(5): 471-5.
[http://dx.doi.org/10.1097/00000372-199510000-00007] [PMID: 8599452]

[17] Gilmour TK, Wilkinson B, Breit SN, Kossard S. Analysis of dendritic cell populations using a revised histological staging of morphoea. Br J Dermatol 2000; 143(6): 1183-92.
[http://dx.doi.org/10.1046/j.1365-2133.2000.03886.x] [PMID: 11122019]

[18] Rapini RP. Special Stains.Practical Dermatopathology. Edinburgh: Elsevier-Saunders 2012; pp. 417-25.
[http://dx.doi.org/10.1016/B978-0-323-06658-7.00030-0]

[19] Dhaliwal CA, MacKenzie AI, Biswas A. Perineural inflammation in morphea (localized scleroderma): Systematic characterization of a poorly recognized but potentially useful histopathological feature. J Cutan Pathol 2014; 41(1): 28-35.
[http://dx.doi.org/10.1111/cup.12242] [PMID: 24117981]

[20] Fontan I, Taïeb A, Guillet G, Rommel A, Fontan D, Maleville J. Immunologic changes in linear scleroderma in children. Apropos of 11 cases. Ann Dermatol Venereol 1988; 115(2): 135-41.
[PMID: 3293512]

[21] Vincent F, Prokopetz R, Miller RAW. Plasma cell panniculitis: A unique clinical and pathologic presentation of linear scleroderma. J Am Acad Dermatol 1989; 21(2): 357-60.
[http://dx.doi.org/10.1016/S0190-9622(89)80034-9] [PMID: 2754069]

[22] Kulthanan K, Jiamton S, Taiyaitiang C, Pinkaew S, Suthipinittharm P. Direct immunofluorescence study in Thai patients with scleroderma. J Med Assoc Thai 2006; 89(10): 1670-6.
[PMID: 17128843]

[23] Sanders MN, Winkelmann RK. Cutaneous reactions to vitamin K. J Am Acad Dermatol 1988; 19(4): 699-704.
[http://dx.doi.org/10.1016/S0190-9622(88)70225-X] [PMID: 2972759]

[24] Alonso-Llamazares J, Ahmed I. Vitamin K1–induced localized scleroderma (morphea) with linear deposition of IgA in the basement membrane zone. J Am Acad Dermatol 1998; 38(2): 322-4.
[http://dx.doi.org/10.1016/S0190-9622(98)70574-2] [PMID: 9486707]

[25] Daoud MS, Daniel Su WP, Leiferman KM, Perniciaro C. Bullous morphea: Clinical, pathologic, and immunopathologic evaluation of thirteen cases. J Am Acad Dermatol 1994; 30(6): 937-43.
[http://dx.doi.org/10.1016/S0190-9622(94)70113-X] [PMID: 8188883]

[26] Minz RW Chhabra S, Singh S, Radotra BD, Kumar B. Direct immunofluorescence of skin biopsy: Perspective of an immunopathologist. Indian J Dermatol Venereol Leprol 2010; 76(2): 150-7.
[http://dx.doi.org/10.4103/0378-6323.60561] [PMID: 20228544]

[27] Draznin M, Fung MA. The line sign. 42nd Annual Meeting of The American Society of Dermatopathology. 80-100.

[28] Perez-Chua TA, Kisel YG, Chang KH, Bhawan J. Morphea and its variants and the floating sign: An additional finding in morphea. Am J Dermatopathol 2014; 36(6): 500-5.
[http://dx.doi.org/10.1097/DAD.0b013e3182924f0a] [PMID: 23823027]

[29] Laga AC, Larson A, Granter SR. Histopathologic Spectrum of Connective Tissue Diseases Commonly Affecting the Skin. Surg Pathol Clin 2017; 10(2): 477-503.
[http://dx.doi.org/10.1016/j.path.2017.01.012] [PMID: 28477892]

[30] Santos-Alarcón S, López-López OF, Flores-Terry MÁ, *et al.* Collagen Anomalies as Clues for Diagnosis: Part 2. Am J Dermatopathol 2018; 40: 79-110.

[31] Kreuter A, Krieg T, Worm M, *et al.* Diagnosis and Therapy of Localized Scleroderma. JDDG J Ger Soc Dermatology 2009; 7: 1-12.

[32] Deza G, Sánchez-Schmidt J, Pujol R. Solitary plaque-type morphea with dystrophic calcinosis cutis. Acta Derm Venereol 2016; 96(3): 418-9.
[http://dx.doi.org/10.2340/00015555-2271] [PMID: 26525184]

[33] Brockman R, Wills A, Greiling TM, Leitenberger S, Fett N. Calcinosis cutis arising in morphea: A

case series. Dermatol Online J 2020; 26(6): 13030.
[http://dx.doi.org/10.5070/D3266049316] [PMID: 32815688]

[34]   McNiff JM, Glusac EJ, Lazova RZ, Carroll CB. Morphea limited to the superficial reticular dermis: An underrecognized histologic phenomenon. Am J Dermatopathol 1999; 21(4): 315-9.
[http://dx.doi.org/10.1097/00000372-199908000-00001] [PMID: 10446770]

[35]   Mosbeh AS, Aboeldahab S, El-Khalawany M. Superficial morphea: Clinicopathological characteristics and a novel therapeutic outcome to excimer light therapy. Dermatol Res Pract 2019; 2019: 1-7.
[http://dx.doi.org/10.1155/2019/1967674] [PMID: 31641348]

[36]   Saleh Z, Arayssi T, Saleh Z, Ghosn S. Superficial morphea: 20-year follow up in a patient with concomitant psoriasis vulgaris. J Cutan Pathol 2009; 36(10): 1105-8.
[http://dx.doi.org/10.1111/j.1600-0560.2008.01234.x] [PMID: 19602063]

[37]   Walters R, Pulitzer M, Kamino H. Elastic fiber pattern in scleroderma/morphea. J Cutan Pathol 2009; 36(9): 952-7.
[http://dx.doi.org/10.1111/j.1600-0560.2009.01201.x] [PMID: 19674200]

[38]   Gallagher TC. Bullous morphea. Dermatol Online J 2002; 8(2): 11.
[http://dx.doi.org/10.5070/D33R74N91Z] [PMID: 12546766]

[39]   Fernandez-Flores A, Gatica-Torres M, Tinoco-Fragoso F, García-Hidalgo L, Monroy E, Saeb-Lima M. Three cases of bullous morphea: Histopathologic findings with implications regarding pathogenesis. J Cutan Pathol 2015; 42(2): 144-9.
[http://dx.doi.org/10.1111/cup.12418] [PMID: 25367438]

[40]   Rencic A, Goyal S, Mofid M, Wigley F, Nousari HC. Bullous lesions in scleroderma. Int J Dermatol 2002; 41(6): 335-9.
[http://dx.doi.org/10.1046/j.1365-4362.2002.01360.x] [PMID: 12100687]

[41]   Sacher C, König C, Scharffetter-Kochanek K, Krieg T, Hunzelmann N. Bullous pemphigoid in a patient treated with UVA-1 phototherapy for disseminated morphea. Dermatology 2001; 202(1): 54-7.
[http://dx.doi.org/10.1159/000051588] [PMID: 11244232]

[42]   Su DWP, Person JR. Morphea profunda. Am J Dermatopathol 1981; 3(3): 251-60.
[http://dx.doi.org/10.1097/00000372-198110000-00003] [PMID: 6172992]

[43]   Wick MR. Panniculitis: A summary. Semin Diagn Pathol 2017; 34(3): 261-72.
[http://dx.doi.org/10.1053/j.semdp.2016.12.004] [PMID: 28129926]

[44]   Bielsa I, Ariza A. Deep Morphea. Semin Cutan Med Surg 2007; 26(2): 90-5.
[http://dx.doi.org/10.1016/j.sder.2007.02.005] [PMID: 17544960]

[45]   Requena L, Yus ES. Panniculitis. Part I. Mostly septal panniculitis. J Am Acad Dermatol 2001; 45(2): 163-86.
[http://dx.doi.org/10.1067/mjd.2001.114736] [PMID: 11464178]

[46]   Torrelo A, Suárez J, Colmenero I, Azorín D, Perera A, Zambrano A. Deep morphea after vaccination in two young children. Pediatr Dermatol 2006; 23(5): 484-7.
[http://dx.doi.org/10.1111/j.1525-1470.2006.00289.x] [PMID: 17014648]

[47]   Touloei K, Wiener A, Glick BP. Solitary morphea profunda following trauma sustained in an automobile accident. Cutis 2015; 95(1): 32-6.
[PMID: 25671442]

[48]   Sayama K, Chen M, Shiraishi S, Miki Y. Morphea Profunda. Int J Dermatol 1991; 30(12): 873-5.
[http://dx.doi.org/10.1111/j.1365-4362.1991.tb04356.x] [PMID: 1816132]

[49]   Peters MS, Su WPD. Eosinophils in lupus panniculitis and morphea profunda. J Cutan Pathol 1991; 18(3): 189-92.
[http://dx.doi.org/10.1111/j.1600-0560.1991.tb00151.x] [PMID: 1918506]

[50]   Snow JL, Daniel Su WP. Lipomembranous (membranocystic) fat necrosis. Clinicopathologic correlation of 38 cases. Am J Dermatopathol 1996; 18(2): 151-5.
[http://dx.doi.org/10.1097/00000372-199604000-00007] [PMID: 8739989]

[51]   Ahn SK, Won JH, Choi EH, Kim SC, Lee SH. Perforating plate-like osteoma cutis in a man with solitary morphoea profunda. Br J Dermatol 1996; 134(5): 949-52.
[http://dx.doi.org/10.1046/j.1365-2133.1996.136871.x] [PMID: 8736344]

[52]   Julian CG, Bowers PW. Osteoma cutis in a lesion of solitary morphoea profunda. Clin Exp Dermatol 2003; 28(6): 673-4.
[http://dx.doi.org/10.1046/j.1365-2230.2003.01353.x] [PMID: 14616844]

[53]   Hamadah IR, Banka N. Autosomal recessive plasma cell panniculitis with morphea-like clinical manifestation. J Am Acad Dermatol 2006; 54(5 Suppl.): S189-91.
[http://dx.doi.org/10.1016/j.jaad.2005.06.032] [PMID: 16631937]

[54]   Tomb R, Soutou B, Chehadi S. Plasma cell panniculitis: A histopathological variant of morphea profunda. Ann Dermatol Venereol 2009; 136(3): 256-9.
[http://dx.doi.org/10.1016/j.annder.2008.04.019] [PMID: 19328308]

[55]   Shiiya C, Iwata H, Imafuku K, Yamane N, Ito E, Shimizu H. Plasma cell panniculitis, a type of morphea profunda, surrounded by congenital nevus spilus. Eur J Dermatol 2016; 26(2): 210-1.
[http://dx.doi.org/10.1684/ejd.2015.2724] [PMID: 26905083]

[56]   Kauer F, Simon JC, Sticherling M. Nodular Morphea. Dermatology 2009; 218(1): 63-6.
[http://dx.doi.org/10.1159/000173976] [PMID: 19005241]

[57]   Ohata C, Yasunaga M, Tsuruta D, *et al.* Nodular morphea (NM): report of a case of concurrent NM and morphea profunda associated with limited type systemic sclerosis, and overview and definition for NM. Eur J Dermatol 2013; 23(1): 87-93.
[http://dx.doi.org/10.1684/ejd.2012.1893] [PMID: 23400240]

[58]   Micalezi C, Parodi A, Rebora A. Morphoea with nodular lesions. Br J Dermatol 1994; 131(2): 298-301.
[http://dx.doi.org/10.1111/j.1365-2133.1994.tb08512.x] [PMID: 7918002]

[59]   Salmon NE, Roberts N, Agnew K. Keloid-like morphoea. Clin Exp Dermatol 2014; 39(1): 90-1.
[http://dx.doi.org/10.1111/ced.12196] [PMID: 23875911]

[60]   Chiu HY, Tsai TF. Keloidal Morphea. N Engl J Med 2011; 364(14): e28.
[http://dx.doi.org/10.1056/NEJMicm1007601] [PMID: 21470006]

[61]   El Khoury J, Salman S, Kibbi AG, Abbas O. Indurated hyperpigmented plaques with overlying fibrotic nodules in an adolescent boy. Pediatr Dermatol 2012; 29(1): 111-2.
[http://dx.doi.org/10.1111/j.1525-1470.2011.01625.x] [PMID: 22256991]

[62]   Taniguchi T, Asano Y, Tamaki Z, *et al.* Histological features of localized scleroderma *en coup de sabre*: A study of 16 cases. J Eur Acad Dermatol Venereol 2014; 28(12): 1805-10.
[http://dx.doi.org/10.1111/jdv.12280] [PMID: 24118540]

[63]   Pierre-Louis M, Sperling LC, Wilke MS, Hordinsky MK. Distinctive histopathologic findings in linear morphea (*en coup de sabre*) alopecia. J Cutan Pathol 2013; 40(6): 580-4.
[http://dx.doi.org/10.1111/cup.12124] [PMID: 23506089]

[64]   Goh C, Biswas A, Goldberg LJ. Alopecia with perineural lymphocytes: A clue to linear scleroderma en coup de sabre. J Cutan Pathol 2012; 39(5): 518-20.
[http://dx.doi.org/10.1111/j.1600-0560.2012.01889.x] [PMID: 22515223]

[65]   Saceda-Corralo D, Nusbaum AG, Romanelli P, Miteva M. A Case of Circumscribed Scalp Morphea with Perineural Lymphocytes on Pathology. Skin Appendage Disord 2017; 3(4): 175-8.
[http://dx.doi.org/10.1159/000471855] [PMID: 29177141]

[66]   Tallon B, Blanchard E, Goldberg LJ. Permanent chemotherapy-induced alopecia: Case report and

review of the literature. J Am Acad Dermatol 2010; 63(2): 333-6.
[http://dx.doi.org/10.1016/j.jaad.2009.06.063] [PMID: 20471136]

[67]   Marzano AV, Menni S, Parodi A, *et al.* Localized scleroderma in adults and children. Clinical and laboratory investigations on 239 cases. Eur J Dermatol 2003; 13(2): 171-6.
[PMID: 12695134]

[68]   Niklander S, Marín C, Martínez R, Esguep A. Morphea en coup de sabre: An unusual oral presentation. J Clin Exp Dent 2017; 9(2): 0.
[http://dx.doi.org/10.4317/jced.53151] [PMID: 28210455]

[69]   Tang MM, Bornstein MM, Irla N, Beltraminelli H, Lombardi T, Borradori L. Oral mucosal morphea: A new variant. Dermatology 2012; 224(3): 215-20.
[http://dx.doi.org/10.1159/000337554] [PMID: 22538799]

[70]   Jablonska S, Blaszczyk M. Is superficial morphea synonymous with atrophoderma Pasini-Pierini? J Am Acad Dermatol 2004; 50(6): 979-80.
[http://dx.doi.org/10.1016/j.jaad.2003.11.088] [PMID: 15153911]

[71]   Jablonska S, Blaszczyk M. Is superficial morphea synonymous with atrophoderma Pasini-Pierini? J Am Acad Dermatol 2004; 50(6): 979-80.
[http://dx.doi.org/10.1016/j.jaad.2003.11.088] [PMID: 15153911]

[72]   Bassi A, Remaschi G, Difonzo EM, *et al.* Idiopathic congenital atrophoderma of Pasini and Pierini. Arch Dis Child 2015; 100(12): 1184.
[http://dx.doi.org/10.1136/archdischild-2015-309498] [PMID: 26374755]

[73]   Kim SK, Rhee SH, Kim YC, Lee ES, Kang HY. Congenital atrophoderma of pasini and pierini. J Korean Med Sci 2006; 21(1): 169-71.
[http://dx.doi.org/10.3346/jkms.2006.21.1.169] [PMID: 16479086]

[74]   Liu S, Oliver F, Agnew K. An unusual infantile rash. Clin Exp Dermatol 2018; 43(7): 835-8.
[http://dx.doi.org/10.1111/ced.13541] [PMID: 29736989]

[75]   Weedon D. Disorders of collagen.Weedon's Skin Pathology. Edinburgh: Churchill Livingstone-Elsevier 2016; pp. 348-79.

[76]   Kamath NV, Ormsby A, Bergfeld WF, House NS. A light microscopic and immunohistochemical evaluation of scars. J Cutan Pathol 2002; 29(1): 27-32.
[http://dx.doi.org/10.1034/j.1600-0560.2002.290105.x] [PMID: 11841514]

[77]   Succaria F, Kurban M, Kibbi AG, Abbas O. Clinicopathological study of 81 cases of localized and systemic scleroderma. J Eur Acad Dermatol Venereol 2013; 27(2): e191-6.
[http://dx.doi.org/10.1111/j.1468-3083.2012.04581.x] [PMID: 22620486]

[78]   Sehgal VN, Srivastava G, Aggarwal AK, Behl PN, Choudhary M, Bajaj P. Localized scleroderma/morphea. Int J Dermatol 2002; 41(8): 467-75.
[http://dx.doi.org/10.1046/j.1365-4362.2002.01469.x] [PMID: 12207760]

[79]   Arif T, Adil M, Amin SS, Mahtab A. Concomitant morphea and Lichen sclerosus (LS) in the same plaque at the site of intramuscular drug injection: An interesting case presentation. Acta Dermatovenerol Alp Panonica Adriat 2018; 27(2): 111-3.
[http://dx.doi.org/10.15570/actaapa.2018.23] [PMID: 29945269]

[80]   Torres JE, Sánchez JL. Histopathologic differentiation between localized and systemic scleroderma. Am J Dermatopathol 1998; 20(3): 242-5.
[http://dx.doi.org/10.1097/00000372-199806000-00003] [PMID: 9650695]

[81]   Walsh N, Rheaume D, Barnes P, Tremaine R, Reardon M. Postirradiation morphea: An underrecognized complication of treatment for breast cancer. Hum Pathol 2008; 39(11): 1680-8.
[http://dx.doi.org/10.1016/j.humpath.2008.04.010] [PMID: 18656234]

[82]   Requena L, Yus ES. Panniculitis. Part II. Mostly lobular panniculitis. J Am Acad Dermatol 2001;

45(3): 325-64.
[http://dx.doi.org/10.1067/mjd.2001.114735] [PMID: 11511831]

[83] Tittelbach J, Peckruhn M, Elsner P. Histopathological patterns in dermatitis artefacta. J Dtsch Dermatol Ges 2018; 16(5): 559-64.
[http://dx.doi.org/10.1111/ddg.13504] [PMID: 29689138]

[84] Onajin O, Wieland CN, Peters MS, Lohse CM, Lehman JS. Clinicopathologic and immunophenotypic features of eosinophilic fasciitis and morphea profunda: A comparative study of 27 cases. J Am Acad Dermatol 2018; 78(1): 121-8.
[http://dx.doi.org/10.1016/j.jaad.2017.06.148] [PMID: 28865864]

[85] Peterson LS, Nelson AM, Su WPD. Classification of morphea (localized scleroderma). Mayo Clin Proc 1995; 70(11): 1068-76.
[http://dx.doi.org/10.4065/70.11.1068] [PMID: 7475336]

[86] Fujimoto M, Basko-Plluska JL, Petronic-Rosic V, Shea CR. Early morphea simulating patch-stage mycosis fungoides. Am J Dermatopathol 2015; 37(5): 409-12.
[http://dx.doi.org/10.1097/DAD.0000000000000271] [PMID: 25768945]

[87] Basir HRG, Alirezaei P, Rezanejad A, Daneshyar S. Early morphea simulating patch-stage mycosis fungoides in two cases. Dermatol Rep 2018; 10(1): 7471.
[PMID: 29760873]

[88] Reggiani C, Massone C, Fink-Puches R, Cota C, Cerroni L. Interstitial mycosis fungoides: A clinicopathologic study of 21 patients. Am J Surg Pathol 2016; 40(10): 1360-7.
[http://dx.doi.org/10.1097/PAS.0000000000000679] [PMID: 27259013]

[89] Su LD, Kim YH, LeBoit PE, Swetter SM, Kohler S. Interstitial mycosis fungoides, a variant of mycosis fungoides resembling granuloma annulare and inflammatory morphea. J Cutan Pathol 2002; 29(3): 135-41.
[http://dx.doi.org/10.1034/j.1600-0560.2002.290302.x] [PMID: 11972709]

[90] Khanna U, North JP. Patch-type granuloma annulare: An institution-based study of 23 cases. J Cutan Pathol 2020; 47(9): 785-93.
[http://dx.doi.org/10.1111/cup.13707] [PMID: 32279342]

[91] Yen PS, Wang KH, Chen WY, Yang YW, Ho WT. The many faces of necrobiosis lipoidica: A report of three cases with histologic variations. Zhonghua Pifuke Yixue Zazhi 2011; 29(2): 67-71.
[http://dx.doi.org/10.1016/j.dsi.2011.05.006]

[92] Delgado JS, Cavalcanti ML, Kac BK, Pires CL. Morphea simulating paucibacillary leprosy clinically and histopathologically. Indian J Dermatol 2013; 58(1): 85.
[http://dx.doi.org/10.4103/0019-5154.105325] [PMID: 23372229]

[93] Nijhawan RI, Bard S, Blyumin M, Smidt AC, Chamlin SL, Connelly EA. Early localized morphea mimicking an acquired port-wine stain. J Am Acad Dermatol 2011; 64(4): 779-82.
[http://dx.doi.org/10.1016/j.jaad.2009.10.017] [PMID: 20850196]

[94] Tannous Z, Rubeiz N, Kibbi AG. Vascular anomalies: Portwine stains and hemangiomas. J Cutan Pathol 2010; 37 (Suppl. 1): 88-95.
[http://dx.doi.org/10.1111/j.1600-0560.2010.01519.x] [PMID: 20482681]

[95] Sung JJ, Chen TS, Gilliam AC, McCalmont TH, Gilliam AE. Clinicohistopathological correlations in juvenile localized scleroderma: Studies on a subset of children with hypopigmented juvenile localized scleroderma due to loss of epidermal melanocytes. J Am Acad Dermatol 2011; 65(2): 364-73.
[http://dx.doi.org/10.1016/j.jaad.2010.02.065] [PMID: 21570153]

CHAPTER 7

Clinical Presentation

Ömer Kutlu[1,*] and **Tasleem Arif**[2,3]

[1] *Department of Dermatology and Venereology, Tokat Gaziosmanpasa University, School of Medicine, Tokat, Turkey*

[2] *Department of Dermatology, STDs, Leprosy and Aesthetics, Dar As Sihha Medical center, Dammam, Saudi Arabia*

[3] *Ellahi Medicare Clinic, Srinagar, Kashmir, India*

Chapter Synopsis.
• All types of morphea usually begin with inflammatory-based processes followed by fibrotic-based stages.
• Circumscribed morphea is the most common clinical presentation of morphea and is subdivided into two subgroups (superficial and deep) based on level of fibrosis.
• Linear morphea is usually seen in children. It is characterized by band-like cutaneous sclerosis that can mostly result in depressed lesions.
• The linear morphea can involve frontoparietal area of the forehead and scalp, which is known as en coup de sabre due to its sword strike-like appearance. The deep involvement of en coup de sabre may imply underlying neurological, ophthalmological, and auditory complications.
• Pansclerotic morphea is a rare presentation of morphea that has been described as an extensive, progressive, full-thickness involvement of the skin including subcutis, muscle, fascia and bone. Pansclerotic morphea predominantly occurs in children and has rapid progression with an aggressive course.
• Generalized morphea has been defined in several ways. One of the widely accepted definition is that it is characterized by plaques of circumscribed morphea (at least four lesions larger than 3 cm) that involve more than two out of seven different anatomical regions (head/neck, two upper extremities, two lower extremities, anterior and posterior sites of trunk).
• Guttate, keloidal/nodal, and bullous morphea are rare forms of morphea.

Keywords: Circumscribed morphea, En coup de sabre, Guttate morphea, Generalized morphea, Ivory-colored, Keloidal/nodular morphea, Linear morphea, Lilac-colored, Lichen sclerosus, Mixed morphea, Pansclerotic morphea, Pseudo-cellulite appearance, Sword strike-like appearance.

* **Corresponding author Ömer Kutlu:** Department of Dermatology and Venereology, Tokat Gaziosmanpasa University, School of Medicine, Tokat, Turkey; E-mail: omerkutlu22@gmail.com

INTRODUCTION

Morphea is characterized by isolated patches/plaques of sclerosed skin. Morphea mostly affects the dermis, but it can also affect subcutaneous fat tissues and in rare cases extend to deeper tissues including fascia, muscle, and bones. There have been several classification systems of morphea and with time newer classifications are evolving [1]. In Chapter 2, various classification systems of morphea in a chronological way have been discussed and their merits and limitations have been highlighted. The list of few chronological classifications of morphea are presented in Fig. (**7.1**) [1, 3]. Circumscribed morphea, generalized morphea and linear morphea are the most common types of morphea while mixed type and keloidal/nodular types are less common clinical variants [2]. A simplified and holistic classification for morphea and 'morphea related disorders' has been presented in (Box **2.1**) (same as in chapter 2). This classification system will be followed throughout this chapter. The reason to follow this simplified and holistic classification in this book has been elaborated in depth in chapter 2. Readers are encouraged to refer to chapter 2 for further details.

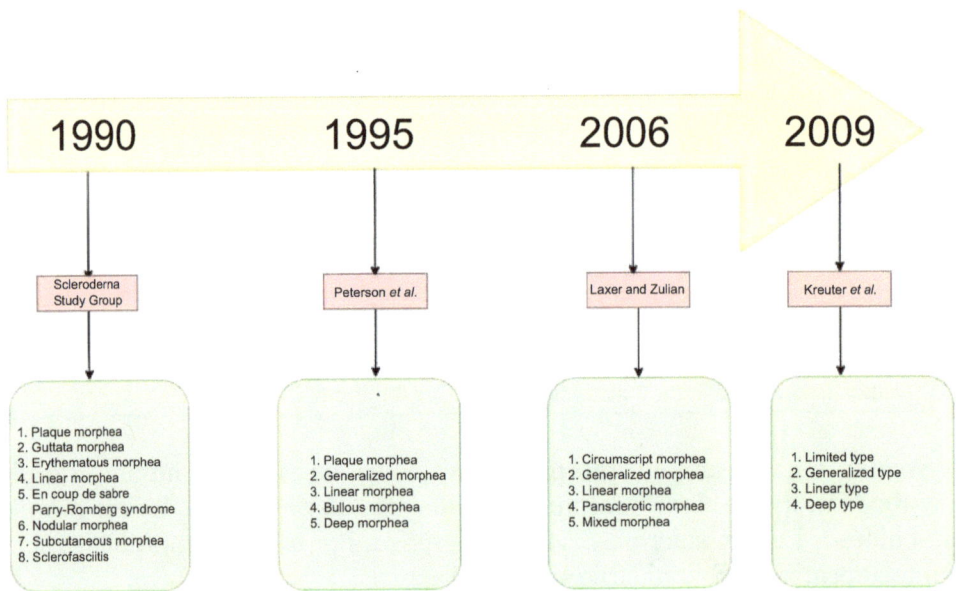

Fig. (7.1). Some chronological classifications of morphea.

Box 2.1. Holistic classification of morphea and related disorders.
I. Morphea
Circumscribed Morphea • Superficial variant • Deep variant **Linear Morphea** • Linear morphea involving trunk/ limbs • En coup de sabre **Generalized morphea.** **Pansclerotic morphea** **Mixed morphea** **Other types:** • Guttate • Bullous • Keloidal/nodular
II. Morphea-Related disorders
Idiopathic atrophoderma of Pasini and Pierini **Lichen sclerosus** **Parry Romberg Syndrome.** **Eosinophilic fasciitis.** **Linear atrophoderma of Moulin**

Morphea usually begins with inflammatory-based processes (Fig. **7.2**) followed by fibrotic-based stages resulting in indurated plaques (Fig. **7.3**). In the late stage, hyper-hypo pigmentation can be seen while lesions undergo atrophy (Fig. **7.4**). Levels of fibrosis in morphea may include subcutaneous fat tissue, muscle, fascia, bone, and even parts of the brain. However, skin softens in the majority of cases of morphea in months to years. In some cases, mild itching or pain can be seen at the site of the disease. Itching may also be related to the dryness of the skin. Morphea may present variably with respect to the type of lesion, color, number and spatial localization. The various clinical possibilities in the evolution of morphea are listed in (Table **7.1**).

Morphea can be seen as Wolf's isotopic response at the site of healed herpes zoster infection [4]. This type of involvement is rare and may imply underlying immunosuppression [5, 6]. Morphea can occur prior to or after the presence of granuloma annulare and autoimmune conditions such as lupus erythematosus, relapsing polychondritis, vitiligo, alopecia areata, and so on [7 - 10]. In addition, coexisting lichen sclerosus et atrophicus may be observed with morphea [11, 12]. Therefore, dermatologic examination of morphea should include signs and symptoms of such cutaneous diseases.

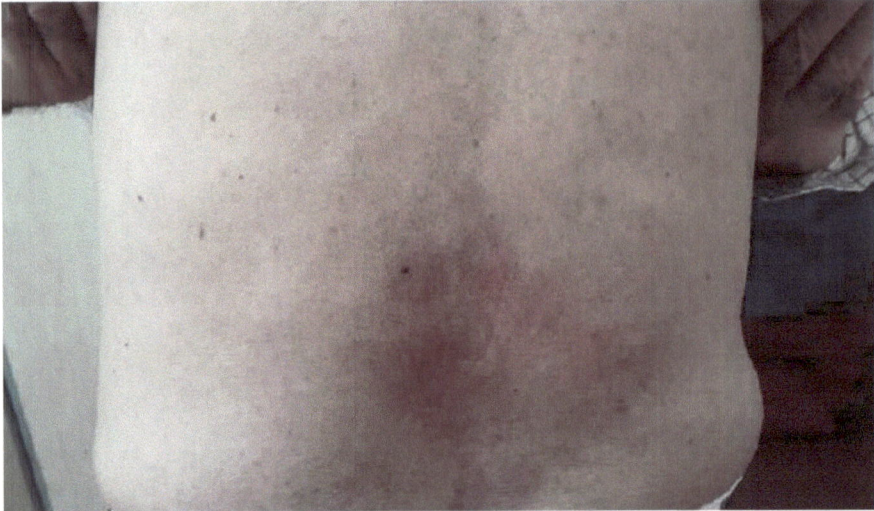

Fig. (7.2). An ill-defined erythematous plaque representing the early inflammatory stage of circumscribed morphea.

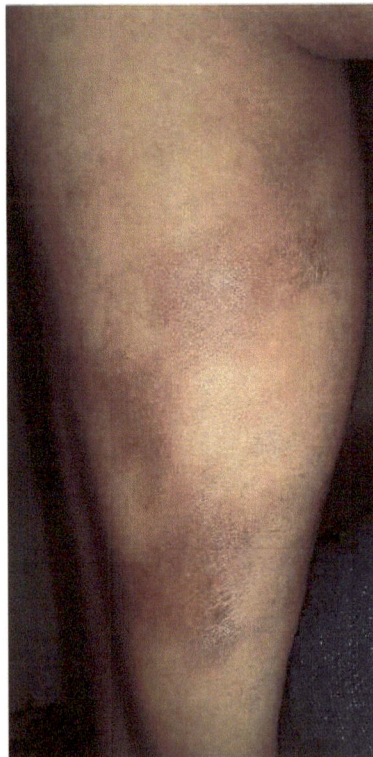

Fig. (7.3). Circumscribed morphea over leg. Multiple ill-defined brownish colored indurated plaques involving leg.

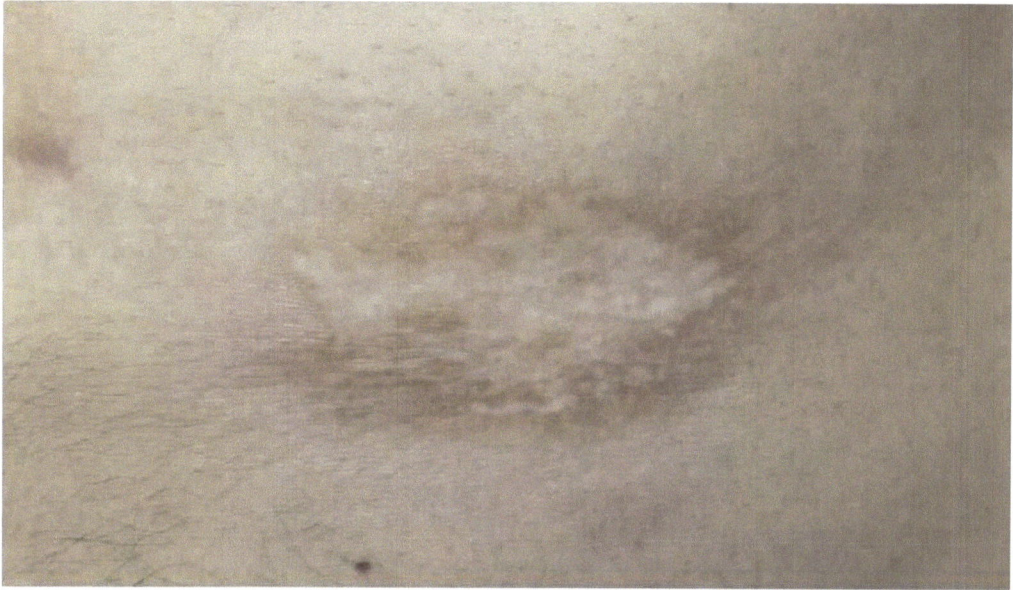

Fig. (7.4). Late stage of morphea characterized by central whitish-yellow sclerotic plaque.

Table 7.1. The clinical appearances of morphea.

Clinical Features	Color	Number and Distribution	Additional Features
Primary	Erythema	Single	Asymptomatic
Macule	Purple (Violaceous)	Multiple	Itching
Patch	Ivory-colored	Unilateral	Pain
Papule (guttate)	White (hypopigmentation)	Bilateral	Scarring alopecia
Plaque	Yellowish-white	Zosteriform	
Nodule	Brown (hyperpigmentation)	Blaschkoid	
Bulla	Shiny		
Keloid-like			
Secondary			
Erosion			
Ulceration			
Atrophy			

CIRCUMSCRIBED MORPHEA

The circumscribed morphea is usually characterized by shiny round or oval-shaped patches or plaques with >1 cm in size. Plaques can occur anywhere but commonly located on the trunk in 41-74% of cases. Although the breast area may be involved in the trunk, nipples and areola are usually spared [3]. In addition, face and neck can also be involved approximately in 13% of the cases [13, 14].

Although, the most common forms of morphea involving the face include en coup de sabre, rare manifestations of circumscribed morphea including bilateral face involvement was reported Fig. (**7.5**) [15, 16]. Circumscribed morphea may resemble some clinical forms of systemic lupus erythematosus including oral mucosal ulcers, facial erythema and pattern loss of hair, [17]. In addition, there are few cases of breast-associated morphea during pregnancy mimicking breast cancer [18]. Conditions mimicking circumscribed morphea have been mentioned in (Box **7.1**). In a case series, it has been reported that a patient who had circumscribed morphea on the breast resolved shortly after giving birth [19].

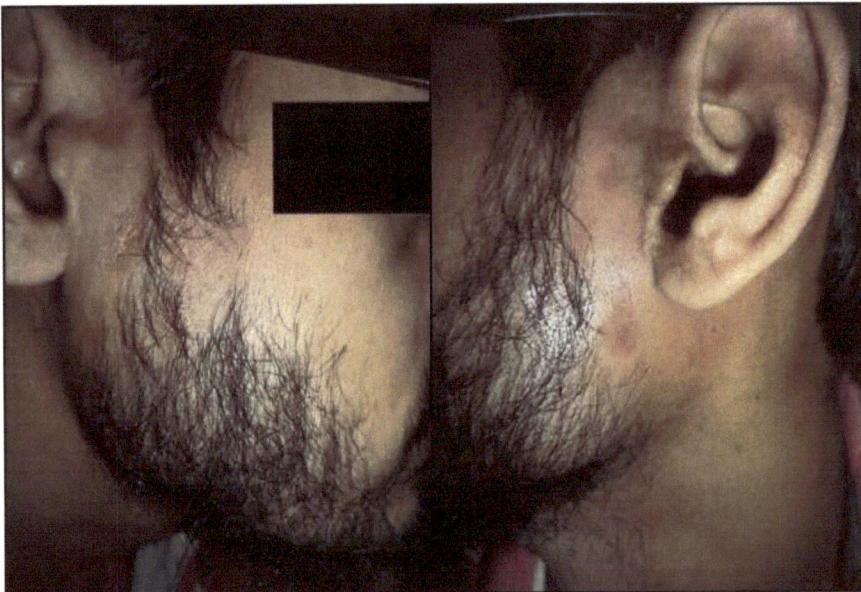

Fig. (7.5). Bilateral facial circumscribed morphea. There are multiple superficial atrophic plaques present on both sides of face.

Box 7.1: Differential diagnosis of circumscribed morphea.
Anetoderma
Systemic lupus erythematosus
Carcinoma breast
Lichen sclerosus et atrophicus
Vitiligo
Pseudoscleroderma
Necrobiosis lipoidica

Circumscribed morphea is the most common clinical presentation of morphea and is subdivided into two subgroups (superficial and deep) based on the level of fibrosis [2].

Superficial Variant of Circumscribed Morphea

Superficial variant of circumscribed morphea includes dermal involvement that is restricted to reticular dermis and reflects patch forms clinically while deep variant of morphea includes subcutis, fascia, *etc* resulting in thickened indurated plaques [1]. In the inflammatory stage, insidious onset of erythematous, edematous lesions occur and develop slowly. The center of the lesion usually becomes thick yellowish-white or ivory-colored and surrounded by lilac-colored erythema or violaceous ring Fig. (**7.6**). Hyperpigmentation often occurs as lesions develop and eventually involute Fig. (**7.7**). The lesions are generally asymptomatic and are recognized by the patients in the late period. As the time progresses, irreversible fibrosis can take place which results in atrophy, loss of hair, sweat, and sebaceous glands. The erosions and ulcers can be observed on morphea plaques in the flexural areas in obese patients Fig. (**7.8**). The lesions can occur in any part of the body but mostly develop on the trunk and it can be either solitary or multiple [2, 13]. The peripheral erythematous and violaceous halo is considered to reflect the inflammatory stage

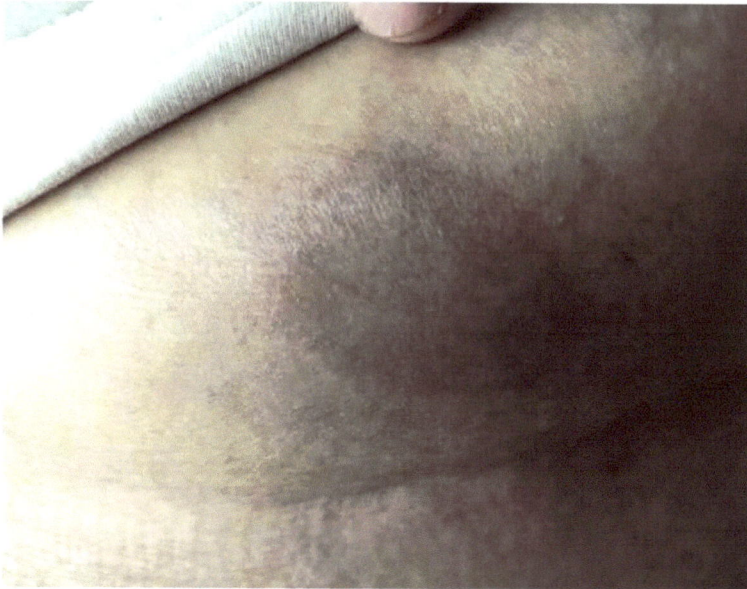

Fig. (7.6). Superficial variant of circumscribed morphea. Yellowish-white center surrounded by lilac-colored erythema.

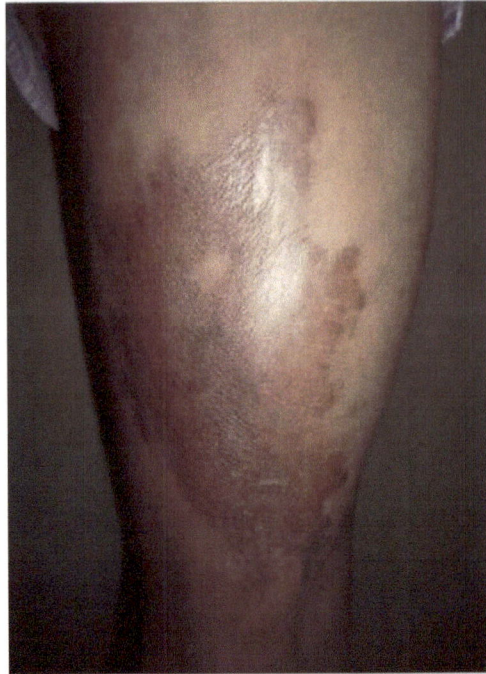

Fig. (7.7). Circumscribed morphea over thigh. Well defined brownish hyperpigmented indurated plaque over thigh.

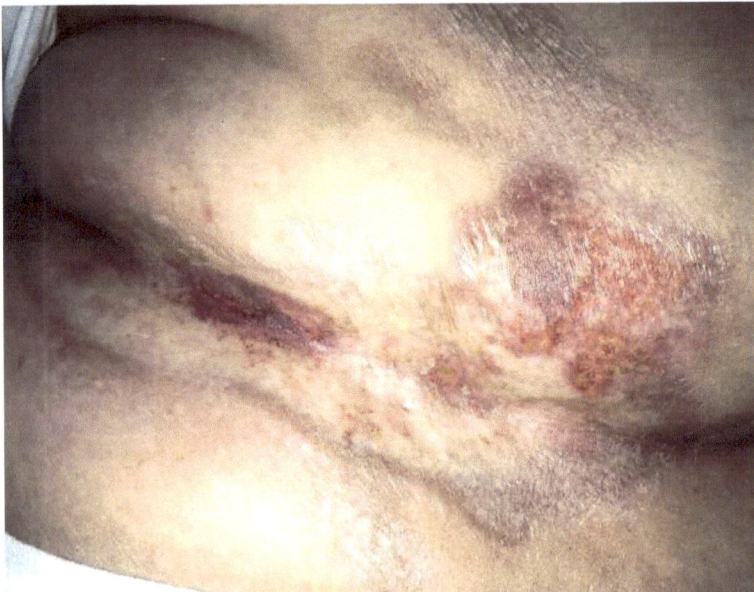

Fig. (7.8). Multiple erosions and ulcers on the atrophic plaques of morphea.

Deep Variant of Circumscribed Morphea

The deep variant of circumscribed morphea is primarily characterized by the involvement of subcutaneous fat and underlying tissues such as fascia and muscle. It was previously referred to as subcutaneous morphea and morphea profunda. Person and Su proposed the term "morphea profunda" when there is involvement of deep dermis, subcutaneous fat, fascia or muscle alone or in any combination [20]. The authors have also previously suggested the term "subcutaneous morphea" for the involvement of morphea in the subcutaneous fat tissue or fascia. Currently, the term "deep variant of circumscribed morphea" has replaced these aforementioned terms. Deep circumscribed morphea may have "pseudo-cellulite" appearance due to the extension of sclerotic process to the subcutaneous fat and underlying structures. The lesions in the deep variant are often hyperpigmented in contrast to the superficial variant in which there are other color changes (Figs. **7.9-7.11**). Thick yellowish-white or ivory-colored plaques and surrounded by lilac-colored erythema or violaceous ring may also be observed as in superficial variant of morphea Fig. (**7.12**). The deep variant that comprises approximately 5% of the morphea cases in both adult and pediatric populations is less common than the superficial variant [11, 14]. The distribution of deep variant is usually symmetric and plaques have poorly defined borders.

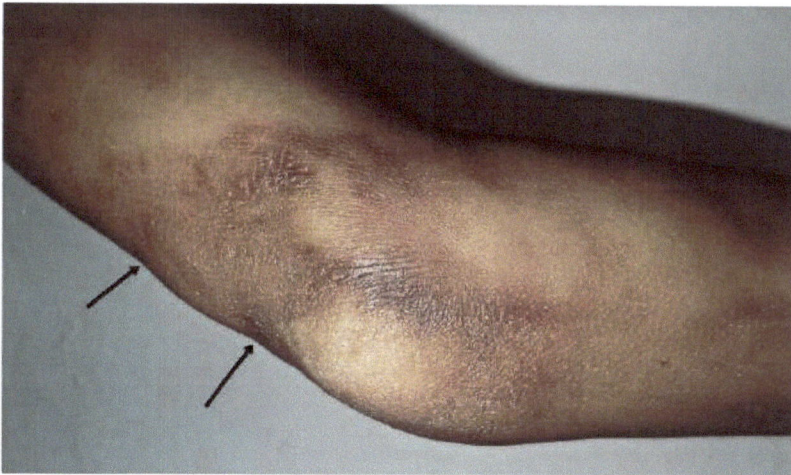

Fig. (7.9). Circumscribed morphea (deep variant). Brownish hyperpigmented indurated plaques over extensor aspect of elbow fixed to underlying muscles. Note the bound down skin (black arrows).

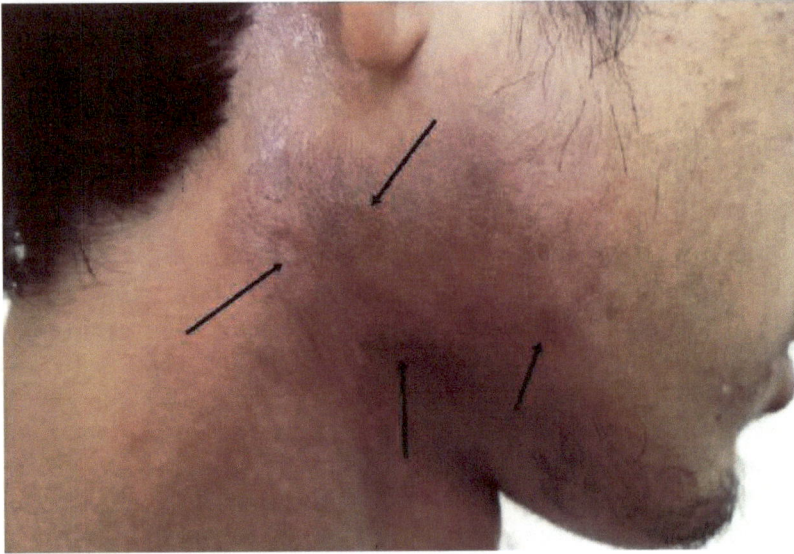

Fig. (7.10). Circumscribed morphea (deep variant): Indurated plaque extending downwards to subcutis and muscle. The main complaint of the patient was difficulty in lateral flexion of the neck. Note the bound down skin (black arrows).

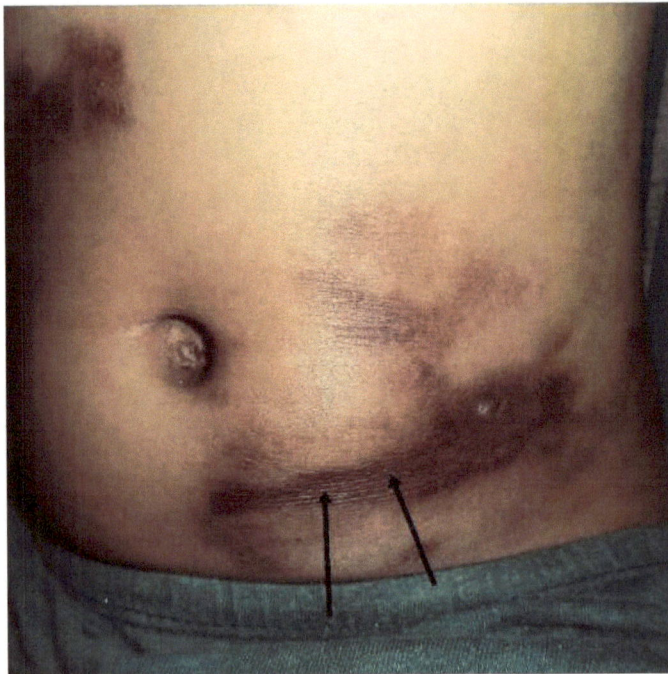

Fig. (7.11). Circumscribed morphea. Deep variant of circumscribed morphea over abdomen and chest. See the dark, brownish indurated plaques with bound down skin (black arrows). Here, sclerosis extended deeper than dermis..

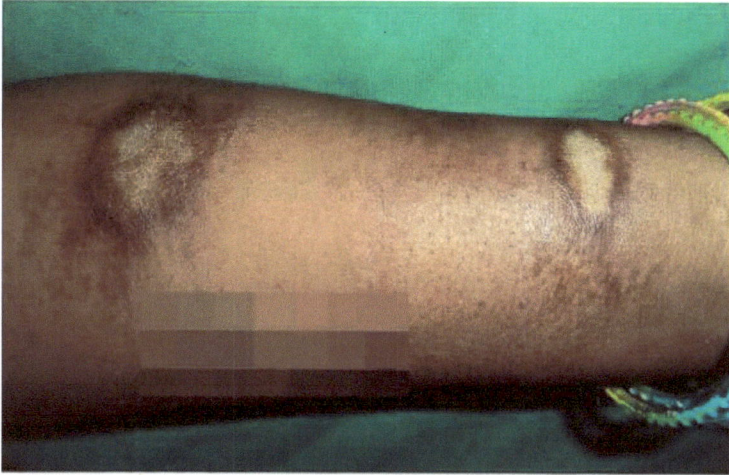

Fig. (7.12). Circunscribed morphea over arm. Two indurated plaques with central ivory white sclerotic areas.

LINEAR MORPHEA

Linear morphea is characterized by band-like cutaneous sclerosis (Fig. **7.13**) that mostly results in depressed lesions. The lesions in linear morphea may be limited to the dermis, but deeper involvement is a common condition. It is usually observed as a unilateral involvement of the body that can follow Blaschko lines

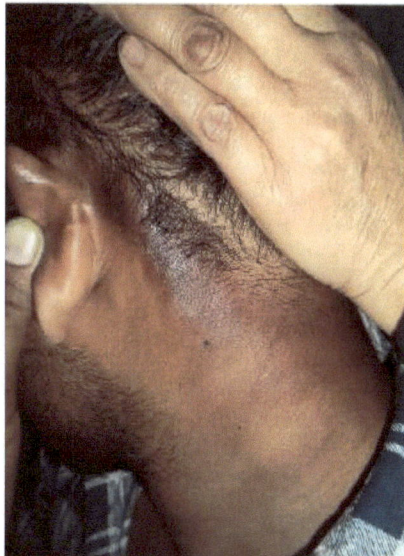

Fig. (7.13). Linear morphea involving left mastoid and post auricular area. There is a linear brownish indurated plaque in which sclerosis extended deeper than dermis. Radiological examination ruled out any bone involvement. Main complaint of the patient was tightening of the skin.

Linear morphea mostly occurs in children and adolescents. In a large series, linear morphea has been found to be the most frequent (65%) subtype in the pediatric population [21]. On the other hand, in adults it has been found to account for approximately 20% of morphea cases [13, 22]. Linear morphea can be accompanied by pregnancy. In a case series of morphea in pregnancy, 3 out of 4 patients have been reported to have a linear form of morphea (2 had en coupe de sabre, one had linear limb morphea) [19].

There are two common clinical involvement sites of linear morphea; trunk/limbs and linear morphea involving head/neck. In head and neck variant, there are mainly two closely related entities namely en coup de sabre (ECDS) and Parry Romberg syndrome (PRS). In this chapter we will discuss only ECDS. There is a separate chapter on PRS (chapter 17) where it has been described in detail.

The Trunk/Limb Variant

The trunk/limb variant of morphea (Figs. **7.14** and **7.15**) usually tends to follow unilaterally along Blaschko lines with typical clinical appearance of morphea lesions. However, in the largest pediatric study, the bilateral involvement of trunk/limb variant has been found in 11% of the morphea cases [23].

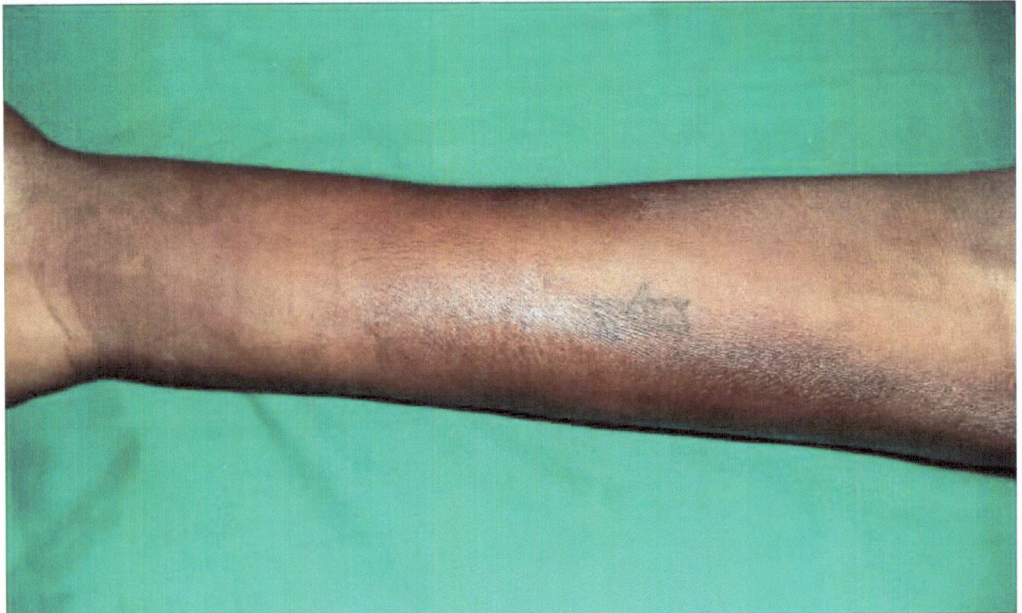

Fig. (7.14). Linear morphea involving forearm. There is linear ill defined brownish hyperpigmented indurated plaque with shiny surface. The skin was fixed and was not mobile. The sclerosis extended deeper than dermis.

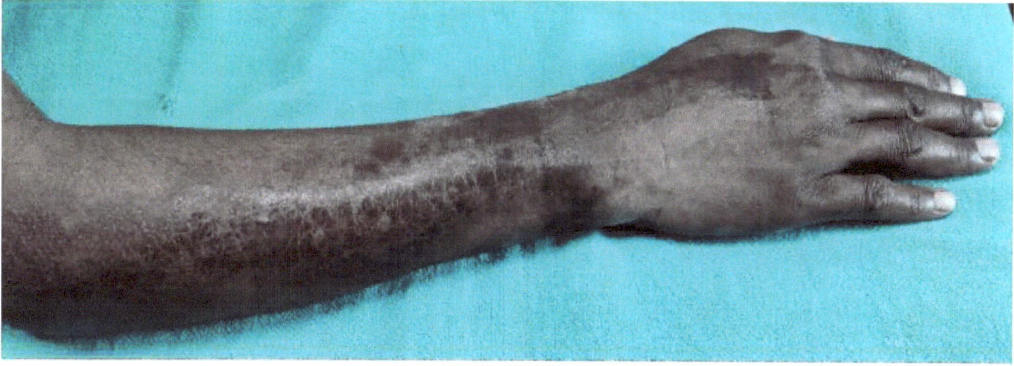

Fig. (7.15). Linear morphea involving forearm and hand. There is linear ill defined brownish hyperpigmented indurated plaque with shiny surface extending from elbow to the middle of the hand. [Image credit: Dr Saima Naaz, Resident, Dept. Of Dermatology, JNMCH, AMU].

The lesions in the trunk/limb variant of linear morphea initially occur as a linear, erythematous band-like appearance, while in some cases the lesions may start as extended linear shapes similar to circumscribed morphea. The linear morphea may have circumferential involvement in extremities (Fig. **7.16**) [24]. Circumscribed morphea especially localized on the trunk can be accompanied by the trunk/limb variant of linear morphea.

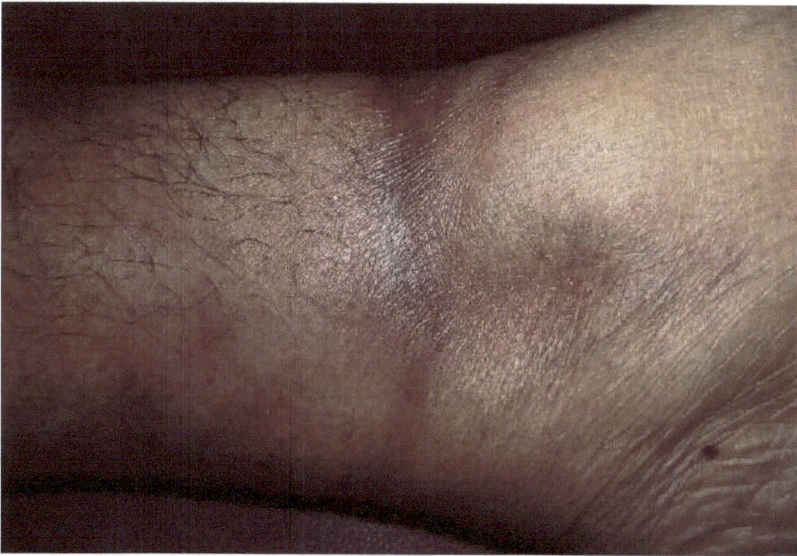

Fig. (7.16). Linear morphea. Brownish linear indurated plaque encircling the distal leg. (Copyright: Arif T, Masood Q, Singh J, Hassan I. Assessment of esophageal involvement in systemic sclerosis and morphea (localized scleroderma) by clinical, endoscopic, manometric and pH metric features: A prospective comparative hospital based study. BMC Gastroenterology 2015; 15:24. / BioMed Central. /CC BY 4.0).

The trunk/limb involvement (54-65%) of morphea occurs more often than head (23-25%) variant. Rarely, the trunk/limb variant is accompanied by head involvement [14, 25].

This variant tends to involve deep tissues such as fascia, muscle, and tendons which can result in contracture. Generalized arthralgias can occur prior to the onset of the limb variant. In addition, edema of the extremity may be a clue for the insidious presence of the disease in that region [13, 26, 27].

The lesion over joints may lead to flexion contractures, restriction of movements and functional impairment. The pain may be observed due to joint contractures and muscle atrophy. Limb length discrepancies can also occur as a complication of limb variant. The limb lenght discrepancies and weakness of involved muscle may lead to decrease in quality of life and psychological morbidities [27, 28].

In the largest pediatric study, it has been reported that contractures developed in 25.6% of the patients with linear morphea involving at least one extremity [23].This type of morphea can have reactivation/recurrence after a prolonged period of clinical inactivity.

En Coup De Sabre

The linear morphea can involve frontoparietal area of the forehead and scalp, which is known as ECDS due to its sword strike-like appearance. ECDS can occur following trauma after years and usually has a unilateral involvement [29] (Fig. **7.17**). There are reports that in rare instances, it extends below the forehead in a downward fashion and in exceedingly rare cases it can reach chin and even submandibular area of neck (Figs. **7.18-7.20**). The mouth and gum involvement in ECDS has also been reported [30, 31].

The clinical appearance of ECDS may be as linear streaks or as a group of coalescence of small plaques. The plaques at first may exhibit erythematous/violaceous color and later become hard/indurated resulting in varying degrees of hypo- hyperpigmented fibrotic plaques. Multiple and bilateral lesions can occur in addition to coexistence with other morphea subtypes especially circumscribed morphea [32, 33].

The ECDS is predominantly seen in pediatric age (2-14 years of age) and female gender.

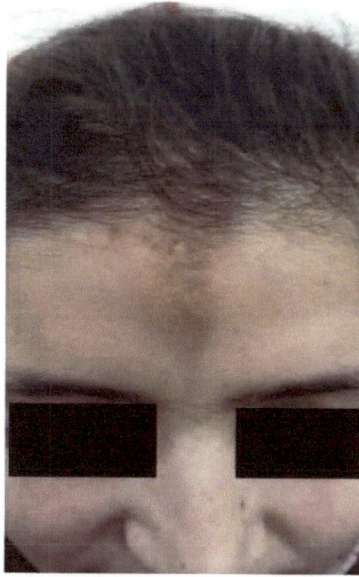

Fig. (7.17). ECDS following trauma.This patient developed en coup de sabre 6 years after receiving trauma at the frontal scalp. There is hyperpigmented brownish indurated plaque with areas of atrophy extending from frontal scalp down to the glabellar area. (Copyright: Arif T, Majid I, Haji MLI. Late onset 'en coup de sabre' following trauma: Rare presentation of a rare disease. Our Dermatol Online 2015; 6(1):49-51).

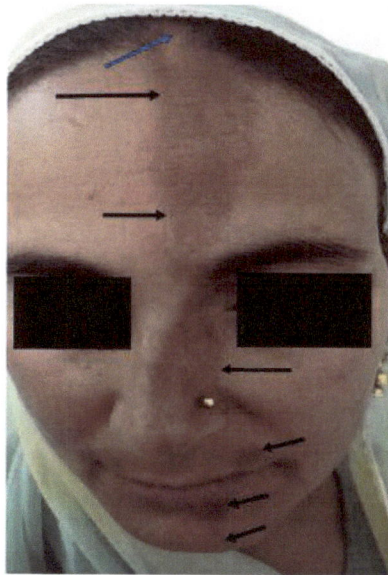

Fig. (7.18). ECDS extending from scalp to chin area which is a very rare presentation. There are well defined, brownish hyper pigmented, mildly indurated plaques over the frontal region of the scalp, forehead extending to the chin (black arrows) in a vertical fashion. Note scarring alopecia (blue arrow) at the frontal scalp [copyright: ©Iranian Journal of Dermatology: Arif T, Majid I. Can lesions of 'en coup de sabre' progress after being quiescent for a decade? Iran J Dermatol 2015; 18: 77-79.].

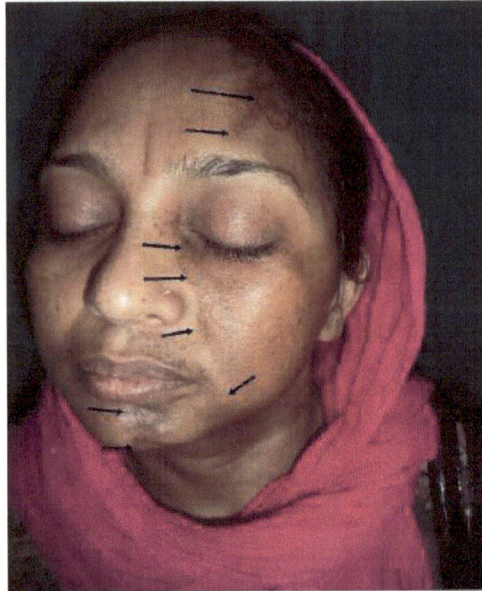

Fig. (7.19). ECDS extending from frontoparietal scalp to neck in a vertical fashion (black arrows) sparing eye lids. She didn't have neurological or any other organ system related manifestations. (copyright: Arif T, Sami M. En coup de sabre' extending from scalp to neck: an extremely rare presentation. J Pak Assoc Derm 2018; 28(3):381-383).

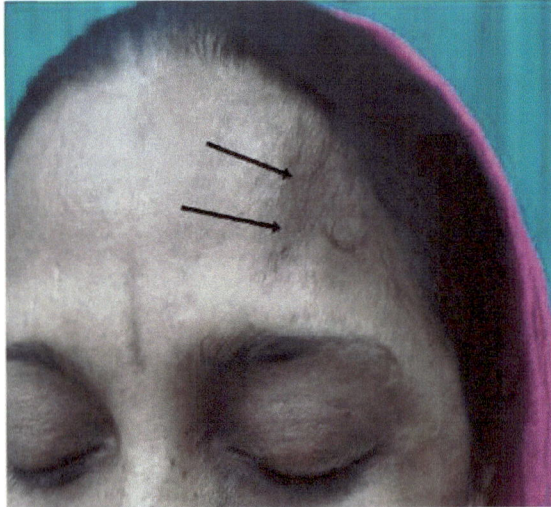

Fig. (7.20). Close view of depressed plaque on forehead in ECDS. (Copyright: Arif T, Sami M. En coup de sabre extending from scalp to neck: an extremely rare presentation. J Pak Assoc Derm 2018; 28(3):381-383).

The spectrum of clinical appearance in linear morphea including ECDS may extend from hypo-hyper pigmentation, atrophy, to scarring alopecia in the site of eyebrows, eyelashes, and scalp (Fig. **7.21**). Involement of bone is another complication of ECDS. Progressive hemifacial atrophy, which is also known as PRS, is one of the diseases most often confused with ECDS. ECDS can be accompanied by PRS.

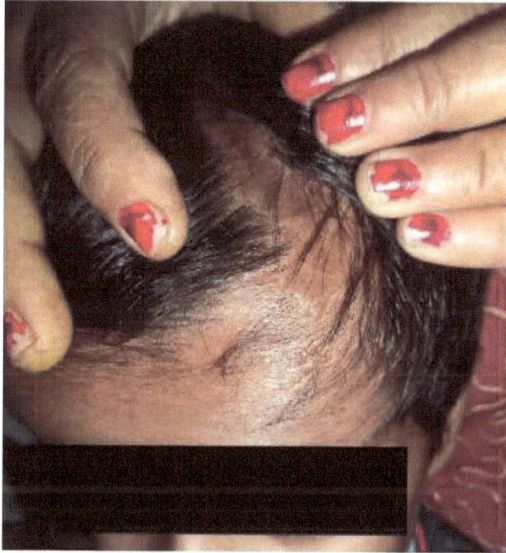

Fig. (7.21). Linear morphea ECDS in a child. Note the scarring alopecia. This patient also had vitiligo with associated leucotrichia.

PRS is characterized by unilateral atrophy of the face including skin, subcutaneous fat tissue, facia, muscle, and underlying bone in the distribution of one of the branches of trigeminal nerve. Chapter 17 has been exclusively dedicated to PRS. Readers are requested to refer to chapter 17 for full details related to PRS.

The deep involvement in linear morphea involving face may imply underlying neurological, ophthalmological, and auditory complications [22, 34, 35]. Therefore, certain consultations should be done in order to rule out aforementioned conditions (Table **7.2**).

Table 7.2. Complications of linear morphea.

Involvement Area	Clinical Findings
Neurological	Epilepsy, trigeminal neuralgia, pseudotumour cerebri, peripheral neuropathy
Ophthalmological	Eyelid abnormalities, ectropion, anterior uveitis, episcleritis, dry eye, refractive error, paralytic strabismus, pupillary mydriasis
Other	Hearing loss, arthritis, Raynaud phenomemon, abnormal pulmonary functions.

Neurological complications include seizures, trigeminal neuralgia, and headache. Most of the patients with neurologic complications in ECDS have magnetic resonance imaging (MRI) abnormalities mostly including white matter hyperintensities in subcortical and periventricular areas [36]. Neurological abnormalities associated with ECDS are usually preceded by the presence of skin lesions months to years. Extracutaneous signs and symptoms may not correlate with cutaneous disease activity.

The active stage of ECDS may last between 2-5 years. However, there is also a concept of latency or subclinical activity or reactivation in morphea in which new lesions can appear after the disease has been clinically in quiescent phase for years or decades [31].

GENERALIZED MORPHEA

There has been a lot of debate about what defines generalized morphea. Peterson *et al.* and Kreuter *et al.* defined generalized morphea as involvement of three or more of the seven following anatomic sites (head/neck, two upper extremities, two lower extremities, anterior and posterior sites of the trunk) [2, 3, 11]. Falanga *et al.*, on the other hand, classified patients as having generalized morphea fullfilling the following criteria: a) five or more than five lesions; b) lesions present bilaterally; and c) clinical evidence of confluence of at least two individual plaques [37].

According to Laxer and Zulian classification, generalized form of morphea is defined as circumscribed morphea plaques (at least four lesions, larger than 3 cm) that involve more than two out of seven different localisations (head/neck, two upper extremities, two lower extremities, anterior and posterior sites of trunk) [1]. The individual plaques may become confluent and spread across the body [2] (Figs. **7.22-7.24**).

The generalized form of morphea occurs in 7-9% of morphea patients. Unlike the linear type, it is more common in adults than children and adolescents.

Sclerotic lesions in generalized morphea are mostly observed on the trunk and extremities. In cases, where the chest wall involvement is severe, breathing difficulties may occur [14, 38]. Although, generalized morphea may course with sclerosis of the hand and fingers; it differs from systemic sclerosis by rare ulceration of fingers and absence of Raynaud's phenomenon and changes in nail folds [39, 40]. However, extensive telangiectasia on palms and nailfold capillary changes can be observed in patients with generalized morphea [41]. Extracutaneous symptoms such as myalgia, arthralgia, and dysphagia have a higher prevalence in these patients while cardiac, pulmonary, renal, and esophageal involvement were rarely reported. The main extracutaneous symptoms in generalized morphea have been mentioned in (Box **7.2**) [38, 39, 42].

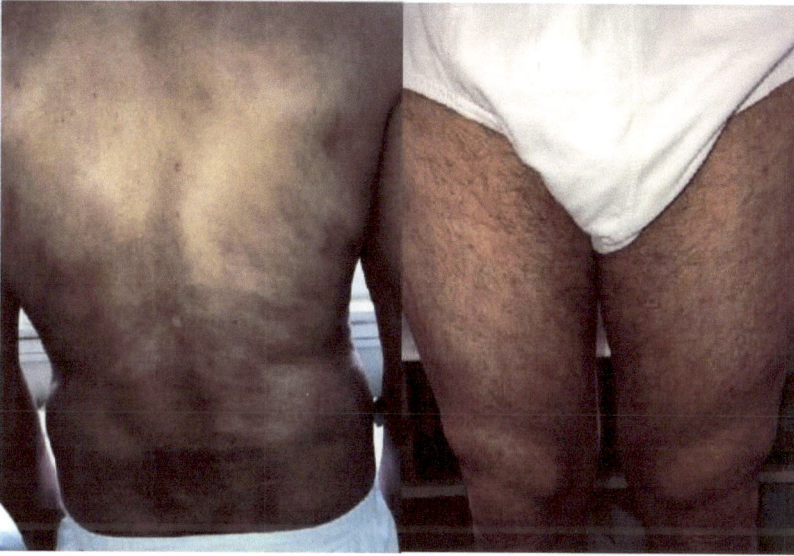

Fig. (7.22). Patient with generalized morphea.

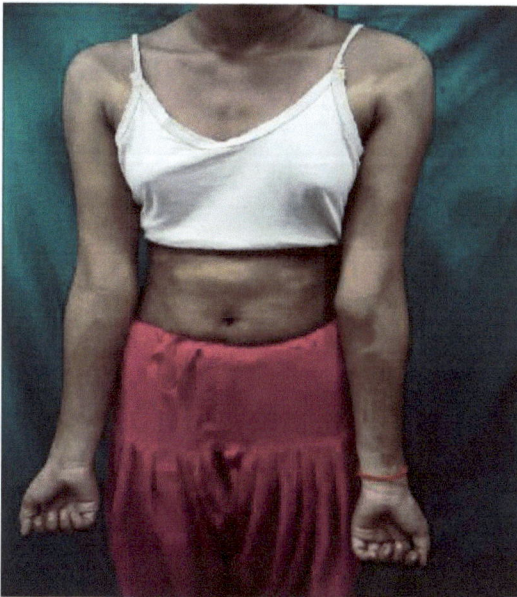

Fig. (7.23). Generalized morphea. This patient had numerous hyperpigmented indurated plaques on neck, chest, abdomen, arms, back and legs to meet the criteria for generalized morphea.

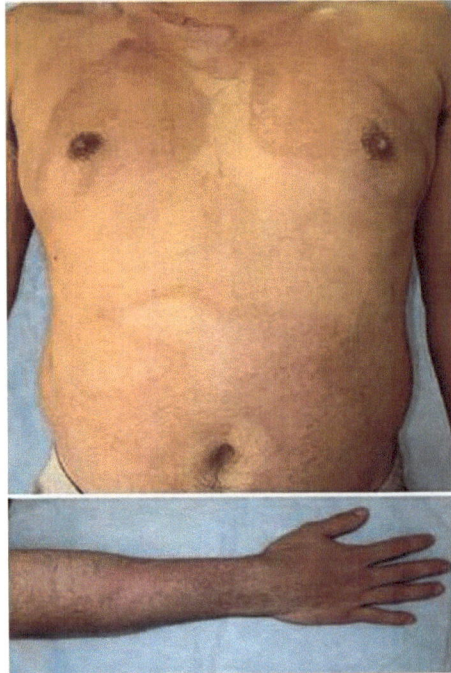

Fig. (7.24). Generalized morphea: Multiple well-defined, indurated plaques on the trunk (**a**) and right forearm (**b**). This patient also had autoimmune hepatitis. [Copyright: Himori C, Kawakami Y, Kariyama K, Oda W, Yamamoto T. A case of generalized morphea complicated by autoimmune hepatitis. Our Dermatol Online. 2021;12(1):99-100. Courtesy: Dr Piotr Brzezinski, MD PhD].

Box 7.2: Extracutaneous symptoms in generalized morphea.
Myalgia
Fatigue
Arthralgia
Limited range of motion
Dysphagia
Dyspnea
Cold fingers

Patients with circumscribed and linear morphea should have a regular follow up since generalized morphea may initially occur with these two types of morphea. In a large study, it has been found that generalized morphea is the most common subtype of morphea (49%) that is associated with rheumatic and other autoimmune disorders in morphea patients and their relatives. Therefore, patients with generalized morphea should be investigated regarding rheumatic and other autoimmune disorders [38].

PANSCLEROTIC MORPHEA

According to Laxer and Zulian classification, pansclerotic morphea has been described as an extensive, progressive, full-thickness involvement of the skin including subcutis, muscle, fascia and bone (Fig. **7.25**) [1]. The trunk, extremities, and head including face and scalp may be involved while fingertips and toes are usually spared.

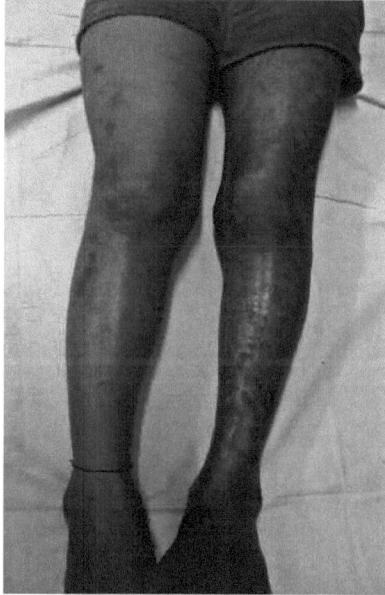

Fig. (7.25). Pansclerotic morphea. Unilateral disabling pansclerotic morphea in a 13 year old female. The sclerosis had a rapid progression and involved the left lower limb completely in a span of 4 months. The limb girth was less in the affected limb compared to the other which is quite visible from the appearance.

Pansclerotic morphea is a rare presentation of morphea that predominantly occurs in children and has rapid progression with an aggressive course. The common complications include contractures of joints with functional impairment and chronic ulcerations. Given high incidence and severe

course of the disease in pediatric age group, pansclerotic morphea is also referred to as disabling pansclerotic morphea of children [44, 45]. Secondary mutilation, ectropion, spontaneous amputation of phalanges and ear, dental malpositions, osteolysis, and ulcerations are among its complications. The ulceration of the lesions can be transformed to squamous cell carcinoma (Box **7.3**) [44, 45].

Box 7.3: Complications of pansclerotic morphea.
Secondary mutilation
Ectropion
Spontaneous amputation of phalanges and ear
Dental malpositions
Osteolysis
Ulcerations
Squamous cell carcinoma

MIXED MORPHEA

Certain clinical types of morphea may be present in the same patient at the same time. According to Laxer and Zulian classification, the presence of two or more subtypes of morphea is known as mixed type morphea [1]. In this context, the clinical appearance of circumscribed, linear, generalized, and pansclerotic forms of morphea can be seen in the same patient. A large series conducted on 245 adult and pediatric cases revealed the frequency of mixed type to account for 13% of all types of morphea. These studies also pointed out the majority of the cases with mixed type morphea were more common in children (23%) than adult (4%) morphea patients [37].

The combination of linear type limb/ trunk morphea and the circumscribed morphea is the most common clinical presentation of mixed morphea (Figs. **7.26** and **7.27**) [46]. In a recent study, generalized mixed type morphea (8.9%) has been observed more frequently than non-generalized mixed type morphea (5%). In addition, it has been reported that non-generalized mixed type morphea is more common in children (15-23%) than adults (4%) [47].

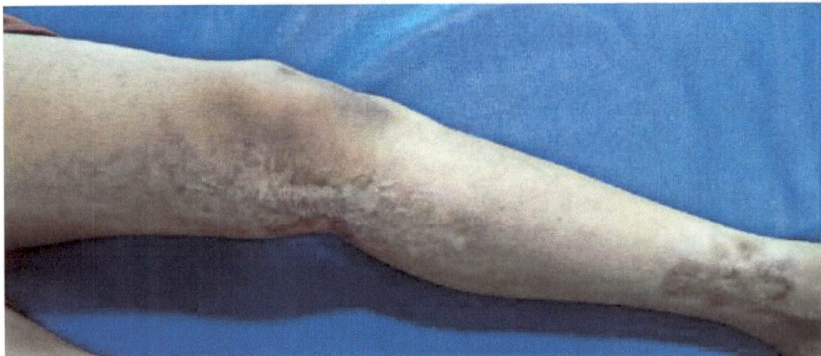

Fig. (7.26). Mixed morphea comprising of linear morphea and circumscribed morphea.

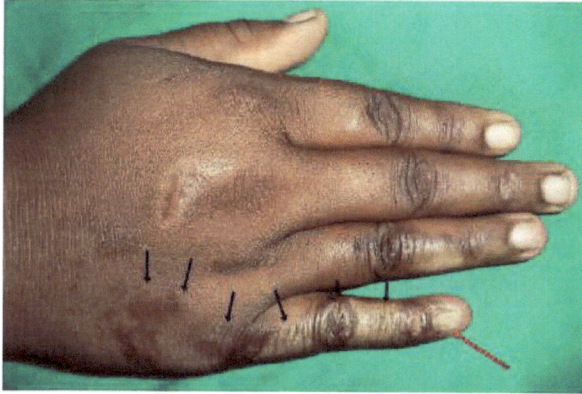

Fig. (7.27). Mixed morphea. Linear morphea involving right little finger (black arrows) and ring finger causing nail dystrophy (red arrows). She also had circumscribed plaques over arm meeting the criteria of mixed morphea.

OTHER CLINICAL TYPES OF MORPHEA

Guttate Morphea

It is characterized by multiple, small (2-10 mm), chalk white, drop-like lesions. These lesions are flat or slightly depressed and not as firm as other types of morphea. The lesions usually occur on the trunk and neck (Figs. **7.28** and **7.29**). In a study, guttate morphea has been found to account for about 1% of the morphea subtypes [37]. It is difficult to distinguish guttate morphea from extragenital lichen sclerosis (LS) and idiopathic atrophoderma of Pasini and Pierini (IAPP). Different from LS, guttate morphea does not have follicular plugging or epidermal atrophy [48, 49]. Moreover, guttate morphea usually resolves with hyperpigmentation. On the other hand, guttate morphea can overlap with extragenital LS.

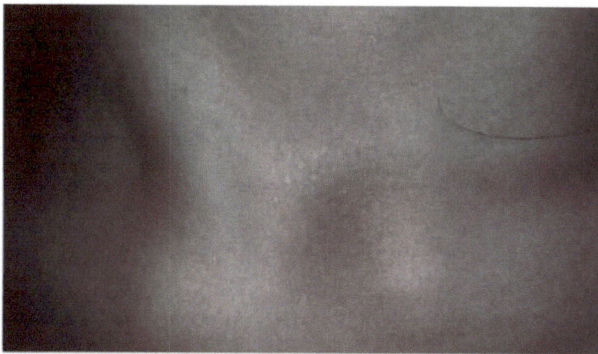

Fig. (7.28). Guttate morphea. Multiple pin point 1-3 mm whitish lesions over neck.

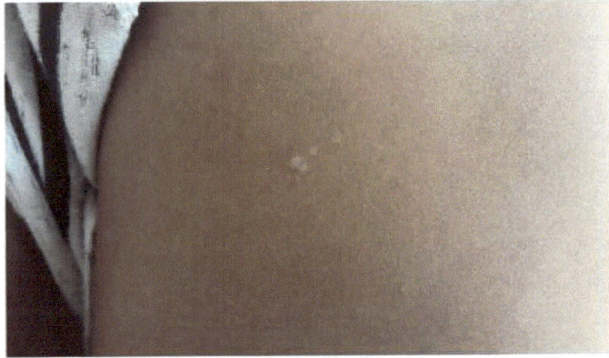

Fig. (7.29). Guttate morphea localized on the trunk.

The superficial shiny plaques of the guttate morphea may resemble IAPP. IAPP usually occurs in childhood age. The lesions start with erythematous patches, afterward, characterized by single or multiple symmetrical, sharply demarcated, hyperpigmented non-indurated plaques with typical cliff drop borders, mostly located on the trunk [50].

Keloidal morphea

Keloidal/nodular morphea is characterized by firm, different sizes (ranging from 2 to 3 cm) of non-tender keloid-like nodular lesions. This type of morphea mostly occurs in the upper part of the body where some lesions may be confluent (Fig. **7.30**) or take place in a linear pattern [47]. Different from other types, keloidal morphea does not have flat or depressed characteristics. Also, the possible coexistence of typical foci of morphea may give some clues in order to make a diagnosis. Previous reports have revealed an increased prevalence of keloidal/nodular morphea which is mostly located on the trunk in patients with systemic sclerosis [51, 52]. In rare cases, the keloidal/nodular morphea was reported to be associated with linear morphea, Steinert disease, and recalcitrant generalized morphea [53, 54].

Bullous Morphea

Bullous morphea is a rare form of morphea that may arise from morphea plaques (Figs. **7.31-7.34**) and characterized by the presence of erosions or blisters. Bullous lesions may develop with all types of morphea, hence, Laxer and Zulian classification didnt include bullous morphea as a distinct entity. In a retrospective series, the frequency of bullous morphea has been found as 1.4% of the morphea cases [55].

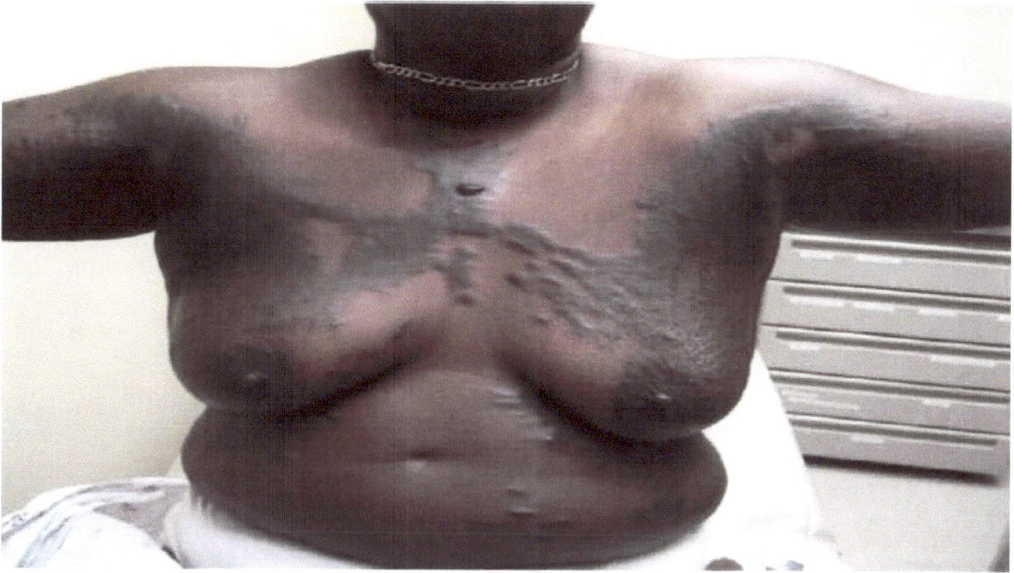

Fig. (7.30). Keloidal morphea. Multiple, scattered, confluent and hyperpigmented plaques and nodules along the trunk and upper extremities. Some nodules of keloidal morphea are discrete over lower abdomen. [Image credit: Kassira S, Jaleel T, Pavlidakey P, Sami N. Keloidal Scleroderma: Case Report and Review. Case Rep Dermatol Med. 2015;2015:635481.].

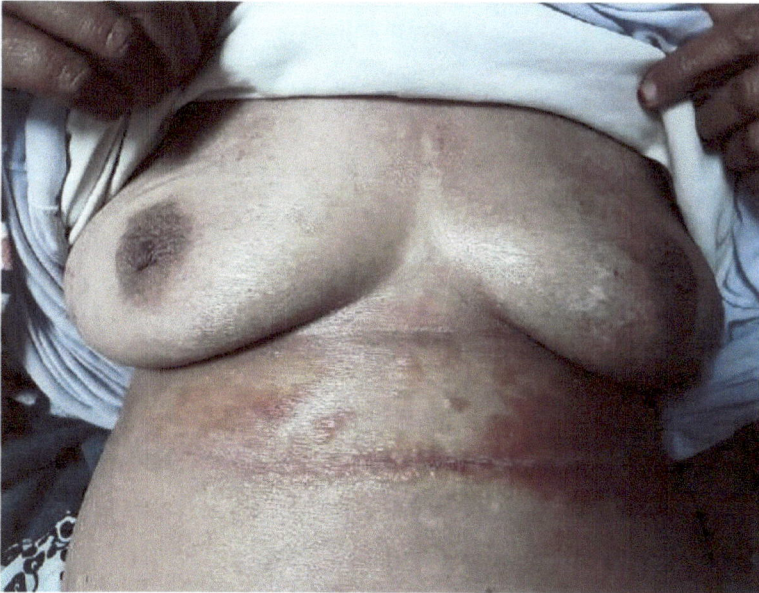

Fig. (7.31). Bullous morphea showing sclerotic plaques over abdomen bordered by tense bullae. [Copyright: Aouali S, Sefraoui S, Sof K, Dikhaye S, Zizi N. Sclerosis and blisters: An uncommon association revealing a new case of bullous morphea. Our Dermatol Online. 2021;12(2):167-168. Courtesy: Dr Piotr Brzezinski, MD, PhD].

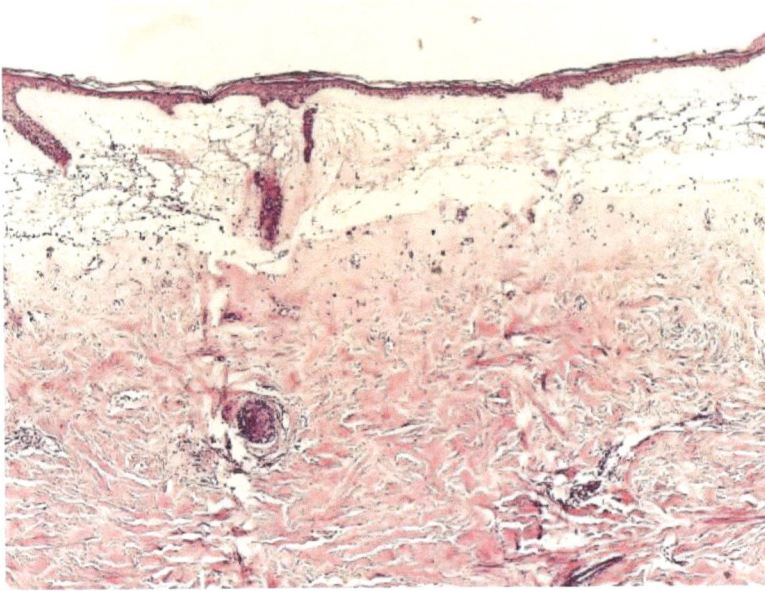

Fig. (7.32). Histopathology of Bullous morphea showing sclerodermiform dermal fibrosis with sub-epidermal blistering. [Copyright: Aouali S, Sefraoui S, Sof K, Dikhaye S, Zizi N. Sclerosis and blisters: An uncommon association revealing a new case of bullous morphea. Our Dermatol Online. 2021;12(2):167-168. Courtesy: Dr Piotr Brzezinski, MD PhD].

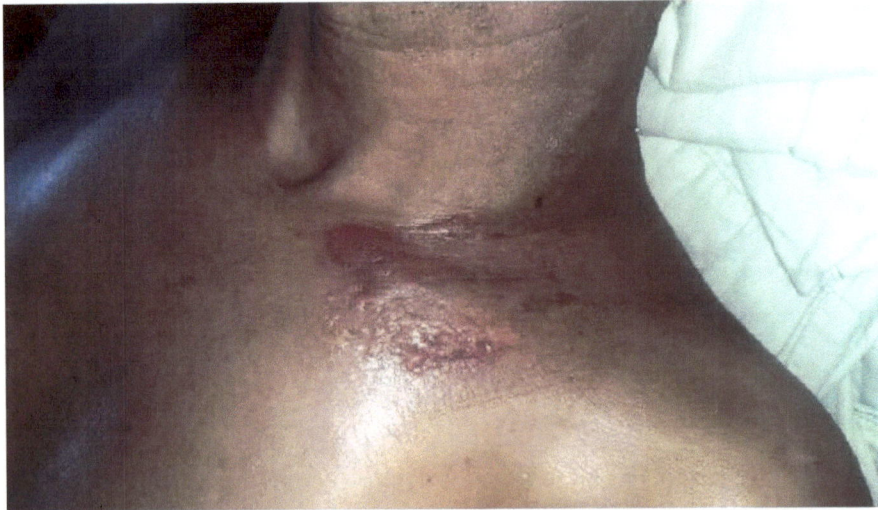

Fig. (7.33). Bullous morphea. Tense bullae with underlying indurated plaques. This patient had generalized cutaneous sclerosis with a very thick and hard skin covering the trunk and the limbs sparing head, face, hands and feet. Raynaud's phenomenon, systemic symptoms and sclerodactyly were absent. Systemic sclerosis was ruled out. Nikolsky's sign was negative. [Copyright: Mai S, Mansouri S, Znati K, Meziane M, Ismaili N, Benzekri L, Senouci K. Generalized bullous morphea. Our Dermatol Online. 2020;11(e):e102.1-e102.3. Courtesy: Dr Piotr Brzezinski, MD PhD].

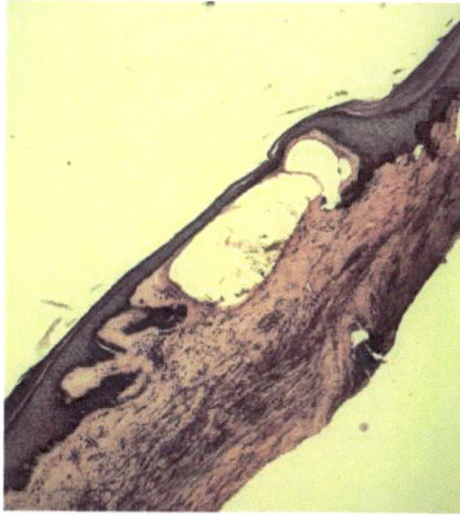

Fig. (7.34). Bullous morphea: Histopathological examination showing a bullae in the papillary dermis (HE stain x20). Direct immunofluorescence test was Negative. Beneath the bullae, there is hyalinization of the collagen and thickening of the collagen bundles in the dermis. [Copyright: Mai S, Mansouri S, Znati K, Meziane M, Ismaili N, Benzekri L, Senouci K. Generalized bullous morphea. Our Dermatol Online. 2020;11(e):e102.1-e102.3. Courtesy: Dr Piotr Brzezinski, MD PhD].

The possible stasis of lymphatic fluid mainly due to sclerosis after radiotherapy, may lead to the presence of bullous morphea formation. Also, the existence of circumscribed morphea lesions in intertriginous areas may induce bullous morphea. The association of LS and bullous morphea has also been documented [56 - 58].

Box 7.4: Learning points.
• Circumscribed morphea, generalized morphea and linear morphea are the commonest types of morphea while mixed type and keloidal/nodular type morphea are less common clinical variants.
• Morphea can be seen as Wolf's isotopic response at the site of healed herpes zoster infection
• The peripheral erythematous and violaceous halo in morphea is considered to reflect the inflammatory stage.
• Linear morphea is the most frequent (65%) subtype in the pediatric age group. The deep involvement in linear morphea involving face may imply underlying neurological, ophthalmological, and auditory complications.
• Generalized morphea may course with sclerosis of the hand and fingers. However, it differs from systemic sclerosis by rare ulceration of fingers and absence of Raynaud's phenomenon and changes in nail folds.
• Secondary mutilation, ectropion, spontaneous amputation of phalanges and ear, dental malpositions, osteolysis, and cutaneous ulcerations are common complications in pansclerotic morphea. The chronic ulcerations may turn in to squamous cell carcinoma.

REFERENCES

[1]   Laxer RM, Zulian F. Localized scleroderma. Curr Opin Rheumatol 2006; 18(6): 606-13.
        [http://dx.doi.org/10.1097/01.bor.0000245727.40630.c3] [PMID: 17053506]

[2]   Arif T, Adil M, Amin SS, *et al.* Clinico-epidemiological Study of Morphea from a Tertiary Care
        Hospital. Curr Rheumatol Rev 2018; 14(3): 251-4.
        [http://dx.doi.org/10.2174/1573397114666180410115553] [PMID: 29637865]

[3]   Peterson LS, Nelson AM, Su WPD. Classification of morphea (localized scleroderma). Mayo Clin
        Proc 1995; 70(11): 1068-76.
        [http://dx.doi.org/10.4065/70.11.1068] [PMID: 7475336]

[4]   Noh TW, Park SH, Kang YS, Lee UH, Park HS, Jang SJ. Morphea developing at the site of healed
        herpes zoster. Ann Dermatol 2011; 23(2): 242-5.
        [http://dx.doi.org/10.5021/ad.2011.23.2.242] [PMID: 21747631]

[5]   Forschner A, Metzler G, Rassner G, Fierlbeck G. Morphea with features of lichen sclerosus et
        atrophicus at the site of a herpes zoster scar: Another case of an isotopic response. Int J Dermatol
        2005; 44(6): 524-5.
        [http://dx.doi.org/10.1111/j.1365-4632.2005.01625.x] [PMID: 15941448]

[6]   Joshi A, Al-Mutairi N. Zosteriform morphea: A new pattern. Acta Derm Venereol 2005; 85(3): 279-
        80.
        [PMID: 16040427]

[7]   Mazori DR, Wright NA, Patel M, *et al.* Characteristics and treatment of adult-onset linear morphea: A
        retrospective cohort study of 61 patients at 3 tertiary care centers. J Am Acad Dermatol 2016; 74(3):
        577-9.
        [http://dx.doi.org/10.1016/j.jaad.2015.09.069] [PMID: 26892661]

[8]   Ben-Amitai D, Hodak E, Lapidoth M, David M. Coexisting morphoea and granuloma annulare-are the
        conditions related? Clin Exp Dermatol 1999; 24(2): 86-9.
        [http://dx.doi.org/10.1046/j.1365-2230.1999.00425.x] [PMID: 10233660]

[9]   Holmes RC, Meara RH. Morphoea, sclerotic panatrophy and disseminated granuloma annulare. Clin
        Exp Dermatol 1983; 8(2): 201-3.
        [http://dx.doi.org/10.1111/j.1365-2230.1983.tb01767.x] [PMID: 6851242]

[10]   Tajima S, Suzuki Y, Inazumi T, Mori N. Systemic scleroderma and perforating granuloma annulare:
        differential diagnosis from calcinosis. Dermatology 1996; 192(3): 271-3.
        [http://dx.doi.org/10.1159/000246383] [PMID: 8726647]

[11]   Kreuter A, Wischnewski J, Terras S, Altmeyer P, Stücker M, Gambichler T. Coexistence of lichen
        sclerosus and morphea: A retrospective analysis of 472 patients with localized scleroderma from a
        German tertiary referral center. J Am Acad Dermatol 2012; 67(6): 1157-62.
        [http://dx.doi.org/10.1016/j.jaad.2012.04.003] [PMID: 22533994]

[12]   Arif T, Adil M, Amin SS, Mahtab A. Concomitant morphea and lichen sclerosus et atrophicus in the
        same plaque at the site of intramuscular drug injection: An interesting case presentation. Acta
        Dermatovenerol Alp Panonica Adriat 2018; 27(2): 111-3.
        [http://dx.doi.org/10.15570/actaapa.2018.23] [PMID: 29945269]

[13]   Christianson HB, Dorsey CS, Kierland RR, O'Leary PA. Localized Scleroderma. AMA Arch Derm
        1956; 74(6): 629-39.
        [http://dx.doi.org/10.1001/archderm.1956.01550120049012] [PMID: 13371921]

[14]   Mertens JS, Seyger MMB, Kievit W, *et al.* Disease recurrence in localized scleroderma: A
        retrospective analysis of 344 patients with paediatric or adult-onset disease. Br J Dermatol 2015;
        172(3): 722-8.
        [http://dx.doi.org/10.1111/bjd.13514] [PMID: 25381928]

[15]   Arif T, Sami M. Bilateral facial circumscribed morphea: The first case report. J Dtsch Dermatol Ges 2018; 16(12): 1480-2.
[http://dx.doi.org/10.1111/ddg.13705] [PMID: 30466150]

[16]   Giri S, Paudel U, Jha A, Gurung D, Parajuli S. Morphoea profunda presenting with atrophic skin lesions in a 26 year old female: A case report. Clin Med Insights Case Rep 2012; 5: CCRep.S9433.
[http://dx.doi.org/10.4137/CCRep.S9433] [PMID: 22661901]

[17]   Wardhana , Datau EA. A patient with plaque type morphea mimicking systemic lupus erythematosus. Acta Med Indones 2015; 47(2): 146-52.
[PMID: 26260557]

[18]   Benchat L, Mernissi FZ. Morphea on the breast and pregnancy. Pan Afr Med J 2013; 16: 22.
[http://dx.doi.org/10.11604/pamj.2013.16.22.3317] [PMID: 24570783]

[19]   Pham AK, Srivastava B, Deng A. Pregnancy-associated morphea: A case report and literature review 2017.
[http://dx.doi.org/10.5070/D3231033691]

[20]   Su DWP, Person JR. Morphea profunda. Am J Dermatopathol 1981; 3(3): 251-60.
[http://dx.doi.org/10.1097/00000372-198110000-00003] [PMID: 6172992]

[21]   Zulian F, Athreya BH, Laxer R, *et al.* Juvenile Scleroderma Working Group of the Pediatric Rheumatology European Society (PRES). Juvenile localized scleroderma: clinical and epidemiological features in 750 children. An international study. Rheumatology 2006; 45(5): 614-20.
[http://dx.doi.org/10.1093/rheumatology/kei251] [PMID: 16368732]

[22]   Peterson LS, Nelson AM, Su WP, Mason T, O'Fallon WM, Gabriel SE. The epidemiology of morphea (localized scleroderma) in Olmsted County 1960-1993. J Rheumatol 1997; 24(1): 73-80.
[PMID: 9002014]

[23]   Christen-Zaech S, Hakim MD, Afsar FS, Paller AS. Pediatric morphea (localized scleroderma): Review of 136 patients. J Am Acad Dermatol 2008; 59(3): 385-96.
[http://dx.doi.org/10.1016/j.jaad.2008.05.005] [PMID: 18571769]

[24]   Arif T, Masood Q, Singh J, Hassan I. Assessment of esophageal involvement in systemic sclerosis and morphea (localized scleroderma) by clinical, endoscopic, manometric and pH metric features: A prospective comparative hospital based study. BMC Gastroenterol 2015; 15(1): 24.
[http://dx.doi.org/10.1186/s12876-015-0241-2] [PMID: 25888470]

[25]   Jue MS, Kim MH, Ko JY, Lee CW. Digital image processing for the acquisition of graphic similarity of the distributional patterns between cutaneous lesions of linear scleroderma and Blaschko's lines. J Dermatol 2011; 38(8): 778-83.
[http://dx.doi.org/10.1111/j.1346-8138.2010.01162.x] [PMID: 21366680]

[26]   Falanga V, Medsger TA Jr, Reichlin M, Rodnan GP. Linear Scleroderma. Ann Intern Med 1986; 104(6): 849-57.
[http://dx.doi.org/10.7326/0003-4819-104-6-849] [PMID: 3486617]

[27]   Larrègue M, Ziegler JE, Lauret P, *et al.* Linear scleroderma in children (apropos of 27 cases). Ann Dermatol Venereol 1986; 113(3): 207-24.
[PMID: 3752860]

[28]   Das S, Bernstein I, Jacobe H. Correlates of self-reported quality of life in adults and children with morphea. J Am Acad Dermatol 2014; 70(5): 904-10.
[http://dx.doi.org/10.1016/j.jaad.2013.11.037] [PMID: 24534655]

[29]   Arif T, Majid I, Ishtiyaq Haji ML. Late onset 'en coup de sabre' following trauma: Rare presentation of a rare disease. Nasza Dermatol Online 2015; 6(1): 49-51.
[http://dx.doi.org/10.7241/ourd.20151.12]

[30]   Arif T, Sami M. En coup de sabre' extending from scalp to neck: An extremely rare presentation. J

Pak Assoc Dermatol 2018; 28: 381-3.

[31]   Arif T, Majid I. Can lesions of 'en coup de sabre' progress after being quiescent for a decade? Iran J Dermatol 2015; 18: 77-9.

[32]   Tollefson MM, Witman PM. En coup de sabre morphea and Parry-Romberg syndrome: A retrospective review of 54 patients. J Am Acad Dermatol 2007; 56(2): 257-63.
[http://dx.doi.org/10.1016/j.jaad.2006.10.959] [PMID: 17147965]

[33]   Rai R, Handa S, Gupta S, Kumar B. Bilateral en coup de sabre-a rare entity. Pediatr Dermatol 2000; 17(3): 222-4.
[http://dx.doi.org/10.1046/j.1525-1470.2000.01757.x] [PMID: 10886757]

[34]   Weibel L, Harper JI. Linear morphoea follows Blaschko's lines. Br J Dermatol 2008; 159(1): 175-81.
[http://dx.doi.org/10.1111/j.1365-2133.2008.08647.x] [PMID: 18503590]

[35]   Zannin ME, Martini G, Athreya BH, *et al.* Juvenile Scleroderma Working Group of the Pediatric Rheumatology European Society (PRES). Ocular involvement in children with localised scleroderma: A multi-centre study. Br J Ophthalmol 2007; 91(10): 1311-4.
[http://dx.doi.org/10.1136/bjo.2007.116038] [PMID: 17475707]

[36]   Doolittle DA, Lehman VT, Schwartz KM, Wong-Kisiel LC, Lehman JS, Tollefson MM. CNS imaging findings associated with Parry–Romberg syndrome and en coup de sabre: correlation to dermatologic and neurologic abnormalities. Neuroradiology 2015; 57(1): 21-34.
[http://dx.doi.org/10.1007/s00234-014-1448-6] [PMID: 25304124]

[37]   Falanga V, Medsger TA Jr, Reichlin M. Antinuclear and anti-single-stranded DNA antibodies in morphea and generalized morphea. Arch Dermatol 1987; 123(3): 350-3.
[http://dx.doi.org/10.1001/archderm.1987.01660270088021] [PMID: 3545090]

[38]   Leitenberger JJ, Cayce RL, Haley RW, Adams-Huet B, Bergstresser PR, Jacobe HT. Distinct autoimmune syndromes in morphea: A review of 245 adult and pediatric cases. Arch Dermatol 2009; 145(5): 545-50.
[http://dx.doi.org/10.1001/archdermatol.2009.79] [PMID: 19451498]

[39]   Bielsa I, Cid M, Herrero C, Cardellach F. Generalized morphea: systemic aspects of a skin disease. Description of 12 cases and review of the literature. Med Clin 1985; 85(5): 171-4.
[PMID: 4021633]

[40]   Dehen L, Roujeau JC, Cosnes A, Revuz J. Internal involvement in localized scleroderma. Medicine 1994; 73(5): 241-5.
[http://dx.doi.org/10.1097/00005792-199409000-00002] [PMID: 7934808]

[41]   Miyagawa F, Ogawa K, Asada H. Generalized morphea with extensive telangiectasia on the palms. J Dermatol 2021; 48(1): e22-3.
[http://dx.doi.org/10.1111/1346-8138.15609] [PMID: 32902882]

[42]   Marzano AV, Menni S, Parodi A, *et al.* Localized scleroderma in adults and children. Clinical and laboratory investigations on 239 cases. Eur J Dermatol 2003; 13(2): 171-6.
[PMID: 12695134]

[43]   Diaz-Perez JL, Connolly SM, Winkelmann RK. Disabling pansclerotic morphea of children. Arch Dermatol 1980; 116(2): 169-73.
[http://dx.doi.org/10.1001/archderm.1980.01640260045011] [PMID: 7356347]

[44]   Wollina U, Buslau M, Heinig B, *et al.* Disabling pansclerotic morphea of childhood poses a high risk of chronic ulceration of the skin and squamous cell carcinoma. Int J Low Extrem Wounds 2007; 6(4): 291-8.
[http://dx.doi.org/10.1177/1534734607308731] [PMID: 18048875]

[45]   Singh A, Singhal K, Choudhary S, Bisati S, Arora M. Adult-onset unilateral disabling pansclerotic morphea. Indian J Dermatol 2014; 59(3): 316.
[http://dx.doi.org/10.4103/0019-5154.131459] [PMID: 24891683]

[46]   Albuquerque JV, Andriolo BN, Vasconcellos MR, Civile VT, Lyddiatt A, Trevisani VF. Interventions for morphea. Cochrane Database Syst Rev 2019; 7(7): CD005027.
[PMID: 31309547]

[47]   Hong JH, Kim JE, Ko JY, Ro YS. A clinicopathologic study of morphea in Korean patients. J Cutan Pathol 2015; 42(12): 929-36.
[http://dx.doi.org/10.1111/cup.12528] [PMID: 25965906]

[48]   Sehgal VN, Srivastava G, Aggarwal AK, Behl PN, Choudhary M, Bajaj P. Localized scleroderma/morphea. Int J Dermatol 2002; 41(8): 467-75.
[http://dx.doi.org/10.1046/j.1365-4362.2002.01469.x] [PMID: 12207760]

[49]   Chung L, Lin J, Furst DE, Fiorentino D. Systemic and localized scleroderma. Clin Dermatol 2006; 24(5): 374-92.
[http://dx.doi.org/10.1016/j.clindermatol.2006.07.004] [PMID: 16966019]

[50]   Jablonska S, Blaszczyk M. Is superficial morphea synonymous with atrophoderma Pasini-Pierini? J Am Acad Dermatol 2004; 50(6): 979-80.
[http://dx.doi.org/10.1016/j.jaad.2003.11.088] [PMID: 15153911]

[51]   Krell JM, Solomon AR, Glavey CM, Lawley TJ. Nodular scleroderma. J Am Acad Dermatol 1995; 32(2): 343-5.
[http://dx.doi.org/10.1016/0190-9622(95)90400-X] [PMID: 7829737]

[52]   Nakazato S, Nomura T, Yamane N, *et al.* Nodular morphoea: A first case associated with linear morphoea. Eur J Dermatol 2016; 26(1): 95-6.
[http://dx.doi.org/10.1684/ejd.2015.2656] [PMID: 26841724]

[53]   Campione E, Ventura A, Garofalo V, *et al.* Nodular morphea in a patient with Steinert disease. G Ital Dermatol Venereol 2019; 154(2): 209-10.
[http://dx.doi.org/10.23736/S0392-0488.17.05624-3] [PMID: 28895373]

[54]   Dadkhahfar S, Asadi Kani Z, Araghi F, Moravvej H. Development of keloidal morphea after treatment with cyclosporine in a case of recalcitrant generalized morphea. Clin Case Rep 2020; 8(5): 837-9.
[http://dx.doi.org/10.1002/ccr3.2776] [PMID: 32477528]

[55]   Venturi M, Pinna AL, Pilloni L, Atzori L, Ferreli C, Rongioletti F. Bullous morphoea: A retrospective study. Clin Exp Dermatol 2017; 42(5): 532-5.
[http://dx.doi.org/10.1111/ced.13127] [PMID: 28543394]

[56]   Lahouel M, Soua Y, Njim L, Belhadjali H, Youssef M, Zili J. An unusual presentation of localized bullous morphea. Dermatol Online J 2020; 26: 13030/qt6hm3k4g9.
[http://dx.doi.org/10.5070/D3266049323]

[57]   Hellen R, Kiely C, Murad A, *et al.* Two cases of dermatoses koebnerizing within fields of previous radiotherapy. Clin Exp Dermatol 2014; 39(8): 900-3.
[http://dx.doi.org/10.1111/ced.12421] [PMID: 25224250]

[58]   Zindanci I, Demirkesen C, Beyhan EKS, Turkoglu Z, Kavala M. Intertriginous bullous morphea: A clue for the pathogenesis? Indian J Dermatol Venereol Leprol 2007; 73(4): 262-4.
[http://dx.doi.org/10.4103/0378-6323.33640] [PMID: 17675738]

CHAPTER 8

Differential Diagnosis

Shazia Jeelani[1,*] and **Tasleem Arif**[2,3]

[1] *Department of Dermatology, STDs and Leprosy, Government Medical College, Srinagar Kashmir, India*

[2] *Department of Dermatology, STDs, Leprosy and Aesthetics, Dar As Sihha Medical Center, Dammam, Saudi Arabia*

[3] *Ellahi Medicare Clinic, Srinagar, Kashmir, India*

Chapter Synopsis.
• Morphea is the localized form of scleroderma characterized by the thickening of the skin and sometimes the underlying subcutaneous tissue.
• Morphea has diverse presentations in different subtypes, in different age groups, and in different stages.
• The differential diagnosis of morphea encompasses a wide spectrum from systemic sclerosis at one end to drug-induced morphea at the other end.
• Detailed history and examination together with histopathology and nail fold capillaroscopy help to differentiate morphea from other close mimics.
• The presence of Raynaud's phenomenon, sclerodactyly, calcinosis cutis, mat-like telangiectasia and autoantibody levels are the features that differentiate systemic sclerosis from morphea.
• Scleromyxedema is characterized by the deposition of mucin mostly in the skin and sometimes in the internal organs. Face, arms, and hands are mostly affected. In contrast to morphea, skin can be pinched and moved over the subcutis as mucin deposition is mainly in the papillary dermis.
• Scleredema is a fibro mucinous connective-tissue disorder associated with antecedent infections, diabetes or plasma cell dyscrasias. It is characterized clinically by woody hard induration of the skin. As compared to morphea, hands, and feet are typically spared in scleredema.

Keywords: Atrophic stage, Autoantibody, Calcinosis cutis, Circumscribed morphea, Comedo-like openings, Differential diagnosis of morphea, Drug-induced morphea, Early inflammatory stage, Generalized morphea, Interstitial mycosis fungoides, Linear morphea, Lilac ring, Morphea, Nail fold capillaroscopy, Neutrophilic panniculitis, Raynaud's phenomenon, Sclerodactyly, Sclerosis, Sclerotic stage, Systemic sclerosis.

* **Corresponding author Shazia Jeelani:** Department of Dermatology, STDs and Leprosy, Government Medical College, Srinagar Kashmir, India; E-mail: shazia46@gmail.com

INTRODUCTION

Morphea is a disorder limited to the skin and subcutaneous tissue, sometimes extending to the deeper underlying structures. It is more prevalent in children and young adults. Clinically, morphea is characterized by one or more circumscribed oval asymmetric plaques. Usually, the lesions are present on the trunk, sometimes, on the limbs. Classically, there is no sclerodactyly, fingers are spared. Linear forms are more common on the limbs. Three different stages of the disease have been delineated.

In the inflammatory phase, the plaque is surrounded by a "lilac ring". In the sclerotic stage, central sclerosis develops which heals with a hypo- or hyperpigmented atrophic stage. Morphea is a clinical diagnosis and there are no definite markers for proper diagnosis, disease activity and prognosis. As morphea encompasses a wide range of clinical phenotypes and has a different presentation in its different stages, it has to be differentiated from a variety of other diagnoses that it mimics.

DIFFERENTIAL DIAGNOSIS OF GENERALISED MORPHEA

Systemic Sclerosis

Generalized morphea may be difficult to differentiate from systemic sclerosis [1]. However, progression to systemic sclerosis is uncommon. Delay in the diagnosis of systemic sclerosis can lead to progressive systemic involvement and can have bad prognostic implications. Pansclerotic and generalized morphea present with diffuse and widespread sclerosis as seen in systemic sclerosis but spares the fingers and toes. Again one has to remember that morphea often called localized scleroderma and systemic sclerosis (systemic scleroderma) is different diseases, and it does not progress to systemic sclerosis over time. In such patients, where there is confusion, they should be evaluated for the presence of Raynaud's phenomenon, sclerodactyly, calcinosis cutis, telangiectasia and auto-antibody levels. Therefore, in systemic sclerosis, there is the presence of these differentiating points (Box **8.1**).

Box 8.1: Salient features of systemic sclerosis differentiating it from morphea.
Internal organ involvement.
Acrosclerosis/sclerodactyly
Raynaud's phenomenon
Nail Fold Capillaroscopic Changes
Antibodies: Anti-centromere, Scl-70, and RNA polymerase-III

DIFFERENTIAL DIAGNOSIS OF CIRCUMSCRIBED MORPHEA

Clinical presentations of circumscribed morphea vary in the different stages- viz., early, sclerotic and atrophic stage, so do the differential diagnosis (Table **8.1**).

Table 8.1. Differential diagnosis of circumscribed morphea.

• Early Lesions	• Sclerodermoid/Atrophic Lesions
Acquired Port wine stain	Idiopathic Atrophoderma of Pasini and Pierini
Granuloma annulare	Lipodermatosclerosis
Mycosis fungoides (interstitial type)	Morpheaform dermatofibrosarcoma protuberans
Early Sweet syndrome	Radiation fibrosis
Interstitial and granulomatous dermatitis	Reflex sympathetic dystrophy
Erythema migrans	Scleromyxedema
Erythema nodosum migrans	Cheiroarthropathy due to diabetes mellitus
Annular lichenoid dermatitis of youth	Carcinoid syndrome
Hypertrophic scars or keloids	Porphyria cutanea tarda (PCT)
Connective tissue nevi	Nephrogenic systemic fibrosis (NSF)
	Pretibial myxedema
	Morpheaform Basal Cell Carcinoma
	Scleredema
	Anetoderma
	Stiff skin syndrome
	Restrictive dermopathy

Early Stage Circumscribed Morphea

Early circumscribed morphea presents as an erythematous plaque without apparent thickening of the underlying structures and without classical histopathological features, so it is not very easy to distinguish it from other common conditions.

Interstitial Mycosis Fungoides (IMF)

In the literature, there are several case reports where the initial histopathological diagnosis of IMF later turned out to be morphea on close follow-up [2]. Initially, the collagen deposition may not be evident in the histopathology and it may be difficult to differentiate morphea from mycosis fungoides which shows cellular proliferation. Immunohistochemistry helps to differentiate between the two disorders as morphea being a reactive disorder shows the presence of CD7 cells when compared to IMF which is a neoplastic disorder.

Acquired Port Wine Stain (APWS)

In a few reported cases, the APWS on years of follow-up turned out to be morphea on the histopathology of the lesions obtained [3]. Morphea especially on the face initially due to its erythematous or violaceous colour may resemble port wine stain in children. Over years of follow-up, the typical clinical features of morphea develop and it becomes easier to diagnose the condition.

Granuloma Annulare (GA)

GA may occasionally be seen as a patch. This uncommon patch variant is mostly found in middle-aged females and clinically can be misdiagnosed as morphea. Morphea and granuloma annulare both cause alterations in collagen and a common etiology (autoimmune/ infectious) has been proposed for both of them, however, classical interstitial granulomatous infiltrate with palisading is seen on the histopathological examination in granuloma annulare [4].

Subcutaneous Variant of Sweet's Syndrome

Subcutaneous variant of sweet's syndrome (acute febrile neutrophilic dermatosis) has been described and may sometimes pose a diagnostic challenge that resembles morphea. Subcutaneous sweets syndrome presents as erythematous subcutaneous dermal nodules usually tender to touch and may mimic early morphea. Like the classical sweets syndrome, it may present with systemic features and on histopathology, it is characterised by neutrophilic panniculitis [5].

Interstitial Granulomatous Dermatitis (IGD)

Differentiating between IGD (a T- cell lymphoma subtype) and the early stages of morphea is not easy as no well-circumscribed granulomas are formed instead of a diffuse interstitial histiocytic inflammatory infiltrate is seen. So, in long-standing cases of morphea not responding to treatment, T-cell lymphoma should always be excluded from histopathology [6]. The detection of a monoclonal T-cell expansion and features of vasculitis in IGD are helpful to differentiate it from morphea [6].

Erythema Migrans

Erythema migrans is the pathognomonic rash of Lyme disease clinically characterised by annular homogenous erythema, which may sometimes be difficult to distinguish from early morphea. Besides both may have *Borrelia* infection as a common causal factor [7].

Erythema Nodosum Migrans

Erythema nodosum migrans (sub-acute nodular migratory panniculitis) is a panniculitis clinically characterized by migrating subcutaneous nodules or plaques and should be kept in mind in the differential diagnosis of any morpheaform centrifugally enlarging plaque, especially in the legs [8]. Lesions tend to be less tender as compared to the classic erythema nodosum and may have a yellowish hue with a morpheaform appearance.

Annular Lichenoid Dermatitis of Youth

Annular lichenoid dermatitis of youth typically presents as asymptomatic rounded, oval, or annular red-brown macules or patches [9]. These start as erythematous macules with a raised border and develop central hypopigmentation as they gradually enlarge and hence may be clinically misdiagnosed as morphea.

Hypertrophic Scars or Keloids

Hypertrophic scars or keloids resemble indurated plaques of morphea. Keloidal or nodular morphea is a rare subtype of morphea in which keloids are seen. Trunk, neck and upper arms are the most common sites. Keloidal morphea may either be due to the combined mechanism with a dermal inflammatory process of sclerosis forming keloidal lesions or a process unrelated to sclerosis. Keloidal/nodular morphea is difficult to differentiate from the simple hypertrophic scars or keloids. Keloidal morphea is very rare. Less than 50 cases of keloidal morphea have been described till date. Most of these cases were associated with systemic sclerosis. However, some of them have been reported in the setting of other types of morphea. Clinically, keloidal morphea is manifested by single or multiple keloidal nodules or plaques that develop in sclerodermatous areas in the absence of preceding trauma or injury. These affect most commonly young and middle-aged women. In general, these firm, elevated, non-tender lesions have different sizes, ranging from 2 to 3 cm. The majority of patients of keloidal morphea have associated sclerodactyly as well as other extracutaneous manifestations of systemic scleroderma like Raynaud's phenomenon and arthritis. Histopathology can help in better differentiating keloidal morphea from hypertrophic scars or keloids. In keloidal morphea, there is a proliferation of myofibroblasts and thickened collagen bundles in dermis. There is a lack of vertically oriented blood vessels and a lack of atrophy of the overlying epidermis which differentiates it from keloids and hypertrophic scars. Elastic fibers within areas of scleroderma are preserved. However, in areas of keloid, these elastic fibers are typically absent (Figs. **8.1** and **8.2**).

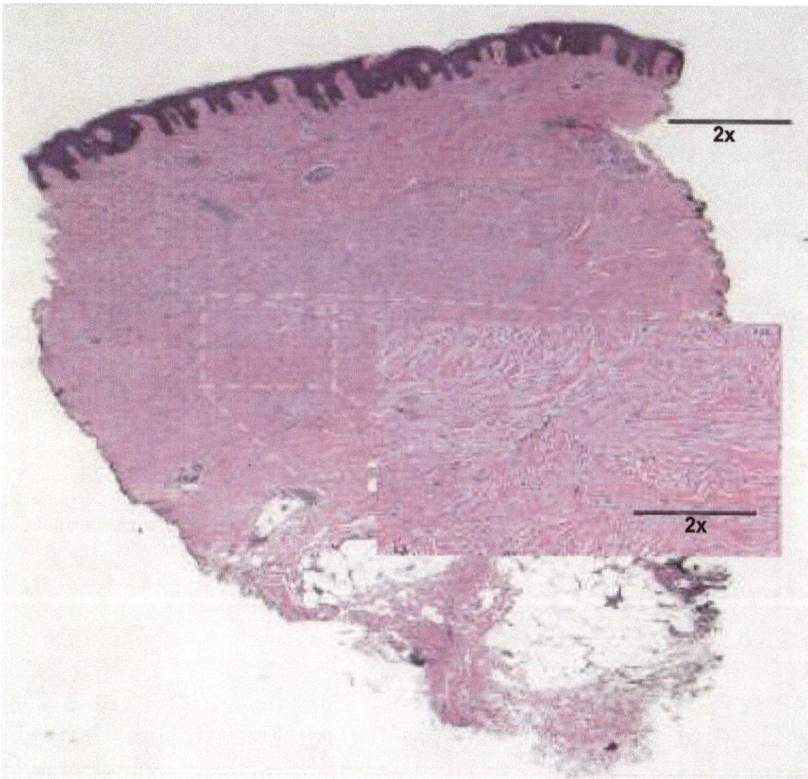

Fig. (8.1). Keloidal morphea. Histologic sections show an acanthotic epidermis with overlying basilar hyperpigmentation. Within the dermis there is a proliferation of myofibroblasts and thickened collagen bundles. There is a lack of vertically oriented blood vessels and a lack of atrophy of the overlying epidermis speaking against that of a keloid or scar. At low power (2x) biopsy has a barrel-shaped appearance. The dermal component is expansile and extends beyond that of the epidermal component. [Image credit: Kassira S, Jaleel T, Pavlidakey P, Sami N. Keloidal Scleroderma: Case Report and Review. Case Rep Dermatol Med. 2015;2015:635481.].

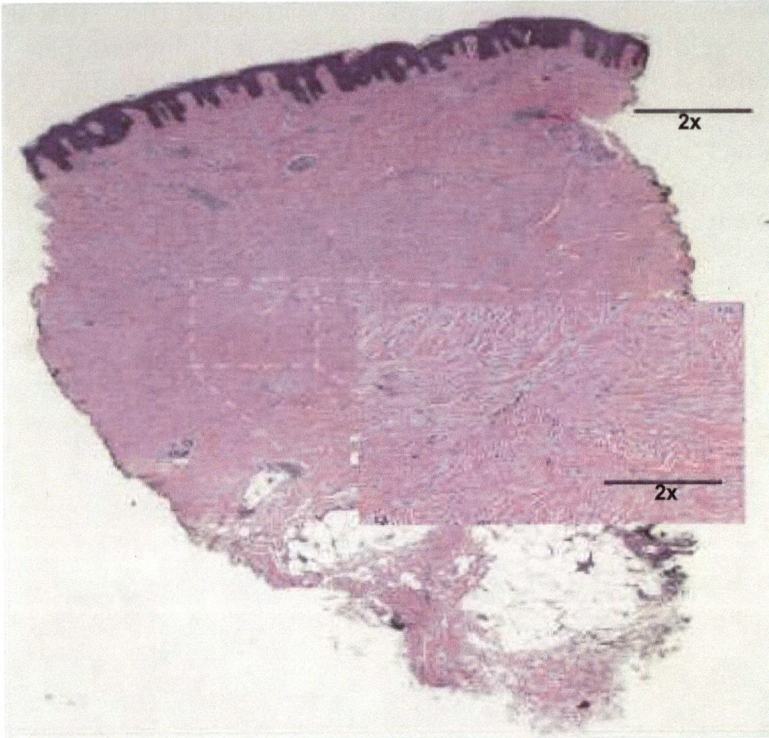

Fig. (8.2). Keloidal morphea. A tissue elastic stain shows preserved elastic fibers within areas of morphea. In keloid, these elastic fibres are typically absent, thus supporting the diagnosis of keloidal morphea and not that of a true keloid. [Image credit: Kassira S, Jaleel T, Pavlidakey P, Sami N. Keloidal Scleroderma: Case Report and Review. Case Rep Dermatol Med. 2015;2015:635481.].

Connective Tissue Nevi

Connective tissue nevi can also resemble morphea from which it can be differentiated by histopathology. They may be hereditary or sporadic and may be associated with certain syndromes. They are made up of extracellular collagen tissue and products of fibroblasts, such as collagen, elastin, and proteoglycans. Clinically, connective tissue nevi are seen as multiple skin-colored or yellowish-thickened papules and plaques. On histopathology, connective tissue nevi show thickened, abundant collagen bundles with or without associated increases in elastic tissue.

Sclerotic/Atrophic Stages

In the sclerotic stage, plaques develop sclerosis which is usually more evident in the centre giving an ivory-white color appearance. This central sclerosis may heal with hypo- or hyperpigmented atrophic stage. Thus practically, any dermatoses which are associated with cutaneous sclerosis can qualify as a differential diagnosis for this stage of morphea.

Idiopathic Atrophoderma of Pasini and Pierini

(IAPP) is a form of dermal atrophy that presents as hyperpigmented, non-indurated patches. Lesions have a classical cliff-drop border with a slightly depressed centre and an abrupt edge, and are usually located on the backs of adolescents or young adults. IAPP as compared to morphea characteristically lacks sclerosis and may present as multiple atrophic lesions that may coalesce over a period of time. There may be a moth-eaten appearance that is not consistent with morphea. The detailed description of IAPP and its differences from morphea have been discussed in chapter 15.

Lipodermatosclerosis (LDS)

Lipodermatosclerosis (LDS) is sclerosing panniculitis characterised by subcutaneous fibrosis and hardening of the skin of lower limbs. It usually results from venous insufficiency and is commonly seen in middle-aged women. In acute stages, it mimics cellulitis or morphea and may be seen as a localized single plaque with induration, edema, pain, and feeling of swelling or heaviness in lower limbs. In the chronic stage, a characteristic inverted champagne bottle appearance of lower limbs is seen. Histopathological examination reveals adipocyte necrosis, pseudo cyst and lipogranuloma formation [10].

Dermatofibrosarcoma Protuberans (DFSP)

Dermatofibrosarcoma protuberans (DFSP) is a malignant mesenchymal tumor of the dermis. Clinically, it is characterised by painless indurated plaque and/or nodule that feels rubbery or firm to touch and is fixed to the underlying skin. In its early stage, DFSP may be non-protuberant and may resemble morphea. Also one of its subtypes is atrophic or morphea-like DFSP. Clinically, it resembles morphea, but is locally infiltrative like the classical variant. There are cases where non-protuberant DFSP has been diagnosed as morphea for as long as 20 years [11].

Radiation Fibrosis Syndrome (RFS)

Radiation fibrosis syndrome (RFS) is the fibrosis of any tissue within the radiation field, including skin, nerves, muscles, blood vessels, bones, tendons, ligaments, or internal organs like the heart or lungs. RFS is characterized by scarring and hardening of tissue inside the body or on the skin and has to be differentiated from a true radiation-induced morphea (RIM) that occurs in only 2 per thousand patients. Radiation-induced morphea is a rare and chronically progressive localized scleroderma after radiation [12].

Reflex Sympathetic Dystrophy (RSD)

Morphea may sometimes be misdiagnosed as RSD, however, the absence of pain, swelling, and vasomotor instability in a patient with the involvement of only a small part of the extremity, should alert clinicians to the diagnosis of linear morphea instead of RSD, which if not treated, may lead to contractures [13]. An early biopsy can help to diagnose morphea in such cases.

Scleromyxedema (SCX)

Scleromyxedema (SCX) is characterized by the deposition of mucin mostly in the skin and sometimes, in the internal organs. Cutaneous mucinosis and fibrosis in SCX are seen on the face, arms, and hands and less commonly over the legs and trunk. SCX is associated with an underlying gammopathy, so these patients require appropriate testing by serum and urine electrophoresis [14]. In contrast to morphea, skin can be pinched and moved over the subcutis as mucin deposition is mainly in the papillary dermis.

Diabetic Cheiroarthropathy

Diabetic cheiroarthropathy is clinically seen as thick, tight, waxy skin resembling systemic sclerosis with the inability to fully flex or extend the fingers [15]. It is caused by increased glycosylation of collagen in the skin and periarticular tissue, decreased collagen degradation, and diabetic microangiopathy.

Carcinoid Syndrome

Carcinoid syndrome may be caused due to metastatic tumours and may clinically present as scleroderma-like lesions on the skin. The exact mechanism of fibrosis is unknown, however, it involves capillary permeability and tissue edema induced by serotonin or other active tumor metabolites. Carcinoid-associated scleroderma can be differentiated from scleroderma as it involves lower limbs more commonly. There is an absence of acral lesions and Raynaud's phenomenon, so lesions tend to resemble morphea more than systemic sclerosis. Associated endocardial fibrosis is usually seen in this entity.

Porphyria Cutanea Tarda (PCT)

Porphyria cutanea tarda (PCT) is clinically characterised by photosensitivity due to porphyrins. It involves photoexposed sites including the face, hands and forearms. Early lesions show fluid-filled blisters progressing to crusted erosions that heal slowly over time. Post-inflammatory pigmentation, milia formation and atrophic scarring lead to a sclerodermoid appearance. Lesions on the face, arms and forearms can be differentiated from morphea by history, increased sensitivity to the sun, evolution of the lesions and laboratory investigations [16].

Nephrogenic Systemic Fibrosis (NSF)

Nephrogenic systemic fibrosis (NSF) is caused by exposure to gadolinium-based contrast agents. Skin lesions are characterised by bound down and shiny plaques like morphea profundus leading to contracture formation. Unlike morphea, skin changes are bilateral and symmetrical. Moreover, NSF has systemic features associated with it [17]. Patients may present with disabling pain in the joints. Fibrosis is usually progressive with deposits in the muscles, lungs, esophagus and the heart causing damage to these organs as well.

Pretibial Myxedema

Pretibial myxedema is a type of diffuse mucinosis and may present as bilateral, firm, non-pitting, asymmetrical plaques or nodules which coalesce to form scaly, thickened and hardened skin areas. Lesions have a peaud'orange (orange peel) appearance. It is differentiated from morphea by the presence of underlying thyroid dysfunction, TSH-R antibodies and the typical site of involvement (pretibial areas or dorsum of the feet) [18]. Histopathology shows adipocyte necrosis, pseudo cyst formation and lipogranuloma formation.

Morpheaform Basal Cell Carcinoma

Morpheaform basal cell carcinoma is a histopathological diagnosis. It is typically found in mid-facial sites with a waxy, scar-like plaque with indistinct borders. Clinically, it may be confused with morphea but has a wide and deep subclinical extension with perineural spread along with other features of BCC [19].

Scleredema

Scleredema is a fibromucinous connective-tissue disorder associated with antecedent infections, diabetes, or plasma cell dyscrasias. It is characterized clinically by woody hard induration of the skin of the upper part of the body that results from excessive mucin deposition between thickened collagen bundles in the dermis. As compared to scleroderma, hands, and feet are typically spared in scleredema, hence it may mimic morphea more than systemic sclerosis [20].

Anetoderma

Anetoderma is an idiopathic atrophy of skin clinically seen as round, soft, thin, wrinkled skin due to the disruption of underlying dermal connective tissue. It may be primary or secondary to some underlying disorders. This dermal atrophic process is easily differentiated by palpation and by histopathological studies. The skin looks normal on routine H&E stains but show minimal or no elastic fibres with special stains. Additionally, on histopathology, it typically shows sparse lymphocytic inflammatory cell infiltrate.

Stiff Skin Syndrome

Stiff skin syndrome is characterized by an early, insidious onset of stony-hard skin, often with associated a contracture-like joint restriction, hypertrichosis, and postural and thoracic wall abnormalities [21]. It is characterised by the absence of visceral or muscle involvement. There are no micro-vascular or immunological changes associated with this disorder when compared with connective tissue disorders.

Restrictive Dermopathy

Restrictive dermopathy is an autosomal recessive fatal type of laminopathy with skin manifestations in the form of rigid, translucent, and tightly adherent skin. Skin erosions at flexural areas, superficial vessels, typical dysmorphism and generalised joint disorders are features of the disease. Respiratory distress secondary to the tight chest wall is noted at birth. On histopathology, the dermis is flat with appendageal hypoplasia, dense collagen bundles, and a paucity of elastic fibres.

DIFFERENTIAL DIAGNOSIS ACCORDING TO THE PIGMENTARY CHANGES

Morphea in children can present as nonspecific hypopigmented or hyperpigmented lesions (Table **8.2**).

Table 8.2. Differential diagnosis according to the pigmentary changes.

Hyper / Hypo pigmented patches	Fixed drug eruption
	Macular Lichen planus
	Post-inflammatory hyperpigmentation
	Vitiligo
	Lichen sclerosis

Fixed Drug Eruption (FDE)

Morphea presenting as hyperpigmented patches may mimic FDE. In such cases, a detailed drug history must be elicited. The histopathological examination helps to differentiate between the two conditions.

Macular Lichen Planus

Macular lichen planus retains its typical histopathological characteristics. Loss of appendages and sclerosis of skin are not seen in the macular form of lichen planus.

Vitiligo

Vitiligo is seen as hypopigmented macules and may sometimes be clinically confused with morphea. Appendageal loss and sclerosis of the skin are not seen in vitiligo. Again typical histopathological changes of morphea are not seen in vitiligo.

Lichen Sclerosus

Extragenital lichen sclerosus (white spot disease) presents as white dry plaques that may be found on the inner thigh, buttocks, lower back, abdomen, infra-mammary areas, and axillae. Affected skin is dry, wrinkled, and atrophic resembling cigarette paper. It is clinically confused with guttate and plaque type of morphea. It may also coexist with morphea when it is known as lichen sclerosus / morphea overlap. On dermoscopic examination, lichen sclerosus has typical comedo-like openings and whitish patches, whereas morphea exhibits fibrotic beams [22].

DIFFERENTIAL DIAGNOSIS OF LINEAR MORPHEA

Linear morphea needs to be differentiated from various other disorders (Box **8.2**) that have linear variants.

Box 8.2: Differential diagnosis of linear morphea.
Linear atrophoderma of Moulin
Linear lupus erythematosus panniculitis
Linear melorheostosis

Linear Atrophoderma of Moulin (LAM)

Linear atrophoderma of moulin (LAM) is characterized by a hyperpigmented atrophoderma that follows the blaschkoid lines. However, it lacks the inflammation and induration associated with linear morphea. There are many clinic-histological similarities between LAM, atrophoderma of Pasini and Pierini (APP), and morphea, and whether these represent the same spectrum of disorders or different disorders is still debatable. The differentiating features between LAM, linear morphea and IAPP have been discussed in detail in chapter 16. Readers are suggested to refer to Table **16.5** of chapter 16.

Linear Form of Cutaneous Lupus Erythematosus (CLE)

Linear form of cutaneous lupus erythematosus (CLE) is very rare. According to the literature review, a little over 100 cases of linear CLE have been reported mostly with discoid lupus erythematosus (DLE) (39.2%), followed by lupus erythematosus panniculitis (LEP) (21.6%), lupus erythematosus tumid (LET) (2.9%), sub-acute lupus erythematosus (SCLE) (2%) and bullous lesions of SLE (1%). Most of the cases occur in children and young adults. In most cases, histopathology and sometimes dermoscopy differentiates between the two types of disorders. Linear DLE mainly occurs in children and young adults [23].

Melorheostosis

Melorheostosis is a rare disorder of bones characterised by the hardening of the skin and tissues around the affected bone and the involved skin may be tense, shiny, reddish, swollen, or with prominent veins. Linear melorheostosis may sometimes coexist with linear morphea. X-ray of the bone shows the characteristic "flowing candle-wax pattern" caused by irregular and wavy sclerotic changes [24].

DIFFERENTIAL DIAGNOSIS OF DEEP MORPHEA

Deep morphea or Morphea profundus has to be differentiated from various types of panniculitis and lipodystrophy (Box **8.3**).

Box 8.3: Differential diagnosis of deep morphea.
Panniculitis- subcutaneous, lipoatrophic types
Lipodystrophy

Subcutaneous Panniculitis-like T-cell Lymphoma

Subcutaneous panniculitis-like t-cell lymphoma is a rare form of non-Hodgkin lymphoma. It presents clinically as panniculitis, with erythematous, firm subcutaneous infiltrates and recurrent papulo-nodules which may resemble morphea clinically, however, repeat biopsy with immunohistochemistry of such lesions which were initially thought to be morphea helps to get to the correct diagnosis [25].

Lipoatrophic Panniculitis

Lipoatrophic panniculitis is seen in young children and presents as localised lipoatrophy on extremities. Initially, there are tender erythematous nodules and plaques which enlarge and leave behind circumferential bands of lipoatrophy. It needs to be differentiated from morphea. There is a need for continuous follow-up with repeat biopsies and the use of immunohistological techniques for early diagnosis of these disorders [26]. On histopathology, there are features of lipophagic panniculitis and absence of vasculitis.

Localized Lipodystrophy

Iatrogenic lipodystrophy (following steroid injections) or vaccinations may occur and may mimic morphea profundus. Usually, lipoatrophy caused by steroid injections resolves spontaneously. There are case reports of morphea developing at the sites of injection and vaccination [27]. Physical injury due to injections or immune response against specifically targeted antigens may be the cause of injection-induced and vaccination-induced morphea respectively. The histopathological examination helps to differentiate between the two.

MORPHEA AS DIFFERENTIAL DIAGNOSIS OF SYSTEMIC DISORDERS

The dermatological manifestations of various systemic disorders (Box **8.4**) may clinically mimic morphea.

Box 8.4. Systemic diseases as a differential diagnosis of morphea.
Eosinophilic fasciitis
Eosinophilia-Myalgia Syndrome
Chronic graft versus host disease
Phenylketonuria (PKU)
POEMS syndrome
Primary systemic amyloidosis

Eosinophilic Fasciitis (EF)

The clinical presentation of EF just like morphea evolves through 3 stages-erythematous, edematous and sclerotic stage [28]. It is a close mimicker of morphea with which it may coexist in 25% of the patients. The atrophoderma of Pasini and Pierini and eosinophilic fasciitis are generally viewed as part of the morphea spectrum. Full-thickness skin biopsies containing muscle as well as fascia are prerequisites for the diagnosis of eosinophilic fasciitis.

Eosinophilia-Myalgia Syndrome (EMS)

In later stages of EMS, sclerodermoid changes occur resulting in skin tightening. However, sclerodactyly and Raynaud's phenomenon and nail fold capillaroscopic changes and visceral involvement are absent. Peripheral eosinophilia is seen in EMS and helps to differentiate from close mimics.

Chronic Graft Versus Host Disease

Chronic graft versus host disease primarily involves the skin and may present as discrete morpheaform plaques, lichen sclerosis, diffuse sclerodermoid changes and eosinophilic fasciitis [29]. Morphea like chronic graft versus host disease is characterised histologically by epidermal apoptotic keratinocytes and dermal sclerosis.

Phenylketonuria (PKU)

Skin involvement in PKU includes fair skin and hair, eczema, light sensitivity and scleroderma-like plaques [30]. PKU is an autosomal recessive disorder with a positive urinary ferric chloride test. Hence PKU should be considered as a differential in young children with sclerodermatous changes.

Polyneuropathy, Organomegaly, Endocrinopathy, Monoclonal Gammopathy, and Skin Changes (POEMS) Syndrome

Polyneuropathy, organomegaly, endocrinopathy, monoclonal gammopathy, and skin changes (POEMS) syndrome is a rare multi-systemic disease that occurs in the setting of a plasma cell dyscrasia. Multiple dermatologic changes have been associated with POEMS syndrome [31]. The most common changes include hyperpigmentation, skin thickening, sclerodermoid changes, and hypertrichosis.

Primary Systemic Amyloidosis (PSA)

The most characteristic skin lesion in PSA consists of waxy papules, nodules, or plaques characteristically seen in the eyelids, retro auricular region, neck, or inguinal and anogenital regions. These plaques may coalesce to form large tumefactive lesions. Diffuse infiltrates may resemble infiltrates of scleroderma or myxedema.

DIFFERENTIAL DIAGNOSIS OF MORPHEA DUE TO EXOGENOUS AGENTS

While scleroderma is frequently attributed to the intake of certain drugs, morphea due to exogenous agents such as drugs is rarely reported. Some drugs like cathepsin K inhibitor balicatib are associated with morphea-like lesions with temporal association to the drug and complete remission on stopping the drug [32]. Other causes of drug-induced morphea include bisoprolol, bleomycin, D-penicillamine, pembrolizumab, interferon beta-1a, and ustekinumab [33 - 36]. Few cases of morphea associated with occupational contact with organic solvents have been reported [37].

Box 8.5. Learning Points.
• Morphea is a clinical diagnosis and encompasses a wide range of clinical phenotypes that have different presentations in their different stages, so need to be differentiated from a myriad of conditions that it mimics.
• Generalized morphea may be difficult to differentiate from systemic sclerosis, however internal organ involvement, sclerodactyly, Raynaud's phenomenon, nail fold capillaroscopy and positive antibodies in the later help to distinguish between the two.
• Clinical presentations vary in the different stages in case of circumscribed morphea - viz; early, sclerotic and atrophic stage, so do the differential diagnosis.

cont.....

• Dermatological manifestations in eosinophilic fasciitis, eosinophilia-myalgia syndrome, chronic graft versus host disease, phenylketonuria (PKU), POEMS syndrome, primary systemic amyloidosis may mimic morphea and need to be differentiated.
• Morphea needs to be differentiated from certain drug and toxin induced skin disorders.

REFERENCES

[1]   Tuffanelli DL. Localized scleroderma. Semin Cutan Med Surg 1998; 17(1): 27-33.
        [http://dx.doi.org/10.1016/S1085-5629(98)80059-X] [PMID: 9512104]

[2]   Nijhawan RI, Bard S, Blyumin M, Smidt AC, Chamlin SL, Connelly EA. Early localized morphea mimicking an acquired port-wine stain. J Am Acad Dermatol 2011; 64(4): 779-82.
        [http://dx.doi.org/10.1016/j.jaad.2009.10.017] [PMID: 20850196]

[3]   Basir HRG, Alirezaei P, Rezanejad A, Daneshyar S. Early morphea simulating patch-stage mycosis fungoides in two cases. Dermatol Rep 2018; 10(1): 7471.
        [PMID: 29760873]

[4]   Cohen PR. Subcutaneous Sweet's syndrome: A variant of acute febrile neutrophilic dermatosis that is included in the histopathologic differential diagnosis of neutrophilic panniculitis. J Am Acad Dermatol 2005; 52(5): 927-8.
        [http://dx.doi.org/10.1016/j.jaad.2005.03.001] [PMID: 15858502]

[5]   Khanna U, North JP. Patch-type granuloma annulare: An institution-based study of 23 cases. J Cutan Pathol 2020; 47(9): 785-93.
        [http://dx.doi.org/10.1111/cup.13707] [PMID: 32279342]

[6]   Rose C, Holl-Ulrich K. Granulomatöses Reaktionsmuster in der Haut. Hautarzt 2017; 68(7): 553-9.
        [http://dx.doi.org/10.1007/s00105-017-4004-6] [PMID: 28608042]

[7]   Vasudevan B, Chatterjee M. Lyme borreliosis and skin. Indian J Dermatol 2013; 58(3): 167-74.
        [http://dx.doi.org/10.4103/0019-5154.110822] [PMID: 23723463]

[8]   Abtahi-Naeini B, Pourazizi M, Mokhtari F. Erythema nodosum migrans successfully treated with indomethacin: A rare entity. Adv Biomed Res 2014; 3(1): 264.
        [http://dx.doi.org/10.4103/2277-9175.148243] [PMID: 25625103]

[9]   Annessi G, Paradisi M, Angelo C, Perez M, Puddu P, Girolomoni G. Annular lichenoid dermatitis of youth. J Am Acad Dermatol 2003; 49(6): 1029-36.
        [http://dx.doi.org/10.1016/S0190-9622(03)02147-9] [PMID: 14639381]

[10]   Miteva M, Romanelli P, Kirsner RS. Lipodermatosclerosis. Dermatol Ther 2010; 23(4): 375-88.
        [http://dx.doi.org/10.1111/j.1529-8019.2010.01338.x] [PMID: 20666825]

[11]   Hanabusa M, Kamo R, Harada T, Ishii M. Dermatofibrosarcoma protuberans with atrophic appearance at early stage of the tumor. J Dermatol 2007; 34(5): 336-9.
        [http://dx.doi.org/10.1111/j.1346-8138.2007.00283.x] [PMID: 17408444]

[12]   Spalek M, Jonska-Gmyrek J, Gałecki J. Radiation-induced morphea: A literature review. J Eur Acad Dermatol Venereol 2015; 29(2): 197-202.
        [http://dx.doi.org/10.1111/jdv.12704] [PMID: 25174551]

[13]   Thng TG, Wong KY. A case of linear morphoea mistaken for reflex sympathetic dystrophy. Singapore Med J 2013; 54(3): e50-2.
        [http://dx.doi.org/10.11622/smedj.2013057] [PMID: 23546034]

[14]   Endo J, Strickland N, Grewal S, *et al.* Correspondence: The association between morphea profunda and monoclonal gammopathy: A case series. Dermatol Online J 2016; 22(3): 13030/qt857261f5.

[15]   Aleppo G, Kanapka LG, Foster NC, *et al.* T1D Exchange Clinic Network. Cheiroarthropathy: A common disorder in patients in the t1d exchange. Endocr Pract 2019; 25(2): 138-43.

[http://dx.doi.org/10.4158/EP-2018-0346] [PMID: 30383489]

[16]	Zemtsov R, Zemtsov A. Porphyria cutanea tarda presenting as scleroderma. Cutis 2010; 85(4): 203-5.
[PMID: 20486461]

[17]	Lunyera J, Mohottige D, Alexopoulos AS, *et al.* Risk for nephrogenic systemic fibrosis after exposure to newer gadolinium agents. Ann Intern Med 2020; 173(2): 110-9.
[http://dx.doi.org/10.7326/M20-0299] [PMID: 32568573]

[18]	Fatourechi V, Pajouhi M, Fransway AF. Dermopathy of Graves disease (pretibial myxedema). Review of 150 cases. Medicine 1994; 73(1): 1-7.
[http://dx.doi.org/10.1097/00005792-199401000-00001] [PMID: 8309359]

[19]	East E, Fullen DR, Arps D, *et al.* Morpheaform Basal Cell Carcinomas With Areas of Predominantly Single-Cell Pattern of Infiltration: Diagnostic Utility of p63 and Cytokeratin. Am J Dermatopathol 2016; 38(10): 744-50.
[http://dx.doi.org/10.1097/DAD.0000000000000541] [PMID: 27043336]

[20]	Venturi M, Damevska K, Ferreli C, *et al.* Scleredema of Buschke associated with lichen sclerosus: Three cases. Indian J Dermatol Venereol Leprol 2020; 86(3): 272-7.
[http://dx.doi.org/10.4103/ijdvl.IJDVL_288_17] [PMID: 30289118]

[21]	Liu T, McCalmont TH, Frieden IJ, Williams ML, Connolly MK, Gilliam AE. The stiff skin syndrome: case series, differential diagnosis of the stiff skin phenotype, and review of the literature. Arch Dermatol 2008; 144(10): 1351-9.
[http://dx.doi.org/10.1001/archderm.144.10.1351] [PMID: 18936399]

[22]	Moinzadeh P, Kreuter A, Krieg T, Hunzelmann N. Morphea/lokalisierte Sklerodermie und extragenitaler Lichen sclerosus. Hautarzt 2018; 69(11): 892-900.
[http://dx.doi.org/10.1007/s00105-018-4266-7] [PMID: 30255259]

[23]	Khelifa E, Masouye I, Pham HC, Parmentier L, Borradori L. Linear sclerodermic lupus erythematosus, a distinct variant of linear morphea and chronic cutaneous lupus erythematous. Int J Dermatol 2011; 50(12): 1491-5.
[http://dx.doi.org/10.1111/j.1365-4632.2011.04936.x] [PMID: 22097995]

[24]	Shivanand G, Srivastava DN. Melorheostosis with scleroderma. Clin Imaging 2004; 28(3): 214-5.
[http://dx.doi.org/10.1016/S0899-7071(03)00149-9] [PMID: 15158228]

[25]	Troskot N, Lugović L, Situm M, Vucić M. From circumscribed scleroderma (morphea) to subcutaneous panniculitis-like T-cell lymphoma: case report. Acta Dermatovenerol Croat 2004; 12(4): 289-93.
[PMID: 15588564]

[26]	Weryńska-Kalemba M, Kalemba M, Filipowska-Grońska A, Lorenc A, Jarząb J, Bożek A. A case of lipoatrophic panniculitis in a 2-year-old boy. Postepy Dermatol Alergol 2016; 2(2): 155-6.
[http://dx.doi.org/10.5114/ada.2016.59165] [PMID: 27279828]

[27]	Liao Y-H, Lo Y, Jee S-H. Concomitant development of morphea and lipoatrophy after local corticosteroid injection. Zhonghua Pifuke Yixue Zazhi 2020; 38(2): 119-20.
[http://dx.doi.org/10.4103/ds.ds_44_19]

[28]	Kroft EBM, de Jong EMGJ, Evers AWM. Physical burden of symptoms in patients with localized scleroderma and eosinophilic fasciitis. Arch Dermatol 2008; 144(10): 1394-5.
[http://dx.doi.org/10.1001/archderm.144.10.1394] [PMID: 18936410]

[29]	White JML, Creamer D, du Vivier AWP, *et al.* Sclerodermatous graft-versus-host disease: clinical spectrum and therapeutic challenges. Br J Dermatol 2007; 156(5): 1032-8.
[http://dx.doi.org/10.1111/j.1365-2133.2007.07827.x] [PMID: 17419693]

[30]	Vockley J, Andersson HC, Antshel KM, *et al.* American College of Medical Genetics and Genomics Therapeutics Committee. Phenylalanine hydroxylase deficiency: diagnosis and management guideline. Genet Med 2014; 16(2): 188-200.

[http://dx.doi.org/10.1038/gim.2013.157] [PMID: 24385074]

[31]   Li Y, Valent J, Soltanzadeh P, Thakore N, Katirji B. Diagnostic challenges in POEMS syndrome presenting with polyneuropathy: A case series. J Neurol Sci 2017; 378: 170-4.
[http://dx.doi.org/10.1016/j.jns.2017.05.019] [PMID: 28566158]

[32]   Peroni A, Zini A, Braga V, Colato C, Adami S, Girolomoni G. Drug-induced morphea: Report of a case induced by balicatib and review of the literature. J Am Acad Dermatol 2008; 59(1): 125-9.
[http://dx.doi.org/10.1016/j.jaad.2008.03.009] [PMID: 18410981]

[33]   Fett N, Werth VP. Update on morphea. J Am Acad Dermatol 2011; 64(2): 217-28.
[http://dx.doi.org/10.1016/j.jaad.2010.05.045] [PMID: 21238823]

[34]   Herrscher H, Tomasic G, Castro Gordon A. Generalised morphea induced by pembrolizumab. Eur J Cancer 2019; 116: 178-81.
[http://dx.doi.org/10.1016/j.ejca.2019.05.018] [PMID: 31202088]

[35]   Peterson E, Steuer A, Franco L, Nolan MA, Lo Sicco K, Franks AG. Morphoea induced by treatment with interferon beta-1a. Br J Dermatol 2020; 182(1): 244-6.
[PMID: 31323114]

[36]   Steuer AB, Peterson E, Lo Sicco K, Franks AG Jr. Morphea in a patient undergoing treatment with ustekinumab. JAAD Case Rep 2019; 5(7): 590-2.
[http://dx.doi.org/10.1016/j.jdcr.2019.05.008] [PMID: 31312709]

[37]   Hanami Y, Ohtsuka M, Yamamoto T. Paraneoplastic eosinophilic fasciitis with generalized morphea and vitiligo in a patient working with organic solvents. J Dermatol 2016; 43(1): 67-8.
[http://dx.doi.org/10.1111/1346-8138.13174] [PMID: 26507670]

CHAPTER 9

Assessment of Disease Severity

Anju George[1,*]

[1] *Department of Dermatology, Christian Medical College, Vellore, Tamil Nadu, India*

Chapter Synopsis.
• As the validation of new outcome measures in morphea are becoming available, however; a good histopathological correlation may provide additional information regarding disease activity and the depth of involvement. Thus, the role of skin biopsy in morphea can't be ignored.
• Several scoring tools have been validated in morphea to elucidate the clinical assessment. This will help in determining the appropriate time for treatment, especially systemic immunosuppressive therapy.
• Infrared thermography (IT) is a non-invasive technique that detects infrared radiation. It provides an image of the temperature distribution across the body surface and has been shown to be of value in the detection of active lesions with high sensitivity (92%).
• Active morphea is universally inflammatory. Features that suggest activity include new onset lesions, peripheral extension of older lesions, erythema and induration, localized warmth, pruritus and lilac ring surrounding the lesions.
• A cutometer measures skin elasticity and relaxation. The measurement is dependent upon anatomic site, age, sex, and edema. The probe measures the rate at which it is able to pull skin in and the rate at which the skin returns to baseline.
• Durometer is a device to measure skin hardness. The measurement is dependent on patient's sex, age, edema and location. The durometer measurements have low inter- and intra-observer variability.
• Cone beam computed tomography (CBCT) is used in linear morphea of the face (especially oral mucosal morphea). The CBCT scanner uses a 2D detector and a cone-shaped X-ray beam which scans the affected region providing both 2D and 3D images. It is cost effective, fast when compared to MRI, and the radiation dose is relatively less than a routine CT.

Keywords: Cone beam computed tomography, Clinical activity, Colour doppler, Cutometer, Durometer, Elasticity, Hardening, High-frequency ultrasound, Infrared thermography, Laser doppler flowmetry, Localized scleroderma.

---

[*] **Corresponding author Anju George:** Department of Dermatology, Christian Medical College, Vellore, Tamil Nadu, India; E-mail: dranjugeo@gmail.com

Tasleem Arif (Ed.)

Localized scleroderma cutaneous assessment tool, Localized scleroderma skin severity index, Localized scleroderma skin damage index, Morphea, Outcome measures, Physician global assessment, Skin scoring tools, Skin thickness, Surface area measurement.

INTRODUCTION

Morphea is an inflammatory skin disorder that is characterised by excessive collagen deposition in the skin, dermis, and/or subcutaneous tissue, leading to skin thickening and hardening, often extending to the fascia, muscles, and even bone. This can result in potential functional and cosmetic sequelae including dyspigmentation, facial deformities, contractures, impaired joint mobility and deformities. In children, this can cause serious growth restrictions of the affected area [1, 2]. The disease may be relatively mild and the clinical presentation can vary from isolated superficial skin lesions to multiple plaques with a deeper component. The pleomorphic presentations can result in numerous subtypes/variants: plaque morphea, linear morphea, bullous morphea, deep morphea, and generalized morphea; also, eosinophilic fasciitis, morphea profunda and pansclerotic morphea of children. The clinical course of morphea may be static or progressive to skin thickening or atrophy [3].

Although the validation of new outcome measures in morphea is valuable, a good histopathological correlation may provide additional information regarding the depth of involvement and activity (inflammation) in cases where the clinical examination is inconclusive and ultrasound or magnetic resonance imaging (MRI) is not readily available [4]. Thus a biopsy in morphea not alone helps in the diagnosis but also in assessment.

It is important to assess the disease severity in a patient with morphea to decide on the appropriate line of management, as the condition carries a huge impact on the quality of life of the affected individual and their families. Morphea is more commonly reported in children than in adults and extracutaneous manifestations are also not rare. In early morphea, the lesions are erythematous, swollen and warmer than the surrounding skin. Gradually the central part of the lesion appears porcelain white with a surrounding lilac ring. In later stages as fibrosis and sclerosis ensue, the lesions are atrophic and hypo- or hyperpigmented, while their temperature is close to that of the surrounding skin [5]. A proper history and clinical examination will give the initial clue in staging the phase of the disease. Several scoring tools have been validated to elucidate the clinical assessment which will help in determining the appropriate time for treatment, especially systemic immunosuppressive therapy.

The commonly used skin scoring tools include the LoSCAT (Localized Scleroderma Cutaneous Assessment Tool) which is a scoring system that includes a Skin Severity Index (LoSSI) and a Skin Damage Index (LoSDI). Although this method does not evaluate the real size of the lesions, it can be performed by physicians in daily practice without the need for special equipment.

Though tried in few studies, the cutometer which measures the cutaneous elasticity, and the durometer which measures the skin's hardness, have their limitations. Infrared rmography (IT) is a non-invasive technique that detects infrared radiation and provides an image of the temperature distribution across the body surface. It has been shown to be of value in the detection of active lesions with high sensitivity (92%) but moderate specificity (68%). High-frequency ultrasound can detect several abnormalities such as increased blood flow related to inflammation as well as increased echogenicity due to fibrosis and loss of subcutaneous fat. The main limits of this tool are its operator dependency and the lack of standardisation [6]. Other methods such as laser Doppler flowmetry and cone beam tomography need better validation to be used as an outcome measuring tool in morphea.

CLINICAL AND HISTOLOGICAL ASSESSMENT OF DISEASE ACTIVITY

The clinical manifestations of morphea are dependent on the subtype, depth of involvement and phase of progression of the lesions. Morphea is characterised by an early or active phase and a late fibrotic phase. A thorough physical examination helps in the assessment of disease activity. Correctly identifying and quantifying disease activity and damage in different subtypes of morphea is essential for its appropriate management [2].

Active Morphea

Active lesions are important to identify as they are highly treatment responsive. Active morphea is universally inflammatory and features suggesting activity include new onset lesions, a peripheral extension of older lesions, erythema and induration, localized warmth, pruritus, and a lilac ring surrounding the lesions [7, 8]. Deep morphea lesions are poorly circumscribed tethered erythematous plaques, with varying amounts of edema/induration, and may not always have surface changes. Linear depressions (groove sign) may be present. Functional impairment and pain also suggest deep involvement. When there is an overlap of sclerotic lesions, the peripheral erythema in such lesions represents activity, while the deeply sclerotic skin represents damage [9].

Inactive Stage

As the inflammation subsides, lesions develop peripheral hyperpigmentation with central sclerosis and a yellow-white color. Sclerosis is followed by the atrophic stage which is characterised by shiny skin, lack of hair growth, prominent underlying vessels, and often a cliff-drop deformity. When lesions extend to the subcutaneous fat, a finely wrinkled, "cobblestone" appearance is noted. The clinical assessment has been summarised in Table **9.1**. Dermoscopy can help in distinguishing erythema from telangiectasia in the inactive stage [9].

Table 9.1. Clinical assessment of disease activity.

Active Lesion	Inactive Lesion
New onset lesions	Peripheral hyperpigmentation
Peripheral extension of older lesions	Central sclerosis
Lilac ring in the periphery	Yellow white colour
Localized warmth	**Atrophic Lesion**
Erythema	Shiny skin
Induration	Lack of hair growth
Pruritus, pain and functional impairment	Prominent underlying vessels
Linear depressions (groove sign)	Cliff-drop deformity and cobblestone appearance

Histological Features of Disease Activity

Early inflammatory skin lesions of morphea are characterized by thickened collagen bundles within the reticular dermis that run parallel to the skin surface along with dense inflammatory infiltrates between the collagen bundles in a peri appendageal/ perivascular pattern. The predominant cells are lymphocytes but plasma cells, histiocytes and eosinophilic granulocytes might be present as well. Late fibrotic lesions usually contain collagen fibres that are tightly packed and are highly eosinophilic. Sweat glands are atrophic or absent. Collagen may replace fat cells in the subcutaneous tissue [10].

Wortsman *et al.* have defined histologic criteria for the assessment of morphea activity in their study as follows [3]:

1. Active lesion

• Inflammatory cellular infiltrates (lymphocytes, histiocytes, plasma cells, or a combination of these).

• Collagen deposition.

2. Inactive lesion

• Increased collagen deposits without inflammatory infiltrates.

3. Atrophic lesion

• Decreased thickness of all cutaneous layers with the disappearance of skin appendages.
• Collagen deposits are arranged into actual bundles (sclerosis).

The presence of a bottom-heavy pattern of sclerosis has been associated with the presence of symptoms like pain (especially perineural location), tightness, and functional impairment in patients with all subtypes of morphea, while patients with top-heavy sclerosis patterns have less frequent symptoms. Hence the pattern of sclerosis and not the clinical subtype alone, predicts the clinical severity of morphea. This also explains the clinical heterogeneity of morphea which ranges from mild cosmetic impairment to extreme pain and disability even within the same subtype. The depth of sclerosis and inflammation definitely helps in the treatment of morphea in that more superficial lesions may respond to skin-directed therapy (phototherapy), while bottom-heavy lesions should be treated systemically or intralesionally [4, 11].

Risk Factors for Recurrence of Disease

Few studies have evaluated the risk factors for recurrence in morphea. Mertens *et al.* studied the risk factors for recurrence in both pediatric and adult-onset disease (Box **9.1**). The chances for recurrence were more in juvenile-onset disease than in adult-onset. Patients with linear morphea of the limbs alone or as part of a mixed subtype of morphea, more frequently develop disease recurrences, independent of the age of disease onset. Morphea en plaque (circumscribed morphea) and generalized morphea, the two most frequently observed subtypes in the adult-onset group, had recurrence rates of 16% and 25% in their study, respectively. The two subtypes with the lowest recurrence rates were en coup de sabre (7%) and atrophoderma (6%) [8].

Box 9.1: Risk factors for disease recurrence.
Juvenile population > adults
Linear morphea of limbs alone or as mixed subtype
Morphea en plaque (16%)
Generalised morphea (25%)
Positive auto antibodies
Elevated cytokines CXCL9 and CXCL10

Laboratory Markers of Disease Severity/ Activity

No definite biomarkers are yet validated to ascertain the activity or severity of morphea. Autoantibody testing in morphea patients is recommended only when signs or symptoms of other autoimmune conditions are present. Although antinuclear, anti-histone, and anti-single stranded DNA antibodies have been associated with morphea severity, they do not correlate with activity and have limited utility due to their infrequency. Recent studies have shown lesional morphea skin to be a source of elevated circulating cytokines CXCL9 and CXCL10, which in the future could be potential markers reflective of disease activity [9, 12, 13].

SKIN SCORING TOOLS

The outcome measuring scores were designed so as to have objective measures of both disease activity and disease damage which can accurately measure the efficacy of therapeutic interventions.

Localized Scleroderma Cutaneous Assessment Tool (LoSCAT)

The 'modified localized scleroderma skin severity index' (mLoSSI) which was introduced in 2009, was the first validated skin score for LS. This score includes parameters such as erythema, skin thickness and development of new skin lesions or lesional extension in 18 anatomical regions. The same group of researchers later introduced a score for skin damage in LS, called 'localized scleroderma skin damage index' (LoSDI). Consequently, it was recommended to combine the LoSSI, LoSDI and the Physician's Global Assessment (PGA) to measure both activity and damage in LS.

The Localized Scleroderma Clinical and Ultrasound Study Group (LOCUS) combined the above together to form the 'localized scleroderma cutaneous assessment tool or the LoSCAT, which currently provides the most adequate assessment in morphea [10]. This was developed and validated by Arkachaisri *et al.* based on clinical examination, and can be easily used in any clinical setting. The LoSCAT, which was initially designed for juvenile LS is the only score that has specific parameters for the assessment of morphea activity (LoSSI) and damage (LoSDI), and has undergone extensive validation studies [5, 11].

The LoSSI (Table **9.2**) is calculated by summing 4 domain scores based on the extent (surface area: enlargement of existing lesions and new lesion development) and intensity (erythema and skin thickness) of the disease in 18 cutaneous surface anatomic sites (head, neck, chest, abdomen, upper back, lower back, right and left — arms, forearms, hands/fingers, buttocks/thighs, legs and feet) [14].

Table 9.2. LoSSI – assessment of morphea activity.

SURFACE AREA SCORE The extent of surface area involvement within each anatomic site is scored from 0 to 3. This is obtained by simple "eyeball" estimation of the whole circumference of the given limbs or entire surface of the anatomic sites of the trunk.	0 = no involvement; 1 = ≤ 1/3, 2 = > 1/3–2/3 3 = > 2/3–3/3 of surface area of site affected.
ERYTHEMA The degree of erythema at the edge of a lesion is scored 0–3	0 = normal or postinflammatory hyper/hypopigmentation 1 = slight erythema/pink 2 = red/clearly erythema 3 = violaceous/marked erythema
SKIN THICKNESS SCORE This is determined at the edge of a lesion and compared to the unaffected contralateral, or nearby ipsilateral skin if symmetrical lesions are present	0 = normal 1 = mild increase in thickness 2 = moderate increase in thickness, difficult to move skin 3 = severe thickness, unable to move skin.
NEW-LESION/LESION EXTENSION A new lesion and/or enlargement of an existing lesion within the past month is scored 3	Score- 3

In mLoSSI, the surface area parameter has been omitted as surface area estimates resulted in poor inter- and intrarater reliability and poor sensitivity to change [15]. This is more reliable in detecting disease activity [16].

Arif T and Sami M have described an innovative technique to calculate the surface area in vitiligo lesions prior to surgery which can also be utilised in measuring the surface area of morphea lesions. The technique requires a graph paper (or an ECG paper), a thin transparent plastic film and a marking pen. Using the marking pen, the boundaries of the lesion are marked after placing the transparent film over the affected area. Place this marked film over the graph paper and secure the edges so that it doesn't slip. Beneath the marked area, count the number of complete large squares. At a few places, the marked area involves half, less than half, or more than half of large squares. In such areas, count the number of small squares. The total area in cm² is given by the following formula:

Area (in cm²) = No. of complete big squares + 1/100 X No. of small squares.

Thus, depending on the number of lesions, individual lesional scores can be combined to give the total surface area affected [17]. This technique is simple, cost-effective and can even be incorporated in the LoSSI.

Three cutaneous damage domains are summated to obtain the LoSDI, as follows (Table **9.3**) [18]:

Table 9.3. LoSDI – Assessment of skin damage in morphea.

DERMAL ATROPHY	0= normal skin 1= mild skin atrophy, *i.e.* shiny skin 2= moderate atrophy, *i.e.* visible blood vessels or mild 'cliff-drop' sign 3= severe skin atrophy, *i.e.* obvious 'cliff-drop' sign
SUBCUTANEOUS ATROPHY	0= normal subcutaneous thickness 1= flattening or 1/3 fat loss 2= obvious concave surface or 1/3 – 2/3 fat loss 3= severe subcutaneous fat loss (>2/3 loss).
DYSPIGMENTATION	0= normal skin pigment 1= mild 2= moderate 3=severe dyspigmentation.

LoSCAT does not include the evaluation of extracutaneous manifestations, such as bone deformities, joint contractures, central nervous system involvement etc. and has some limitations also in detecting changes in deeper layers [16].

Physician's Global Assessment of Disease Activity (PGA-A) and Damage (PGA-D)

Both PGA-A and PGA-D are assessed using a 100mm visual analog scale, being "not active" at the 0 point and "very active" at the 100 point [14]. In the assessment of PGA-A, only those clinical variables with considerable importance in the determination of disease activity (erythema, enlargement of pre-existing lesion, development of new lesions), along with elevated erythrocyte sedimentation rate and C-reactive protein, are included. Studies have shown that PGA-A is a feasible alternative to ultrasound and biopsy for the determination of activity and response to therapy.

The following clinical variables are considered in the assessment of PGA-D: facial atrophy, skeletal muscle atrophy, physical disability, joint contracture, bone atrophy, cataract or glaucoma, limb length discrepancy, central nervous system symptoms (seizures), abnormal brain MRI, psychosocial impairment, dermal atrophy, subcutaneous atrophy, and dyspigmentation. Successful treatment will stabilize the score over time as the PGA-D score measures damage, which is irreversible. However, this is an objective method and does not evaluate the real size or extent of lesions [11].

DIET SCORE

The DIET score, an acronym that stands for Dyspigmentation, Induration, Erythema and Telangiectasia, was previously utilised in many studies and clinical trials. Each parameter is rated on a scale of 0 (none) to 3 (severe). The advantage of this scoring tool is that it includes a wider range of skin manifestations present in different phases of morphea. However, the exact extension of the lesions and the body surface area are not included. Besides, telangiectasias though common in systemic sclerosis are quite rare in morphea, especially in pediatric morphea [19, 20].

COMPUTERISED SKIN SCORE (CSS)

In 2007, Zulian *et al.* described a computerized method for assessing the skin lesions of morphea (Box **9.2**). In this method, a Tegaderm film is applied atop the morphea lesion. The indurated border of the lesion is then outlined with a marker onto the Tegaderm. The surrounding erythema or violaceous hue is also assessed and outlined on the Tegaderm with a different color marker. Specialized computer software delineates between the two color zones and thus calculates the surface area of the total lesion, and of the active and inactive zones.

Box 9.2: Computerised skin score (CSS).
Indurated border and erythematous border are separately outlined onto a tegaderm or plastic film.
Specialized computer software delineates between the two color zones and calculates the surface area of the total lesion, and of the active and inactive zones.
Standardized-CSS (s-CSS) = CSS/BSA in cm^2.
Useful in evaluating disease progression.
Saves time and calculates the actual surface area.
Advantageous in pediatric morphea.
Insensitive in assessing improvement of lesions.
Dyspigmentation and erythema assessment also needs further validation.

The standardized-CSS (s-CSS) can be calculated using the software which is the ratio of CSS/BSA in cm^2. This parameter is quite useful to evaluate the disease progression during childhood. In fact, the observation of an enlarged lesion, over the time, does not mean necessarily disease progression but can be related just to the natural growth process of the child. The s-CSS, calculated at different times, allows to establish if a skin lesion is enlarging or not. This method has been validated for good inter-rater and intra-rater reliability. CSS saves time and calculates surface area instead of relying on an estimation of the surface area. However, because morphea lesions do not shrink as they resolve, it is likely to be insensitive to improvement [15, 19].

The CSS just requires a plastic adhesive film, a scanner and a personal computer. It represents a simple, reliable and widely applicable method to assess disease progression in morphea and may be helpful in multicentre trial studies. This is focused on skin induration alone and represents the first method to measure the real extension of sclerotic lesions and is easily applicable in growing body as in childhood. Dyspigmentation and erythema may also be possibly measured by CSS, which needs further validation [19].

CUTOMETER

A cutometer is a handheld device that, when connected to a computer with the appropriate software, is capable of measuring skin elasticity and relaxation. The measurement is dependent upon anatomic site, age, sex, and edema. The probe measures the rate at which it is able to pull skin in and the rate at which the skin returns to the baseline. Although cutometer readings reported in morphea studies appear to be sensitive to change, cutometer measurements have not been validated in morphea [15, 21].

DUROMETER

A durometer is a handheld device that measures skin hardness. The measurement is dependent on edema, location, and patient's sex and age. Seyger *et al.* evaluated the durometer as an outcome measure in patients with morphea. The durometer measurements had low inter- and intra-observer variability; however, they found poor correlation between durometer scores and a non-validated modified skin score (0.5). Although the durometer's high reliability makes it a potential outcome measure, its poor correlation with clinical skin scores and low sensitivity limit its use [15, 22].

INFRARED THERMOGRAPHY

Thermography is the process of capturing infrared radiation emitted by the body and procuring images representative of the surface temperature of the skin [23]. This technique requires a temperature-controlled room, a 15-minute time period to calibrate patient's skin temperature, an infrared camera, and a trained operator. A positive area is considered to be 0.5°C warmer than the surrounding tissue. The criterion standard by which thermography is calibrated is the clinical appearance of the lesion and the lesion's behavior over time. Using the clinical examination as the criterion standard, Birdi *et al.* reported a sensitivity of 100% and a specificity of 80%, and Martini *et al.* reported a sensitivity of 92% and a specificity of 68%. The authors speculate that the loss of subcutaneous tissue resulted in increased thermal conductivity of the epidermis, and reflects the underlying vascular plexus and not the disease activity [15]. Thermography has been found to yield false positive results in the evaluation of older lesions of morphea [24].

HIGH-FREQUENCY ULTRASOUND (HFUS)

Noninvasive color Doppler ultrasound has been in use for decades and now recent studies have shown that it is almost an equal counterpart to histologic examination in the assessment of morphea lesion activity, thus minimizing the need for multiple skin biopsies. The depth of penetration obtained in HFUS is inversely proportional to the frequency of the probe used. The dermis affected by morphea lesions can be studied using a 20 MHz probe whereas frequencies of 8 to 15 MHz may be needed to assess the subcutaneous tissue, fascia, and muscle [25 - 27].

Technique of HFUS in Morphea

Sonographic imaging using HFUS is done along both the transverse and longitudinal axis of the lesion. The lesion should always be compared to the normal contralateral side as there can be variations in the parameters depending on the site and age of the individual. The important sonographic parameters considered are dermal thickness, dermal and subcutaneous tissue echogenicities, and vascularity for which a color doppler is essential. Dermal hypoechogenicity (suggestive of inflammation) is categorized into focal (partial thickness) or diffuse (full thickness). Lesional blood flow and maximum peak systolic velocity in the feeding arterial vessels can be determined by color Doppler examination. In the sonographic report, morphea activity level is categorized for each individual lesion and body segment [3].

Wortsman *et al.* have put forth the sonographic criteria for the assessment of morphea activity as shown in Table **9.4** [3]:

Table 9.4. Sonographic criteria for assessment of morphea activity.

ACTIVE LESION (evidence of inflammation)	Increased dermal thickness.
	Decreased dermal echogenicity (focal or diffuse).
	Increased subcutaneous tissue echogenicity.
	Increased cutaneous blood flow (dermal or subcutaneous tissue).
	Active lesions require two or more of the first 3 criteria, whereas increased cutaneous blood flow by itself is considered a marker of activity.
INACTIVE LESION	Incomplete criteria for active lesion (assessment by default).
ATROPHIC LESION	Decreased dermal and subcutaneous thickness.
	Blood flow is not increased.

Merits and demerits of HFUS

Ultrasound is a safe, cost-effective outcome tool in morphea that can be easily used in children and adults (Box **9.3**). Latent lesions can also be detected which may not always be clinically evident. The signs with the highest sensitivity and specificity for disease activity include increased cutaneous blood flow and subcutaneous tissue hyper echogenicity. Isolated dermal thickening and decreased dermal echogenicity are highly sensitive, but also seen with photoaging and thus, much less specific. In contrast, the phase of atrophy can be easily recognized on the sonogram. Subcutaneous thickness also correlates with disease activity, but is not included among the diagnostic criteria as it is sensitive to body weight and probe pressure.

Box 9.3: Disadvantages of HFUS.
Unable to detect lesions <0.1mm deep
Not useful for face and scalp lesions
Highly operator dependent
Expensive
Lack of standardisation of procedure and definitions
Better validation required

HFUS cannot detect lesions less than 0.1 mm in depth [3]. Also, it may not be very useful for facial or scalp lesions as the tissue is relatively thin [28]. The technique is highly operator-dependent and larger trials are required before it can be used as a reliable validated outcome measure. The technique requires a universal standardization for the acquisition of images, technical aspects involving machine settings, and regions of interest to be imaged and measured, as there can be subjective variation depending on the expertise of the performing clinician. The definition of dermal and subcutaneous tissue thickness as measured by HFUS also needs to be defined clearly [29].

LASER DOPPLER FLOWMETRY (LDF)

LDF is a noninvasive method for the measurement of cutaneous microcirculation (Box **9.4**). Besides its use in inflammatory skin disorders, it has been widely tried in vascular disorders, and neuropathies and to monitor the microcirculation in skin flaps or grafts following surgical procedures [24]. LDF helps to discriminate disease activity in morphea, and is more accurate for this purpose than thermography.

Box 9.4: Laser Doppler Flowmetry (LDF).
Aids in functional assessment of cutaneous microcirculation.
Elevated blood flow is noted in clinically active scleroderma lesions.
Superior to thermography in monitoring disease activity in children.
Disease progression or latent ongoing inflammation can lead to increased blood flow in clinically inactive lesions, which is a demerit.
Evaluates only a small skin area.
Measurements are susceptible to motion artefacts.

Principle of LDF

Laser Doppler flowmetry (LDF) aids in the functional assessment of the cutaneous microcirculation, including not only the capillaries but also the deeper dermal vessels. A single probe that is in contact with the skin emits the laser beam. The moving particles such as red blood cells in the circulation reflects the laser beam (known as the Doppler effect). The shifted frequencies are detected by the receiving optical fiber in the same probe and the resulting photocurrent is processed to quantify the skin's blood perfusion [30].

LDF has been shown to be superior to thermography in detecting and monitoring disease activity in children with morphea. Blood flow is elevated in clinically active scleroderma lesions. However, studies have shown slightly higher blood flow in clinically inactive lesions which could be due to persistent changes in the microcirculation caused by disease progression or due to latent ongoing inflammation. LDF can be used to investigate only a small skin area, and measurements are susceptible to motion artifacts. The more recently developed technique of laser Doppler imaging (LDI) allows the evaluation of blood flow over a specific area of skin while avoiding contact with the skin surface. Nevertheless, current LDI devices are of limited use in children, because of their slow scanning times [24].

CONE BEAM COMPUTED TOMOGRAPHY (CBCT)

Isolated oral mucosal morphea without cutaneous involvement has been reported and CBCT helps in such cases to assess the extent of odontostomatologic involvement [31] (Box **9.5**). CBCT is largely used in dentistry and maxillofacial surgery with a good sensitivity to assess changes in soft and bony tissues. It is often used in linear morphea of the face, which is more common in the juvenile population. The CBCT scanner uses a 2D detector and a cone-shaped X-ray beam that scans the affected region, reproducing a digital volume, thus providing both 2D and 3D images. The benefits of this technique are that it is fast when compared to MRI, cost-effective and the radiation dose is relatively less than a routine computed tomography (CT) with even better spatial resolution. However, forehead lesions are difficult to evaluate as the conical beam has a low affinity in this area and hence the image definition is inaccurate [32].

Box 9.5: Cone Beam Computed Tomography (CBCT).
Aids in assessing the extent of odontostomatologic involvement in oral mucosal morphea.
Sensitive to changes in soft and bony tissue
Useful in juvenile linear morphea of face.
Advantages of being fast, cost-effective and emits less radiation when compared to a routine CT.
Better spatial resolution.

Box 9.6. Learning points.
• Assessment of disease severity is very important to decide on the activity of the disease and the treatment modality to be initiated, failing which can result in disastrous sequelae.
• Clinical and histological correlation are still the mainstay in correlating the disease severity.
• The LoSCAT, which was initially designed for juvenile morphea is the only score that has specific parameters for assessment of morphea activity (LoSSI) and damage (LoSDI) and has undergone extensive validation studies.
• High-frequency ultrasound is also being widely used as it obviates the need for repeated biopsies; however, it is operator dependent and needs better standardization
• Computerised skin scores, cutometer and durometer have limited potential as outcome measures.
• Laser doppler flowmetry has been shown to be more accurate and hence superior to thermography in activity assessment especially in pediatric morphea.
• It is important to have larger trials so that the newer techniques can be better validated.

REFERENCES

[1]   Kim A, Marinkovich N, Vasquez R, Jacobe H. Clinical features of morphea patients with the pansclerotic subtype: A cross-sectional study from the Morphea in Adults and Children (MAC cohort). J Rheumatol 2014; 41: 106-12.
[http://dx.doi.org/10.3899/jrheum.130029] [PMID: 24293577]

[2]   Abbas L, Joseph A, Kunzler E, Jacobe HT. Morphea: progress to date and the road ahead. Ann Transl Med 2020; 1-16.
[PMID: 33842658]

[3]   Wortsman X, Wortsman J, Sazunic I, Carreño L. Activity assessment in morphea using color Doppler ultrasound. J Am Acad Dermatol 2011; 65(5): 942-8.
[http://dx.doi.org/10.1016/j.jaad.2010.08.027] [PMID: 21550692]

[4]   Walker D, Susa JS, Currimbhoy S, Jacobe H. Histopathological changes in morphea and their clinical correlates: Results from the Morphea in Adults and Children Cohort V. J Am Acad Dermatol 2017; 76(6): 1124-30.
[http://dx.doi.org/10.1016/j.jaad.2016.12.020] [PMID: 28285783]

[5]   Ranosz-Janicka I, Lis-Święty A, Skrzypek-Salamon A, Brzezińska-Wcisło L. Detecting and quantifying activity/inflammation in localized scleroderma with thermal imaging. Skin Res Technol 2019; 25(2): 118-23.
[http://dx.doi.org/10.1111/srt.12619] [PMID: 30030915]

[6]   Zulian F, Culpo R, Sperotto F, *et al.* Consensus-based recommendations for the management of juvenile localised scleroderma. Ann Rheum Dis 2019; 78(8): 1019-24.

[http://dx.doi.org/10.1136/annrheumdis-2018-214697] [PMID: 30826775]

[7]   George R, George A, Kumar TS. Update on management of morphea (Localized Scleroderma) in children. Indian Dermatol Online J 2020; 11(2): 135-45.
[http://dx.doi.org/10.4103/idoj.IDOJ_284_19] [PMID: 32477969]

[8]   Mertens JS, Seyger MMB, Kievit W, *et al.* Disease recurrence in localized scleroderma: A retrospective analysis of 344 patients with paediatric- or adult-onset disease. Br J Dermatol 2015; 172(3): 722-8.
[http://dx.doi.org/10.1111/bjd.13514] [PMID: 25381928]

[9]   Florez-Pollack S, Kunzler E, Jacobe HT. Morphea: Current concepts. Clin Dermatol 2018; 36(4): 475-86.
[http://dx.doi.org/10.1016/j.clindermatol.2018.04.005] [PMID: 30047431]

[10]   Knobler R, Moinzadeh P, Hunzelmann N, *et al.* European Dermatology Forum S1-guideline on the diagnosis and treatment of sclerosing diseases of the skin, Part 1: localized scleroderma, systemic sclerosis and overlap syndromes. J Eur Acad Dermatol Venereol 2017; 31(9): 1401-24.
[http://dx.doi.org/10.1111/jdv.14458] [PMID: 28792092]

[11]   Nouri S, Jacobe H. Recent developments in diagnosis and assessment of morphea. Curr Rheumatol Rep 2013; 15(2): 308.
[http://dx.doi.org/10.1007/s11926-012-0308-9] [PMID: 23307579]

[12]   Torok KS, Kurzinski K, Kelsey C, *et al.* Peripheral blood cytokine and chemokine profiles in juvenile localized scleroderma: T-helper cell-associated cytokine profiles. Semin Arthritis Rheum 2015; 45(3): 284-93.
[http://dx.doi.org/10.1016/j.semarthrit.2015.06.006] [PMID: 26254121]

[13]   O'Brien JC, Rainwater YB, Malviya N, *et al.* Transcriptional and Cytokine Profiles Identify CXCL9 as a Biomarker of Disease Activity in Morphea. J Invest Dermatol 2017; 137(8): 1663-70.
[http://dx.doi.org/10.1016/j.jid.2017.04.008] [PMID: 28450066]

[14]   Arkachaisri T, Vilaiyuk S, Li S, *et al.* Localized Scleroderma Clinical and Ultrasound Study Group. The localized scleroderma skin severity index and physician global assessment of disease activity: A work in progress toward development of localized scleroderma outcome measures. J Rheumatol 2009; 36(12): 2819-29.
[http://dx.doi.org/10.3899/jrheum.081284] [PMID: 19833758]

[15]   Fett N, Werth VP. Update on morphea. J Am Acad Dermatol 2011; 64(2): 231-42.
[http://dx.doi.org/10.1016/j.jaad.2010.05.046] [PMID: 21238824]

[16]   Agazzi A, Fadanelli G, Vittadello F, Zulian F, Martini G. Reliability of LoSCAT score for activity and tissue damage assessment in a large cohort of patients with Juvenile Localized Scleroderma. Pediatr Rheumatol Online J 2018; 16(1): 37.
[http://dx.doi.org/10.1186/s12969-018-0254-9] [PMID: 29914516]

[17]   Arif T, Sami M. Calculating area of graft required for vitiliginous areas during split-thickness skin grafting: A simple, accurate, and cost-effective technique. J Cutan Aesthet Surg 2017; 10(3): 160-2.
[http://dx.doi.org/10.4103/JCAS.JCAS_45_17] [PMID: 29403189]

[18]   Kelsey CE, Torok KS. The Localized Scleroderma Cutaneous Assessment Tool: Responsiveness to change in a pediatric clinical population. J Am Acad Dermatol 2013; 69(2): 214-20.
[http://dx.doi.org/10.1016/j.jaad.2013.02.007] [PMID: 23562760]

[19]   Zulian F, Meneghesso D, Grisan E, *et al.* A new computerized method for the assessment of skin lesions in localized scleroderma. Rheumatology 2007; 46(5): 856-60.
[http://dx.doi.org/10.1093/rheumatology/kel446] [PMID: 17264088]

[20]   Dytoc M, Ting PT, Man J, Sawyer D, Fiorillo L. First case series on the use of imiquimod for morphoea. Br J Dermatol 2005; 153(4): 815-20.
[http://dx.doi.org/10.1111/j.1365-2133.2005.06776.x] [PMID: 16181467]

[21] Andres C, Kollmar A, Mempel M, Hein R, Ring J, Eberlein B. Successful ultraviolet A1 phototherapy in the treatment of localized scleroderma: A retrospective and prospective study. Br J Dermatol 2010; 162(2): 445-7.
[http://dx.doi.org/10.1111/j.1365-2133.2009.09438.x] [PMID: 19785603]

[22] Seyger MMB, van den Hoogen FHJ, Boo T, de Jong EMGJ. Reliability of two methods to assess morphea: Skin scoring and the use of a durometer. J Am Acad Dermatol 1997; 37(5): 793-6.
[http://dx.doi.org/10.1016/S0190-9622(97)70121-X] [PMID: 9366834]

[23] Murray A, Moore T, Manning J, *et al.* Non-invasive Imaging of Localised Scleroderma for Assessment of Skin Blood Flow and Structure. Acta Derm Venereol 2016; 96(5): 641-4.
[http://dx.doi.org/10.2340/00015555-2328] [PMID: 26695444]

[24] Weibel L, Howell KJ, Visentin MT, *et al.* Laser Doppler flowmetry for assessing localized scleroderma in children. Arthritis Rheum 2007; 56(10): 3489-95.
[http://dx.doi.org/10.1002/art.22920] [PMID: 17907196]

[25] Li SC, Liebling MS, Haines KA, Weiss JE, Prann A. Initial evaluation of an ultrasound measure for assessing the activity of skin lesions in juvenile localized scleroderma. Arthritis Care Res 2011; 63(5): 735-42.
[http://dx.doi.org/10.1002/acr.20407] [PMID: 21557528]

[26] Wortsman X, Wortsman J. Clinical usefulness of variable-frequency ultrasound in localized lesions of the skin. J Am Acad Dermatol 2010; 62(2): 247-56.
[http://dx.doi.org/10.1016/j.jaad.2009.06.016] [PMID: 19962214]

[27] Aranegui B, Jiménez-Reyes J. Morphea in Childhood: An Update. Actas Dermosifiliogr 2018; 109(4): 312-22.
[http://dx.doi.org/10.1016/j.ad.2017.06.021] [PMID: 29248149]

[28] Shahidi-Dadras M, Abdollahimajd F, Jahangard R, Javinani A, Ashraf-Ganjouei A, Toossi P. Magnetic Resonance Imaging Evaluation in Patients with Linear Morphea Treated with Methotrexate and High-Dose Corticosteroid. Dermatol Res Pract 2018; 2018: 1-6.
[http://dx.doi.org/10.1155/2018/8391218] [PMID: 30057597]

[29] Ch'ng SS, Roddy J, Keen HI. A systematic review of ultrasonography as an outcome measure of skin involvement in systemic sclerosis. Int J Rheum Dis 2013; 16(3): 264-72.
[http://dx.doi.org/10.1111/1756-185X.12106] [PMID: 23981746]

[30] Melsens K, Van Impe S, Paolino S, Vanhaecke A, Cutolo M, Smith V. The preliminary validation of laser Doppler flowmetry in systemic sclerosis in accordance with the OMERACT filter: A systematic review. Semin Arthritis Rheum 2020; 50(2): 321-8.
[http://dx.doi.org/10.1016/j.semarthrit.2019.08.007] [PMID: 31526595]

[31] Tang MM, Bornstein MM, Irla N, Beltraminelli H, Lombardi T, Borradori L. Oral mucosal morphea: A new variant. Dermatology 2012; 224(3): 215-20.
[http://dx.doi.org/10.1159/000337554] [PMID: 22538799]

[32] Di Giovanni C, Puggina S, Meneghel A, Vittadello F, Martini G, Zulian F. Cone beam computed tomography for the assessment of linear scleroderma of the face. Pediatr Rheumatol Online J 2018; 16(1): 1-5.
[http://dx.doi.org/10.1186/s12969-017-0218-5] [PMID: 29298697]

Associated Diseases

Ola Ahmed Bakry[1,*]

[1] *Department of Dermatology, Andrology and STDs, Faculty of Medicine, Menoufiya University, Menoufiya Governorate, Shabeen El-kom, Egypt*

Chapter synopsis.
• Morphea is a skin disorder characterized by early inflammation followed by fibrosis.
• It has been thought that morphea is a disease confined only to the skin. However, several reports demonstrated the association between morphea and other cutaneous and systemic disorders.
• Diseases associated with morphea may be autoimmune or inflammatory, cutaneous or extracutaneous disorders.
• Various concomitant inflammatory/autoimmune diseases that have been reported in morphea patients include psoriasis, vitiligo, alopecia areata, inflammatory bowel disorders, type I diabetes mellitus, Meniere's disease, multiple sclerosis, systemic lupus erythematosus, rheumatoid arthritis, Sjogren's syndrome, mixed connective tissue disease, and antiphospholipid syndrome.
• Concomitant familial disorders which have been described in cases of morphea include rheumatoid arthritis, scleroderma, systemic lupus erythematosus (SLE), psoriasis, vitiligo, lichen sclerosus et atrophicus, thyroiditis, insulin-dependent diabetes mellitus, inflammatory bowel disease, myasthenia gravis, multiple sclerosis and sarcoidosis.
• Psoriasis, vitiligo and SLE are more prevalent in morphea cases than in the general population.

Keywords: Adult morphea, Antihistone antibodies, Anti-ssDNA antibodies, Antinuclear antibodies, Associated diseases, Autoimmune diseases, Autoantibodies, Childhood morphea, Connective tissue disorders, Familial, Family history, Fibrosis, Generalized morphea, Inflammation, Localized scleroderma, Morphea, Morphea and vitiligo, Morphea and psoriasis, Rheumatologic diseases, Rheumatoid factor, Scleroderma.

INTRODUCTION

Morphea is generally thought to be a self-limited benign disease confined to the skin with musculoskeletal involvement typically including growth defects with

---

[*] **Corresponding author Ola Ahmed Bakry:** Department of Dermatology, Andrology and STDs, Faculty of Medicine, Menoufiya University, Menoufiya Governorate, Shabeen El-kom, Egypt; E-mail: olabakry8@gmail.com

Tasleem Arif (Ed.)

shortening of the affected limb, scoliosis, thorax asymmetry and muscle atrophy [1 - 4]. However, there are many reports that described morphea as a systemic autoimmune condition which has manifestations outside the skin [5 - 7]. Several case reports describe morphea coexisting with other autoimmune diseases [8 - 12]. These may underscore the postulation that morphea and systemic sclerosis are two ends of a continuous disease spectrum [7].

The prevalence of systemic and autoimmune or inflammatory diseases associated with morphea had been studied with different outcomes in different populations. The presence of concomitant diseases may affect patient management because many patients are untreated or are treated with skin-directed therapy despite being candidates for systemic therapy.

DISEASES ASSOCIATED WITH MORPHEA

Concomitant Autoimmune/Inflammatory Diseases

Concomitant rheumatic or other autoimmune diseases were reported in 18% of cases with morphea in a cohort study involving 245 cases. These concomitant diseases were more prevalent in adults and in cases with generalized morphea than in children and patients with other morphea subtypes respectively [1]. It is unknown whether children with morphea will develop autoimmune disorders at an increased rate as they grow older [6].

Concomitant autoimmune diseases included psoriasis, vitiligo, alopecia areata, inflammatory bowel disorders, type I diabetes mellitus, Menier's Disease and multiple sclerosis. Concomitant rheumatic diseases included systemic lupus erythematosus (SLE), rheumatoid arthritis, Sjogren's syndrome, mixed connective tissue disease and antiphospholipid syndrome (Table **10.1**). The association of morphea with primary biliary cirrhosis, myasthenia gravis and Hashimoto's thyroiditis has also been reported [1, 5 - 7, 10 - 12].

Table 10.1. Concomitant autoimmune and rheumatic diseases reported in morphea cases.

• Autoimmune Diseases	• Rheumatic Diseases
Psoriasis	Systemic lupus erythematosus
Vitiligo	Rheumatoid arthritis
Alopecia areata	Sjogren's syndrome
Inflammatory bowel disease	Mixed connective tissue disease
Type I diabetes mellitus	Antiphospholipid syndrome
Menier's disease	Spondyloarthropathy

(Table 10.1) cont.....

• Autoimmune Diseases	• Rheumatic Diseases
Multiple sclerosis	Still's disease
Coeliac disease	
Autoimmune thyroiditis	
Primary biliary cirrhosis	

Several disorders occurred with greater frequency in morphea patients compared to published population-based prevalence estimates including psoriasis (1.5 to 4.5 fold increase), SLE (5.8 fold increase), multiple sclerosis (7-8 fold increase), and vitiligo (3.5 fold increase) [13 - 15].

The association between morphea and non-segmental vitiligo has rarely been reported [16 - 20]. In addition, the co-occurrence of linear morphea and homolateral segmental vitiligo has also been reported [21]. A possible mechanism explaining this finding is cutaneous mosaicism as linear morphea following Blaschko's lines has been previously reported [22]. A decrease in T-regulatory cells leading to loss of tolerance can also be a common link [23].

Kim *et al.*, reported a case who had generalized morphea lesions on the right and left sides of the back and linear morphea on the left side of the forehead, which was on the same side of the body where segmental vitiligo was located [24].

Van Geel *et al*, have also described a case with the simultaneous presence of segmental vitiligo, alopecia areata, psoriasis and a halo nevus and postulated a shared autoimmune-mediated process as the underlying mechanism [25]. Similarly, Bonilla-Abadía *et al.*, postulated an autoimmune mechanism to explain the association of morphea, vitiligo, autoimmune hypothyroidism, pneumonitis, autoimmune thrombocytopenic purpura, and central nervous system vasculitis [19]. In these reports, morphea becomes part of a multiple autoimmune syndrome (MAS), where there are three or more well-defined autoimmune diseases present in a single patient [26]. Therefore, it may be imperative to screen and follow up morphea cases for the development of other autoimmune diseases in the future.

Hydroxychloroquine was reported to be effective in blocking the progression of scleroderma and treating vitiligo. Hydroxychloroquine sulfate (200 mg/day) was used in a case with concurrent morphea and vitiligo. Skin lesions of morphea and vitiligo stabilized within 6 weeks. In addition, the vitiliginous lesions showed 70% repigmentation after 5 months from the start of medication. Skin lesions of morphea also showed no more progression. The patient tolerated the 7-month treatment period with no side effects [24].

The incidence of concurrent morphea and psoriasis is unknown and scarcely twenty cases have been recorded in the literature [27]. Psoriasis vulgaris is the most common skin disease associated with morphea and generally affects adults with widespread morphea [1]. Although the etiopathogenesis of these two diseases is still unclear, an underlying genetic basis, immunological T-cell defects, autoimmunity and trauma can play a role in both morphea and psoriasis [27]. Both conditions may have a common immunological base, since although morphea has been related to the Th2 pathway, those of Th1 and Th17 would also be essentially involved in initial stages [28].

Steur *et al.* reported a case of morphea in a patient undergoing treatment with ustekinumab for psoriasis. The ability of ustekinumab to alter the Th17 pathway of inflammation is critical to its utility in psoriasis and may also help explain the progression of morphea while under treatment with this drug [29].

On the other hand, Belin *et al.* reported a case of morphea and psoriasis that improved with acitretin treatment. They noticed improvement of the morphea lesions which may be due to an immunomodulatory effect of the drug or a decrease in collagen production by dermal fibroblasts due to retinoic acid [30].

The association between morphea and lichen sclerosus (LS) has been reported. Genital LS is significantly more frequent in patients with morphea than in unaffected individuals. Forty-five percent of patients with plaque morphea have associated LS. Complete clinical examination, including careful inspection of genital mucosa, should therefore be mandatory in patients with morphea because genital LS bears a risk of evolution into squamous cell carcinoma [31].

Moreover, although up to 12% of patients with systemic sclerosis have features of lupus erythematosus (LE), the association between cutaneous morphea and Systemic LE is extremely rare [32].

In the overlap of cutaneous LE and morphea, there is a predilection for young women, photo-distributed lesions, linear morphology clinically, and positivity along the dermoepidermal junction on direct immunofluorescence. Most patients had a good response to antimalarials, topical steroids, or systemic steroids [33].

Familial Autoimmune/rheumatic Diseases

In a study involving adult and pediatric cases, 16.3% reported positive family history of autoimmune disorders in the first or second-degree relatives. Positive family history was significantly higher in children than in adults. In adults, the generalized subtype had the highest frequency of familial disorders [1]. In another report involving only pediatric cases with morphea, the family history of rheumatic and autoimmune diseases was present in 12% of cases [6]. Reported disorders (Table **10.2**) included rheumatoid arthritis which was the most frequently encountered, followed by scleroderma and SLE. Cutaneous autoimmune diseases consisted of psoriasis, vitiligo and lichen sclerosus. Autoimmune diseases involving internal organs were represented by thyroiditis, insulin-dependent diabetes mellitus, and inflammatory bowel disease and, to a lesser extent, myasthenia gravis, multiple sclerosis and sarcoidosis [1 - 6].

Table 10.2. Familial autoimmune and rheumatic diseases reported in morphea cases.

• **Autoimmune Diseases**	• **Rheumatic Diseases**
Psoriasis	Rheumatoid arthritis
Vitiligo	Systemic lupus erythematosus
Lichen sclerosus et atrophicus	Scleroderma
Inflammatory bowel disease	Raynaud's phenomenon
Type I diabetes mellitus	Polymyositis
Autoimmune thyroiditis	Dermatomyositis
Multiple sclerosis	Acute rheumatic fever
Sarcoidosis	
Myasthenia Gravis	

Vancheeswaran *et al.* found a positive family history for autoimmune diseases in 12.7% of 47 patients with pediatric morphea but the type of disease was not specified [34]. Another study reported other cases of morphea in the families of five patients, with an overall prevalence of 2.6% [35]. Morphea was described in two generations of families and in one parent and daughter [36 - 38]. Affected monozygotic twins were also reported [39].

A positive family history for various autoimmune conditions in one out of eight pediatric morphea patients could support the hypothesis that the genetic background contributes to susceptibility to clinically distinct autoimmune/inflammatory diseases. A non-random clustering of non-MHC candidate loci, already shown in other conditions such as multiple sclerosis, Crohn's disease, familial psoriasis, asthma and type-1 diabetes, may explain this overlapping susceptibility [40]. On the other hand, the lack of similarity in disease expression within a family, the low incidence of multicase families and the data on twins seem to indicate that non-hereditary factors may play a major role in the pathogenesis of the disease [6].

Leitenberger *et al.,* found a positive family history of scleroderma in 1% of their studied subjects while Peterson *et al.*, reported a prevalence of 0.2% [1, 41]. Multicase families with morphea have been described independently in the literature and, were in a non-Mendelian pattern suggestive of a multifactorial, polygenic inheritance [37, 42].

Extracutaneous Manifestations

Morphea as discussed above shouldn't be considered as exclusively limited to the skin but as a disease which may have possible extracutaneous manifestations. Several extracutaneous manifestations have been reported in morphea which include gastrointestinal, articular, neurologic, vascular, respiratory and ocular involvement. Extracutaneous manifestations have been described in detail in chapter 11.

AUTOANTIBODIES

Several autoantibodies have been demonstrated in morphea patients which include antinuclear, antihistone, anti-ssDNA antibodies and rheumatoid factor. Antibodies to centromere, Scl-70, nuclear RNP, Sm, and SS-B antigens were seldom detected in patients with morphea [43]. A detailed description of autoantibodies and their significance in morphea has been provided in chapter 5.

Box 10.1. Learning points.
• Morphea seems to be a disease which is not necessarily confined to skin. It may rather have associations with other systemic inflammatory disorders.
• Concomitant diseases which have occurred more frequently with morphea may be inflammatory, autoimmune, rheumatic, or other extracutaneous systemic disorders.
• Most cases of morphea should be carefully examined to look for possible associated disorders.
• A positive family history for various autoimmune conditions in one out of eight pediatric morphea patients supports the view that the genetic background contributes to susceptibility to clinically distinct autoimmune/inflammatory diseases.
• Genital LS is significantly more frequent in patients with morphea. Careful inspection of genital mucosa, should therefore be mandatory in patients with morphea as genital LS carries a risk of evolution into squamous cell carcinoma.

REFERENCES

[1]   Leitenberger JJ, Cayce RL, Haley RW, Adams-Huet B, Bergstresser PR, Jacobe HT. Distinct autoimmune syndromes in morphea: A review of 245 adult and pediatric cases. Arch Dermatol 2009; 145(5): 545-50.
[http://dx.doi.org/10.1001/archdermatol.2009.79] [PMID: 19451498]

[2]   Christen-Zaech S, Hakim MD, Afsar FS, Paller AS. Pediatric morphea (localized scleroderma): Review of 136 patients. J Am Acad Dermatol 2008; 59(3): 385-96.
[http://dx.doi.org/10.1016/j.jaad.2008.05.005] [PMID: 18571769]

[3]   Marzano AV, Menni S, Parodi A, *et al.* Localized scleroderma in adults and children. Clinical and laboratory investigations on 239 cases. Eur J Dermatol 2003; 13(2): 171-6.
[PMID: 12695134]

[4]   Uziel Y, Krafchik BR, Silverman ED, Thorner PS, Laxer RM. Localized scleroderma in childhood: A report of 30 cases. Semin Arthritis Rheum 1994; 23(5): 328-40.
[http://dx.doi.org/10.1016/0049-0172(94)90028-0] [PMID: 8036522]

[5]   Harrington C, Dunsmore IR. An investigation into the incidence of auto-immune disorders in patients with localized morphoea. Br J Dermatol 1989; 120(5): 645-8.
[http://dx.doi.org/10.1111/j.1365-2133.1989.tb01350.x] [PMID: 2757929]

[6]   Zulian F, Athreya BH, Laxer R, *et al.* Juvenile Scleroderma Working Group of the Pediatric Rheumatology European Society (PRES). Juvenile localized scleroderma: clinical and epidemiological features in 750 children. An international study. Rheumatology 2006; 45(5): 614-20.
[http://dx.doi.org/10.1093/rheumatology/kei251] [PMID: 16368732]

[7]   Zulian F, Vallongo C, Woo P, *et al.* Juvenile Scleroderma Working Group of the Pediatric Rheumatology European Society (PRES). Localized scleroderma in childhood is not just a skin disease. Arthritis Rheum 2005; 52(9): 2873-81.
[http://dx.doi.org/10.1002/art.21264] [PMID: 16142730]

[8]   Majeed M, Al-Mayouf SM, Al-Sabban E, Bahabri S. Coexistent linear scleroderma and juvenile systemic lupus erythematosus. Pediatr Dermatol 2000; 17(6): 456-9.
[http://dx.doi.org/10.1046/j.1525-1470.2000.01820.x] [PMID: 11123778]

[9]   González-López MA, Drake M, González-Vela MC, Armesto S, Llaca HF, Val-Bernal JF. Generalized morphea and primary biliary cirrhosis coexisting in a male patient. J Dermatol 2006; 33(10): 709-13.
[http://dx.doi.org/10.1111/j.1346-8138.2006.00165.x] [PMID: 17040502]

[10]   Khalifa M, Ben Jazia E, Hachfi W, Sriha B, Bahri F, Letaief A. Autoimmune hepatitis and morphea: A rare association. Gastroenterol Clin Biol 2006; 30(6-7): 917-8.
[http://dx.doi.org/10.1016/S0399-8320(06)73344-9] [PMID: 16885881]

[11]   Dervis E, Acbay O, Barut G, Karaoglu A, Ersoy L. Association of vitiligo, morphea, and Hashimoto's thyroiditis. Int J Dermatol 2004; 43(3): 236-7.
[http://dx.doi.org/10.1111/j.1365-4632.2004.01973.x] [PMID: 15009403]

[12]   Parra V, Driban N, Bassotti A. Localized morphea and myasthenia gravis. J Am Acad Dermatol 2008; 49: 1-5.

[13]   Spritz RA. The genetics of generalized vitiligo and associated autoimmune diseases. Pigment Cell Res 2007; 20(4): 271-8.
[http://dx.doi.org/10.1111/j.1600-0749.2007.00384.x] [PMID: 17630960]

[14]   Lawrence RC, Helmick CG, Arnett FC, *et al.* Estimates of the prevalence of arthritis and selected musculoskeletal disorders in the United States. Arthritis Rheum 1998; 41(5): 778-99.
[http://dx.doi.org/10.1002/1529-0131(199805)41:5<778::AID-ART4>3.0.CO;2-V] [PMID: 9588729]

[15]   Hoffman RW, Greidinger EL. Mixed connective tissue disease. Curr Opin Rheumatol 2000; 12(5): 386-90.
[http://dx.doi.org/10.1097/00002281-200009000-00006] [PMID: 10990174]

[16]   Soylu S, Gül Ü, Gönül M, Klç A, Çakmak SK, Demiriz M. An uncommon presentation of the co-existence of morphea and vitiligo in a patient with chronic hepatitis B virus infection: is there a possible association with autoimmunity? Am J Clin Dermatol 2009; 10(5): 336-8.
[http://dx.doi.org/10.2165/11310800-000000000-00000] [PMID: 19658447]

[17]   Arif T, Hassan I, Nisa N. Morphea and vitiligo-A very uncommon association. Nasza Dermatol Online 2015; 6(2): 232-4.
[http://dx.doi.org/10.7241/ourd.20152.62]

[18]   Yorulmaz A, Kilic S, Artuz F, Kahraman E. Concomitant appearance of morphea and vitiligo in a patient with autoimmune thyroiditis. Postepy Dermatol Alergol 2016; 4(4): 314-6.
[http://dx.doi.org/10.5114/ada.2016.61610] [PMID: 27605907]

[19]   Bonilla-Abadía F, Muñoz-Buitrón E, Ochoa CD, Carrascal E, Cañas CA. A rare association of localized scleroderma type morphea, vitiligo, autoimmune hypothyroidism, pneumonitis, autoimmune thrombocytopenic purpura and central nervous system vasculitis. Case report. BMC Res Notes 2012; 5(1): 689.
[http://dx.doi.org/10.1186/1756-0500-5-689] [PMID: 23256875]

[20]   Lee JS, Park H, Cho S, Yoon HS. Concurrence of Circumscribed Morphea and Segmental Vitiligo: A Case Report. Ann Dermatol 2018; 30(6): 708-11.
[http://dx.doi.org/10.5021/ad.2018.30.6.708] [PMID: 33911512]

[21]   Bonifati C, Impara G, Morrone A, Pietrangeli A, Carducci M. Simultaneous occurrence of linear scleroderma and homolateral segmental vitiligo. J Eur Acad Dermatol Venereol 2006; 20(1): 63-5.
[http://dx.doi.org/10.1111/j.1468-3083.2005.01336.x] [PMID: 16405610]

[22]   Soma Y, Fujimoto M. Frontoparietal scleroderma (en coup de sabre) following Blaschko's lines. J Am Acad Dermatol 1998; 38(2): 366-8.
[http://dx.doi.org/10.1016/S0190-9622(98)70586-9] [PMID: 9486719]

[23]   Yadav P, Garg T, Chander R, Nangia A. Segmental vitiligo with segmental morphea: An autoimmune link? Indian Dermatol Online J 2014; 5(5 Suppl. 1): 23.
[http://dx.doi.org/10.4103/2229-5178.144517] [PMID: 25506558]

[24]   Kim HJ, Shin D, Oh SH. A Case of Segmental Vitiligo with Generalized Morphea Stabilized by Antimalarial Medication. Ann Dermatol 2016; 28(2): 249-50.
[http://dx.doi.org/10.5021/ad.2016.28.2.249] [PMID: 27081277]

[25]   van Geel N, Mollet I, Brochez L, *et al.* New insights in segmental vitiligo: case report and review of theories. Br J Dermatol 2012; 166(2): 240-6.
[http://dx.doi.org/10.1111/j.1365-2133.2011.10650.x] [PMID: 21936857]

[26]   Anaya JM, Castiblanco J, Rojas-Villarraga A, *et al.* The multiple autoimmune syndromes. A clue for the autoimmune tautology. Clin Rev Allergy Immunol 2012; 43(3): 256-64.
[http://dx.doi.org/10.1007/s12016-012-8317-z] [PMID: 22648455]

[27]   Corral Magaña O, Escalas Taberner J, Escudero Góngora MM, Giacaman Contreras A. Morphea in a patient with psoriasis on treatment with ustekinumab: Comorbidity or adverse effect? Actas Dermo-Sifiliográficas 2017; 108(5): 487-9.
[http://dx.doi.org/10.1016/j.adengl.2017.03.021] [PMID: 28110825]

[28]   Harrison B, Herrick A, Griffiths C. Psoriasis and diffuse systemic sclerosis: A report of three patients. Rheumatology (Oxford) 2000; 39(2): 213-5.
[http://dx.doi.org/10.1093/rheumatology/39.2.213] [PMID: 10725077]

[29]   Steuer AB, Peterson E, Lo Sicco K, Franks AG Jr. Morphea in a patient undergoing treatment with ustekinumab. JAAD Case Rep 2019; 5(7): 590-2.
[http://dx.doi.org/10.1016/j.jdcr.2019.05.008] [PMID: 31312709]

[30]   Bilen N, Apaydin R, Erçin C, Harova G, Başdaş F, Bayramgürler D. Coexistence of morphea and psoriasis responding to acitretin treatment. J Eur Acad Dermatol Venereol 1999; 13(2): 113-7.
[http://dx.doi.org/10.1111/j.1468-3083.1999.tb00863.x] [PMID: 10568490]

[31]   Tremaine R, Adam JE, Orizaga M. Morphea coexisting with lichen sclerosus et atrophicus. Int J Dermatol 1990; 29(7): 486-9.
[http://dx.doi.org/10.1111/j.1365-4362.1990.tb04840.x] [PMID: 2228375]

[32] García-Arpa M, Flores-Terry MA, Ramos-Rodríguez C, Franco-Muñoz M, González-Ruiz L, Ramírez-Huaranga MA. Cutaneous lupus erythematosus, morphea profunda and psoriasis: A case report. Reumatología Clínica (English Edition) 2020; 16(2): 180-2.
[http://dx.doi.org/10.1016/j.reumae.2018.02.009] [PMID: 29625815]

[33] Pascucci A, Lynch PJ, Fazel N. Lupus erythematosus and localized scleroderma coexistent at the same sites: A rare presentation of overlap syndrome of connective-tissue diseases. Cutis 2016; 97(5): 359-63.
[PMID: 27274545]

[34] Vancheeswaran R, Black CM, David J, *et al.* Childhood-onset scleroderma: Is it different from adult-onset disease? Arthritis Rheum 1996; 39(6): 1041-9.
[http://dx.doi.org/10.1002/art.1780390624] [PMID: 8651969]

[35] Christianson HB, Dorsey CS, Kierland RR, O'Leary PA. Localized Scleroderma. AMA Arch Derm 1956; 74(6): 629-39.
[http://dx.doi.org/10.1001/archderm.1956.01550120049012] [PMID: 13371921]

[36] Wadud MA, Bose BK, Al Nasir T. Familial localised scleroderma from Bangladesh: Two case reports. Bangladesh Med Res Counc Bull 1989; 15(1): 15-9.
[PMID: 2818409]

[37] Kass H, Hanson V, Patrick J, Centeno LM, Moore ME. Scleroderma in childhood. J Pediatr 1966; 68(2): 243-56.
[http://dx.doi.org/10.1016/S0022-3476(66)80156-7]

[38] Rees RB, Bennett J. Localized scleroderma in father and daughter. AMA Arch Derm Syphilol 1953; 68(3): 360-1.
[PMID: 13079320]

[39] De Keyser F, Peene I, Joos R, Naeyaert JM, Messiaen L, Veys EM. Occurrence of scleroderma in monozygotic twins. J Rheumatol 2000; 27(9): 2267-9.
[PMID: 10990246]

[40] Becker KG, Simon RM, Bailey-Wilson JE, *et al.* Clustering of non-major histocompatibility complex susceptibility candidate loci in human autoimmune diseases. Proc Natl Acad Sci 1998; 95(17): 9979-84.
[http://dx.doi.org/10.1073/pnas.95.17.9979] [PMID: 9707586]

[41] Peterson LS, Nelson AM, Su WP, Mason T, O'Fallon WM, Gabriel SE. The epidemiology of morphea (localized scleroderma) in Olmsted County 1960-1993. J Rheumatol 1997; 24(1): 73-80.
[PMID: 9002014]

[42] Pham CM, Browning JC. Morphea affecting a father and son. Pediatr Dermatol 2010; 27(5): 536-7.
[http://dx.doi.org/10.1111/j.1525-1470.2010.01277.x] [PMID: 21182646]

[43] Khatri S, Torok KS, Mirizio E, Liu C, Astakhova K. Autoantibodies in Morphea: An Update. Front Immunol 2019; 10: 1487-22.
[http://dx.doi.org/10.3389/fimmu.2019.01487] [PMID: 31354701]

CHAPTER 11

Extracutaneous Manifestations

Abid Keen[1,*] and Tasleem Arif[2,3]

[1] Dermatology Clinic, Esthetica Skin, Hair and Dental Institute, Nai Basti, Anantnag, Kashmir, India

[2] Department of Dermatology, STDs, Leprosy and Aesthetics, Dar As Sihha Medical center, Dammam, Saudi Arabia

[3] Ellahi Medicare Clinic, Srinagar, Kashmir, India

Chapter synopsis.
• Some patients with morphea have extra-cutaneous manifestations. Morphea should not be considered as exclusively limited to the skin but as a disease that may have other organ system involvement.
• Musculoskeletal manifestations have been reported in morphea. These include arthralgia, flexion contractures, arthritis, *etc.* MRI may be a useful tool for the detection of musculoskeletal involvement.
• Gastroesophageal manifestations are rarely reported in morphea. Most authors believe that routine workup for gastroesophageal manifestations is justified only in SSC. However, morphea patients symptomatic for gastroesophageal symptoms or having autoantibodies may be referred to a gastroenterologist.
• Cardiac involvement is common in SSC but it is exceedingly rare in morphea. Isolated cases of pericarditis and incomplete right bundle branch block have been reported in morphea.
• Ophthalmological involvement is not uncommon in pediatric morphea especially with linear morphea involving the face. Ocular monitoring is mandatory in those with skin lesions on the face and/or concomitant CNS involvement. Common ocular manifestations include eyelid abnormalities, eyelash abnormalities, lacrimal gland abnormalities, anterior uveitis, secondary glaucoma, episcleritis, strabismus, *etc.*
• Neurological symptoms and signs in linear morphea involving the face are protean and include seizures, headache, focal neurologic deficits, and movement disorders as well as neuropsychiatric symptoms and intellectual deterioration.

Keywords: Arthralgia, Arthritis, Autoimmune disease, Autoimmune thyroiditis, Cardiac manifestations, Dental anomalies, Epilepsy, Extra-cutaneous manifestations, Focal neurologic deficits, Flexion contractures, Gastrointestinal manifestations, Gastroesophageal reflux, Headache, Linear morphea ECDS, Morphea, Musculoskeletal manifestations, Neurological manifestations, Ocular manifestations, Squamous cell carcinoma, Thyroid abnormalities.

* **Corresponding author Abid Keen:** Dermatology Clinic, Esthetica Skin, Hair and Dental Institute, Nai Basti, Anantnag, Kashmir, India; E-mail: keenabid31@gmail.com

INTRODUCTION

Several patients with morphea have extra-cutaneous manifestations and associated autoimmune diseases. Morphea should not be considered as exclusively limited to the skin but as a disease that may potentially develop systemic involvement. These patients should be studied more thoroughly and followed with close collaboration between the dermatologist and rheumatologist and other allied specialities.

EXTRACUTANEOUS MANIFESTATIONS

Though morphea is known as a dermatologic disease, in the literature the possibility of visceral involvement has also been reported, in the case of overlap with other autoimmune diseases or as possible evolution towards a systemic form; the latter possibility was described anecdotally in pediatric cases [1, 2]. Various extracutaneous manifestations of morphea have been discussed below:

Musculoskeletal Manifestations

Musculoskeletal complications (Box **11.1**) are reported in up to 40% of cases with morphea [3]. These include arthralgia, flexion contractures, arthritis and considerable impairment [4]. In recent years, the first data documenting a high prevalence of musculoskeletal involvement in patients with morphea have been published [3, 5, 6]. Furthermore, musculoskeletal manifestations may be an important argument for systemic rather than topical therapy. The recent German Society of Dermatology guidelines for the management of patients with morphea recommends treatment with methotrexate and prednisolone if the patient has a deep, linear or generalized form of morphea or if fasciae, muscles or bones are involved [7]. It has been shown that in patients with morphea, magnetic resonance imaging (MRI) is a useful tool for the detection of musculoskeletal manifestations [8]. MRI provides complementary information about the depth of involvement of underlying morphologic structures, contrary to the clinical examination, which generally reveals information about the superficial involvement in this disorder. The use of MRI makes it possible to objectively evaluate changes in fascial, muscular and joint disease.

Box 11.1: Musculoskeletal involvement in morphea.
Reported in 40 % cases of morphea.
The presence of musculoskeletal manifestations may indicate systemic therapy.
Arthralgia, flexion contractures, and arthritis are the usual presentations.

(Table 11.1) cont.....

In case of fascial, muscle or bone involvement, a combination of methotrexate and systemic steroids is recommended.
MRI is recommended for the detection of musculoskeletal manifestations.
MRI objectively evaluates changes in fascial, muscular and joint disease.

Gastrointestinal Manifestations

There is a scarcity of data regarding gastrointestinal involvement (Box **11.2**) in morphea. Zulian *et al.* [5] in their study reported gastroesophageal reflux in 1.6% of the patients. Zaninotto *et al.* [9] in their study recommended that esophageal tests may be useful in the evaluation of SSC; however, they did not recommend its routine use in cases of morphea. Esophageal involvement has been seen in some patients with pediatric morphea [10]. Patients of pediatric morphea who are symptomatic for gastroesophageal symptoms or having autoantibodies can be subjected to a meticulous history regarding gastroesophageal symptoms and referral to a gastroenterologist can be considered based on the patient's clinical profile [11].

Box 11.2: Gastrointestinal involvement in morphea.
Data regarding gastrointestinal involvement in morphea is scarce.
Gastroesophageal reflux has been reported in 1.6% of the patients in some case series while others have not found such abnormality.
Meticulous work-up for the gastroesophageal system is justified in SSC but seems to be unjustified in morphea.
Morphea patients who are symptomatic for gastroesophageal symptoms or having autoantibodies may be subjected to gastroesophageal evaluation.

Need for Upper GI Evaluation?

Esophageal manometry has been performed in children with morphea, showing nonspecific alterations without any changes typical of SSC [5]. Arif *et al.* [12] in their study concluded that esophageal involvement in SSC is very frequent while its involvement in morphea is very insignificant. In their study, they mentioned that every case of SSC needed a meticulous upper GI evaluation, whether symptomatic or not, however, such an evaluation in morphea seemed to be unjustified [12]. These facts and the lack of information on the natural history of this abnormality in asymptomatic children hardly support the recent recommendation for an extensive gastrointestinal evaluation of all patients with morphea [13].

Cardiac Manifestations

Primary cardiac involvement (Box **11.3**), in SSC, may manifest as myocardial damage, fibrosis of the conduction system, pericardial and, less frequently, as valvular disease [14]. Although cardiac involvement in morphea is rarely seen, Zulian *et al* [5] studied the prevalence and clinical features of extracutaneous manifestations in a large cohort of children with pediatric morphea. In their study, they noticed cardiac involvement in 2 children (0.3%) [5]. One had acute pericarditis soon after the onset of linear morphea, and the other had arrhythmias (incomplete right bundle branch block) [5]. Although pericarditis is rare in children with pediatric morphea, electrocardiographic abnormalities, mainly represented by incomplete right bundle branch block, have been reported in both children as well as in adults [15, 16].

Box 11.3: Cardiac involvement in morphea.
Cardiac involvement is well known in SSC but it is exceedingly rare in morphea.
In morphea, cardiac involvement has been reported in 0.3% of cases.
Pericarditis
Incomplete right bundle branch block

Ocular Manifestations

Ocular abnormalities (Box **11.4**) are not unusual in patients with pediatric morphea. Careful ophthalmic monitoring is recommended for every patient with pediatric morphea, but is mandatory in those with skin lesions on the face and/or concomitant CNS involvement [17]. Linear morphea of the face, also known as "en coup de sabre" (ECDS) because it resembles the strike of a sword, affects the frontoparietal area of the head and often involves the ocular adnexa and even the eye [18]. The data on ocular involvement in morphea consist essentially of single case reports of adult patients with a wide variability of manifestations [19 - 22]. Zanin *et al.* [17] evaluated the frequency and characteristics of ocular involvement in a large cohort of children with pediatric morphea from a multi-centre international data collection. Twenty-four patients (3.2%) had significant ocular involvement in the form of eyelid abnormalities, eyelash abnormalities, lacrimal gland abnormalities, anterior uveitis, secondary glaucoma, episcleritis, papillary mydriasis, strabismus, refractive errors, pseudopailloedema, neuroretinits, and enophthalmos [17]. In their study, they recommended an ophthalmic screening every 3–4 months for the first 3 years and then only in case of relapse [17].

Box 11.4: Ocular manifestations in morphea (mainly in linear morphea involving face).
Eyelid abnormalities
Eyelash abnormalities
lacrimal gland abnormalities
Anterior uveitis
Secondary glaucoma
Episcleritis
Papillary mydriasis
Strabismus
Refractive errors
Pseudopapilloedema
Neuroretinits
Enophthalmos
Keratitis
Xerophthalmia

Zulian *et al.* [5] reported ocular involvement, which was seen in 2.1% of patients, almost exclusively in those with linear morphea involving the face. Ocular complications consisted of anterior uveitis episcleritis, and keratitis. Other conditions like xerophthalmia and glaucoma were explained on the basis of a fibrotic process involving the anterior segment of the eye or the lacrimal glands [5].

Neurological Manifestations

Linear morphea ECDS has been associated with a variety of neurologic abnormalities (Box **11.5**) and typically is preceded by the development of cutaneous disease in months to years [23 - 26]. Nervous system involvement is usually not correlated to skin activity and may present years after the disease's initial symptomatology [26]. In 16% of cases, neurologic symptoms predate the cutaneous manifestations [27]. Neurological symptoms and signs in ECDS are protean and include epilepsy [28], headache [29], focal neurologic deficits, and movement disorders [30], as well as neuropsychiatric symptoms and intellectual deterioration [31, 32].

Epilepsy is a frequently reported manifestation of ECDS. Complex partial seizures have been reported most frequently, followed by tonic-clonic, absence seizures, as well as status epilepticus [28]. Electroencephalography analyses show abnormalities in the majority of patients. Some authors advocate that brain lesions of morphea are more epileptogenic than those of other autoimmune disorders [33].

Computed tomography (CT) and MRI studies have shown central nervous system abnormalities in ECDS patients. Neurologic findings are more frequently ipsilateral to the skin lesions, but contralateral involvement has been described [34]. Neurologic symptoms should not be used as a predictor for MRI abnormalities because neurologic lesions have been discovered in asymptomatic patients [35]. Moreover, symptomatic patients were sometimes proven to have a normal radiologic examination. Cerebral angiograms and magnetic resonance angiogram studies showed vascular involvement suggestive of vasculitis. Reports of cerebral aneurysms and other vascular malformations, such as brain cavernomas, exist and could represent late sequelae of the vasculitic process [36, 37].

Box 11.5: Neurological manifestations in morphea (mainly in linear morphea involving face).
Seizures of various types
Headache
Focal neurologic deficits
Movement disorders
Intellectual deterioration
Vasculitis
Cerebral aneurysms
Brain cavernomas
Neuropsychiatric symptoms

D-penicillamine, methylprednisolone, mycophenolate mofetil, and methotrexate might be considered in the treatment of neurologic involvement of ECDS [38]. In reported cases combination of methotrexate or mycophenolate mofetil and steroids appeared to have an impact on controlling intractable seizures and stabilizing central nervous system damage [39, 40].

Renal Manifestations

Zulian *et al.* [5] studied the prevalence and clinical features of extracutaneous manifestations in a large cohort of children with pediatric morphea. In their study, they noticed proteinuria and haematuria in 2 patients, but neither of these patients experienced renal failure in the follow-up period.

Respiratory Manifestations

Although the distinction between SSC and morphea is restricted to the presence or absence of internal organ disease; in some cases, organ involvement has been demonstrated in morphea; though patients were asymptomatic and involvement was mild [41]. The literature describes a few cases of extrapulmonary disease secondary to morphea due to the involvement of muscles and subcutaneous tissue of the chest wall [42, 43]. A case of interstitial lung involvement in ECDS has also been reported [44]. Zulian *et al.* [5] in their study reported respiratory involvement in 5 patients (0.5%), all of them having moderate dyspnea and/or persistent cough, with 1 patient having pulmonary insufficiency. Results of pulmonary function tests showed a restrictive pattern in 3 patients and abnormalities in diffusing capacity for carbon monoxide (DLCO) in 2 patients [5]. Persistent basal infiltrates on chest radiography and high-resolution computed tomography were observed in 2 patients [5]. Similar findings were previously reported in patients with linear morphea who underwent routine respiratory function tests and chest radiography [45].

Oral Manifestations

Oral involvement in morphea is very rare, with less than 20 reports noted in the literature [46]. Linear morphea of the oral cavity typically involves the mucosal lip and upper anterior teeth [47 - 49]. Depending on the stage of progression at the time of diagnosis, these patients may present with varying degrees of gingival recession, alveolar bone loss, atrophy of the tongue, and loosening of the teeth [47 - 49]. Most of these patients have been treated successfully with an initial combination of oral or intramuscular methotrexate as well as systemic corticosteroids for at least 1 year before a subsequent taper [50, 51]. A cross-sectional, multicentre study performed in Denmark showed a higher incidence of odontostomatologic abnormalities in patients with linear morphea of the face [52]. In that study, 16 patients were investigated and all these patients reported at least one of the following odontostomatologic complications: malocclusion, overgrowth tendency of the anterior lower third of the face, gnatologic alterations, dental anomalies, skeletal asymmetry, bone involvement, and temporomandibular joint involvement [53].

It is important for the clinician to keep morphea in the differential diagnosis when evaluating the oral cavity, as untreated linear morphea may lead to atrophy of the tongue papillae, demineralization and loosening of teeth, and recession of oral gingivae (Box **11.6**) [46]. Prompt treatment of this inflammatory disease with immunosuppressive medications allows for the prevention of these possible complications and the need for further trauma to the affected area with maxillofacial reconstructive efforts [46].

Box 11.6: Oral manifestations in morphea (mainly in linear morphea involving the face).
Malocclusion
Overgrowth tendency of the anterior lower third of the face
Gnatologic alterations
Dental anomalies
Skeletal asymmetry
Alveolar bone loss
Temporomandibular joint involvement
Atrophy of the tongue papillae
Teeth demineralization
Loosening of teeth
Gingival Recession

Thyroid Abnormalities

The association of thyroid dysfunction with morphea has not yet been established and only a few studies and case reports are available in the literature [53]. Thyroid hormones act on nuclear receptors of human fibroblasts and intermediate the regulation of collagen synthesis and degradation [54]. The co-existence of two autoimmune diseases in patients may not have occurred by chance, but could be attributed to autoimmune reactions elicited by the recognition of common antigens. The existence of a separate subset of scleroderma with autoimmune thyroiditis is another possibility that has to be seriously explored [54].

Malignant Complications

Morphea is a localized form of scleroderma that occasionally leads to chronic erosions and ulcerations of the skin. Morphea is therefore, a rare, but established risk factor for cutaneous squamous cell carcinoma (SCC) [55]. The pathophysiological sequence that triggers cutaneous SCC in morphea patients may start with an increased tendency of skin areas affected by fibrosis to develop erosions and ulcers [55]. Fibrosis leads to reduced skin elasticity, diminished resistance to shear forces as well as poor nutrient and oxygen supply of the involved tissue, resulting in increased skin vulnerability [55]. Several authors have described the development of cutaneous SCC, the second most frequent type of skin cancer, on long-standing lesions of generalized morphea [56 - 58]. SCC has been reported to present as malignant ulcers in pansclerotic morphea of childhood in a 16-year-old boy [59].

So, it becomes imperative for the clinicians carrying out follow-up examinations to be well aware of possible tumor development on long-standing morphea lesions [55]. Moreover, common therapeutic strategies for morphea, such as immunosuppressive medication and phototherapy, should be viewed critically in light of their potential carcinogenic side effects [55]. A careful risk-benefit analysis should be performed when considering the application of such therapies for patients suffering from morphea [55].

CONCLUSION

In conclusion, patients with morphea who have extracutaneous manifestations represent a newly described subset of patients with peculiar clinical and laboratory features. In these patients, organ impairment is milder than that seen in patients with SSC and is not life-threatening.

Box 11.7: Learning points.
• Though morphea primarily involves skin but there may be extracutaneous manifestations associated with it.
• Among extracutaneous manifestations, musculoskeletal findings are the commonest.
• In case of linear morphea involving face, neurological and ocular manifestations are common and it becomes imperative to screen for the same. In such cases oral and dental manifestations should also be looked for.
• Current evidence doesn't recommend routine work up for gastroesophageal system. However, morphea patients symptomatic for gastroesophageal symptoms or having autoantibodies may require evaluation.
• Rarely, extrapulmonary disease secondary to morphea due to the involvement of muscles and subcutaneous tissue of the chest wall can occur which may cause restrictive lung disease.

REFERENCES

[1]   Birdi N, Laxer RM, Thorner P, Fritzler MJ, Silverman ED. Morphea progressing to systemic disease. Case report and review of the literature. Arthritis Rheum 1993; 36: 410-5.
       [http://dx.doi.org/10.1002/art.1780360318] [PMID: 8452586]

[2]   Mayorquin FJ, McCurley TL, Levernier JE, *et al.* Progression of childhood linear scleroderma to fatal systemic sclerosis. J Rheumatol 1994; 21(10): 1955-7.
       [PMID: 7837166]

[3]   Christen-Zaech S, Hakim MD, Afsar FS, Paller AS. Pediatric morphea (morphea): Review of 136 patients. J Am Acad Dermatol 2008; 59: 385-96.
       [http://dx.doi.org/10.1016/j.jaad.2008.05.005] [PMID: 18571769]

[4]   Tekin NS, Altinyazar HC, Tekin IO, Keskin SI, Kucukoglu R, Onsun N. Disabling pansclerotic morphoea: A case report. Int J Clin Pract 2010; 64(1): 99-101.

[http://dx.doi.org/10.1111/j.1742-1241.2006.01039.x] [PMID: 20089019]

[5]   Zulian F, Vallongo C, Woo P, *et al.* Morphea in childhood is not just a skin disease. Arthritis Rheum 2005; 52: 2873-81.
[http://dx.doi.org/10.1002/art.21264] [PMID: 16142730]

[6]   Leitenberger JJ, Cayce RL, Haley RW, Adams-Huet B, Bergstresser PR, Jacobe HT. Distinct autoimmune syndromes in morphea: A review of 245 adult and pediatric cases. Arch Dermatol 2009; 145(5): 545-50.
[http://dx.doi.org/10.1001/archdermatol.2009.79] [PMID: 19451498]

[7]   Kreuter A, Krieg T, Worm M, *et al.* Deutsche Dermatologische Gesellschaft AWMF Guideline no. 013/066. Diagnosis and therapy of circumscribed scleroderma. J Dtsch Dermatol Ges 2009; 7 (Suppl. 6): S1-S14.
[PMID: 19660073]

[8]   Schanz S, Fierlbeck G, Ulmer A, *et al.* Morphea: MR findings and clinical features. Radiology 2011; 260: 817-24.
[http://dx.doi.org/10.1148/radiol.11102136] [PMID: 21693661]

[9]   Zaninotto G, Peserico A, Costantini M, Salvador L, Rondinone R. Oesophageal motility and lower oesophageal sphincter competence in progressive SSC and morphea. Scand J Gastroenterol 1989; 24: 95-102.
[http://dx.doi.org/10.3109/00365528909092245] [PMID: 2928728]

[10]   Guariso G, Conte S, Galeazzi F, Vettorato MG, Martini G, Zulian F. Esophageal involvement in juvenile morphea: a pilot study. Clin Exp Rheumatol 2007; 25: 786-9.
[PMID: 18078634]

[11]   Arif T. Screening for esophageal involvement in morphea: Is it needed? JPAD 2018; 28: 395-7.

[12]   Arif T, Masood Q, Singh J, Hassan I. Assessment of esophageal involvement in systemic sclerosis and morphea (localized scleroderma) by clinical, endoscopic, manometric and pH metric features: a prospective comparative hospital based study. BMC Gastroenterol 2015; 15(1): 24.
[http://dx.doi.org/10.1186/s12876-015-0241-2] [PMID: 25888470]

[13]   Weber P, Ganser G, Frosch M, Roth J, Hülskamp G, Zimmer KP. Twenty-four hour intraesophageal pH monitoring in children and adolescents with scleroderma and mixed connective tissue disease. J Rheumatol 2000; 27(11): 2692-5.
[PMID: 11093455]

[14]   Lambova S. Cardiac manifestations in systemic sclerosis. World J Cardiol 2014; 6(9): 993-1005.
[http://dx.doi.org/10.4330/wjc.v6.i9.993] [PMID: 25276300]

[15]   Rokicki W, Dukalska M, Rubisz-Brzezinska J, Gasior Z. Circulatory system in children with morphea. Pediatr Cardiol 1997; 18: 213-7.
[http://dx.doi.org/10.1007/s002469900153] [PMID: 9142712]

[16]   Targa L, Cardin G, Cozzi F. ECG abnormalities in the various clinical subtypes of scleroderma. G Clin Med 1990; 71: 17-24.
[PMID: 2142111]

[17]   Zannin ME, Martini G, Athreya BH, *et al.* Juvenile Scleroderma Working Group of the Pediatric Rheumatology European Society (PRES). Ocular involvement in children with localised scleroderma: a multi-centre study. Br J Ophthalmol 2007; 91(10): 1311-4.
[http://dx.doi.org/10.1136/bjo.2007.116038] [PMID: 17475707]

[18]   Peterson LS, Nelson AM, Su WPD. Classification of morphea (morphea). Mayo Clin Proc 1995; 70: 1068-76.
[http://dx.doi.org/10.4065/70.11.1068] [PMID: 7475336]

[19]   Rees TD. Facial atrophy. Clin Plast Surg 1976; 3(4): 637-46.
[PMID: 788999]

[20] West RH, Barnett AJ. Ocular involvement in scleroderma. Br J Ophthalmol 1979; 63(12): 845-7.
[http://dx.doi.org/10.1136/bjo.63.12.845] [PMID: 526467]

[21] Muchnick RS, Aston SJ, Rees TD. Ocular manifestations and treatment of hemifacial atrophy. Am J Ophthalmol 1979; 88(5): 889-97.
[http://dx.doi.org/10.1016/0002-9394(79)90567-1] [PMID: 507167]

[22] Blaszczyk M, Królicki L, Krasu M, Glinska O, Jablonska S. Progressive facial hemiatrophy: central nervous system involvement and relationship with scleroderma en coup de sabre. J Rheumatol 2003; 30(9): 1997-2004.
[PMID: 12966605]

[23] Katsumoto TR, Whitfield ML, Connolly MK. The pathogenesis of systemic sclerosis. Annu Rev Pathol 2011; 6(1): 509-37.
[http://dx.doi.org/10.1146/annurev-pathol-011110-130312] [PMID: 21090968]

[24] Marzano AV, Menni S, Parodi A, *et al.* Morphea in adults and children: clinical and laboratory investigations of 239 cases. Eur J Dermatol 2003; 13: 171-6.
[PMID: 12695134]

[25] Stone J, Franks AJ, Guthrie JA, Johnson MH. Scleroderma en coup de sabre: pathological evidence of intracerebral inflammation. J Neurol Neurosurg Psychiatry 2001; 70(3): 382-5.
[http://dx.doi.org/10.1136/jnnp.70.3.382] [PMID: 11181863]

[26] Menni S, Marzano AV, Passoni E. Neurologic abnormalities in two patients with facial hemiatrophy and sclerosis coexisting with morphea. Pediatr Dermatol 1997; 14(2): 113-6.
[http://dx.doi.org/10.1111/j.1525-1470.1997.tb00216.x] [PMID: 9144696]

[27] Kister I, Inglese M, Laxer RM, Herbert J. Neurologic manifestations of morphea: A case report and literature review. Neurology 2008; 71: 1538-45.
[http://dx.doi.org/10.1212/01.wnl.0000334474.88923.e3] [PMID: 18981376]

[28] Flores-Alvarado DE, Esquivel-Valerio JA, Garza-Elizondo M, Espinoza LR. Linear scleroderma en coup de sabre and brain calcification: is there a pathogenic relationship? J Rheumatol 2003; 30(1): 193-5.
[PMID: 12508412]

[29] David J, Wilson J, Woo P. Scleroderma en coup de sabre. Ann Rheum Dis 1991; 50(4): 260-2.
[http://dx.doi.org/10.1136/ard.50.4.260] [PMID: 1903032]

[30] Unterberger I, Trinka E, Engelhardt K, *et al.* Linear scleroderma en coup de sabre coexisting with plaque-morphea: neuroradiological manifestation and response to corticosteroids. J Neurol Neurosurg Psychia 2003; 74(5): 661-4.
[http://dx.doi.org/10.1136/jnnp.74.5.661] [PMID: 12700315]

[31] Carreño M, Donaire A, Barceló MI, *et al.* Parry Romberg syndrome and linear scleroderma in coup de sabre mimicking Rasmussen encephalitis. Neurology 2007; 68(16): 1308-10.
[http://dx.doi.org/10.1212/01.wnl.0000259523.09001.7a] [PMID: 17438222]

[32] Shah JR, Juhász C, Kupsky WJ, *et al.* Rasmussen encephalitis associated with Parry–Romberg syndrome. Neurology 2003; 61(3): 395-7.
[http://dx.doi.org/10.1212/WNL.61.3.395] [PMID: 12913207]

[33] Amaral TN, Marques Neto JF, Lapa AT, Peres FA, Guirau CR, Appenzeller S. Neurologic involvement in scleroderma en coup de sabre. Autoimmune Dis 2012; 2012: 1-6.
[http://dx.doi.org/10.1155/2012/719685] [PMID: 22319646]

[34] Obermoser G, Pfausler BE, Linder DM, Sepp NT. Scleroderma en coup de sabre with central nervous system and ophthalmologic involvement: Treatment of ocular symptoms with interferon gamma. J Am Acad Dermatol 2003; 49(3): 543-6.
[http://dx.doi.org/10.1067/S0190-9622(03)00901-0] [PMID: 12963929]

[35]   Appenzeller S, Montenegro MA, San Juan Dertkigil S, *et al.* Neuroimaging findings in scleroderma *en coup de sabre.* Neurology 2004; 62(9): 1585-9.
        [http://dx.doi.org/10.1212/01.WNL.0000124518.25087.18] [PMID: 15136686]

[36]   Fain ET, Mannion M, Pope E, Young DW, Laxer RM, Cron RQ. Brain cavernomas associated with en coup de sabre linear scleroderma: Two case reports. Pediatr Rheumatol Onl J 2011; 9(1): 18.
        [http://dx.doi.org/10.1186/1546-0096-9-18] [PMID: 21801349]

[37]   Catala M, Mellinger JF, Atkinson JLD. Progressive intracranial aneurysmal disease in a child with progressive hemifacial atrophy (Parry-Romberg disease): Case report. Neurosurgery 1998; 42(5): 1195-6.
        [http://dx.doi.org/10.1097/00006123-199805000-00161] [PMID: 9588570]

[38]   Holland KE, Steffes B, Nocton JJ, Schwabe MJ, Jacobson RD, Drolet BA. Linear scleroderma ECDS with associated neurologic abnormalities. Pediatrics 2006; 117(1): e132-6.
        [http://dx.doi.org/10.1542/peds.2005-0470]

[39]   Paprocka J, Jamroz E, Adamek D, Marszal E, Mandera M. Difficulties in differentiation of Parry–Romberg syndrome, unilateral facial sclerodermia, and Rasmussen syndrome. Childs Nerv Syst 2006; 22(4): 409-15.
        [http://dx.doi.org/10.1007/s00381-005-1262-x] [PMID: 16247619]

[40]   Sartori S, Martini G, Calderone M, Patrizi A, Gobbi G, Zulian F. Severe epilepsy preceding by four months the onset of scleroderma en coup de sabre. Clin Exp Rheumatol 2009; 27(3) (Suppl. 54): 64-7.
        [PMID: 19796565]

[41]   Dehen L, Roujeau JC, Cosnes A, Revuz J. Internal involvement in morphea. Medicine 1994; 73: 241-5.
        [http://dx.doi.org/10.1097/00005792-199409000-00002] [PMID: 7934808]

[42]   Aguayo S, Richardson C, Roman J. Severe extrapulmonary thoracic restriction caused by Morphea, a form of morphea. Chest 1993; 104: 1304-5.
        [http://dx.doi.org/10.1378/chest.104.4.1304] [PMID: 8404222]

[43]   Nagai Y, Hattori T, Ishikawa O. Unilateral generalized morphea in childhood. J Dermatol 2002; 29(7): 435-8.
        [http://dx.doi.org/10.1111/j.1346-8138.2002.tb00301.x] [PMID: 12184643]

[44]   Pérez J, Fernández O. Lung Disease Secondary to Morphea ECDS, a Form of Morphea. Arch Bronconeumol 2009; 45(8): 411-6.
        [http://dx.doi.org/10.1016/S1579-2129(09)72941-6] [PMID: 19398256]

[45]   Bourgeois-Droin C, Touraine R. [Scleroderma in plaques. Immunological and visceral disturbances (author's transl)]. Ann Med Interne 1978; 129(2): 107-12.
        [PMID: 305741]

[46]   Lopez Pineiro M, Lee K, Pinney S. A case of linear morphea involving the oral cavity. JAAD Case Rep 2019; 5(2): 144-6.
        [http://dx.doi.org/10.1016/j.jdcr.2018.10.024] [PMID: 30733981]

[47]   Hørberg M, Lauesen SR, Daugaard-Jensen J, Kjær I. Linear scleroderma en coup de sabre including abnormal dental development. Eur Arch Paediatr Dent 2015; 16(2): 227-31.
        [http://dx.doi.org/10.1007/s40368-014-0148-6] [PMID: 25355303]

[48]   Niklander S, Marín C, Martínez R. Morphea ECDS: An unusual oral presentation. J Clin Exp Dent 2017; 9: 315-8.

[49]   Baxter AM, Roberts A, Shaw L. Morphea in a 12-year-old girl presenting as gingival recession. A case report and literature review. Dent Update 2001; 28: 458-62.
        [http://dx.doi.org/10.12968/denu.2001.28.9.458] [PMID: 11806189]

[50]   Barton DH, Henderson HZ. Oral-facial characteristics of circumscribed scleroderma: Case report. J

Clin Pediatr Dent 1993; 17(4): 239-42.
[PMID: 8217889]

[51]   Wang P, Guo W, Liu S. A rare case of juvenile morphea with intra-oral and dental involvement. Exp Ther Med 2015; 10: 2213-5.
[http://dx.doi.org/10.3892/etm.2015.2791] [PMID: 26668618]

[52]   Trainito S, Favero L, Martini G, *et al.* Odontostomatologic involvement in juvenile localised scleroderma of the face. J Paediatr Child Health 2012; 48(7): 572-6.
[http://dx.doi.org/10.1111/j.1440-1754.2012.02435.x] [PMID: 22409322]

[53]   Lee HJ, Kim MY, Ha SJ, Kim JW. Two cases of morphea associated with Hashimoto's thyroiditis. Acta Derm Venereol 2002; 82(1): 58-9.
[http://dx.doi.org/10.1080/000155502753600920] [PMID: 12013202]

[54]   Hiremath NC, Madan Mohan NT, Srinivas C, Sangolli PM, Srinivas K, Vrushali VD. Juvenile morphea with autoimmune thyroid disorder. Indian J Dermatol 2010; 55: 308-9.
[http://dx.doi.org/10.4103/0019-5154.70701] [PMID: 21063540]

[55]   Heck J, Olk J, Kneitz H, Hamm H, Goebeler M. Long-standing morphea and the risk of squamous cell carcinoma of the skin. J Dtsch Dermatol Ges 2020; 18(7): 669-73.
[http://dx.doi.org/10.1111/ddg.14096] [PMID: 32364667]

[56]   Michalowski R. Diffuse morphoea with calcinosis cutis and squamous-cell carcinoma. Br J Dermatol 1967; 79(8-9): 453-5.
[http://dx.doi.org/10.1111/j.1365-2133.1967.tb11532.x] [PMID: 6039630]

[57]   Gréco M, Kupfer-Bessaguet L, Delahaye JF, Plantin P. Multiple cutaneous squamous cell carcinomas arising in a patient with generalized morphea. Eur J Dermatol 2006; 16(1): 90-1.
[PMID: 16436352]

[58]   Saleh DB, Williams AM, Smith IM. Cutaneous squamous cell carcinoma arising within generalised morphea. J Plast Reconstr Aesthet Surg 2011; 64(6): e149-52.
[http://dx.doi.org/10.1016/j.bjps.2011.01.019] [PMID: 21420372]

[59]   Wollina U, Buslau M, Weyers W. Squamous cell carcinoma in pansclerotic morphea of childhood. Pediatr Dermatol 2002; 19(2): 151-4.
[http://dx.doi.org/10.1046/j.1525-1470.2002.00033.x] [PMID: 11994182]

CHAPTER 12

Disease Prognosis

Adriana Polańska[1,*], Aleksandra Dańczak-Pazdrowska[2], Ryszard Żaba[1] and **Zygmunt Adamski[2]**

[1] *Department of Dermatology and Venereology, University of Medical Sciences, Poznan, Poland*

[2] *Department of Dermatology, University of Medical Sciences, Poznan, Poland*

Chapter synopsis.
• Morphea is a chronic and relapsing skin disease; its course depends on the specific clinical variant.
• The typical course of morphea is self-limited and takes approximately 3- 5 years.
• The morphea prognosis is good, however, the disease may relapse. The relapsing course of the morphea is mainly observed in linear and generalized variants.
• The rapid progression of the disease is observed among patients suffering from generalized morphea and disabling pansclerotic morphea.
• The factor significantly associated with worse outcomes may be related to the prolonged time from diagnosis to treatment.
• Morphea affects the patient's quality of life, especially in adult and female patients.

Keywords: Circumscribed morphea, En coup de sabre, Extracutaneous complications, Generalized morphea, Functional disabilities, Joint contractures, linear morphea, Morphea course, Morphea prognosis, Morphea recurrence, Morphea relapse, Morphea plaque, Musculoskeletal complications, Pansclerotic morphea, Progression of morphea, Quality of life, Relapsing course of morphea, Unpredictable course, Worse prognosis.

INTRODUCTION

Morphea belongs to chronic and relapsing skin disorders [1]. The natural course of morphea, especially in localized forms, is usually mild and predictable, leading to mainly cosmetic consequences (dyspigmentation and/or telangiectasia which

* **Corresponding author Adriana Polańska:** Department of Dermatology and Venereology, University of Medical Sciences, Poznan, Poland; E-mail: adriana-polanska@wp.pl

Tasleem Arif (Ed.)

can be also of post-steroidal origin) [2]. However, its course and prognosis are mainly related to its clinical subtypes. Unpredictable course and worse prognosis may concern deep, linear forms as well pansclerotic morphea.

Morphea which involves subcutaneous tissue, muscle tissue and bones may lead to functional disabilities including joint contractures and limb length discrepancies. Approximately 20-40% of children may present extracutaneous complications, and musculoskeletal manifestations are the commonest [3, 4]. Internal organ involvement is rare, however possible, especially associated with the involvement of the central nervous system and the organ of vision. The aspects related to extracutaneous manifestations in morphea are described in detail in Chapter 11.

MORPHEA COURSE

The usual course of morphea is self-limited and takes approximately 3- 5 years [3, 4]. The typical plaque changes the morphology over time. In the initial active phase of morphea, it is characterized by an erythematous, violaceous border (lilac ring) and central induration, which becomes discolored and often turns into a yellowish-white (ivory) color [5]. Inactive lesions of morphea are mainly characterized by atrophy and dyspigmentation. Deeper skin involvement may be accompanied by hair loss. Although the disappearance of the erythema indicates that the inflammatory phase has subsided, what takes usually several months, sclerosis may resolve within years. The softening of the skin lesions in plaque morphea may take approximately 2.7 years after diagnosis and occurs in half of the patients. However, this process in deep forms of morphea may take even up to 5.5 years [6]. The decrease in induration indicates an improvement in the clinical condition, similarly to hair regrowth [2]. In deep and linear forms of morphea, tissue damage and atrophy appear at the beginning and may remain stable over time, despite the treatment. To limit and stabilize the disease, treatment should be introduced as early as possible [7, 8].

Adults with pediatric-onset morphea are less likely to present with active disease and are characterized by higher disease damage [measured by Physician Global Assessment of Disease Activity (PGA-A)] [9]. The most aggressive disease course was observed among children with linear subtypes and more than 10% of them presented with persistent activity lasting longer than 10 years [7]. In Parry-Romberg syndrome, the disease usually presents with a slow progression over a highly variable course ranging from 2 to 20 years [10]. The factor significantly associated with worse outcomes could be the prolonged time from diagnosis to treatment [7].

The rapid progression of the disease is observed among patients suffering from generalized morphea and disabling pansclerotic morphea [2, 4, 5]. According to Alimova *et al.* the generalized morphea as the initial presentation and positive baseline ANA may be associated with the worsening course of the disease [11]. Due to the progressive, extensive and deep sclerosis, the disease may lead to disability in a short period of time [12]. Hard-to-heal ulcers and calcification can be associated with dermatogenic contractures. Moreover, the occurrence of squamous cell carcinoma in the area of ulcers has also been described, especially within the lower extremities [13]. In (Box **12.1**) characteristic features of morphea related to its course are listed.

Box 12.1: Characteristic features of morphea course.
The usual course lasts 3-5 years.
The morphology changes over time.
The softening of skin lesions may take 2.7 – 5.5 years.
In linear and deep morphea, the disease damage may persist despite the treatment.
The most aggressive disease course regarding children is with linear subtype and may present with persistent disease activity.
The slow progression usually occurs in Parry-Romberg syndrome.
The rapid progression is usually seen in generalized morphea and disabling pansclerotic morphea.

MORPHEA RECURRENCE

Although long-term studies evaluating the recurrence risk in morphea are limited, especially in the adult population, the disease shows significant relapse tendency [1, 9, 14 - 16]. Florenz-Pollack *et al.* conducted a prospective study on a group of children and adults [17]. 66% of patients treated with methotrexate and 41% with UVA1 had achieved a complete response in a 1-year follow-up period. In that group of patients, almost one-third experienced disease flare-ups at an average of 1.7 years after remission [17]. The longer periods between remission and relapse have been reported by other researchers [7, 16]. Martens *et al.* observed that recurrence occurs more frequently in the juvenile population than in adult one (27% vs.17%, respectively) and the median time for morphea relapse was 26 -27 months. Moreover, they considered linear morphea of the limbs as the most frequently recurrent variant [16]. In other studies, the higher recurrence rate was related to generalized morphea [16]. After 5 years, the recurrence was observed in 44% of patients as a new activity in the area of previous morphea plaque [16]. In the study of Saxton-Daniels *et al.* the percentage of new or expanded lesions was even higher and accounted for 89% [14].

The recurrent course of morphea may indicate necessary life-long evaluation even after a prolonged period of inactivity [14, 18]. A relatively high relapse rate was seen after the completion of a full course of treatment with systemic medications [18]. However, it is worth emphasizing that the recurrence rate after UVA1 phototherapy may be higher than after methotrexate, which can be related to the shorter duration of phototherapy [1, 17]. One of the largest studies in juvenile morphea describing both clinical course and long-term outcomes was presented by the Italian group [7] and also shows that flare occurrence can not be inhibited by systemic treatment. They found lowered relapse rate than detected in previous studies (22%); however, they reported multiple reactivations despite the introduction of systemic treatment [7]. In (Box **12.2**), the summary of morphea recurrence is presented.

Box 12.2: Characteristic features of morphea recurrence.
Morphea has a tendency to relapse.
Morphea relapses can occur years after remission and despite systemic treatment.
The linear morphea of the limbs and generalised subtype are the most frequently recurring variants.
The long-term follow-up of morphea patients should be practiced.

MORPHEA PSYCHOLOGIC COMPLICATIONS

There are several studies analyzing the impact of morphea on quality of life (QoL) but they show inconsistent data [19 - 25]. Most of them showed that QoL is disturbed to a mild and medium degree and may be lower than in patients with non-melanoma skin cancers, vitiligo or alopecia [26]. A negative impact on QoL was described especially in adult patients who presented physical disability suffering from a linear subtype of morphea as well as in patients with generalized type and eosinophilic fasciitis [23 - 27]. Children with morphea have good coping strategies and present better QoL than adults [23, 27]. Although, there are studies describing no influence of the severity of the disease as well as no relation of disease-induced skin damage on QoL [23, 27]. The pain and pruritus may also influence QoL, but also sociodemographic characteristics like older age, female gender and living conditions may also impair it [19, 23, 28, 29]. According to some authors, the evaluation of QoL in morphea patients is challenging and there is a need for further investigations in that field and searching for new assessment methods dedicated to these patients [23]. (Box **12.3**) highlights the important aspects of the quality of life of morphea patients.

Box 12.3: Morphea and quality of life.

Morphea may influence a patient's quality of life.

The linear, generalized types of morphea and eosinophilic fasciitis have the strongest impact on quality of life.

Worse quality of life is observed among female patients.

The subjective symptoms as well as sociodemographic conditions have an impact on the quality of morphea patients.

Box 12.4: Learning points.

• Although the disappearance of the erythema indicates that the inflammatory phase of morphea has subsided, which takes usually several months, sclerosis may resolve within years after discontinuation of the treatment.

• Morphea shows a significant relapse tendency (especially linear and generalized variants) which is also possible after the completion of a full course of treatment with systemic medications.

• A negative impact on the quality of life was described especially in adult patients having a physical disability and suffering from a linear subtype of morphea as well as in patients with generalized type and eosinophilic fasciitis.

REFERENCES

[1]   Vasquez R, Jabbar A, Khan F, Buethe D, Ahn C, Jacobe H. Recurrence of morphea after successful ultraviolet A1 phototherapy: A cohort study. J Am Acad Dermatol 2014; 70(3): 481-8.
[http://dx.doi.org/10.1016/j.jaad.2013.10.018] [PMID: 24365168]

[2]   Florez-Pollack S, Kunzler E, Jacobe HT. Morphea: Current concepts. Clin Dermatol 2018; 36(4): 475-86.
[http://dx.doi.org/10.1016/j.clindermatol.2018.04.005] [PMID: 30047431]

[3]   Christianson HB, Dorsey CS, Kierland RR, O'Leary PA. Localized scleroderma. AMA Arch Derm 1956; 74(6): 629-39.
[http://dx.doi.org/10.1001/archderm.1956.01550120049012] [PMID: 13371921]

[4]   Mertens JS, Seyger MMB, Thurlings RM, Radstake TRDJ, de Jong EMGJ. Morphea and eosinophilic fasciitis: An update. Am J Clin Dermatol 2017; 18(4): 491-512.
[http://dx.doi.org/10.1007/s40257-017-0269-x] [PMID: 28303481]

[5]   Fett N. Scleroderma: Nomenclature, etiology, pathogenesis, prognosis, and treatments: Facts and controversies. Clin Dermatol 2013; 31(4): 432-7.
[http://dx.doi.org/10.1016/j.clindermatol.2013.01.010] [PMID: 23806160]

[6]   Peterson LS, Nelson AM, Su WPD. Classification of morphea (localized scleroderma). Mayo Clin Proc 1995; 70(11): 1068-76.
[http://dx.doi.org/10.4065/70.11.1068] [PMID: 7475336]

[7]   Martini G, Fadanelli G, Agazzi A, Vittadello F, Meneghel A, Zulian F. Disease course and long-term outcome of juvenile localized scleroderma: Experience from a single pediatric rheumatology Centre and literature review. Autoimmun Rev 2018; 17(7): 727-34.
[http://dx.doi.org/10.1016/j.autrev.2018.02.004] [PMID: 29729451]

[8]   Fett N, Werth VP. Update on morphea. J Am Acad Dermatol 2011; 64(2): 231-42.
[http://dx.doi.org/10.1016/j.jaad.2010.05.046] [PMID: 21238824]

[9]   Condie D, Grabell D, Jacobe H. Comparison of outcomes in adults with pediatric-onset morphea and those with adult-onset morphea: A cross-sectional study from the morphea in adults and children cohort. Arthritis Rheumatol 2014; 66(12): 3496-504.
[http://dx.doi.org/10.1002/art.38853] [PMID: 25156342]

[10]   Wong M, Phillips CD, Hagiwara M, Shatzkes DR. Parry romberg syndrome: 7 cases and literature review. AJNR Am J Neuroradiol 2015; 36(7): 1355-61.
[http://dx.doi.org/10.3174/ajnr.A4297] [PMID: 26066627]

[11]   Alimova E, Farhi D, Plantier F, *et al.* Morphoea (localized scleroderma): Baseline body surface involvement and antinuclear antibody may have a prognostic value. Clin Exp Dermatol 2009; 34(7): e491-2.
[http://dx.doi.org/10.1111/j.1365-2230.2009.03557.x] [PMID: 19747327]

[12]   Maragh SH, Davis MDP, Bruce AJ, Nelson AM. Disabling pansclerotic morphea: Clinical presentation in two adults. J Am Acad Dermatol 2005; 53(2 Suppl. 1): S115-9.
[http://dx.doi.org/10.1016/j.jaad.2004.10.881] [PMID: 16021158]

[13]   Heck J, Olk J, Kneitz H, Hamm H, Goebeler M. Long□standing morphea and the risk of squamous cell carcinoma of the skin. J Dtsch Dermatol Ges 2020; 18(7): 669-73.
[http://dx.doi.org/10.1111/ddg.14096] [PMID: 32364667]

[14]   Saxton-Daniels S, Jacobe HT. An evaluation of long-term outcomes in adults with pediatric-onset morphea. Arch Dermatol 2010; 146(9): 1044-5.
[http://dx.doi.org/10.1001/archdermatol.2010.239] [PMID: 20855712]

[15]   Piram M, McCuaig CC, Saint-Cyr C, *et al.* Short and long-term outcome of linear morphoea in children. Br J Dermatol 2013; 169(6): 1265-71.
[http://dx.doi.org/10.1111/bjd.12606] [PMID: 24032480]

[16]   Mertens JS, Seyger MMB, Kievit W, *et al.* Disease recurrence in localized scleroderma: A retrospective analysis of 344 patients with paediatric or adult-onset disease. Br J Dermatol 2015; 172(3): 722-8.
[http://dx.doi.org/10.1111/bjd.13514] [PMID: 25381928]

[17]   Florez-Pollack S, O'Brien JC, Jacobe HT. 2547 Long-term response to treatment and disease recurrence in a prospective cohort of morphea patients. J Clin Transl Sci 2018; 2(S1): 43-4.
[http://dx.doi.org/10.1017/cts.2018.170]

[18]   Kurzinski K, Zigler C, Torok D. Prediction of disease relapse in a cohort of juvenile localized scleroderma patients. Br J Dermatol 2019; 180: 1183-9.

[19]   Lis-Święty A, Skrzypek-Salamon A, Ranosz-Janicka I, Brzezińska-Wcisło L. Health-related quality of life and its influencing factors in adult patients with localized scleroderma: A cross-sectional study. Health Qual Life Outcomes 2020; 18(1): 133.
[http://dx.doi.org/10.1186/s12955-020-01386-0] [PMID: 32398135]

[20]   Kroft EBM, de Jong EMGJ, Evers AWM. Physical burden of symptoms in patients with localized scleroderma and eosinophilic fasciitis. Arch Dermatol 2008; 144(10): 1394-5.
[http://dx.doi.org/10.1001/archderm.144.10.1394] [PMID: 18936410]

[21]   Kroft EBM, de Jong EMGJ, Evers AWM. Psychological distress in patients with morphea and eosinophilic fasciitis. Arch Dermatol 2009; 145(9): 1017-22.
[http://dx.doi.org/10.1001/archdermatol.2009.202] [PMID: 19770441]

[22]   Das S, Bernstein I, Jacobe H. Correlates of self-reported quality of life in adults and children with morphea. J Am Acad Dermatol 2014; 70(5): 904-10.
[http://dx.doi.org/10.1016/j.jaad.2013.11.037] [PMID: 24534655]

[23]   Klimas NK, Shedd AD, Bernstein IH, Jacobe H. Health-related quality of life in morphoea. Br J Dermatol 2015; 172(5): 1329-37.
[http://dx.doi.org/10.1111/bjd.13572] [PMID: 25483169]

[24]   Bali G, Kárpáti S, Sárdy M, Brodszky V, Hidvégi B, Rencz F. Association between quality of life and clinical characteristics in patients with morphea. Qual Life Res 2018; 27(10): 2525-32.
[http://dx.doi.org/10.1007/s11136-018-1897-1] [PMID: 29922914]

[25]   Szczęch J, Samotij D, Jaworecka K, Tobiasz A, Reich A. Quality of life in patients with morphea: A cross-sectional study and a review of the current literature. BioMed Res Int 2020; 2020: 1-8.
[http://dx.doi.org/10.1155/2020/9186274] [PMID: 32258158]

[26]   Dehen L, Roujeau JC, Cosnes A, Revuz J. Internal involvement in localized scleroderma. Medicine 1994; 73(5): 241-5.
[http://dx.doi.org/10.1097/00005792-199409000-00002] [PMID: 7934808]

[27]   Szramka-Pawlak B, Dańczak-Pazdrowska A, Rzepa T, Szewczyk A, Sadowska-Przytocka A, Żaba R. Quality of life and optimism in patients with morphea. Appl Res Qual Life 2014; 9(4): 863-70.
[http://dx.doi.org/10.1007/s11482-013-9273-3] [PMID: 25400708]

[28]   Baildam EM, Ennis H, Foster H, *et al.* Influence of childhood scleroderma on physical function and quality of life. J Rheumatol 2011; 38(1): 167-73.
[http://dx.doi.org/10.3899/jrheum.100447] [PMID: 21041272]

[29]   Orzechowski NM, Davis DM, Mason TG III, Crowson CS, Reed AM. Health-related quality of life in children and adolescents with juvenile localized scleroderma. Rheumatology 2009; 48(6): 670-2.
[http://dx.doi.org/10.1093/rheumatology/kep059] [PMID: 19336577]

CHAPTER 13

Investigations

Yasmeen Jabeen Bhat[1,*] and **Safia Bashir**[2]

[1] *Department of Dermatology, Venereology, and Leprology, Government Medical College Srinagar, University of Kashmir, Srinagar, Jammu & Kashmir, India*

[2] *Jammu & Kashmir Health Services, Kashmir. Jammu & Kashmir, India*

Chapter synopsis.
• Clinical findings are usually sufficient to make a presumptive diagnosis of morphea. Several procedures and investigations are employed to confirm the diagnosis and to assess the depth of involvement, disease severity, and activity.
• Autoantibodies especially Anti-nuclear antibodies (ANA), Antihistone antibodies (AHA) and Anti single-stranded DNA (a-ssDNA) antibodies have been implicated as potential markers of disease severity. These antibodies are however infrequently present even in patients with severe forms of morphea.
• Skin biopsy shows a prominent lymphoplasmacytic inflammatory infiltrate at the dermal-adipose tissue interphase in early lesions and a more characteristic replacement of normal dermal and subcutaneous structures by abnormal collagen.
• Radiographic studies might be abnormal and are especially helpful if deeper tissues are involved.
• Infrared thermography, durometer and cutometer measurements are being investigated as outcome measures in morphea.

Keywords: Antinuclear antibody, Anti-histone antibodies, Collagen deposition, Cutometer, Durometer, Dermoscopy, Eosinophilia, High eccrine glands, Hypervascularity, Infrared thermography, Line sign, Magnetic resonance imaging, Mucinosis, Skin biopsy, Ultrasonography.

INTRODUCTION

In most patients of morphea, the diagnosis can be made based on the clinical findings alone. However, the significance of investigative studies to confirm the diagnosis and to determine the severity of the disease cannot be underestimated. Early clinical diagnosis of morphea is pivotal in minimizing functional and cosm-

---

[*] **Corresponding author Yasmeen Jabeen Bhat:** Department of Dermatology, Venereology, and Leprology, Government Medical College Srinagar, University of Kashmir, Srinagar, Jammu & Kashmir, India; E-mail: yasmeenasif76@gmail.com

Tasleem Arif (Ed.)

etic impairment that may occur in severe forms of morphea. Unlike systemic sclerosis, no specific serological parameters have been defined in morphea and screening for antibodies is probably relevant only if the presence of another autoimmune disease is clinically suspected. Also, there are no disease activity indicators for morphea. Monitoring of disease activity relies mainly on clinical findings. Some parameters have recently been defined as indicators of disease activity in morphea and may be utilized for assessment of disease activity on case to case basis. Histopathology would be relevant in cases with unclear clinical presentation. In addition, diagnostic techniques like ultrasonography, laser Doppler measurements, cutometer and durometer have been used for assessing the course of the disease and for assessing therapeutic efficacy in clinical studies. Such diagnostic techniques for the assessment of disease activity as well as disease severity have been already discussed in detail in chapter 9. In this chapter, only a brief overview of such techniques will be presented.

ROUTINE LABORATORY INVESTIGATIONS

Complete Blood Count

Blood counts are usually normal. However, patients in the early inflammatory phase of morphea and those with deep morphea may exhibit peripheral eosinophilia.

Erythrocyte Sedimentation Rate (ESR) and C-reactive Protein (CRP)

ESR and CRP may be elevated in patients with active disease or those with extensive involvement.

Creatinine Kinase and Aldolase

Creatinine kinase levels in morphea are especially relevant in patients with suspected concomitant myositis. Elevated creatinine kinase and aldolase levels may indicate disease activity in juvenile localized scleroderma and are usually elevated in patients with new active skin lesions. In an observational analysis of children with juvenile localized scleroderma, creatinine levels were also found to be associated with muscle atrophy and extremity shortening [1].

AUTOANTIBODIES

The role of autoantibodies in morphea is not very clear but serological biomarkers in the form of autoantibodies may be used as a valid means to classify and differentiate morphea. The commonly used antibody markers in morphea include:

Antinuclear Antibody (ANA)

Antinuclear antibodies are found in 23-68% of patients with morphea [2]. Speckled and homogenous patterns are the most common. Although ANA positivity does not appear to vary with the different clinical subtypes of morphea, it does seem to be associated with disease severity with respect to the extent and depth of lesions, presence of extracutaneous manifestations and probability of disease relapses [3 - 5]. ANA can thus act as a potential biomarker for disease stratification and management in morphea.

Antihistone Antibodies (AHA)

Antihistone antibodies can be detected in 47-87% of patients with morphea. Similar to antinuclear antibodies, a positive correlation with the disease severity with respect to the number and size of lesions has been observed [6, 7]. Also noteworthy is the frequent association of AHA with the linear morphea subtype where it may correlate significantly with the extent of involvement and disease activity [3, 7, 8]. AHA do not appear to be predictive of disease relapses, unlike ANA.

Anti-single Stranded DNA Antibodies (a-ssDNA)

They are detected in nearly 50% of patients with morphea being most common in patients with generalized morphea and least in the circumscribed form. Anti-ssDNA antibodies may have a positive correlation with disease activity as well as severity. Musculofascial involvement and joint contractures have also been found more commonly in patients with antibodies to single-stranded DNA [9, 10].

Rheumatoid Factor (RF)

RF has been detected in 15 – 60% of patients with morphea, being more common in children with linear morphea. The presence of RF may correlate positively with arthritis and musculoskeletal involvement in morphea and should mandate clinical monitoring of such patients for the development of any musculoskeletal abnormalities or arthritis [11].

Antibodies to Extractable Nuclear Antigens (ENAs)

In 1-15% of patients with morphea, antibodies against the extractable nuclear antigens like anti-double stranded DNA (ds DNA), anti-SSA/SSB, anti-

Smith/Ribonucleoprotein (RNP), anti-ScL70 and anti- centromere antibodies [2] may be seen. The clinical significance of these antibodies in morphea is not well defined.

Others

In addition to the aforementioned ones, antibodies to matrix metalloproteinase (MMP)-1, antiphospholipid antibodies, cardiolipin antibodies (IgM and IgG), anti-topoisomerase II alpha antibodies, lupus anticoagulant, anti-Cu/Zn - superoxide dismutase antibodies may be seen in patients with morphea [12 - 15].

Emerging Antibody Markers

Autoantibodies to the dense fine-speckled 70 kDa antigen (Anti-DFS70) are being investigated for their association with rheumatic disease. They have been found to be more common in those whose disease is not ANA associated. Anti-DFS70 antibody positivity in morphea has also been reported [16].

Despite the frequent association between certain autoantibodies and disease severity and activity in morphea, autoantibody testing in morphea is of limited clinical utility. The prognostic significance of autoantibodies in morphea also remains unclear. Hence, routine testing for autoantibodies is not indicated in the absence of any clues to suggest the association of other autoimmune diseases. The detailed description of auto-antibodies in morphea and their clinical correlation has been given in chapter 5. Readers are referred to chapter 5 for in-depth details about autoantibodies.

SKIN BIOPSY

A diagnostic skin biopsy in morphea is recommended in case of an unclear clinical presentation as well as to determine the depth of involvement for categorization into morphea subtypes. While a deep punch biopsy involving subcutaneous fat is usually sufficient in superficial lesions of morphea (circumscribed and generalized), an incisional biopsy extending up to the muscle is required for linear and deep morphea. The histopathological changes observed in the inflammatory border will be different from those in the central sclerotic area. Therefore, it is imperative to note the site of biopsy at the time of specimen collection.

Histopathological changes observed in the biopsied lesion depend on the stage and morphological type of morphea. While the epidermis is normal in most cases, some advanced cases do demonstrate flattening of the rete ridges. In most cases, morphological changes are best observed in the transition area between the dermis and subcutaneous tissue [17]. The in-depth account of histopathology in morphea has been discussed in chapter 6. Here only a brief overview of histopathological findings will be presented.

Early Inflammatory Stage

Histopathological changes in early inflammatory lesions are not specific to morphea and do not provide a definitive diagnosis. Depending on the depth of involvement, interstitial and perivascular inflammatory cell infiltrate of variable density is observed in the reticular dermis and / or the subcutaneous tissue. Lymphocytes and plasma cells are the predominant inflammatory cell types while eosinophilia may occasionally be present. Mast cells and macrophages may also be found. In addition, blood vessels demonstrate endothelial cell edema. The deposition of new collagen fibers and thickening of the pre-existing collagen bundles are also seen [17, 18]. (Figs. **13.1** & **13.2**).

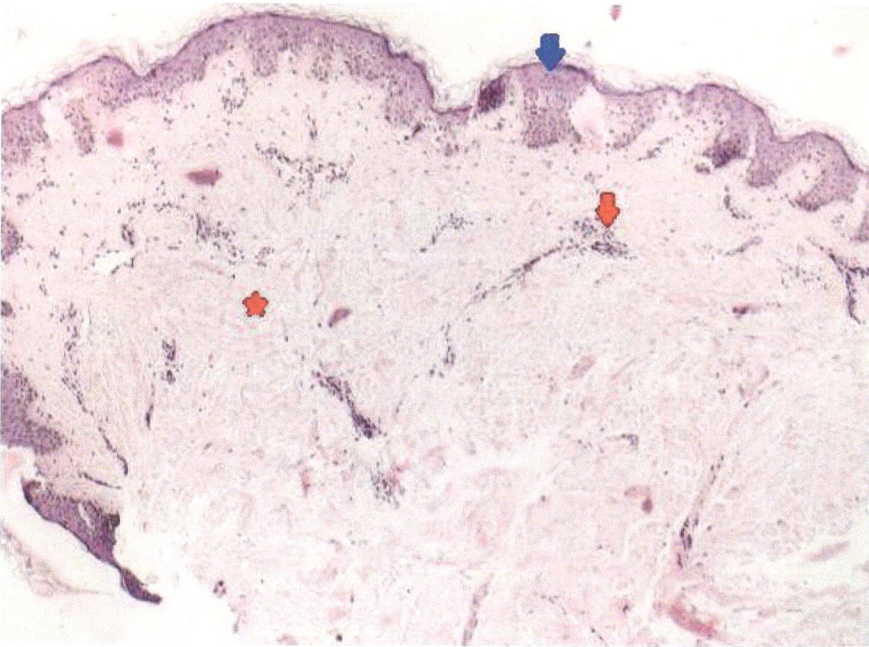

Fig. (13.1). Histopathological image of morphea showing hyperkeratosis and epidermal atrophy (blue arrow), chronic perivascular inflammation (red arrow) and increased dermal collagen (red star) with the absence of adnexae in the sections examined (H&E, X100).

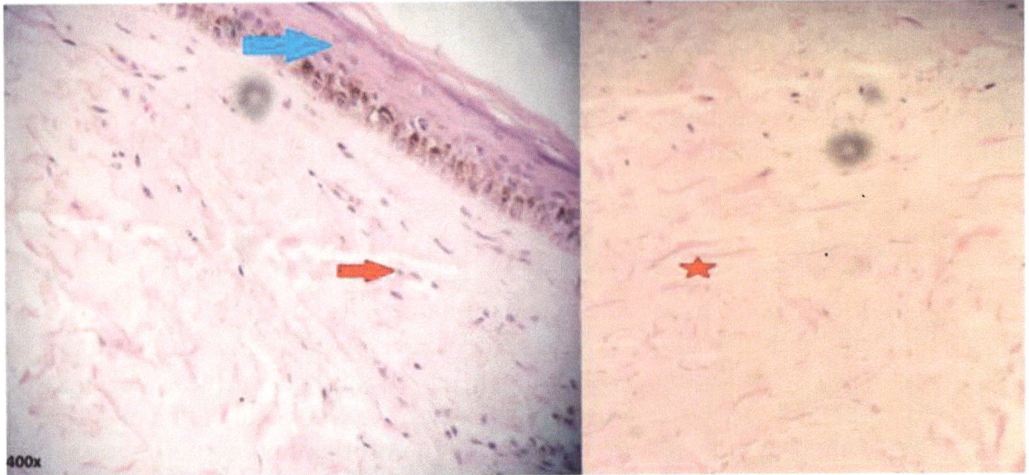

Fig. (13.2). Histopathological image of the same patient showing thinned epidermis with flattened rete ridges (blue arrow), minimal chronic perivascular inflammation (red arrow) with the absence of adnexa in the sections examined (H&E X400) a). Thick, closely packed collagen bundles in reticular dermis and subcutis with hyalinisation (red star) (H&E X400) (b). (Copyright @Bhat YJ, Akhtar S, Hassan I. Dermoscopy of morphea. Indian Dermatol Online J 2019;10:92-3)

Late sclerotic stage

Inflammatory infiltrate is typically absent in this stage although a few cases may exhibit discrete peri-adnexal infiltrate [17]. This stage is characterized by the homogenization of the papillary dermis with thickening and hyalinization of collagen bundles in the reticular dermis and subcutaneous tissue. As subcutaneous fat gets replaced by collagen and fat around eccrine glands diminishes, the glands appear atrophic and trapped within the thickened dermis. The replacement of adipose tissue by collagen is best assessed by comparing it with a skin biopsy from the contralateral side. Blood vessels are diminished and have fibrotic walls and narrow lumina. Appendageal structures are also progressively lost. Eccrine glands may be located higher in the dermis due to excessive deposition of collagen beneath them. Secondary cutaneous mucinosis between the collagen bundles may be noted [19]. Sclerotic changes in superficial morphea are limited to the papillary and superficial reticular dermis whereas in deep morphea sclerosis involves the deep reticular dermis and may extend to the subcutis and fascia. Different patterns of sclerosis defined in morphea include [20]:

1. Top heavy pattern: Hyalinized collagen bundles are localised to the papillary and superficial reticular dermis.
2. Bottom-heavy pattern: Hyalinized collagen bundles are present in the deep dermis and subcutaneous tissue.

3. Full thickness pattern: Here the hyalinized collagen bundles are distributed throughout the dermis.

Atrophic Stage

This stage is characterised by the complete absence of appendageal structures. Inflammatory cell infiltrate is absent and decreased sclerosis is observed in this stage.

Few histological clues at scanning magnification can facilitate rapid diagnosis of morphea. These have been designated specific names and are enumerated in Table **13.1.**

Table 13.1. Named signs in histopathology of morphea [21].

Line sign	Prominent, straight/linear interface between the subcutis and adjacent collagen of the reticular dermis.
Cookie cutter sign	Straight and parallel lateral edges of the biopsy section.
Square biopsy sign	The four corners of the biopsy have an approximate 90° angle between them.
High eccrine glands	The upper 2/3rd of the dermis shows the presence of eccrine glands.

'High eccrine glands' appear to be a very sensitive feature in biopsy specimens of morphea whereas the 'line sign' has been found to be highly specific but has a very low sensitivity for the diagnosis of morphea [22].

IMAGING STUDIES

Radiography

In cases of deep and linear morphea, radiography can help determine the involvement of underlying bone and can also be used for the recognition of any growth defects in children with morphea.

Ultrasonography (USG)

USG in morphea supports the diagnosis as well as aids in the assessment of activity and severity of the disease. 10-25 MHz ultrasound probes are ideal. An ultrasound can easily be used for detection of structural changes like tissue thickening, atrophy and other alterations in the tissue architecture [23]. Detection of lesion size is also more accurate than clinical examination as lesion borders are readily detected (by changes in the thickness or appearance of subcutaneous fat)

[24]. Ultrasonography can monitor any changes in skin lesions during the course of treatment and changes seen on sequential ultrasounds have been found to correlate with the clinical findings. This allows easy documentation of treatment response [24]. Figs. (**13.3** & **13.4**). A detailed account of high frequency ultrasound (HFUS) in morphea has been presented in chapter 9.

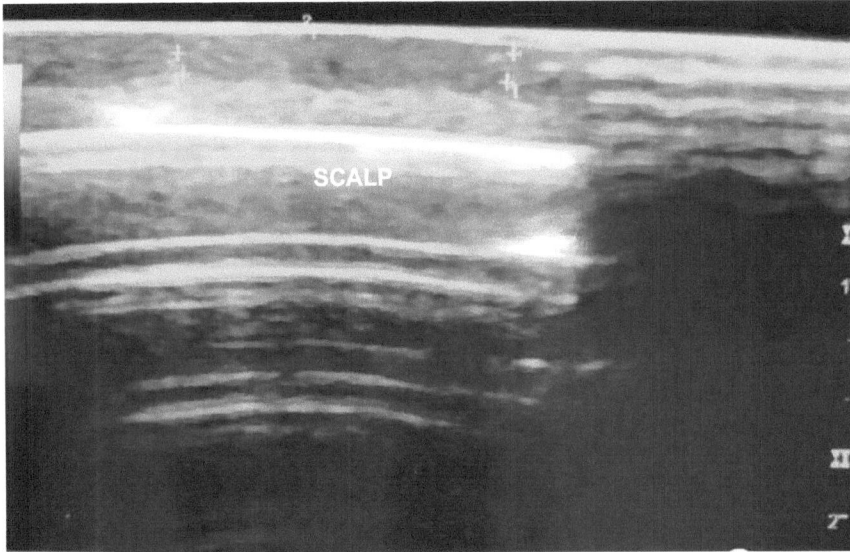

Fig. (13.3). USG of scalp lesion which shows increased echogenicity and decreased subcutaneous fat.

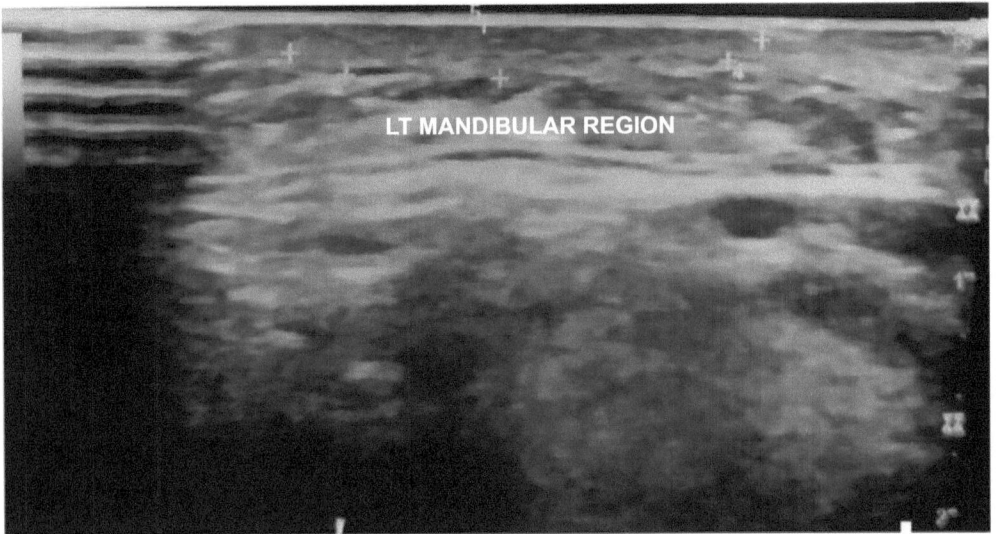

Fig. (13.4). USG of left sub mandibular area showing increased echogenicity and decreased subcutaneous fat.

Colour doppler ultrasonography represents a beneficial counterpart to histological examination in morphea. It can avoid the difficulties and complications of taking a skin biopsy, especially those of repeated biopsies for disease monitoring. Changes seen on a colour doppler ultrasound in different phases of morphea are given in Table **13.2** [25, 26].

Table 13.2. Colour doppler ultrasonographic findings in morphea.

Inflammatory phase	• Loss of definition of dermal-subcutis border • Increased echogenicity of the subcutaneous tissue • Increased dermal and subcutaneous vascularity • Thickening and decreased echogenicity of the dermis
Atrophic phase	• Thinning of the dermis and subcutis • Absence of subcutaneous fat • Increased echogenicity of the dermis and subcutaneous fat

Magnetic Resonance Imaging (MRI)

MR imaging yields information on musculoskeletal involvement in morphea. Any abnormalities of the muscles, tendons, fasciae, and bones can easily be detected on MR imaging. It may also detect subclinical changes where patients are devoid of any physical findings suggestive of musculoskeletal involvement.

MRI findings in morphea are given in (Box **13.1**) [27].

Box 13.1. MRI findings in morphea.
Thickening of the dermis
Loss of subcutaneous tissue
Subcutaneous septal thickening
Fascial and perifascial enhancement
Articular synovitis
Tenosynovitis
Myositis
Enthesitis
Bone marrow involvement

MRI of the brain has also been recommended for patients with morphea affecting the face, head, and neck [28]. Changes like cerebral atrophy, intracranial calcifications, white matter abnormalities and vascular abnormalities have been reported [29]. Patients with severe neurological symptoms may also have infratentorial lesions and cerebellar hemiatrophy [30].

OTHER INVESTIGATIONS

Dermoscopy

Dermoscopy is an *in vivo* non-invasive, diagnostic method based on optics & microscopy that is gaining importance as its simple, rapid and repetitive to perform. It is based on the principle of transillumination of the lesion and studying it with high magnification to visualize subtle clinical patterns of skin lesions and subsurface skin structures as deep as in the reticular dermis. In order to reduce the reflection of light, the cross-polarized lens absorbs all the scattered light and hence allows light to pass in a single plane only, thereby visualising deeper structures. All the modern dermoscopes are hybrid, having both non-polarised and polarised modes, the former visualises surface features like scales and follicular openings better and the latter, the vessels, pigment and fibrotic areas.

The dermoscopy of inflammatory disorders of the skin is known as inflammoscopy. Dermoscopic evaluation of the inflammatory disorders includes vessels (arrangement and morphology), background hue, scales, follicles and special clues as their dermoscopic features. It can be used as a diagnostic tool in morphea. The most common dermoscopic features of morphea include white clouds/fibrotic beams or ill-defined dull white globules, red structureless areas, linear branching vessels, and loss of appendages [31, 32]. White clouds that were previously described as fibrotic beams correspond to the increased and thickened collagen bundles in the reticular dermis and are considered a hallmark of morphea. Shiny white streaks can be seen which are due to the increased dermal collagen density [31]. Dermoscopic findings in morphea correlate well with the histopathological findings and may be used as a non-invasive and simpler alternative to skin biopsy for diagnosis and disease monitoring [31, 33]. Erythematous background and pigmentary structures in the form of structureless brown areas, reticular brown areas, and brown dots may also be seen Figs. (**13.5 - 13.9**).

Dermoscopic findings may vary in different phases of morphea. The 'inflammatory' findings seen are erythematous areas and red-focussed vessels; the 'sclerotic' findings are white clouds and crystalline structures; the 'The follicular atrophic' findings are unfocussed purplish vessels and white structureless areas. The follicular findings are very rarely seen, differentiating it from lichen sclerosus atrophicus which shows white bright patches also due to superficial fibrosis. Dermoscopy has high accuracy in monitoring inflammation and fibrosis regression by showing a reduction in vessels and white areas, respectively [34].

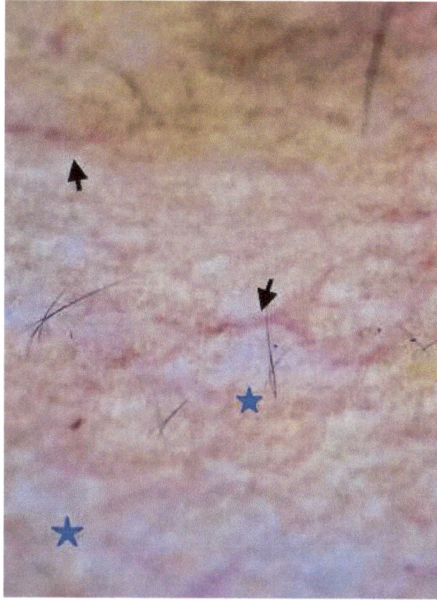

Fig. (13.5). White fibrotic beams or cloud like areas (blue star) crossed by linear branching vessels (black arrows). (polarized mode, Dermlite DL3N, California USA, 10X) (Copyright @Bhat YJ, Akhtar S, Hassan I.Dermoscopy of morphea. Indian Dermatol Online J 2019;10:92-3)

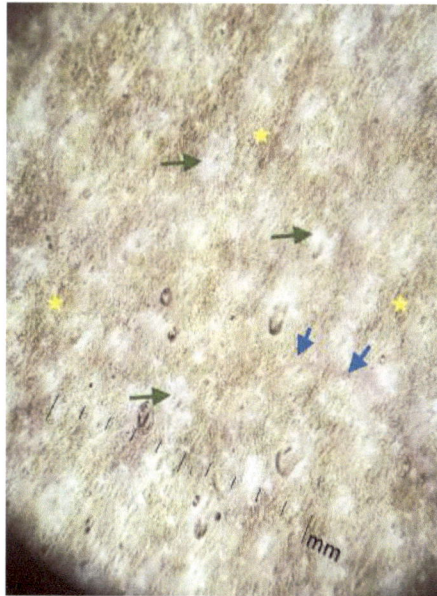

Fig. (13.6). Dermoscopy of morphea showing white fibrotic beams (green arrows), crossed by linear branching vessels (blue arrows), loss of appendages and reticular brown areas (yellow stars). (Dermlite DL3N 10X, polarized mode). (Copyright@Bhat YJ, Jha AK. Dermatoscopy of inflammatory diseases in the skin of colour. Indian Dermatol Online J 2021;12:45-57)

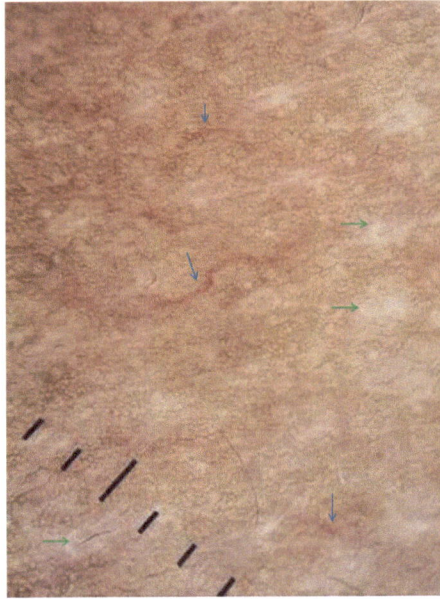

Fig. (13.7). Dermoscopy of morphea in inflammatory phase showing less number of ill-defined dull white globules (green arrows), multiple linear branching vessels (blue arrows) (Dermlite DL4 10X, polarized mode).

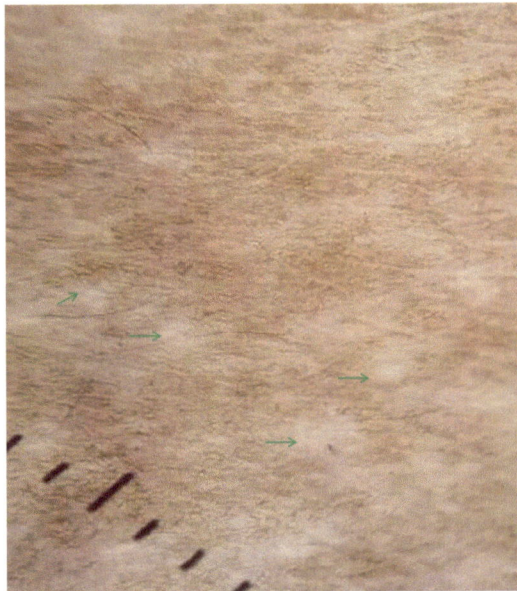

Fig. (13.8). Dermoscopy of morphea in late phase showing more white cloudy areas (green arrows) and absence of vessels and appendages (Dermlite DL4 10X, polarized mode).

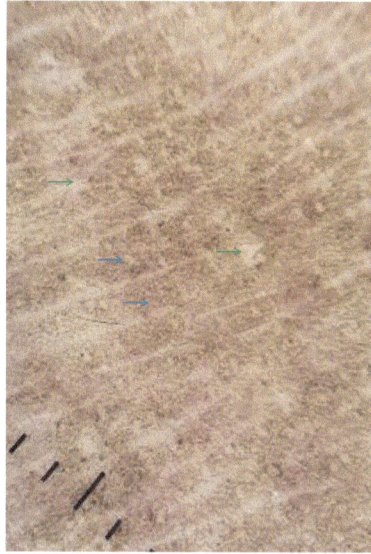

Fig. (13.9). Dermoscopy of morphea showing background erythema, ill-defined dull white globules (green arrows), reticular brown areas and brown dots (blue arrows) (Dermlite DL4 10X, polarized mode).

Infrared thermography (IRT)

It is a non-invasive, non-contact technique which provides an indirect measure of tissue perfusion and microcirculation. IRT can be used for quantifying the degree of inflammation and disease activity in the erythematous lesions of morphea. Thermography is carried out in a temperature-controlled room and uses an infrared camera. Areas 0.5°C warmer than the surrounding tissue are considered positive. The distinction between active and quiescent lesions is generally not possible by infrared thermography [35]. Also, refer to chapter 9 for Infrared thermography.

Durometer

Durometer is a handheld device used to measure skin hardness. Durometry has a low inter and intra-observer variability but may be of limited clinical utility as the durometer scores correlate poorly with skin scores [36]. Also, see chapter 9 for the durometer.

Cutometer

It is a handheld device used to measure skin elasticity and relaxation. The rate at which the probe is able to pull the skin and the rate at which it relaxes to baseline is measured [37]. Also, see chapter 9 for the cutometer.

Laser Doppler flowmetry (LDF)

It is a non-invasive method for the measurement of cutaneous microcirculation and has been used for the detection of active lesions of morphea [38]. LDF has been described in detail in chapter 9.

OUTCOME MEASURES

To characterize improvement and for meaningful data collection, it is important to have validated outcome measures in a disease. In addition to skin scores, some investigations which are being studied as outcome measures in morphea are given in (Box **13.2**) [37]. The various outcome measures in morphea and their principle and applications have been discussed in detail in chapter 9.

Box 13.2. Some of the outcome measures in morphea.
Cutometer measurements
Durometer measurements
Infrared Thermography
Ultrasound measurements

Diagnostic algorithms in morphea are highly variable among different patients. This can be attributed to the lack of validated methods for the assessment of severity and disease activity in morphea. This also translates into the lack of evidence-based therapies for morphea. Thus the development of appropriate diagnostic algorithms and outcome measures with minimum inter and intraobserver variability is the need of the hour.

Box 13.3. Learning points.
• Elevated creatinine kinase and aldolase levels may indicate disease activity in morphea and are usually elevated in patients with new active skin lesions.
• Role and clinical application of autoantibodies in morphea is not clear and autoantibody testing may be more relevant when concurrent rheumatic and other autoimmune diseases are suspected.
• Skin biopsy is the gold standard of diagnosis and is especially valuable in cases where the clinical examination is inconclusive and ultrasound or MRI are not readily available.
• In linear morphea en coup de sabre and progressive facial hemiatrophy, a cranial MRI is imperative to rule out CNS involvement.
• Dermoscopic findings in morphea correlate well with the histopathological findings and may be used as a noninvasive and simpler alternative to skin biopsy for diagnosis and disease monitoring
• Durometer, cutometer, ultrasonography, and infrared thermography have been used as outcome measures in morphea but have questionable clinical utility.

REFERENCES

[1]   Wu EY, Li SC, Torok KS, Virkud Y, Fuhlbrigge R, Rabinovich CE. A28: Description of the juvenile localized scleroderma subgroup of the CARRA registry. Arthritis Rheumatol 2014; 66: S43-4.
        [http://dx.doi.org/10.1002/art.38444]

[2]   Khatri S, Torok KS, Mirizio E, Liu C, Astakhova K. Autoantibodies in morphea: An update. Front Immunol 2019; 10: 1487.
        [http://dx.doi.org/10.3389/fimmu.2019.01487] [PMID: 31354701]

[3]   Warner Dharamsi J, Victor S, Aguwa N, *et al.* Morphea in adults and children cohort III: Nested case-control study the clinical significance of autoantibodies in morphea. JAMA Dermatol 2013; 149(10): 1159-65.
        [http://dx.doi.org/10.1001/jamadermatol.2013.4207] [PMID: 23925398]

[4]   Zulian F, Vallongo C, Woo P, *et al.* Juvenile Scleroderma Working Group of the Pediatric Rheumatology European Society (PRES). Localized scleroderma in childhood is not just a skin disease. Arthritis Rheum 2005; 52(9): 2873-81.
        [http://dx.doi.org/10.1002/art.21264] [PMID: 16142730]

[5]   Kurzinski KL, Zigler CK, Torok KS. Prediction of disease relapse in a cohort of paediatric patients with localized scleroderma. Br J Dermatol 2019; 180(5): 1183-9.
        [http://dx.doi.org/10.1111/bjd.17312] [PMID: 30315656]

[6]   Sato S, Ihn H, Soma Y, *et al.* Antihistone antibodies in patients with localized scleroderma. Arthritis Rheum 1993; 36(8): 1137-41.
        [http://dx.doi.org/10.1002/art.1780360815] [PMID: 8343189]

[7]   Arkachaisri T, Fertig N, Pino S, Medsger TA Jr. Serum autoantibodies and their clinical associations in patients with childhood- and adult-onset linear scleroderma. A single-center study. J Rheumatol 2008; 35(12): 2439-44.
        [http://dx.doi.org/10.3899/jrheum.080098] [PMID: 19004036]

[8]   Torok KS, Kurzinski K, Kelsey C, *et al.* Peripheral blood cytokine and chemokine profiles in juvenile localized scleroderma: T-helper cell-associated cytokine profiles. Semin Arthritis Rheum 2015; 45(3): 284-93.
        [http://dx.doi.org/10.1016/j.semarthrit.2015.06.006] [PMID: 26254121]

[9]   Falanga V, Medsger TA Jr, Reichlin M, Rodnan GP. Linear scleroderma. Ann Intern Med 1986; 104(6): 849-57.
        [http://dx.doi.org/10.7326/0003-4819-104-6-849] [PMID: 3486617]

[10]   Takehara K, Sato S. Localized scleroderma is an autoimmune disorder. Br J Rheumatol 2005; 44(3): 274-9.
        [http://dx.doi.org/10.1093/rheumatology/keh487] [PMID: 15561734]

[11]   Zulian F, Athreya BH, Laxer R, *et al.* Juvenile scleroderma working group of the pediatric rheumatology european society (PRES). Juvenile localized scleroderma: clinical and epidemiological features in 750 children. An international study. Rheumatology 2006; 45(5): 614-20.
        [http://dx.doi.org/10.1093/rheumatology/kei251] [PMID: 16368732]

[12]   Tomimura S, Ogawa F, Iwata Y, *et al.* Autoantibodies against matrix metalloproteinase-1 in patients with localized scleroderma. J Dermatol Sci 2008; 52(1): 47-54.
        [http://dx.doi.org/10.1016/j.jdermsci.2008.04.013] [PMID: 18565735]

[13]   Lis-Święty A, Brzezińska-Wcisło L, Arasiewicz H, Bergler-Czop B. Antiphospholipid antibodies in localized scleroderma: the potential role of screening tests for the detection of antiphospholipid syndrome. Postepy Dermatol Alergol 2014; 2(2): 65-70.
        [http://dx.doi.org/10.5114/pdia.2014.40978] [PMID: 25097470]

[14]   Hayakawa I, Hasegawa M, Takehara K, Sato S. Anti-DNA topoisomerase II? autoantibodies in localized scleroderma. Arthritis Rheum 2004; 50(1): 227-32.

[http://dx.doi.org/10.1002/art.11432] [PMID: 14730620]

[15]   Nagai M, Hasegawa M, Takehara K, Sato S. Novel autoantibody to Cu/Zn superoxide dismutase in patients with localized scleroderma. J Invest Dermatol 2004; 122(3): 594-601.
[http://dx.doi.org/10.1111/j.0022-202X.2004.22333.x] [PMID: 15086540]

[16]   Schmeling H, Mahler M, Levy DM, *et al.* Autoantibodies to dense fine speckles in pediatric diseases and controls. J Rheumatol 2015; 42(12): 2419-26.
[http://dx.doi.org/10.3899/jrheum.150567] [PMID: 26472409]

[17]   Careta MF, Romiti R. Localized scleroderma: clinical spectrum and therapeutic update. An Bras Dermatol 2015; 90(1): 62-73.
[http://dx.doi.org/10.1590/abd1806-4841.20152890] [PMID: 25672301]

[18]   George R, George A, Kumar TS. Update on management of morphea (Localized Scleroderma) in children. Indian Dermatol Online J 2020; 11(2): 135-45.
[http://dx.doi.org/10.4103/idoj.IDOJ_284_19] [PMID: 32477969]

[19]   Weedon D. Weedon's Skin Pathology. China: Churchill Livingstone Elsevier 2010; pp. 304-29.

[20]   Walker D, Susa JS, Currimbhoy S, Jacobe H. Histopathological changes in morphea and their clinical correlates: Results from the Morphea in Adults and Children Cohort V. J Am Acad Dermatol 2017; 76(6): 1124-30.
[http://dx.doi.org/10.1016/j.jaad.2016.12.020] [PMID: 28285783]

[21]   Yang S, Draznin M, Fung MA. The line sign a rapid and efficient diagnostic test for morphea: Clinicopathological study of 73 cases. Am J Dermatopathol 2018; 40(12): 873-8.
[http://dx.doi.org/10.1097/DAD.0000000000001177] [PMID: 30475273]

[22]   Chauhan P, Jindal R, Shirazi N. Histopathology of morphea: Sensitivity of various named signs, a retrospective study. Indian J Pathol Microbiol 2020; 63(4): 600-3.
[http://dx.doi.org/10.4103/IJPM.IJPM_67_20] [PMID: 33154313]

[23]   Li SC, Liebling MS. The use of doppler ultrasound to evaluate lesions of localized scleroderma. Curr Rheumatol Rep 2009; 11(3): 205-11.
[http://dx.doi.org/10.1007/s11926-009-0028-y] [PMID: 19604465]

[24]   Li SC, Liebling MS, Haines KA. Ultrasonography is a sensitive tool for monitoring localized scleroderma. Rheumatology 2007; 46(8): 1316-9.
[http://dx.doi.org/10.1093/rheumatology/kem120] [PMID: 17526926]

[25]   Wortsman X, Carreño LMC. Inflammatory diseases of the skin. In: Wortsman X, Jamec G, Eds. Dermatologic ultrasound with clinical and histologic correlations. 1st Ed.. New York: Springer 2013; pp. 73-117.
[http://dx.doi.org/10.1007/978-1-4614-7184-4_4]

[26]   Wortsman X, Wortsman J, Sazunic I, Carreño L. Activity assessment in morphea using color Doppler ultrasound. J Am Acad Dermatol 2011; 65(5): 942-8.
[http://dx.doi.org/10.1016/j.jaad.2010.08.027] [PMID: 21550692]

[27]   Schanz S, Fierlbeck G, Ulmer A, *et al.* Localized scleroderma: MR findings and clinical features. Radiology 2011; 260(3): 817-24.
[http://dx.doi.org/10.1148/radiol.11102136] [PMID: 21693661]

[28]   Zulian F, Culpo R, Sperotto F, *et al.* Consensus-based recommendations for the management of juvenile localised scleroderma. Ann Rheum Dis 2019; 78(8): 1019-24.
[http://dx.doi.org/10.1136/annrheumdis-2018-214697] [PMID: 30826775]

[29]   Amaral TN, Marques Neto JF, Lapa AT, Peres FA, Guirau CR, Appenzeller S. Neurologic involvement in scleroderma en coup de sabre. Autoimmune Dis 2012; 2012: 1-6.
[http://dx.doi.org/10.1155/2012/719685] [PMID: 22319646]

[30]   Kister I, Inglese M, Laxer RM, Herbert J. Neurologic manifestations of localized scleroderma: A case

report and literature review. Neurology 2008; 71(19): 1538-45.
[http://dx.doi.org/10.1212/01.wnl.0000334474.88923.e3] [PMID: 18981376]

[31]   Wang YK, Hao JC, Liu J, Liu YH, Jin HZ. Dermoscopic features of morphea and extragenital lichen sclerosus in Chinese patients. Chin Med J 2020; 133(17): 2109-11.
[http://dx.doi.org/10.1097/CM9.0000000000000977] [PMID: 32769495]

[32]   Bhat Y, Akhtar S, Hassan I. Dermoscopy of morphea. Indian Dermatol Online J 2019; 10(1): 92-3.
[http://dx.doi.org/10.4103/idoj.IDOJ_350_17] [PMID: 30775314]

[33]   Shim WH, Jwa SW, Song M, *et al.* Diagnostic usefulness of dermatoscopy in differentiating lichen sclerous et atrophicus from morphea. J Am Acad Dermatol 2012; 66(4): 690-1.
[http://dx.doi.org/10.1016/j.jaad.2011.06.042] [PMID: 22421117]

[34]   Errichetti E, Lallas A, Apalla Z, Di Stefani A, Stinco G. Dermoscopy of morphea and cutaneous lichen sclerosus: Clinicopathological correlation study and comparative analysis. Dermatology 2017; 233(6): 462-70.
[http://dx.doi.org/10.1159/000484947] [PMID: 29237158]

[35]   Chojnowski M. Infrared thermal imaging in connective tissue diseases. Reumatologia 2017; 55(1): 46-51.
[http://dx.doi.org/10.5114/reum.2017.66686] [PMID: 28386141]

[36]   Seyger MMB, van den Hoogen FHJ, Boo T, de Jong EMGJ. Reliability of two methods to assess morphea: Skin scoring and the use of a durometer. J Am Acad Dermatol 1997; 37(5): 793-6.
[http://dx.doi.org/10.1016/S0190-9622(97)70121-X] [PMID: 9366834]

[37]   Fett N, Werth VP. Update on morphea. J Am Acad Dermatol 2011; 64(2): 231-42.
[http://dx.doi.org/10.1016/j.jaad.2010.05.046] [PMID: 21238824]

[38]   Weibel L, Howell KJ, Visentin MT, *et al.* Laser Doppler flowmetry for assessing localized scleroderma in children. Arthritis Rheum 2007; 56(10): 3489-95.
[http://dx.doi.org/10.1002/art.22920] [PMID: 17907196]

CHAPTER 14

Treatment

Ozge Askin[1,*] and **Tasleem Arif**[2,3]

[1] *Department of Dermatology, Cerrahpasa Medicine Faculty İstanbul University-Cerrahpaşa, İstanbul, Turkey*

[2] *Department of Dermatology, STDs, Leprosy and Aesthetics, Dar As Sihha Medical center, Dammam, Saudi Arabia*

[3] *Ellahi Medicare Clinic, Srinagar, Kashmir, India*

Chapter synopsis.
• The choice of therapy for morphea should be based on several factors: Relative activity of the disease, depth and the localization of involvement, and course. Subcutaneous involvement, rapid progression, and involvement of functionally/cosmetically sensitive areas or large body surface areas are all indications of systemic treatment.
• Although no specific therapy for morphea exists, a variety of therapeutic options are available. The treatment aimed at reducing inflammatory activity in early, active disease is more successful than attempts to decrease sclerosis in well-established or older lesions.
• Treatment options may be divided into topical and systemic therapy as well as ultraviolet (UV) phototherapy.
• Topical and UV phototherapy are usually appropriate in plaque-type morphea with limited extension, whereas generalized, linear, or deep types usually require systemic therapy.

Keywords: Adverse drug effect, Azathioprine, Broadband ultraviolet A, Calcineurin inhibitors, Calcipotriol, Corticosteroids, D-Penicillamine, Imiquimod, Interferon gamma, Localized scleroderma, Methotrexate, Morphea, Narrowband ultraviolet B, Mycophenolate mofetil, Phototherapy, Systemic treatment, Topical treatment, Tacrolimus, Ultraviolet A1, Vitamin D analogues.

INTRODUCTION

There are various therapeutic modalities for morphea; however, evidence in support of many of these therapies is limited. The activity of the disease, depth and extent of involvement, and the presence of functional impairment or cosmetic deformity determine the most appropriate treatment. The severity of the disease varies and is unpredictable, but the prognosis is usually good. Most morphea pati-

---
[*] **Corresponding author Ozge Askin:** Department of Dermatology, Cerrahpasa Medicine Faculty İstanbul University-Cerrahpaşa, İstanbul, Turkey; E-mail: ozgee_karakus@hotmail.com

Tasleem Arif (Ed.)

ents might be successfully treated with topical therapy and phototherapy but the severe and progressive form of the disease might require systemic anti-inflammatory and immunosuppressive agents [1].

Treatment options for morphea might be divided into topical, phototherapy, and systemic therapy. The extent and severity of the disease should be taken into account before planning the treatment. All the treatments are more effective in the active, early phase of the disease Fig. (**14.1**).

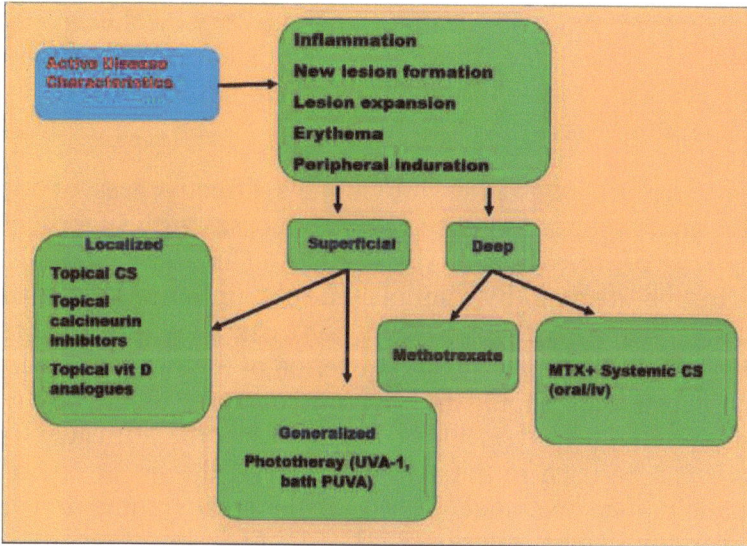

Fig. (14.1). Treatment options during the active phase of the disease.

TOPICAL THERAPY

Topical treatment is useful for the limited and superficial forms of morphea, such as plaque (circumscribed) morphea. Topical corticosteroids, vitamin D analogues, and topical calcineurin inhibitors are the mainstay of topical treatment, however, topical imiquimod, intralesional (IL) interferon gamma might be an alternative choice of treatment as well (Table **14.1**) [2, 3].

Table 14.1. Main topical treatment options in morphea and their mechanism of action.

Corticosteroids	Anti-inflammation, immunosuppression.
Calcipotriene	Antiproliferation, antiinflammation
Tacrolimus, pimecrolimus	Immunmodulator, immunsupression
Imiquimod	Immune response modifier
IFN-gamma	Antifibrosis

Topical/ Intralesional Corticosteroids

Once entered into the cell, topical corticosteroids bind to the cytoplasmic glucocorticoid receptor and are transported to the nucleus. The complex topical corticosteroid-glucocorticoid receptor binds to glucocorticoid response elements in the promoter region of a number of genes and modulates the transcription of a number of genes by inducing or inhibiting the transcription of specific mRNA and protein synthesis. These effects lead to the suppression of synthesis and release of prostaglandins and other inflammation mediators; release of the anti-inflammatory proteins; reduced release of inflammatory cytokines; inhibition of T cell activation; changes in the function of endothelial cells, granulocytes, mast cells, and Langerhans cells; and inhibition of the mitotic activity of epidermal cells and dermal fibroblasts.

Even though there are no studies proving the effectiveness of topical or IL corticosteroids in morphea, they are still used in cases with superficial lesions in the active phase of the disease (Box **14.1**). They can inhibit the further progression of the disease by diminishing the inflammation and softening sclerotic lesions. Therapy with high-potent corticosteroids should be performed in the active phase of disease for a maximum period of 3 months. Longer application of topical corticosteroids should be given as an interval therapy. Application under occlusion might be considered to increase the efficacy. Intralesional corticosteroids can be used in the active margin of the linear en coup de sabre subtype. Triamcinolone acetonide (40 mg) is the most commonly used agent by diluting 1:2 or 1:4 ratio with lidocain [2, 4].

Box 14.1. Topical corticosteroids for morphea.
Paucity of studies proving the effectiveness of topical corticosteroids.
Suited for the superficial lesions in the active phase of the disease.
Primarily act by their anti-inflammatory role. They can inhibit further progression of the disease by inhibiting inflammation and soften sclerotic lesion.
Moderate- to high-potent corticosteroids should be used in the active phase of disease and their application should be restricted to a total of 3 months.
Longer time therapy if needed, should be given as interval therapy.
Topical steroids under occlusion may increase the efficacy of treatment.
Intralesional corticosteroids may be used in the active margin of the linear morphea en coup de sabre.

Topical Vitamin-D Analogues

Vitamin D may exert inhibitory effects on fibroblast proliferation, collagen synthesis, and T lymphocyte activation. Topical treatment with calcipotriene

(0.005%) is effective for superficial plaque type (circumscribed) morphea and appears to work better when occluded, with an early and inflammatory lesion. Calcipotriene should be used twice daily for at least three months (Box **14.2**) [3, 5].

Box 14.2. Topical vitamin-D analogues for morphea.
Inhibitory effects on T lymphocyte activation, fibroblast proliferation and collagen synthesis.
Effective for superficial circumscribed morphea with minimal sclerosis.
Topical application under occlusion has shown better outcome.
The efficacy of fixed dose combination of calcipotriol with betamethasone dipropionate in morphea is supported by level IIB evidence
Therapy should be continued at least 3 months with twice daily application.

In an open-label study, 12 patients resistant to highly potent corticosteroids and in some cases also refractory to systemic medication, calcipotriene ointment application (0.005%, under occlusion, twice daily for 3 months) resulted in a significant reduction of erythema, dyspigmentation, telangiectasis, and induration in all patients without any side effects [6].

Topical Calcineurin Inhibitors

Topical calcineurin inhibitors (CI) suppress the synthesis of pro-inflammatory cytokines, and cause alterations in epidermal antigen-presenting dendritic cells that may result in decreased immunologic response to antigens.

Data on topical tacrolimus therapy are limited, and no studies on pimecrolimus for morphea are published so far. Two pilot studies and several case reports described the successful use of tacrolimus 0.1% under occlusion in morphea. In a trial that included 10 patients with morphea, two lesions on each patient were randomly assigned to either tacrolimus ointment or petrolatum, both applied twice daily for 12 weeks. Regression of erythema and reduction of sclerosis occurred in lesions treated with tacrolimus [7, 8].

Tacrolimus can be used for longer time than corticosteroids in morphea but side effects such as pruritus, burning, or erythema should be taken into consideration. It is not advised to use tacrolimus in patients with post-irradiation morphea, because of a higher risk of radiation-recalled dermatitis occurrence (Box **14.3**) [4].

Box 14.3. Topical calcineurin inhibitors (CI) for morphea.
They suppress the synthesis of pro-inflammatory cytokines, and cause alterations in epidermal antigen-presenting dendritic cells that decrease the immunologic response to antigens.
Topical tacrolimus has improved morphea in terms of changes in erythema, surface area and induration.
Tacrolimus 0.1% formulation under occlusion has been successfully used in morphea.
The efficacy of topical tacrolimus in morphea is supported by level IB evidence.
CI can be used for longer time durations than corticosteroids as they lack atrophogenic side effects.
They should be avoided in patients with post-irradiation morphea, because of a higher risk of radiation-recalled dermatitis.

Imiquimod

Imiquimod is a topical immune response modifier stimulating the synthesis of IFN-α and IFN-γ, that causes the inhibition of transforming growth factor beta (TGF-β), and thus inhibits collagen synthesis. There are few case reports, one small case series, and an open-labelled prospective study that showed the efficacy of imiquimod in the treatment of morphea [3, 4]. In a prospective study of 12 patients, the application of imiquimod 3 times a week was shown to be effective in reducing the erythema and induration of the plaques of morphea. The most common side effects of imiquimod were irritation, hypopigmentation, and ulceration (Box **14.4**) [9]. A trial in which nine children were treated for 36 weeks with imiquimod 5% cream, showed that it was effective in decreasing the thickening of plaques of morphea. Imiquimod can be an alternative treatment of morphea in the pediatric age group [10].

Box 14.4. Topical imiquimod for morphea.
Stimulates synthesis of IFN-α and IFN-γ, causing the inhibition of transforming growth factor beta (TGF-β), and thus inhibits collagen synthesis.
The application of imiquimod 3 times a week is effective in reducing the erythema and induration of the plaques of morphea.
Common side effects of imiquimod include irritation, hypopigmentation and ulceration.
Can be used as an alternative treatment for morphea in the pediatric age group.
The use of topical imiquimod for the treatment of morphea is supported by level IIB evidence.

Intralesional Interferon Gamma

Interferon-gamma (IFN-γ) participates in immuno-regulation by enhancing the oxidative metabolism of macrophages; it also enhances antibody-dependent cellular cytotoxicity, activates natural killer cells, and has a role in the expression of Fc receptors and major histocompatibility antigens. Despite the potential antifibrotic effect of interferon-γ, randomised placebo-controlled research did not prove the effectiveness of such treatment [3].

PHOTOTHERAPY

Ultraviolet (UV) light therapy is used for the treatment of morphea since the 1990s. Phototherapy is one of the most effective treatment modalities for morphea by antiinflammatory and antifibrotic effects, decreasing the synthesis of collagen. The most common side effects of phototherapy are erythema, hyperpigmentation, pruritus, burning, photoaging, and an increased risk of skin cancers [3, 7, 11].

The effect of UV on the skin depends on the wavelength. The UVB (280-320 nm) radiation affects keratinocytes and Langerhans cells in the upper layers of the skin. The UVA (320-400 nm) radiation affects deeper in the skin layer, like fibroblasts, dendritic cells, vascular epithelium, and inflammatory cells. It leads to the apoptosis of dermal T cells, and Langerhans cells, and modulation of various proinflammatory cytokines. Phototherapy with psoralen (PUVA) also activate metalloproteinase-1 which is important in collagen breakdown [3, 7].

Ultraviolet A1 (UVA-1), broadband ultraviolet A (BB-UVA), PUVA, and narrowband ultraviolet B (NB-UVB) light therapy have all been found effective in morphea patients (Box **14.5**). NB-UVB is more effective in the early phase of superficial dermal lesions. BB-UVA/UVA-1 is more appropriate for deeper lesions. Randomized controlled trials assessing morphea therapeutics have concluded that high-dose UVA-1 light is likely the most effective ultraviolet light therapy for morphea [5, 12, 13].

Box 14.5. Phototherapy for the treatment of morphea.
Ultraviolet A1, broadband ultraviolet A, PUVA, and narrowband ultraviolet B light therapy have all been found effective in morphea patients
UVB radiation affects keratinocytes and Langerhans cells in the upper layers of the skin. The UVA radiation affects deeper in the skin layer leading to the apoptosis of dermal T cells, Langerhans cells, and modulation of various proinflammatory cytokines. PUVA also activates metalloproteinase-1.
For UVA-1, all the 3 regimens are effective though medium-dose therapy has been found to score more.
Bath PUVA phototherapy may be considered for pediatric patients especially for the early inflammatory stage.
The efficacy of NB-UVB has been found comparable to low-dose UVA-1 phototherapy.
The level of evidence for BB-UVA, UVA-1, PUVA, and NB-UVB light phototherapy is IIB.

UVA-1

There are three different dose regimens: low-dose UVA-1 (10–29 J/cm^2), medium-dose UVA-1 (30–59 J/cm^2), and high-dose UVA-1 (60– 130 J/cm^2). All three regimens are used in the treatment of morphea. UVA-1 is usually performed 3–5 times weekly for a minimum of 30 sessions [2].

The long wavelength of UVA-1 penetrates the dermis and induces the expression of matrix metalloproteinase-1, depletes T cells, Langerhans cells and mast cells in the dermis, and stimulates the neovascularization of endothelial cells. Due to these effects, UVA-1 is the first treatment choice for morphea. It reverses skin sclerosis even after the end of the treatment [14, 15]. Despite the high dose and medium dose regimens being considered as the ideal options at first, it was shown that low dose regimen was also found effective as well in previous studies in the treatment of morphea [2, 14].

The only randomized controlled study that compared the efficacy of narrowband UVB, low-dose UVA-1, and medium-dose UVA-1 in 64 morphea patients, showed that medium-dose UVA1 was significantly more effective than NB-UVB and low-dose UVA-1 [16]. The response of darker skin type patients to UVA-1 is unclear. In a retrospective study, it was revealed that Fitzpatrick skin type did not significantly influence the efficacy of UVA1 phototherapy and suggested UVA-1 should be considered as a therapeutic option in more darkly pigmented patients [17].

PUVA

In psoralen plus ultraviolet A (PUVA) therapy, photosensitizing psoralens are either given orally or applied topically. 8-methoxy psoralen (8-MOP) should be taken orally at doses of 0.4 to 0.6 mg/kg one to two hours before exposure to ultraviolet A (UVA) radiation. Topical PUVA consists of direct application to the skin of psoralens in creams, ointments, or lotions followed by exposure to UVA radiation for localized diseases. In bath PUVA therapy, the patient takes a 15-3--minute bath in 8-methoxy psoralen-containing water at 37°C. Pruritus, erythema, skin pain, subacute phototoxicity, reactivation of herpes simplex, the requirement for posttreatment eye protection, cataract, and an increased long-term risk of squamous cell carcinoma are the side effects of PUVA. In addition to these, gastrointestinal intolerance and nausea are also common in oral PUVA therapy [18, 19].

The treatment should consist of approximately 30 sessions, performed 2-3 times a week. Bath PUVA phototherapy may be a choice for children patients especially for the early inflammatory phase of limited morphea [3, 18].

Broadband UVA

There are three prospective studies that have been published on the use of BB-UVA (320–400 nm) in morphea. Among these, El-Mofty *et al.* (2004) showed that a satisfactory response was obtained with early indurated lesions with the three doses of 5, 10, and 20 J/cm^2 of BB-UVA. It is suggested to start as early as possible to minimize residual deformity because of the poor response of the late, fibrotic, sclerotic plaques [20].

Narrowband UVB

NB-UVB phototherapy (311 to 313 nm) is preferred in the treatment of inflammatory and T-cell mediated dermatoses such as psoriasis, atopic dermatitis, vitiligo, and mycosis fungoides. NB-UVB may also be effective in treating cutaneous graft-versus-host disease, which is a condition that shares common features with scleroderma. The success of NB-UVB in treating skin conditions previously controlled with UVA phototherapy makes it also a good candidate therapy for morphea [21].

A study that compared low-dose UVA-1(20 J/cm2), medium-dose UVA-1 (50 J/cm2), and NB-UVB (1,3-1,5j/cm^2), in morphea patients, showed no significant differences between low-dose UVA-1 and NB-UVB. In all three regimens, medium dose UVA-1 was more effective but all three groups showed improvement [16].

SYSTEMIC THERAPY

Patients with subcutaneous involvement, that fail to improve with topical and phototherapy or with rapid progression, and cause functional impairment or cosmetically disfigurement are all candidates for systemic treatment [5]. Several clinical assessment methods have been used such as depigmentation, induration, erythema, and telangiectasia score (DIET); modified Rodnan skin score (MRSS); and the Localized scleroderma skin severity index (LoSSI). All these methods assess the activity of the disease and the damage to patients together [1]. These methods have been fully discussed in chapter 9.

Although there is no consensus on the treatment of morphea, a variety of therapeutic options have been proposed. Most of the studies are case reports or series. There are very few placebo-controlled studies. Methotrexate and systemic corticosteroids can be used with topical agents for generalized and deep morphea or forms that are unresponsive to phototherapy. Mycophenolate mofetil might be effective in some cases. Penicillamine, penicillin, oral calcitriol, colchicine, hydroxychloroquine, cyclosporine, bosentan, infliximab, tofacitinib, retinoids, and intravenous immunoglobulins have been used in the recalcitrant cases in the literature (Table **14.2**).

Table 14.2. Systemic treatments in morphea.

First Line	Second Line	Third Line
Methotrexate	Mycophenolate mofetil	Colchicine
Systemic corticosteroids		Hydroxychloroquine
Combination of Methotrexate and corticosteroids		Calcitriol
		Azathioprine
		Penicillin

Methotrexate

Of all the systemic therapeutic agents, methotrexate (MTX) has been the most studied as a treatment option for morphea. It is a folic acid antagonist that inhibits dihydrofolate reductase. MTX is considered to reduce skin fibrosis by its anti-inflammatory effect on the skin fibroblasts. MTX can be used either as monotherapy or in combination with systemic glucocorticoids both in children and adults. Methotrexate doses ranged from 0.3 to 0.4 mg/kg/week in children and 15 to 25 mg/week in adults [22, 23].

There are three prospective and four retrospective studies that showed the efficacy of MTX both in children and adults. In a randomized, double-blind, placebo-controlled trial, 70 children with active morphea were randomized to receive oral methotrexate (15 mg/m^2, maximum:20 mg) or placebo. Oral prednisone (1 mg/kg/day, maximum: 50 mg) was added to both groups for 3 months. Reduction of the clinical scores was observed within the first 6 months in both the groups. At follow-up of 12 months, a significant reduction in the clinical scores was seen only in the methotrexate-treated group [24].

In four prospective studies that included 34 patients altogether (24 adults and 10 children) treated with a combination of intravenous methylprednisolone and MTX, significant improvement was observed in all the adults and in nine of the children. In three retrospective studies that included 119 patients (52 patients with MTX monotherapy and 67 patients with combined MTX and corticosteroid therapy), 97% of patients showed improvement in these trials [3].

Advantages of MTX include a weekly dosage schedule, low cost, and a relatively safe profile. Nausea, vomiting, fatigue, and mucositis are common side effects. Hepatotoxicity, pulmonary damage, and myelosuppression may be seen with the use of MTX but are not usually frequent and not life-threatening in the low-dose regimen that is used for morphea treatment. However, frequent blood monitoring is required [22].

Methotrexate is the current first-line treatment for subtypes of morphea with severe skin affection or musculoskeletal involvement (Box **14.6**). The duration of methotrexate therapy should be at least 12 months, and a reduction of dosage can be considered after first signs of clinical improvement [2].

Box 14.6. Methotrexate for the treatment of morphea.
Most studied systemic treatment option for morphea.
MTX reduces skin fibrosis by its anti-inflammatory effect on skin fibroblasts.
MTX has been used as monotherapy as well as in combination with systemic corticosteroids both in children and adults.
The usual dose ranges from 0.3 to 0.4 mg/kg/week in children and 15 to 25 mg/week in adults.
MTX is considered the first-line treatment for morphea with severe skin affection or musculoskeletal involvement.
Duration of MTX therapy should be at least one year and a dose reduction may be considered after first signs of clinical improvement.
The use of MTX in collaboration with systemic steroids is supported by level IIB evidence.

Systemic Corticosteroids

Glucocorticoids are a mainstay of dermatologic therapy because of their potent immunosuppressive and anti-inflammatory properties. Systemic corticosteroids (CS) are safe and effective in the acute phase of the disease, both as mono- and combination therapy. But they could be administered for a short time in the early acute phase of severe forms of morphea due to the side effects [2, 3].

Systemic CS affect rapidly and when the disease is under control, these can be rapidly tapered. They can be used orally, intravenously or as intravenous (IV) pulse therapy. Adults are usually administered 500-1000mg IV daily of methylprednisolone on three consecutive days, whereas the dose in children is 30mg/kg IV daily of methylprednisolone on three consecutive days per month for a 3- 6 months duration (Box **14.7**). Prednisone may be given 0.5–2 mg/kg orally (maximum 60 mg) for 2-4 weeks, followed by gradual dose tapering [3, 8]. A study with 36 morphea patients that were treated with MTX and CS combination, suggested continuous therapy was more effective than intermittent CS, either oral alternate-day or IV-pulse regimen. Combination therapy with MTX is more effective and has fewer recurrence rates than monotherapy with oral glucocorticoids [25].

Box 14.7. Systemic steroids for the treatment of morphea.
They are safe and effective both as mono- and combination therapy in the acute phase of the disease.
Their response is rapid and when the disease is under control, they can be rapidly tapered.
Their advantage lies in the fact that they can be used orally, intravenously or as IV pulse therapy.
Methylprednisolone pulse therapy in adults is usually administered as 500-1000mg IV daily on three consecutive days per month for a 3- 6 months duration.
For the pediatric population, methylprednisolone is given at 30mg/kg IV daily in a similar fashion as adults.
Combined therapy with MTX is more effective and has lower recurrence rates than monotherapy with oral glucocorticoids.
The combined use of systemic steroids with MTX in morphea is supported by level IIB evidence.

Mycophenolate Mofetil

Mycophenolate mofetil (MMF) is a prodrug of mycophenolic acid (MPA), an inhibitor of inosine-5'-monophosphate dehydrogenase. MPA inhibits the proliferation of T and B lymphocytes, thereby suppressing cell-mediated immune responses and antibody formation.

MMF should be considered as an alternative immunosuppressant therapy in MTX- and corticosteroid-refractory cases of morphea (Box **14.8**). MMF inhibits the proliferation of lymphocytes, smooth muscle cells and fibroblasts. The dose of MMF ranges from 600 to 1200 mg/m^2 given twice a day. In 2009, a case series of seven methotrexate-resistant morphea patients treated with MMF, has shown improvement in skin sclerosis and inflammation [2, 3].

In a retrospective cohort study, 77 patients with morphea who were treated with MMF, showed that MMF was a well-tolerated and effective treatment in recalcitrant, severe morphea. Gastrointestinal adverse effects were the most common. Cytopenia and infection also were seen [26]. The efficacy of treatment with MMF in morphea is supported by level III evidence.

Box 14.8. Mycophenolate mofetil (MMF) for the treatment of morphea.
Inhibits enzyme inosine-5'-monophosphate dehydrogenase which leads to inhibition of proliferation of T and B lymphocytes, thereby suppressing cell-mediated immune responses and antibody formation.
Alternative immunosuppressant in MTX- and corticosteroid-refractory cases of morphea.
The usual dose of MMF ranges from 600 to 1200 mg/m^2 given twice a day.
Studies though limited have shown improvement in cutaneous inflammation and sclerosis in resistant cases of morphea.
Gastrointestinal adverse effects, cytopenia, and infections are the common side effects.
The efficacy of MMF in the treatment of morphea is supported by level III evidence.

Penicillamine

Penicillamine chelates with lead, copper, mercury and other heavy metals to form stable, soluble complexes that are excreted in urine; depresses circulating IgM rheumatoid factor, depresses T-cell but not B-cell activity. For many years, penicillamine has been used for the treatment of systemic sclerosis. There are several case series that showed efficacy in morphea with penicillamine (2-5 mg/kg/day). Because of the adverse effects such as proteinuria, nephrotic syndrome, headache, epigastric pain, nausea, pancreatitis, stomatitis (gingivostomatitis), and diarrhea, and limited efficacy, it is not recommended for the treatment of morphea anymore [5, 13].

Other Treatments

Penicillin, oral calcitriol, colchicine, hydroxychloroquine, cyclosporine, bosentan, infliximab, abatacept, retinoids, extracorporeal photopheresis, plasmapheresis, and intravenous immunoglobulins have been used in morphea with variable results [2, 3].

There are two case reports of the benefit of cyclosporine in the treatment of morphea in children in the literature [13].

In a retrospective study of 84 patients who had morphea and were treated with hydroxychloroquine monotherapy for at least 6 months, 43% of the patients had a complete response to hydroxychloroquine; 38% had a partial response greater than 50%; 12% had a partial response less than or equal to 50%; and 7% had no response [27].

Retinoic acid showed to have anti-fibrotic effects by modulating collagen. Retinoic acid has been studied for the treatment of patients suffering from sclerotic skin diseases and has shown promising results with minimal side effects. Acitretin, and etretinate were used in the case reports that showed efficacy [28].

In a case report with generalized deep morhea patient, tofacitinib (10 mg/day then 20 mg/day) was added to MTX and prednisone (40 mg daily) therapy, and the patient showed improvement in the cutaneous induration markedly [29].

In a randomized, double-blind, placebo-controlled study including 27 patients (20 morphea, 7 systemic sclerosis), calcitriol was found to be not more effective than placebo in patients with morphea [30].

These treatments should be a choice for severe cases that are unresponsive to the standard therapy. In many cases, there is insufficient evidence to support the use of these treatments, so more controlled studies are needed to verify the data about the efficacy of these agents in the treatment of morphea.

PHYSICAL THERAPY AND SURGICAL THERAPY

Although there are no studies on physical therapy in morphea, physical therapy is a crucial component in daily clinical practice, especially in patients with linear, generalized, deep, and mixed forms of morphea in the sclerotic stage. Connective tissue massage and manual lymphatic drainage may be added to systemic therapy once or twice a week for a period of at least three months [3].

Surgical therapy is predominantly indicated in linear types of morphea in the inactive stage of the disease. Epiphysiodesis of the healthy extremity to adjust leg length inequality can be considered by orthopedicians during the pre-puberty growth spurt. Plastic surgery procedures and/or implantations (Autologous fat transplant, filler) can be applied for cosmetic reasons in linear morphea'en coup de sabre' or Parry Romberg syndrome [2].

TREATMENT IN THE PEDIATRIC POPULATION

Topical tacrolimus 0.1%, topical steroids, calcipotriol, and imiquimod have been used in the topical therapy of juvenile morphea (Box **14.9**). MTX, or MTX-systemic corticosteroid combination is the systemic treatment that has sufficient evidence of efficacy in the pediatric group. The treatment of morphea in pediatric patients has been described in detail in chapter 19.

Box 14.9. Treatment of pediatric morphea.
Phototherapy (UVA-1, narrow band UVB, bath PUVA)
Methotrexate
Methotrexate + Systemic corticosteroids
Topical calcipotriol
Topical corticosteroid
Topical tacrolimus

In active, solitary, superficial small-sized plaques, topical steroids may be used in children. Generally, improvement is seen after 6-12 weeks. To avoid adverse effects of topical steroids, they should not be used continuously and for too long [31].

A study including 19 children (range 3-13 years) with morphea indicated that a combined therapy with calcipotriol ointment (twice daily) and low-dose UVA1 phototherapy is highly effective in childhood morphea [32].

Methotrexate is often used to treat the different forms of morphea in the pediatric population at a dose of 0.3-0.6 mg/kg orally or subcutaneously. In the early active phase of the disease, MTX is combined with pulsed intravenous corticosteroid and/or oral prednisone. This combination therapy has been found to be more effective than monotherapy with MTX or corticosteroids [33]. In a retrospective study that included 34 children, the combination therapy resulted in significant clinical improvement (100% of the patients) of lesions and stopped the progression of the disease (94% of the patients) [34].

UVA1, narrow band UVB, and bath PUVA can be used in the treatment of children >12 years with superficial, non-progressive morphea that does not involve deeper structures like subcutis or fascia, or muscle [31].

Mycophenolate mofetil may be used to treat severe MTX-refractory or MTX-intolerant juvenile morphea patients. The dose of MMF is 600–1200 mg/m2 twice daily [35].

TREATMENT ACCORDING TO CLINICAL TYPES

A therapeutic algorithm depending upon the clinical subtype of morphea has been presented in Fig (**14.2**).

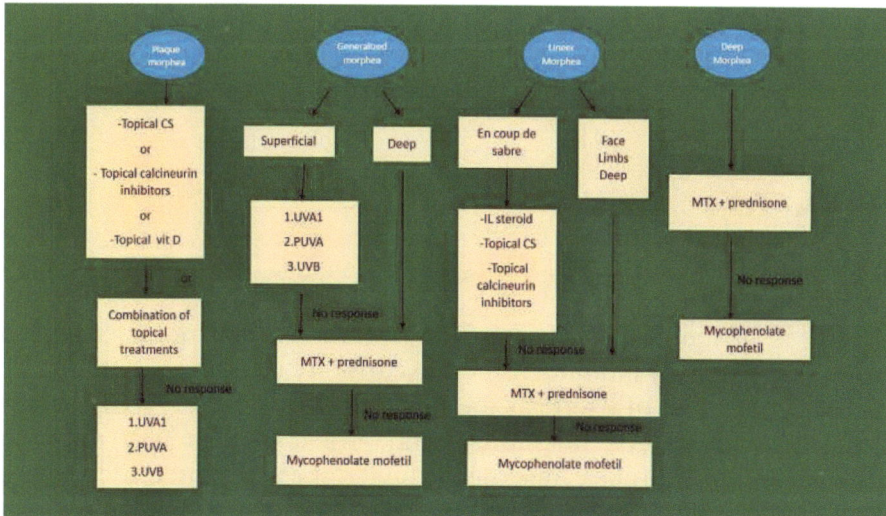

Fig. 14.2. Treatment algorithm for different clinical forms of morphea.

To indicate one treatment modality, we should consider the extent and depth of the disease and the limitations it may cause with the mobility and contractures.

In plaque morphea, if it is superficial, the first choice is the topical treatment. Topical corticosteroids, calcineurin inhibitors and calcipotriene can be used for 4-8 weeks. If there is no enough response, combination therapy with topical CS and calcipotriene, or imiquimod might be effective. Phototherapy with UVA1, PUVA, or UVB might be added to recalcitrant plaque morphea [1, 36].

In generalized morphea, if it is superficial and there is no joint contractures, phototherapy (UVA1, PUVA, or UVB) should be the first-line treatment. If there is no response after 40 sessions, Mtx (15-25 mg/week) with or without prednisone (0,5-1 mg/kg/day) should be preferred. Therapy should be continued for at least 12 months with a reduction of dosage after first signs of clinical improvement. MMF might be an alternative agent for recalcitrant cases with generalized morphea [1, 36, 37].

Linear morphea that affects face and limbs with the possibility of contractures, should be treated with systemic agents such as MTX and CS (prednisone or methylprednisolone). MMF is an alternative agent in this form of morphea for nonresponsive patients. Intralesional steroid therapy might be performed in morphea en coup de saber that affects mainly children. Topical calcipotriol 0.005% (twice daily) and tacrolimus 0.1% ointment under occlusion should be considered for active inflammatory superficial types of en coup de saber with a low degree of sclerosis [1, 37].

Combination of MTX and systemic CS are the first line treatment for deep morphea. When MTX failed, MMF was shown to improve skin sclerosis and inflammation in patients with refractory morphea.

NEWER DRUGS

Phosphodiesterase-4 (PDE-4) Inhibitors

Crisaborole is a boron containing anti-inflammatory, non-steroidal phosphodiesterase-4 (PDE-4) inhibitor which is currently also under investigation for its role in the treatment of psoriasis and atopic dermatitis [38]. A Phase 2, pilot study, to assess the safety, tolerability and efficacy of using crisaborole 2% ointment for adult morphea has been undertaken recently. There were 8 participants in the study of which 7 completed the study. Crisaborole 2% ointment was applied twice daily, on affected plaques for 12 weeks. A 4 mm skin punch biopsy was performed at baseline and at 12 weeks, on the same affected plaque.

Dermal thickness was measured and compared before and at the end of treatment which formed the primary outcome measure. Secondary outcome measures included the percentage of reduction in DIET (dyspigmentation, induration, erythema, and telangiectasias) score of sentinel plaque, percentage of reduction in LoSCAT (localized scleroderma cutaneous assessment tool) score, percentage of reduction in skindex-29 score and change in dermal thickness of sentinel plaque by ultrasonography. 5 patients had a change in dermal thickness on skin biopsy, and there was a significant reduction in DIET, LoSCAT and Skindex-29 Scores [39].

Apremilast is an orally available inhibitor of PDE-4 enzyme. It was approved for the treatment of moderate/severe psoriasis and psoriatic arthritis in 2014. Its mechanism of action is likely related to the modulation of several inflammatory cytokines via increasing the cellular levels of cyclic adenosine monophosphate (c-AMP) [40]. As we know, the exact pathogenesis of morphea is not completely understood; it is partly related to inflammation and immune dysregulation via T helper 2 (TH-2) cell-related cytokines, including interleukin 4 (IL-4) and interleukin 4 (IL-6), that drive fibrosis [41]. In a recent study by Maier *et al.*, they showed that PDE-4 blockade with apremilast had antifibrotic effects on skin fibrosis in animal models. By limiting M2 macrophage (M2 polarised macrophages) differentiation and IL-6 release, apremilast reversed fibrosis and prevented its progression. This study suggested that PDE-4 inhibitors might be helpful in treating inflammation-driven fibrosis in morphea [42].

Most recently, Koschitzky and Khattri (2022) have tried apremilast in 5 patients with biopsy-proven morphea. These patients had inadequate therapeutic responses to other treatment modalities or had intolerable side effects. There was a reduction in erythema and the size of morphea lesions, cessation of the appearance of new lesions, softening of indurated plaques, and decreased atrophy of the dermis. Out of 5 patients, 4 patients reported improvement in one month or less [43].

JAK-STAT Inhibitors

The Janus kinase-signal transducer and activator of transcription (JAK-STAT) pathway is essential for intracellular cytokine signaling mediated by type I and type II cytokine receptors. There are 4 types of JAK kinases (JAK-1, JAK-2, JAK-3, and tyrosine kinase 2 [Tyk-2]) and 7 STAT proteins (STAT-1, STAT-2, STAT-3, STAT-4, STAT-5A, STAT5-B, and STAT-6) that bind directly to the intracellular domain of type I and type II cytokine receptors [44]. Upon binding to their respective ligands, JAKs get phosphorylated and activated. The activated forms of JAKs then phosphorylate STAT proteins, which subsequently get dimerized and translocate to the nucleus. In the nucleus, they directly bind to

DNA segments and regulate the transcription of several genes. There are several cytokines whose synthesis is mediated by the JAK-STAT signaling pathway. Some of them include interleukin (IL) 2, IL-4, IL-5, IL-6, IL-12, IL-13, IL-21, IL-22, IL-23, and interferon alpha/beta/gamma,etc [45, 46]. Thus, it is clear that the activation of the JAK-STAT pathway contributes to a number of inflammatory dermatoses. This means that the inhibitors of JAK-STAT pathway can be employed for the treatment of a variety of dermatologic conditions. Currently, JAK-STAT inhibitors are being investigated for the treatment of several diseases like atopic dermatitis, psoriasis, lichen planus, lichen planopilaris, hidradenitis suppurativa, graft-versus-host disease, alopecia areata, vitiligo, chronic actinic dermatitis, granulomatous disorders, morphea and Eosinophilic fasciitis, dermatomyositis, systemic lupus erythematosus, etc [47].

Inhibition of IL-4 and TGF-beta signaling by JAK-STAT inhibitors may inhibit collagen production and fibroblast-derived extracellular matrix proteins in scleroderma. JAK inhibitor, Tofacitinib, in a dose of 5 mg twice a day, improved a patient with diffuse morphea who had a significant reduction in cutaneous induration after 1 year of treatment along with oral prednisone. The second patient with eosinophilic fasciitis had marked an improvement in skin induration on tofacitinib 5 mg twice daily and low dose weekly (10 mg/week) methotrexate as well as oral prednisolone [30].

CONCLUSION

It is important for patients to know that morphea is not life-threatening and does not progress to systemic sclerosis. Patients also need to recognize that the involved skin will never look completely normal after the treatments, and recurrences may happen after cessation of the therapy. It should be known that the aim of the treatment is preventing the enlargement of the existing lesions and the development of new lesions.

Topical glucocorticosteroids, calcipotriol, and calcineurin inhibitors can be used in the active stage of patients with limited types of morphea. Patients with linear morphea of the head and neck or limbs are at significant risk of facial deformity, limb length discrepancy and contractures and should, therefore, be treated with systemic therapy. Methotrexate in combination with a short course of systemic steroids is the first-line therapy in the active, deep involvement of the disease. If the patient does not show improvement after 2–3 months, therapy can be switched to phototherapy (NB-UVB, PUVA, UVA or UVA-1) based on availability.

Patients with generalized morphea may have superficial or deep variants. In patients without lesions that cross joints, phototherapy is an appropriate first option. There is not enough data to recommend one type of phototherapy over another, but medium-dose UVA1 may be more effective as a first choice. Alternatively, bath-PUVA or narrowband UVB phototherapy can be considered. Phototherapy has a more favorable side-effect profile than methotrexate and systemic steroids.

Box 14.10. Learning points.
• Methotrexate in combination with systemic steroids and ultraviolet-A1 light phototherapy has the most evidence of efficacy in the treatment of severe morphea.
• In the active stage of the disease, concomitant treatment with systemic corticosteroids should be performed if contraindications are absent, especially in severe cases (linear or deep morphea) or in cases with extracutaneous involvement. Alternatively, MMF should be considered in cases with failure or contraindications to methotrexate.
• The first choice of phototherapy for limited types of LS is medium-dose UVA1. Alternatively, bath-PUVA or cream-PUVA, and narrowband UVB can be considered in the generalized superficial morphea.
• Physiotherapy and manual therapy should be added to topical and systemic therapy in all types of morphea that result in restrictions of motion.
• Clinical follow-up visits (at least once a year) and a multidisciplinary approach should be performed in morphea with a high risk for recurrences after successful treatment, and a high rate of extracutaneous involvement. Children, especially those with linear or mixed types of morphea, are particularly affected by the recurrent disease.

REFERENCES

[1]   Careta MF, Romiti R. Localized scleroderma: Clinical spectrum and therapeutic update. An Bras Dermatol 2015; 90(1): 62-73.
[http://dx.doi.org/10.1590/abd1806-4841.20152890] [PMID: 25672301]

[2]   Knobler R, Moinzadeh P, Hunzelmann N, *et al*. European Dermatology Forum S1-guideline on the diagnosis and treatment of sclerosing diseases of the skin, Part 1: localized scleroderma, systemic sclerosis and overlap syndromes. J Eur Acad Dermatol Venereol 2017; 31(9): 1401-24.
[http://dx.doi.org/10.1111/jdv.14458] [PMID: 28792092]

[3]   Kreuter A, Krieg T, Worm M, *et al*. German guidelines for the diagnosis and therapy of localized scleroderma. J Dtsch Dermatol Ges 2016; 14(2): 199-216.
[http://dx.doi.org/10.1111/ddg.12724] [PMID: 26819124]

[4]   Narbutt J, Hołdrowicz A, Lesiak A. Morphea selected local treatment methods and their effectiveness. Reumatologia 2017; 55(6): 305-13.
[http://dx.doi.org/10.5114/reum.2017.72628] [PMID: 29491539]

[5]   Zwischenberger BA, Jacobe HT. A systematic review of morphea treatments and therapeutic algorithm. J Am Acad Dermatol 2011; 65(5): 925-41.
[http://dx.doi.org/10.1016/j.jaad.2010.09.006] [PMID: 21645943]

[6]   Cunningham BB, Landells IDR, Langman C, Sailer DE, Paller AS. Topical calcipotriene for morphea/linear scleroderma. J Am Acad Dermatol 1998; 39(2): 211-5.
[http://dx.doi.org/10.1016/S0190-9622(98)70077-5] [PMID: 9704831]

[7]   Valančienė G, Jasaitienė D, Valiukevičienė S. Pathogenesis and treatment modalities of localized scleroderma. Medicina 2010; 46(10): 649-56.
[http://dx.doi.org/10.3390/medicina46100092] [PMID: 21393982]

[8]   Bielsa Marsol I. Update on the classification and treatment of localized scleroderma. Actas Dermo-Sifiliográficas 2013; 104(8): 654-66.
[http://dx.doi.org/10.1016/j.adengl.2012.10.012] [PMID: 23948159]

[9]   Dytoc M, Ting PT, Man J, Sawyer D, Fiorillo L. First case series on the use of imiquimod for morphoea. Br J Dermatol 2005; 153(4): 815-20.
[http://dx.doi.org/10.1111/j.1365-2133.2005.06776.x] [PMID: 16181467]

[10]   Pope E, Doria AS, Theriault M, Mohanta A, Laxer RM. Topical imiquimod 5% cream for pediatric plaque morphea: a prospective, multiple-baseline, open-label pilot study. Dermatology 2011; 223(4): 363-9.
[http://dx.doi.org/10.1159/000335560] [PMID: 22327486]

[11]   Albuquerque JV, Andriolo BN, Vasconcellos MR, Civile VT, Lyddiatt A, Trevisani VF. Interventions for morphea. Cochrane Database Syst Rev 2019; 16(7): CD005027.
[http://dx.doi.org/10.1002/14651858.CD005027.pub5]

[12]   Hassani J, Feldman SR. Phototherapy in scleroderma. Dermatol Ther 2016; 6(4): 519-53.
[http://dx.doi.org/10.1007/s13555-016-0136-3] [PMID: 27519050]

[13]   Fett N, Werth VP. Update on morphea. J Am Acad Dermatol 2011; 64(2): 231-42.
[http://dx.doi.org/10.1016/j.jaad.2010.05.046] [PMID: 21238824]

[14]   Pereira N, Santiago F, Oliveira H, Figueiredo A. Low-dose UVA1 phototherapy for scleroderma: what benefit can we expect? J Eur Acad Dermatol Venereol 2012; 26(5): 619-26.
[http://dx.doi.org/10.1111/j.1468-3083.2011.04137.x] [PMID: 21635565]

[15]   Zandi S, Kalia S, Lui H. UVA1 phototherapy: A concise and practical review. Skin Therapy Lett 2012; 17(1): 1-4.
[PMID: 22358227]

[16]   Kreuter A, Hyun J, Stücker M, Sommer A, Altmeyer P, Gambichler T. A randomized controlled study of low-dose UVA1, medium-dose UVA1, and narrowband UVB phototherapy in the treatment of localized scleroderma. J Am Acad Dermatol 2006; 54(3): 440-7.
[http://dx.doi.org/10.1016/j.jaad.2005.11.1063] [PMID: 16488295]

[17]   Jacobe HT, Cayce R, Nguyen J. UVA1 phototherapy is effective in darker skin: A review of 101 patients of Fitzpatrick skin types I-V. Br J Dermatol 2008; 159(3): 691-6.
[http://dx.doi.org/10.1111/j.1365-2133.2008.08672.x] [PMID: 18544076]

[18]   Pasić A, Ceović R, Lipozencić J, *et al.* Phototherapy in pediatric patients. Pediatr Dermatol 2003; 20(1): 71-7.
[http://dx.doi.org/10.1046/j.1525-1470.2003.03016.x] [PMID: 12558852]

[19]   Morison WL. Psoralen UVA therapy for linear and generalized morphea. J Am Acad Dermatol 1997; 37(4): 657-9.
[http://dx.doi.org/10.1016/S0190-9622(97)70193-2] [PMID: 9344214]

[20]   El-Mofty M, Mostafa W, El-Darouty M, *et al.* Different low doses of broad-band UVA in the treatment of morphea and systemic sclerosis. A clinico-pathologic study. Photodermatol Photoimmunol Photomed 2004; 20(3): 148-56.
[http://dx.doi.org/10.1111/j.1600-0781.2004.00081.x] [PMID: 15144393]

[21]   Brownell I, Soter NA, Jr AGF. Familial linear scleroderma (en coup de sabre) responsive to antimalarials and narrowband ultraviolet B therapy. Dermatol Online J 2007; 13(1): 11.
[http://dx.doi.org/10.5070/D383K6X3TB] [PMID: 17511944]

[22]   Platsidaki E, Tzanetakou V, Kouris A, Stavropoulos P. Methotrexate: an effective monotherapy for refractory generalized morphea. Clin Cosmet Investig Dermatol 2017; 10: 165-9.
[http://dx.doi.org/10.2147/CCID.S134879] [PMID: 28507446]

[23]   Fett N. Morphea: Evidence-based recommendations for treatment. Indian J Dermatol Venereol Leprol

2012; 78(2): 135-41.
[http://dx.doi.org/10.4103/0378-6323.93628] [PMID: 22421642]

[24] Zulian F, Martini G, Vallongo C, *et al.* Methotrexate treatment in juvenile localized scleroderma: A randomized, double-blind, placebo-controlled trial. Arthritis Rheum 2011; 63(7): 1998-2006.
[http://dx.doi.org/10.1002/art.30264] [PMID: 21305525]

[25] Torok KS, Arkachaisri T. Methotrexate and corticosteroids in the treatment of localized scleroderma: A standardized prospective longitudinal single-center study. J Rheumatol 2012; 39(2): 286-94.
[http://dx.doi.org/10.3899/jrheum.110210] [PMID: 22247357]

[26] Arthur M, Fett NM, Latour E, *et al.* Evaluation of the effectiveness and tolerability of mycophenolate mofetil and mycophenolic acid for the treatment of morphea. JAMA Dermatol 2020; 156(5): 521-8.
[http://dx.doi.org/10.1001/jamadermatol.2020.0035] [PMID: 32236497]

[27] Kumar AB, Blixt EK, Drage LA, el-Azhary RA, Wetter DA. Treatment of morphea with hydroxychloroquine: A retrospective review of 84 patients at Mayo Clinic, 1996-2013. J Am Acad Dermatol 2019; 80(6): 1658-63.
[http://dx.doi.org/10.1016/j.jaad.2019.01.040] [PMID: 30703458]

[28] Thomas RM, Worswick S, Aleshin M. Retinoic acid for treatment of systemic sclerosis and morphea: A literature review. Dermatol Ther 2017; 30(2)e12455
[http://dx.doi.org/10.1111/dth.12455] [PMID: 28032675]

[29] Kim SR, Charos A, Damsky W, Heald P, Girardi M, King BA. Treatment of generalized deep morphea and eosinophilic fasciitis with the Janus kinase inhibitor to facitinib. JAAD Case Rep 2018; 4(5): 443-5.
[http://dx.doi.org/10.1016/j.jdcr.2017.12.003] [PMID: 29984277]

[30] Hulshof MM, Bavinck JNB, Bergman W, *et al.* Double-blind, placebo-controlled study of oral calcitriol for the treatment of localized and systemic scleroderma. J Am Acad Dermatol 2000; 43(6): 1017-23.
[http://dx.doi.org/10.1067/mjd.2000.108369] [PMID: 11100017]

[31] George R, George A, Kumar TS. Update on management of morphea (Localized Scleroderma) in children. Indian Dermatol Online J 2020; 11(2): 135-45.
[http://dx.doi.org/10.4103/idoj.IDOJ_284_19] [PMID: 32477969]

[32] Kreuter A, Gambichler T, Avermaete A, *et al.* Combined treatment with calcipotriol ointment and low-dose ultraviolet A1 phototherapy in childhood morphea. Pediatr Dermatol 2001; 18(3): 241-5.
[http://dx.doi.org/10.1046/j.1525-1470.2001.018003241.x] [PMID: 11438008]

[33] Aranegui B, Jiménez-Reyes J. Morphea in Childhood: An Update. Actas Dermosifiliogr 2018; 109(4): 312-22.
[http://dx.doi.org/10.1016/j.ad.2017.06.021] [PMID: 29248149]

[34] Weibel L, Sampaio MC, Visentin MT, Howell KJ, Woo P, Harper JI. Evaluation of methotrexate and corticosteroids for the treatment of localized scleroderma (morphoea) in children. Br J Dermatol 2006; 155(5): 1013-20.
[http://dx.doi.org/10.1111/j.1365-2133.2006.07497.x] [PMID: 17034534]

[35] Zulian F, Culpo R, Sperotto F, *et al.* Consensus-based recommendations for the management of juvenile localised scleroderma. Ann Rheum Dis 2019; 78(8): 1019-24.
[http://dx.doi.org/10.1136/annrheumdis-2018-214697] [PMID: 30826775]

[36] Mertens JS, Seyger MMB, Thurlings RM, Radstake TRDJ, de Jong EMGJ. Morphea and eosinophilic fasciitis: An update. Am J Clin Dermatol 2017; 18(4): 491-512.
[http://dx.doi.org/10.1007/s40257-017-0269-x] [PMID: 28303481]

[37] Ferreli C, Gasparini G, Parodi A, Cozzani E, Rongioletti F, Atzori L. Cutaneous manifestations of scleroderma and scleroderma-like disorders: A comprehensive review. Clin Rev Allergy Immunol 2017; 53(3): 306-36.

[http://dx.doi.org/10.1007/s12016-017-8625-4] [PMID: 28712039]

[38] Cheape AC, Murrell DF. 2% Crisaborole topical ointment for the treatment of mild-to-moderate atopic dermatitis. Expert Rev Clin Immunol 2017; 13(5): 415-23.
[http://dx.doi.org/10.1080/1744666X.2017.1304820] [PMID: 28290219]

[39] Cardones A. National Library of Medicine. (March 10). Pilot Study Evaluating the Efficacy of a Topical PDE4 Inhibitor for Morphea. Identifier NCT03351114. 2018. Available at: https://clinicaltrials.gov/ct2/show/results/NCT03351114 (Accessed on: September 1 2020).

[40] Li H, Zuo J, Tang W. Phosphodiesterase-4 inhibitors for the treatment of inflammatory diseases. Front Pharmacol 2018; 9: 1048.
[http://dx.doi.org/10.3389/fphar.2018.01048] [PMID: 30386231]

[41] Saracino AM, Denton CP, Orteu CH. The molecular pathogenesis of morphoea: from genetics to future treatment targets. Br J Dermatol 2017; 177(1): 34-46.
[http://dx.doi.org/10.1111/bjd.15001] [PMID: 27553363]

[42] Maier C, Ramming A, Bergmann C, *et al.* Inhibition of phosphodiesterase 4 (PDE4) reduces dermal fibrosis by interfering with the release of interleukin-6 from M2 macrophages. Ann Rheum Dis 2017; 76(6): 1133-41.
[http://dx.doi.org/10.1136/annrheumdis-2016-210189] [PMID: 28209630]

[43] Koschitzky M, Khattri S. Apremilast as a treatment for morphea: A case series. JAAD Case Rep 2022; 19: 58-63.
[http://dx.doi.org/10.1016/j.jdcr.2021.11.009] [PMID: 34917727]

[44] Schwartz DM, Kanno Y, Villarino A, Ward M, Gadina M, O'Shea JJ. Erratum: JAK inhibition as a therapeutic strategy for immune and inflammatory diseases. Nat Rev Drug Discov 2018; 17(1): 78.
[http://dx.doi.org/10.1038/nrd.2017.267] [PMID: 29282366]

[45] Furumoto Y, Gadina M. The arrival of JAK inhibitors: advancing the treatment of immune and hematologic disorders. BioDrugs 2013; 27(5): 431-8.
[http://dx.doi.org/10.1007/s40259-013-0040-7] [PMID: 23743669]

[46] Schwartz DM, Bonelli M, Gadina M, O'Shea JJ. Type I/II cytokines, JAKs, and new strategies for treating autoimmune diseases. Nat Rev Rheumatol 2016; 12(1): 25-36.
[http://dx.doi.org/10.1038/nrrheum.2015.167] [PMID: 26633291]

[47] Chapman S, Kwa M, Gold LS, Lim HW. Janus kinase inhibitors in dermatology: Part I. A comprehensive review. J Am Acad Dermatol 2022; 86(2): 406-13.
[http://dx.doi.org/10.1016/j.jaad.2021.07.002] [PMID: 34246698]

CHAPTER 15

Idiopathic Atrophoderma of Pasini and Pierini

Tasleem Arif[1,2,*]

[1] *Department of Dermatology, STDs, Leprosy and Aesthetics, Dar As Sihha Medical center, Dammam, Saudi Arabia*

[2] *Ellahi Medicare Clinic, Srinagar, Kashmir, India*

Chapter synopsis.
• Idiopathic atrophoderma of Pasini and Pierini (IAPP) is a rare disease of unknown etiology characterized by the presence of single or multiple well-defined atrophic plaques having an abrupt edge forming "cliff-drop" borders.
• The etiology is unknown. Genetic factors, neurogenic causes, immunological factors, somatic mosaicism, *B. burgdorferi,* and abnormal metabolism of dermatan sulphate have been proposed.
• IAPP usually affects individuals during the second or third decades of life and predominantly affects females. However, it can rarely occur in infancy or old age.
• Histopathologically, it is characterized by a normal epidermis with increased pigmentation in the basal layer. There is a mild perivascular mononuclear cell infiltrate and melanophages in the upper dermis. Collagen in the deeper dermis is edematous, clumped, and homogenized. The elastic tissue may show a spectrum that ranges from normal to severe diminution with the fragmentation of elastic fibers.
• The absence of signs of inflammation, 'lilac ring' appearance, sclerosis and induration in the lesions of IAPP differentiates it from morphea. Sclerosis which is prominent in morphea is absent or minimal in IAPP.
• IAPP has a benign course and lacks the complications seen in some forms of morphea. New lesions may develop while the existing lesions may enlarge variably over the next 10-20 years. However, existing lesions do not involute in IAPP.
• Several treatment options have been tried in IAPP but none have been found to be consistently effective. Oral tetracyclines, penicillin, hydroxychloroquine, standard recommended therapy for Lyme disease, potassium aminobenzoate, calcineurin inhibitors, PUVA, retinoids, steroids and phototherapy have shown variable efficacy.

Keywords: Abrupt borders, Anetoderma, Atrophoderma, Atrophy, Atrofodermia idiopatica progressive, Atrophic plaques, Atrophic scleroderma d'emblee, Atrophoscleroderma, Atrophoderma elastolytica discreta, Atrophic-scleroderma superficialis circumscripta, Atypical lilac-colored and non-indurated scleroderma.

[*] **Corresponding author Tasleem Arif:** Department of Dermatology, STDs, Leprosy and Aesthetics, Dar As Sihha Medical center, Dammam, Saudi Arabia and Ellahi Medicare Clinic, Srinagar, Kashmir, India; E-mail: dr_tasleem_arif@yahoo.com

Blaschkoid idiopathic atrophoderma of Pasini and Pierini, Borrellia burgdorferi, Cliff- drop borders, Dermatan sulphate, Dyschromic and atrophic variation of scleroderma, Footprint in snow appearance, Fragmentation of elastic fibers, Idiopathic atrophoderma of Pasini and Pierini, Intra-collagenous edema, Inverted plateau, Linear atrophoderma of Moulin, Morphea, Morphea with an unusual degree of atrophy, Morphea plana atrophica, Mosaicism, Skin glycosaminoglycans, Sclerosis, Swiss cheese, Tetracycline.

INTRODUCTION

Idiopathic atrophoderma of Pasini and Pierini (IAPP) is a rare disease of unknown etiology which is characterized by the presence of single or multiple well-defined atrophic plaques. These plaques are characterized by slight depression of the skin with an abrupt edge causing what is known as "cliff-drop" borders. In contrast to morphea, these plaques do not show signs of inflammation, sclerosis, and induration [1]. The most commonly affected site is the trunk especially the back and abdomen. Proximal extremities can also get affected. Most commonly, plaques are present in a bilaterally symmetrical distribution, although lesions involving the body in an asymmetrical distribution have also been reported [2]. The plaques are generally round or ovoid in shape with their long axis parallel to the lines of cleavage and having a tendency to coalesce to form large, irregular-shaped plaques with convex borders [3].

HISTORICAL BACKGROUND

The history (Table **15.1**) of IAPP dates back to 1902-1904, when Brocq *et al.* termed it "atrophic scleroderma d'emblee" and Thibierge described a "dyschromic and atrophic variation of scleroderma" [4, 5]. In 1923, Pasini described a case report of a 21-year-old woman with a 4-year history of brownish-grey, "cyanotic" lesions on the trunk that was published in an Italian dermatology journal. These lesions were oval to round in shape. They were depressed below the surrounding normal skin. There was no associated inflammation. The lesions had spread from the upper back to the lower part of the back, flanks, and sacral regions. In addition, the patient had some lesions on the chest and a few lesions were present around the waistline. These plaques were flat, smooth, atrophic and depressed 1-2 mm below the surrounding normal skin. There was no induration and the sclerosis was absent. Follicular openings were fewer than normal. The affected skin was appearing thinner because of which one can view the deeper blood vessels. The border of the lesions had an irregular, slightly wavy shape and showed an abrupt transition from normal to diseased skin. He termed this entity "Atrofodermia idiopatica progressiva" designating it as a separate entity from that of morphea or scleroderma [6]. This term by Pasini has been translated into English as "progressive idiopathic atrophoderma". Thirteen years later, in 1936, in Argentina, Pierini and Vivoli described a 19-year-old woman with similar lesions. She presented with multiple bluish, non-indurated patches of 3 years duration. These lesions were present on the right side of her chest and back in a zosteriform distribution. These skin lesions remained completely unaltered for the next 10 years [7]. Subsequently, Pierini observed over 50 such cases. His cases and several reports by other researchers can be seen in the Argentine literature [2]. Pierini classified this disorder into two types, a primary idiopathic form of atrophy and an atrophoscleroderma that was secondary to morphea. Since then, it has been described in the literature by various confusing terms such as "atrophoscleroderma superficialis circumscripta," "morphea with an unusual degree of atrophy," "morphea plana atrophica," and "atypical lilac-colored and non-indurated scleroderma" [2].

Table 15.1. Historical background of Idiopathic atrophoderma of Pasini and Pierini.

1902-1904	Brocq *et al.* coined the term "atrophic scleroderma d'emblee" and Thibierge described a "dyschromic and atrophic variation of scleroderma".
1923	Pasini described a case of a 21-year-old woman with a 4-year history of brownish-grey, "cyanotic" lesions on the trunk without inflammation, induration or sclerosis and termed it as 'Atrofodermia idiopatica progressiva'.
1936	Pierini and Vivoli described a 19-year-old woman with multiple bluish, non-indurated patches of 3 years duration present on the right side of her chest and back in a zosteriform distribution that remained completely unaltered for the next 10 years.
1958	Canizares *et al.*, introduced the entity into the American dermatologic literature and proposed the term "idiopathic atrophoderma of Pasini and Pierini". They suggested that this disease was unique and differed sufficiently from *morphea* and classified it as a separate entity.
2000	Yokoyama *et al.*, showed that skin glycosaminoglycans extracted from the lesions of patients with IAPP were different from those seen in typical lesions of morphea thus supporting the view that IAPP is different from morphea.

In 1958, it was Canizares *et al.*, who first introduced this entity into the American dermatologic literature. He reviewed findings achieved by Pierini and proposed the term "idiopathic atrophoderma of Pasini and Pierini". Canizares *et al.* suggested that the disease was unique and differed sufficiently from morphea and classified it as a distinct entity. Since the two authors deserve the credit for making the greatest contribution to the knowledge of this entity, hence the name IAPP [8]. In 2000, Yokoyama *et al.* investigated the skin glycosaminoglycans extracted from the lesions of patients with IAPP. They concluded that glycosaminoglycans in IAPP were different from those seen in typical lesions of morphea. This further added to the support that IAPP is different from morphea [9].

ETIOPATHOGENESIS

The etiology of IAPP is not known. Various authors have put forth several factors in its etiopathogenesis (Box **15.1**). Genetic factors have been implicated in its pathogenesis. This has been supported by a report where the disease occurred in two brothers [10]. In addition, it has been augmented by another case where IAPP and discoid lupus erythematosus were seen in a patient having hereditary C2 complement deficiency which has been associated with a particular HLA haplotype [11]. Some authors have suggested a neurogenic cause in view of the apparent zosteriform distribution of lesions in few cases [7, 8]. The underlying mechanism for such zosteriform distribution of lesions includes a predisposing defect in the migration of neural crest cells during embryonic life or a defect in the local peripheral nerves. Cells with aberrant T-cell phenotypes have been incriminated as a cause of collagen fiber destruction [12]. Somatic mosaicism in IAPP can be explained by the development of lesions along the blaschko lines in a few reported cases including the one reported by the author and his colleagues. This raises the possibility of a developmental abnormality in such IAPP cases [1].

Box 15.1. Possible factors involved in etiopathogenesis of IAPP.
Genetic factors
Neurogenic cause
Somatic mosaicism
Borrellia burgdorferi
Immunological factors
Abnormal metabolism of dermatan sulphate
Cells with aberrant T-cell phenotype

The role of spirochete *Borrelia burgdorferi* in the pathogenesis of some cases of IAPP has been discussed. Buechner and Rufi investigated the sera of 26 patients with typical lesions of IAPP. About 53% of patients had immunoglobulin G anti–*B burgdorferi* antibodies while only 14% of the control subjects demonstrated such antibodies. However, no immunoglobulin M antibodies were found [13]. Kencka *et al.* found IgG antibodies against *B. burgdorferi* in 5 out of 8 patients [14]. Immunological factors have also revealed some evidence of pathogenesis. Direct immunofluorescence of the skin biopsy from the IAPP patient has revealed strong positive staining of dendritic cells, possibly Langerhans cells, in the epidermis with anti-IgM. Immunoperoxidase staining has shown that the perivascular inflammatory infiltrate seen in IAPP patients was composed of T cells (CD-3+) and macrophages (CD-14+). The majority of the T cells were of the helper/inducer subset (CD-4+) while suppressor/ cytotoxic cells (CD-8+) were sparse. Most of the T cells expressed two pan-T antigens viz., CD-2 and CD-3, in approximately equal numbers. However, CD-7 (another pan-T antigen) expression was not seen while a slight loss of expression of CD-5 was present. Indirect immunofluorescence did not show circulating anto-antibodies. Serum immunoglobulin and serum complement levels (C3 and C4) were normal. CH50 assay revealed normal functional activity of the complement cascade. Flow cytometric analysis revealed an increased circulating population of activated T lymphocytes expressing HLA-DR and CD-25 [12, 15]. The abnormal metabolism of dermatan sulphate has been implicated by a few authors in its pathogenesis [15, 16].

CLINICAL PRESENTATION

IAPP usually affects individuals during the second or third decade of life. However, it can occur in infancy and old age. It predominantly affects females [13]. The author could search four published cases of congenital IAPP [17]. The onset is usually insidious, with the majority of patients being asymptomatic. However, some patients may experience tingling or warmth in the involved areas, but upon testing, sensation is normal in the involved skin. The most commonly affected site is the trunk especially the back and abdomen. Proximal extremities can also get affected. Most commonly, the lesions are present in a bilaterally symmetrical distribution, although lesions involving the body in an asymmetrical distribution have also been reported. Some cases where lesions are present in a zosteriform distribution (Figs. **15.1** and **15.2**) have been described [3, 13, 18, 19].

Less frequently, lesions may involve extremities. A study done by Saleh *et al.* on 16 patients of IAPP showed that extremities were involved in all the patients with the lower and upper extremities affected in 62.5% and 50% of the patients, respectively. Surprisingly, involvement of the trunk was seen in only 31.3% of the patients [20]. Rarely, facial involvement has been reported [21].

The lesions are usually round or ovoid in shape with their long axis parallel to the lines of cleavage ranging in size from a few millimeters to several centimeters. Sometimes they may coalesce, forming large, irregularly shaped plaques with convex borders (Fig. **15.3**).

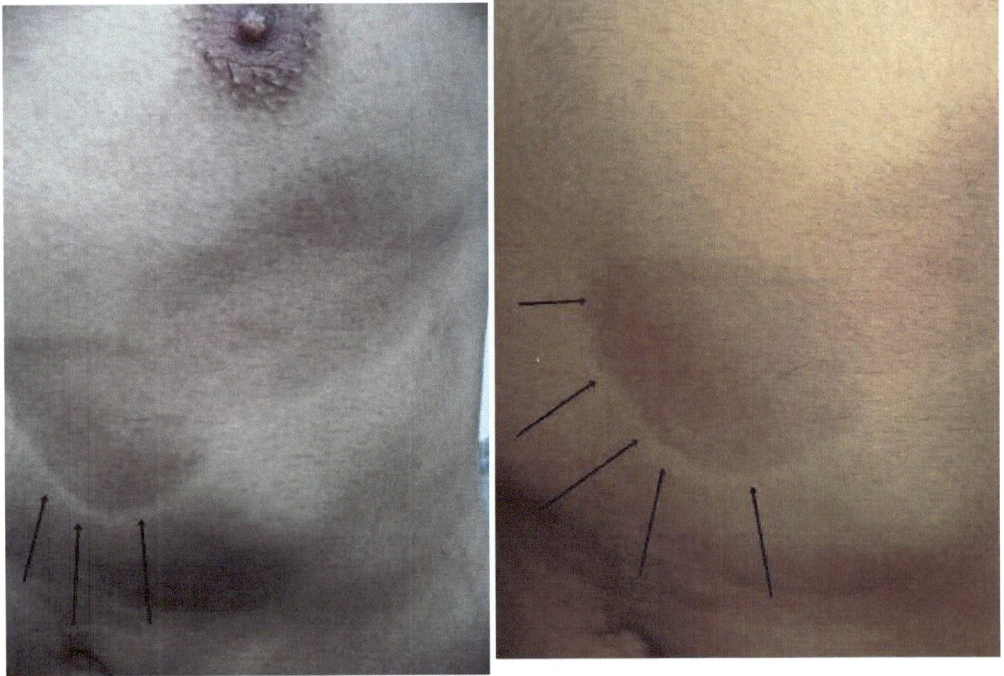

Fig. (15.1 and 15.2). Light-brownish colored, atrophic plaque distributed in a zosteriform pattern on the chest and abdomen not crossing the midline. The affected skin of the plaque is depressed compared to the surrounding normal skin (inverted plateau appearance). Note the sharply defined cliff drop borders of the plaque (black arrows) giving the appearance of "footprint in snow" to the depressed plaques. [Copyright: Arif T. Zosteriform idiopathic atrophoderma of Pasini and Pierini. Indian J Paediatr Dermatol 2019;20:60-3.].

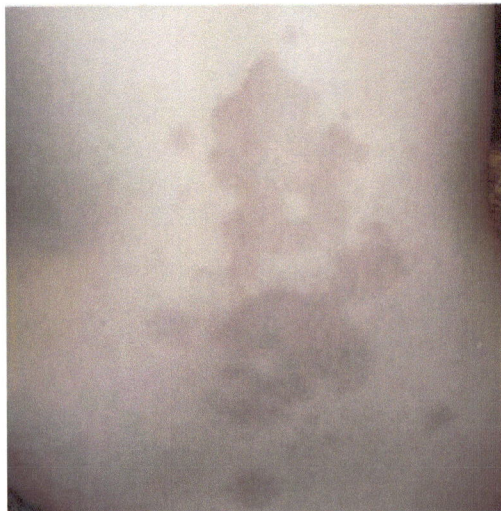

Fig. (15.3). Multiple depressed plaques on the back of a 16 year old caucasian woman with typical cliff drop borders. (Image Credit: Leith C Jones –own work/ English Wikipedia / CC BY 3.0)

Palm sized lesions have been commonly reported. The lesions are characteristically bluish violet to slate-grey or brown in color. Passive hyperemia has been suggested for the "cyanotic" hue of the lesions. Hypopigmented variety has also been described. In fact in a study of 16 patients, nine had hypopigmented, four skin colored and only three had hyperpigmented lesions [20]. The deeper blood vessels may be faintly visible through the thinned out skin and may give a blurred appearance. No telangiectasias are seen. The affected skin of the plaques is depressed compared to the surrounding normal skin, giving the appearance of an "inverted plateau." In some cases where multiple patches are present on the back of a patient, the appearance of the patient's back resembles that of "Swiss cheese" in architecture. The sharply defined, abrupt borders of the plaques give a "cliff-drop" appearance to the lesions (Fig. **15.4**). This depression at the borders usually ranges from 2 to 8 mm. However, this transition is usually less abrupt in the plaques present on the abdomen. These depressed plaques have also been described as resembling "footprint in snow" appearance.

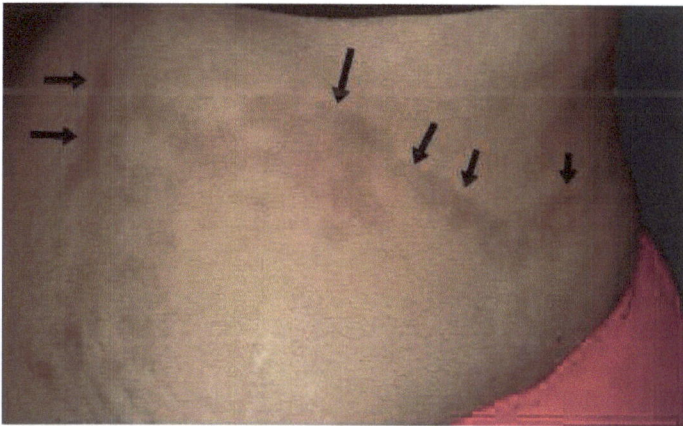

Fig. (15.4). Multiple ill-defined depressed plaques slightly brownish in color present over left half of trunk in a female patient in a blaschkoid pattern. The plaques were non-indurated and were having cliff drop borders (black arrows). The clinical course and the histopathology of the lesions were more in favor of IAPP than Linear atrophoderma of Moulin which was a close differential for this case.

The surface of affected skin itself is smooth without epidermal atrophy or hyperkeratosis. Palpation of the lesions reveals no induration, edema, thickening, or leathery feeling. The "hernia" phenomenon which occurs in the macular atrophies (anetoderma) is not appreciated in IAPP. Signs of inflammation are absent. An erythematous or "lilac-ring" border which is characteristic of morphea, does not occur in IAPP. Some authors have identified two clinical types of IAPP. The first type is comprised of round to oval shaped well defined blue-brown to brown atrophic plaques. The second type consists of superficial mild atrophic macules that coalesce with each other to form larger hyperpigmented lesions [22]. Less commonly, concomitant sclerodermatous changes have been reported in the previous atrophic patches of IAPP. Such sclerodermatous changes usually appear in the center of the plaque and manifest as shiny white indurated area resembling that of morphea. Rarely, in IAPP, sclerodermatous lesions may either predate or occur simultaneously with atrophic lesions and thus become difficult to be differentiated from early edematous lesions of morphea. However, a lilac ring is not present [8, 23]. Contrary to linear atrophoderma of Moulin, IAPP tends to be progressive, with new lesions developing and enlarging variably over the next 10-20 years. Finally, a state is reached at which progression ceases. However, it should be remembered that the existing lesions in IAPP characteristically do not involve [2, 3, 6 - 8].

HISTOPATHOLOGY

Histopathology in IAPP is not diagnostic and most of the times there are only mild changes that may be easily missed unless an elliptical biopsy including both the affected and normal skin is taken perpendicular to the edge of the lesion and deep enough to include the subcutaneous tissue layer [15]. On routine hematoxylin and eosin stain examination, IAPP is characterized by a normal epidermis with increased pigmentation (Figs. **15.5** and **15.6**) in the basal layer (Box **15.2**).

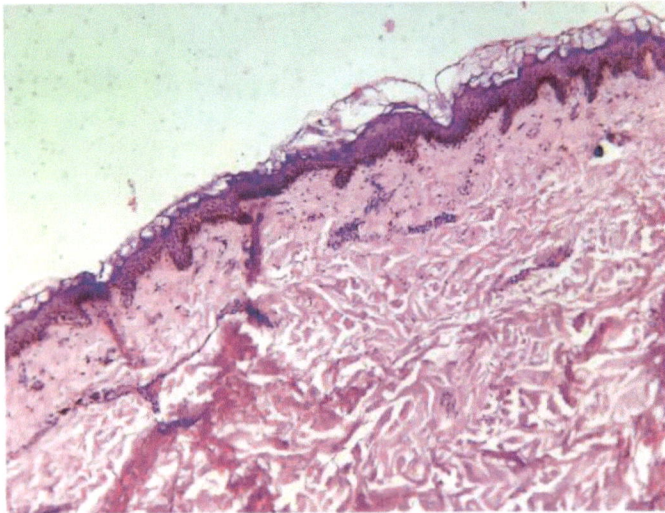

Fig. (15.5). The epidermis is normal with increased pigmentation of the basal layer. There is scanty mononuclear cell infiltrate in the upper dermis. Dermis is filled with homogenized and thickened collagen bundles. Sweat glands and pilosebaceous units are intact. (H and E, ×10).

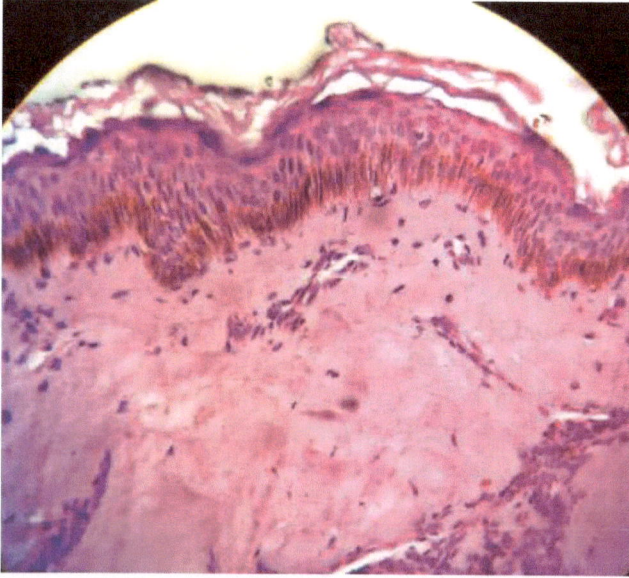

Fig. (15.6). The epidermal thickness is normal with increased pigmentation of the basal layer. There is sparse mononuclear cell infiltrate and homogenized collagen bundles in the upper dermis (H and E, ×40).

Box 15.2: Histopathology in IAPP.
Normal epidermis with increased basal layer pigmentation.
Perivascular mononuclear cell infiltrate.
Melanophages in the upper dermis.
Edematous, clumped and homogenized collagen in the mid and deeper dermis.
Intact appendageal structures and subcutaneous tissue.
Variable changes in elastic tissue ranging from normal to severe reduction and fragmentation of elastic fibers (atrophoderma elastolytica discreta).
Direct immunofluorescence can be negative or nonspecific.

In the upper dermis, there is a mild perivascular mononuclear cell infiltrate and melanophages. Collagen in the deeper dermis is edematous, clumped and homogenized [13]. The appendages and subcutaneous tissue are intact [8]. Though the elastic tissue stain of lesional skin has been essentially normal, there are some reports in which a decreased amount of elastic fibers in the dermis has been described [13, 23 - 25]. Some authors have found variable changes in elastic fibers on Verhoeff-van Gieson and/or orcein- Giemsa stains within a spectrum that ranged from normal to severe diminution with the fragmentation of elastic fibers. In one study, 35.3% of IAPP cases showed moderate to severe decrease in fragmentation in the elastic fibers [20]. The term "atrophoderma elastolytica discreta" has been proposed by Carrington *et al.* to account for the classical lesions of atrophoderma that reveal on histopathology reduction and fragmentation of elastic fibers similar to anetoderma [26]. Hence elastic fibers in IAPP may show a wide spectrum from being completely normal to absent as is seen in anetoderma. Such a variation in the pathology of elastic fibers should be accepted as part of the histological continuum of IAPP [20]. In such cases having significant elastic fiber reduction, clinicopathologic correlation carries prime importance in differentiating those cases from anetoderma. Anetoderma in contrast to IAPP is characterized by wrinkled macules/patches that bulge like pouches and herniate into the skin upon palpation producing sac-like protrusions. Making such a distinction between the two conditions has clinical significance because anetoderma may be associated with HIV infection and certain prothrombotic abnormalities *e.g.*, systemic lupus erythematosus and antiphospholipid syndrome that are not seen with IAPP [27 - 30]. The direct immunofluorescence may be negative or nonspecific [12]. With the use of magnetic resonance imaging, Franck *et al.* demonstrated that skin depression in IAPP lesions is solely because of atrophy in the dermis [31]. An ultrasound analysis using 13-MHz B-mode was conducted by Abe *et al.* to evaluate the cutaneous atrophy in IAPP. They found that the dermal thickness on the sonogram was decreased by 46%-55% and hypodermis by 10%-18% in affected skin in comparison to normal skin in the same patients. However, no associated change in echogenicity was visualized on ultrasonography [32]. Thus it seems that dermal atrophy is more pronounced in IAPP than in the subcutaneous tissue. More studies are needed to establish the actual level of atrophy in IAPP which at present is seen mainly as dermal atrophy in contrast to LAM where the subcutaneous layer is the site of atrophy.

DIFFERENTIAL DIAGNOSIS

There are some disorders from which IAPP needs to be differentiated. These include morphea, linear atrophoderma of Moulin (LAM), and anetoderma (Table **16.5**, chapter 16). The absence of signs of inflammation, 'lilac ring', sclerosis and induration in the lesions of IAPP differentiates it from morphea. Sclerosis which is prominent in morphea is absent or minimal in IAPP. Elastic tissue changes which have been described above in IAPP are not seen in morphea [2]. IAPP needs to be distinguished from LAM by the latter's earlier onset, non-progressive course, and distribution of lesions along Blaschko lines [1]. IAPP is primarily considered as a dermal atrophy while as the atrophy in LAM is because of the reduction of subcutaneous fat [1, 33]. In addition, IAPP is rarely seen to follow Blaschko's lines [1]. Cases of IAPP with significant elastic fiber reduction need to be differentiated from anetoderma. The lesions of anetoderma are characterized by wrinkled macules or patches that protrude and herniate into the skin upon palpation (sac-like protrusions) [27]. Additionally, IAPP shows no erythema and on histopathological examination, the degeneration of elastic tissue is more marked in anetoderma and more superficial in the location in comparison to IAPP [8, 24, 34].

TREATMENT

At present, there is no effective treatment available for IAPP. Several treatment options have been tried, however, none has been found to be consistently effective for IAPP (Box **15.3**). Some researchers have tried oral tetracyclines to prevent the emergence of new lesions in patients of IAPP who had a positive test for the presence of IgG antibodies to *B. burgdorferi* [35, 36]. The early-stage of IAPP, especially those patients who are having a positive *B. burgdorferi* antibody serology, the standard recommended therapy for Lyme disease has been suggested. A 35-year-old woman with IAPP and elevated *B. burgdorferi* antibody titer showed clinical improvement with doxycycline (200 mg/d) for 6 weeks [35].

Box 15.3. Treatment of IAPP.
Oral tetracycline
Oral penicillin
Standard recommended therapy for Lyme disease in early IAPP associated with *B burgdorferi*
Hydroxychloroquine
Potassium aminobenzoate
Topical calcineurin inhibitors.
Q-switched alexandrite laser (755nm)
Psoralen and UVA (PUVA)
Retinoids
Topical and systemic steroids
Phototherapy
D-Penicillamine

A retrospective study involving 25 patients of IAPP who were treated with either oral penicillin (2 million IU per day) or oral tetracycline (500 mg three times per day) for 2-3 weeks showed clinical improvement in 20 patients with no new active lesions [13]. Carter *et al.* in 2006 have reported a patient who was treated with 400-mg per day of hydroxychloroquine. The patient showed dramatic response. He was having positive antinuclear antibody and rheumatoid factor but was negative for Lyme disease related antibodies. There was marked improvement in all the lesions after five months of therapy and complete clearance of trunk and facial lesions was achieved after 1 year [37]. A report of a patient treated with potassium aminobenzoate for three months showed subjective improvement while the new lesions ceased to appear [38]. The variable response has been shown by topical calcineurin inhibitors [37]. Arpey *et al.* tried a Q-switched alexandrite laser (755nm) in the treatment of IAPP. The hyperpigmentation associated with IAPP showed response, however, the laser did not help atrophy [39]. Other treatments that have been tried include psoralen and UVA (PUVA), retinoids, topical and systemic steroids, phototherapy and D-penicillamine with variable results [37, 40]. Aggressive treatment is not needed as most of the times, the disease has a benign course.

PROGNOSIS

IAPP tends to be progressive. New lesions may develop while the existing lesions may enlarge variably over next 10-20 years. Finally, a stage is reached at which further disease progression stops. However, it is important to note that the existing lesions do not involute in IAPP which distinguishes it from morphea [8]. Recently, extramedullary plasmacytoma and papillary carcinoma of the thyroid gland have been reported in association with IAPP [41, 42]. Whether these reports were a coincidence or association needs further reports. In addition, these reports also oblige us to have a thorough follow up of such IAPP patients as well as it implies that we should look for more predisposing factors related to this entity. Progression of IAPP to systemic sclerosis has not been discussed. However, a single case of a 42-year-old woman reported by Bisaccia *et al.* in 1982 has been published. She had typical lesions of IAPP on her back and developed systemic sclerosis with sclerodactyly, Raynaud's phenomenon and lung fibrosis [43].

RELATIONSHIP BETWEEN IAPP AND MORPHEA

There has been a lot of controversy regarding the relationship between IAPP and morphea. Authors differ in opinion as to whether IAPP is a variant of morphea or a separate disease entity. Historically, two school of thoughts have been recognized regarding the same. The first group of researchers who consider IAPP to be a subtype of morphea include Miller, Kogoj, Jablonska and Szczepanski, and Brunauer [24, 34, 44, 45]. They have proposed that IAPP is an abortive form of morphea. Miller *et al.* proposed that the transition from either IAPP to morphea or vice versa can occur at any time during the course of the disease [34]. Thus they are of this opinion that IAPP is an abortive subtype of morphea in which induration fails to occur [12, 14, 24, 34]. The second school of thought who project IAPP as a "separate disease entity" includes Canizares *et al.*, Grupper and

Stevanovic [8, 46, 47]. The Argentine concept for the disease suggested by authors like Pierini and Borda, is that there exist two subtypes of IAPP: (1) A "true" form of IAPP that remains unaltered for many years; and (2) A second type that is closely related to morphea either clinically or histopathologically or both. It is in this type where sclerotic changes can appear after several years following the onset of atrophic lesions [8, 48].

It is important to understand the similarities as well as differences between the two disease entities so as to arrive at a decision. It is because of these similarities and differences which have created controversy among global researchers and led to the division of concepts regarding their relationship. In the following text, the author will elaborate on them so that the readers have a clear and broad vision regarding the two entities.

IAPP as a Subtype of Morphea

The facts which are in favor of IAPP being a variant of morphea are discussed below:

The end stage morphea lesions usually turn atrophic and develop histological changes similar to lesions of IAPP [24].

Induration similar to that of morphea has been described in the long-standing lesions of IAPP [8, 13, 24].

Clumped and homogenized collagen in the dermis and mild sclerosis have been reported in some cases of IAPP [8, 34].

Typical morphea plaques have co-occurred with IAPP lesions in the same patient [8, 14, 19, 23, 24, 34].

A single case of a 42-year-old woman has been reported who had typical lesions of IAPP on her back and developed systemic sclerosis with sclerodactyly, Raynaud's phenomenon and lung fibrosis [43].

IAPP as a Distinct Entity

The Arguments that favor IAPP to be a separate entity and not being a subtype of morphea are discussed below:

Age of Onset

The age of onset for IAPP is earlier than morphea. Usually, IAPP occurs around 10-30 years which is earlier than morphea (20-50 years) [13].

Disease Course

IAPP has a protracted course and may last for 10-20 years before getting stabilized. On the contrary, morphea has a shorter disease duration about 3-5 years [2, 22].

Cliff Drop Border

IAPP lesions are depressed compared to the surrounding normal skin, giving the appearance of an "inverted plateau". The sharply defined, abrupt borders of the plaques give a "cliff-drop" appearance to the lesions. However, such features are not seen in morphea.

Lilac Ring

The initial inflammatory stage of the morphea is characterized by the appearance of a purplish-blue ring around the lesions, and when it is present, it is considered pathognomonic for morphea. Such a ring is not seen in IAPP.

Clinical Sequence of Manifestations

IAPP and morphea have contrasting clinical features when their progression and sequence are studied. IAPP starts as atrophic lesions and hence it has been regarded primarily as dermal atrophy. Long-standing lesions of IAPP may later develop induration which usually appears in the center of the plaque and manifest as a shiny white indurated area resembling that of morphea. On the contrary, morphea starts with inflammation and induration and later progresses to atrophy. Hence the sequence of events is reversed in the two entities [8, 34].

Complications

The natural course of the IAPP lesions is usually benign and most of the times, aggressive therapy is not required. Most often such lesions do not pose any threat of complications [13, 14]. On the contrary, certain types of morphea if left untreated, can cause significant cosmetic and functional morbidity. Morphea itself doesn't seem to increase the chance of mortality; however, it can cause significant morbidity as a result of flexion contractures, limb and facial asymmetry, extracutaneous manifestations, CNS and eye involvement [49 - 51]. The lesions in IAPP do not involute, however, the involution of lesions does occur in morphea [8].

Histopathological Changes

There are many differences in the histopathological findings between IAPP and morphea. Firstly, sclerosis is prominent in morphea and is considered one of the characteristic features of scleroderma. On the contrary, it is minimal or absent in IAPP [2, 8]. Secondly, variable changes in elastic tissue ranging from normal to severe reduction and fragmentation of elastic fibers have been described in IAPP [20]. However, such changes are not seen in morphea. Thirdly, intra-collagenous edema in IAPP occurs in the mid and deep dermis while edema of collagen in morphea extends from the upper to the mid dermis [2]. Fourthly, the appendageal system is preserved in IAPP while appendages may be partially or completely lost in morphea.

Autoimmunity

In children with morphea, 2- 5% have a concomitant autoimmune disease while in case of adults with morphea, the value is higher around 30% [49]. Patients having morphea commonly possess autoantibodies on serology testing. The prevalence of positive ANA titers in morphea patients have been described in the range of 20% to 80% [49]. Several antibodies that have been reported from morphea patients include homogeneous ANA, single-stranded antibody, and rheumatoid factor and anti-histone antibodies. Antitopoisomerase II alpha antibody has been reported in 76% of all morphea patients and 85% of generalized morphea patients [52]. However such findings haven't been reported in IAPP.

Skin Glycosaminoglycans

Yokoyama *et al.*, have studied the disaccharide analysis of skin glycosaminoglycans in IAPP patients. They concluded that skin glycosaminoglycans extracted from the lesions of IAPP patients were different from those seen in typical lesions of morphea. This supports the view that IAPP is distinct from morphea [9].

Thus, from the above facts, it is clear that IAPP has far more differences from morphea than having similarities. Even the magnitude of differences seems stronger than what is holding it as a variant of morphea. At the same time we can't completely ignore the similarities. Probably, the Argentine concept of the IAPP may offer some plausible explanation. It proposes that there are two subtypes of IAPP: A "true/classical" form of IAPP that remains unaltered for many years; and the second type that is closely related to morphea either clinically or histopathologically or both. According to them, it is in this second type where sclerotic changes can appear after several years following the onset of atrophic lesions [8, 48]. Following this concept we can explain IAPP better as a distinct entity as well as related to morphea. However, the author is of the opinion that IAPP must be considered as a separate disease entity distinct from morphea. IAPP is primarily dermal atrophy while morphea is an inflammatory/sclerotic disorder with different etiopathogenesis, the pattern of clinical progression, prognosis and treatment. This is the reason why the author/editor has kept a separate chapter for IAPP.

Box 15.4. Learning points.
• IAPP is a dermal atrophy where the atrophy in plaques is mainly seen in the dermis. Magnetic resonance imaging has demonstrated that skin depression in IAPP is solely because of loss of the dermis.
• Skin glycosaminoglycans from the lesions of IAPP patients are different from those seen in typical lesions of morphea. This supports the concept that IAPP is distinct from morphea.
• Sclerodermatous changes have been reported in the long-standing atrophic lesions of IAPP. Such changes usually appear in the center of the plaque and manifest as a shiny white indurated area resembling that of morphea.
• Variable changes in elastic tissue have been reported in IAPP that range from normal to severe diminution with the fragmentation of elastic fibers. Such cases need to be differentiated from anetoderma.
• In early-stage of IAPP, especially those patients having a positive *B. burgdorferi* antibody serology, the standard therapy for Lyme disease has been recommended.
• Though IAPP shares some similarities with morphea, however, there is more robust clinical, etiopathogenetic, prognostic and therapeutic evidence that set IAPP apart from morphea and obliges us to consider IAPP as a distinct entity.

REFERENCES

[1]   Arif T, Adil M, Amin SS, Ahmed M. Atrophoderma of pasini and pierini in a blaschkoid pattern. J Dtsch Dermatol Ges 2017; 15(6): 663-4.
[http://dx.doi.org/10.1111/ddg.13198] [PMID: 28346752]

[2]   Pullara TJ, Lober CW, Fenske NA. Idiopathic atrophoderma of pasini and pierini. Int J Dermatol 1984; 23(10): 643-5.
[http://dx.doi.org/10.1111/j.1365-4362.1984.tb01222.x] [PMID: 6396245]

[3]   Arif T. Zosteriform idiopathic atrophoderma of pasini and pierini. Indian J Paediatr Dermatol 2019; 20(1): 60-3.

[http://dx.doi.org/10.4103/ijpd.IJPD_85_18]

[4]   Ehrmann S, Brunauer SR. Sclerodermie. In: Jadasshon J, Ed. Handbuch der Haut-und Geschlechtskrankkeiten. Berlin: Springer 1931; p. 717.

[5]   Thibierge G. Sclerodermie. In: Besnier E, Brocq L, Jacqut LMC, Eds. La Pratique Dermatologique. Paris: Masson 1904; p. 253.

[6]   Pasini A. Atrofodermia idiopatica progressiva. G Ital Dermatol 1923; 58: 785.

[7]   Pierini LE, Vivoli D. Atrofodermia idiopatica progressiva (Pasini). G Ital Dermatol 1936; 77: 403-9.

[8]   Canizares O, Sachs PM, Jaimovich L, Torres VM. Idiopathic atrophoderma of pasini and pierini. Arch Dermatol 1958; 77(1): 42-58.
        [http://dx.doi.org/10.1001/archderm.1958.01560010044007] [PMID: 13486933]

[9]   Yokoyama Y, Akimoto S, Ishikawa O. Disaccharide analysis of skin glycosaminoglycans in atrophoderma of pasini and pierini. Clin Exp Dermatol 2000; 25(5): 436-40.
        [http://dx.doi.org/10.1046/j.1365-2230.2000.00682.x] [PMID: 11012603]

[10]   Weiner MA, Gant JQ Jr. Idiopathic atrophoderma of Pasini and Pierini occurring in two brothers. Arch Dermatol 1959; 80(2): 195-7.
        [http://dx.doi.org/10.1001/archderm.1959.01560200063006] [PMID: 13669745]

[11]   Bracco MM, Bianchi CA, Bianchi O, Stringa SG. Hereditary complement (C2) deficiency with discoid lupus erythematosus and idiopathic atrophoderma. Int J Dermatol 1979; 18(9): 713-7.
        [http://dx.doi.org/10.1111/j.1365-4362.1979.tb05007.x] [PMID: 315933]

[12]   Berman A, Berman GD, Winkelmann RK. Atrophoderma (pasini-pierini). Int J Dermatol 1988; 27(7): 487-90.
        [http://dx.doi.org/10.1111/j.1365-4362.1988.tb00927.x] [PMID: 3065258]

[13]   Buechner SA, Rufli T. Atrophoderma of Pasini and Pierini. Clinical and histopathologic findings and antibodies to *Borrelia burgdorferi* in thirty-four patients. J Am Acad Dermatol 1994; 30(3): 441-6.
        [http://dx.doi.org/10.1016/S0190-9622(94)70053-2] [PMID: 8113457]

[14]   Kencka D, Blaszczyk M, Jabłońska S. Atrophoderma pasini-pierini is a primary atrophic abortive morphea. Dermatology 1995; 190(3): 203-6.
        [http://dx.doi.org/10.1159/000246685] [PMID: 7599381]

[15]   Kernohan NM, Stankler L, Sewell HF. Atrophoderma of pasini and pierini. An immunopathologic case study. Am J Clin Pathol 1992; 97(1): 63-8.
        [http://dx.doi.org/10.1093/ajcp/97.1.63] [PMID: 1728865]

[16]   Tajima S, Sakuraoka K. A case of atrophoderma of Pasini and Pierini: analysis of glycosaminoglycan of the lesional skin. J Dermatol 1995; 22(10): 767-9.
        [http://dx.doi.org/10.1111/j.1346-8138.1995.tb03918.x] [PMID: 8586758]

[17]   Bassi A, Remaschi G, Difonzo EM, *et al.* Idiopathic congenital atrophoderma of pasini and pierini. Arch Dis Child 2015; 100(12): 1184.
        [http://dx.doi.org/10.1136/archdischild-2015-309498] [PMID: 26374755]

[18]   Iriondo M, Bloom RF, Neldner KH. Unilateral atrophoderma of pasini and pierini. Cutis 1987; 39(1): 69-70.
        [PMID: 3802912]

[19]   Murphy PK, Hymes SR, Fenske NA. Concomitant unilateral idiopathic atrophoderma of Pasini and Pierini (IAPP) and morphea. Observations supporting IAPP as a variant of morphea. Int J Dermatol 1990; 29(4): 281-3.
        [http://dx.doi.org/10.1111/j.1365-4362.1990.tb02562.x] [PMID: 2370118]

[20]   Saleh Z, Abbas O, Dahdah MJ, Kibbi AG, Zaynoun S, Ghosn S. Atrophoderma of pasini and pierini: A clinical and histopathological study. J Cutan Pathol 2008; 35(12): 1108-14.
        [http://dx.doi.org/10.1111/j.1600-0560.2008.00986.x] [PMID: 18616761]

[21] Daniels F Jr. For diagnosis: Scleroderma? Idiopathic atrophoderma of pacini and pierini? Arch Dermatol 1965; 91(4): 410-2.
[http://dx.doi.org/10.1001/archderm.91.4.410] [PMID: 9626098]

[22] Chu CY, Hsiao GH, Hsiao CH. Atrophoderma of Pasini and Pierini: A variant of morphea-Report of a case and review of literature. Zhonghua Pifuke Yixue Zazhi 2000; 18: 273-9.

[23] Kee C, Brothers WS, New W. Idiopathic atrophoderma of Pasini and Pierini with coexistent morphea. A case report. Arch Dermatol 1960; 82(1): 100-3.
[http://dx.doi.org/10.1001/archderm.1960.01580010106019] [PMID: 14405101]

[24] Jabłońska S, Szczepański A. Atrophoderma Pasini-Pierini: Is it an entity? Dermatology 1962; 125(4): 226-42.
[http://dx.doi.org/10.1159/000254989] [PMID: 13957175]

[25] Miteva L, Kadurina M. Unilateral idiopathic atrophoderma of Pasini and Pierini. Int J Dermatol 2006; 45(11): 1391-3.
[http://dx.doi.org/10.1111/j.1365-4632.2006.03033.x] [PMID: 17076744]

[26] Carrington PR, Altick JA, Sanusi ID. Atrophoderma elastolytica discreta. Am J Dermatopathol 1996; 18(2): 212-7.
[http://dx.doi.org/10.1097/00000372-199604000-00017] [PMID: 8739999]

[27] Sparsa A, Piette JC, Wechsler B, Amoura Z, Francès C. Anetoderma and its prothrombotic abnormalities. J Am Acad Dermatol 2003; 49(6): 1008-12.
[http://dx.doi.org/10.1016/S0190-9622(03)02110-8] [PMID: 14639377]

[28] de Souza EM, Daldon PÉC, Cintra ML. Anetoderma associated with primary antiphospholipid syndrome. J Am Acad Dermatol 2007; 56(5): 881-2.
[http://dx.doi.org/10.1016/j.jaad.2006.10.046] [PMID: 17184875]

[29] Bilen N, Bayramgürler D, Sikar A, Erçin C, Yilmaz A. Anetoderma associated with antiphospholipid syndrome and systemic lupus erythematosus. Lupus 2003; 12(9): 714-6.
[http://dx.doi.org/10.1191/0961203303lu431cr] [PMID: 14514137]

[30] Mastrolorenzo A, Tiradritti L, Vichi F, Ketabchi S, Supuran CT, Zuccati G. Primary anetoderma and HIV infection: A case report. AIDS Read 2006; 16(2): 92-6.
[PMID: 16471275]

[31] Franck JM, MacFarlane D, Silvers DN, Katz BE, Newhouse J. Atrophoderma of Pasini and Pierini: Atrophy of dermis or subcutis? J Am Acad Dermatol 1995; 32(1): 122-3.
[http://dx.doi.org/10.1016/0190-9622(95)90208-2] [PMID: 7822501]

[32] Abe I, Ochiai T, Kawamura A, Muto R, Hirano Y, Ogawa M. Progressive idiopathic atrophoderma of Pasini and Pierini: the evaluation of cutaneous atrophy by 13-MHz B-mode ultrasound scanning method. Clin Exp Dermatol 2006; 31(3): 462-4.
[http://dx.doi.org/10.1111/j.1365-2230.2006.02091.x] [PMID: 16681608]

[33] Lis-Święty A, Bierzyńska-Macyszyn G, Arasiewicz H, Brzezińska-Wcisło L. Bilateral atrophoderma linearis: A relationship between atrophoderma linearis Moulin and atrophoderma Pasini-Pierini? Int J Dermatol 2016; 55(3): 339-41.
[http://dx.doi.org/10.1111/ijd.12893] [PMID: 26220360]

[34] Miller RF. Idiopathic atrophoderma. Arch Dermatol 1965; 92(6): 653-60.
[http://dx.doi.org/10.1001/archderm.1965.01600180045007] [PMID: 5846320]

[35] Lee Y, Oh Y, Ahn S, Park H, Choi EH. A case of atrophoderma of Pasini and Pierini associated with borrelia burgdorferi infection successfully treated with oral doxycycline. Ann Dermatol 2011; 23(3): 352-6.
[http://dx.doi.org/10.5021/ad.2011.23.3.352] [PMID: 21909207]

[36] Lohrer R, Barran L, Kellnar S, Belohradsky BH. Pasini and Pierini idiopathic and progressive

atrophoderma in childhood. Monatsschr Kinderheilkd 1986; 134(12): 878-80.
[PMID: 3493428]

[37]   Carter JD, Valeriano J, Vasey FB. Hydroxychloroquine as a treatment for atrophoderma of Pasini and Pierini. Int J Dermatol 2006; 45(10): 1255-6.
[http://dx.doi.org/10.1111/j.1365-4632.2006.03021.x] [PMID: 17040461]

[38]   Stoner MF, Dixon SL. Purple depressions on the trunk and extremities. Atrophoderma of Pasini and Pierini. Arch Dermatol 1990; 126(12): 1644a.
[http://dx.doi.org/10.1001/archderm.1990.01670360109023] [PMID: 2256692]

[39]   Arpey CJ, Patel DS, Stone MS, Qiang-Shao J, Moore KC. Treatment of atrophoderma of Pasini and Pierini-associated hyperpigmentation with the Q-switched alexandrite laser: A clinical, histologic, and ultrastructural appraisal. Lasers Surg Med 2000; 27(3): 206-12.
[http://dx.doi.org/10.1002/1096-9101] [PMID: 11013382]

[40]   Pragya N, Jhabuawala M, Gupta M. Atrophoderma of Pasini and Pierini: A case report. J Clin Biomed Sci 2013; 3(1)

[41]   Ravic-Nikolic A, Djurdjevic P, Mitrovic S, Milicic V, Petrovic D. Atrophoderma of Pasini and Pierini associated with extramedullary plasmacytoma. Clin Exp Dermatol 2016; 41(7): 837-9.
[http://dx.doi.org/10.1111/ced.12906] [PMID: 27443586]

[42]   Kopeć-Medrek M, Kotulska A, Zycińska-Debska E, Widuchowska M, Kucharz EJ. Exacerbated course of atrophoderma of Pasini and Pierini in patient with papillary cancer of the thyroid gland. Wiad Lek 2010; 63(1): 24-6.
[PMID: 20701027]

[43]   Bisaccia EP, Scarborough DA, Lowney ED. Atrophoderma of Pasini and Pierini and systemic scleroderma. Arch Dermatol 1982; 118(1): 1-2.
[http://dx.doi.org/10.1001/archderm.1982.01650130005002] [PMID: 7059194]

[44]   Kogoj F. Qu'est-ce que c'est *que* la maladie de Pasini-Pierini? Ann Dermatol Syphiligr 1961; 88: 247.
[PMID: 13757552]

[45]   Brunauer SR. Zur Terminologie der sogenannten Idiopatischen Progressiven Atrophodermie von Pasini and Pierini sowre uber die Stellung dieser Affektion in System der Dermatogen. Hautarzt 1964; 15: 108.
[PMID: 14171199]

[46]   Stevanovic OF. L'Atrophodermie idiopathique (Pasini et Pierini). Ann Dermatof Syphiligr 1963; 90: 163.

[47]   Grupper C. La maladie de Pasini et Pierini. Bull Soc Fr Dermatol Syphiligr 1959; 66: 433.
[PMID: 13829881]

[48]   Poché GW. Progressive idiopathic atrophoderma of Pasini and Pierini. Cutis 1980; 25(5): 503-6.
[PMID: 7379582]

[49]   Fett N, Werth VP. Update on morphea. J Am Acad Dermatol 2011; 64(2): 217-28.
[http://dx.doi.org/10.1016/j.jaad.2010.05.045] [PMID: 21238823]

[50]   Fett N, Werth VP. Update on morphea. J Am Acad Dermatol 2011; 64(2): 231-42.
[http://dx.doi.org/10.1016/j.jaad.2010.05.046] [PMID: 21238824]

[51]   Fett N. Scleroderma: Nomenclature, etiology, pathogenesis, prognosis, and treatments: Facts and controversies. Clin Dermatol 2013; 31(4): 432-7.
[http://dx.doi.org/10.1016/j.clindermatol.2013.01.010] [PMID: 23806160]

[52]   Hayakawa I, Hasegawa M, Takehara K, Sato S. Anti-DNA topoisomerase II alpha autoantibodies in localized scleroderma. Arthritis Rheum 2004; 50(1): 227-32.
[http://dx.doi.org/10.1002/art.11432] [PMID: 14730620]

CHAPTER 16

Linear Atrophoderma of Moulin

Tasleem Arif[1,2,*]

[1] *Department of Dermatology, STDs, Leprosy and Aesthetics, Dar As Sihha Medical center, Dammam, Saudi Arabia*

[2] *Ellahi Medicare Clinic, Srinagar, Kashmir, India*

Chapter synopsis.
• Linear atrophoderma of Moulin (LAM) is a rare dermatologic disorder characterized by hyperpigmented atrophic plaques following the lines of Blaschko.
• Most of the reported cases have disease onset during childhood or adolescence. However, it can occur at any age.
• The etiopathogenesis of LAM is not clear. It is believed to be caused by a somatic mutation taking place early in embryogenesis resulting in a genotypic and phenotypic mosaicism. However, no gene responsible for LAM has been reported till date.
• Most often, lesions of LAM are not associated with preceding inflammation, induration, or sclerosis. Trunk has been the most common affected site followed by upper and lower limbs. Face and neck involvement occur rarely.
• Histologically, hyperpigmentation of the basal layer is the most characteristic finding. However, newer findings have been reported which include perivascular lymphocytic infiltrates, epidermal atrophy, decreased elastic tissue, altered dermal collagen, dermal atrophy, acanthosis, plasma cell infiltrate, and dilated dermal blood vessels.
• No definitive treatment for LAM exists. Several treatments have been tried with unsatisfactory results like oral potassium aminobenzoate (12g/day), penicillin, topical corticosteroids, heparin, phototherapy, combined PUVA and penicillin; vitamin E (400 IU/day) and topical clobetasol propionate.

Keywords: Altered dermal collagen, Atrophoderma, Atrophy, Atrophic plaques, Basal hyperpigmentation, Blaschko lines, Blaschkose, Blaschkoid lichen planus, Hyperpigmented bands, Idiopathic atrophoderma of Pasini and Pierini, Linear atrophoderma of Moulin, Linear morphea, Mosaicism, Perivascular lymphocytic infiltrate, Postzygotic mutation, Potassium aminobenzoate, Skin biopsy, Skin ultrasound, Subcutaneous tissue, Twin spotting.

* **Corresponding author Tasleem Arif:** Department of Dermatology, STDs, Leprosy and Aesthetics, Dar As Sihha Medical center, Dammam, Saudi Arabia and Ellahi Medicare Clinic, Srinagar, Kashmir, India; E-mail: dr_tasleem_arif@yahoo.com

INTRODUCTION AND HISTORICAL BACKGROUND

Linear atrophoderma of Moulin (LAM) is a rare dermatological disorder characterized by hyperpigmented depressed plaques following the lines of Blaschko [1]. It was first reported by Moulin *et al.* in 1992. They reported five patients in good health who were having unilateral hyperpigmented atrophic plaques along Blaschko lines (BL) which they couldn't attribute to any known skin disorder. The lesions were having variable amount of pigmentation and atrophy that exactly followed BL. The onset of the lesions was during childhood or adolescence falling in the age group of 6-20 years. All the five patients had unilateral lesions and were present on the trunk forming a recumbent "S" pattern. The lesions started from a point 3 to 6 cm away from the posterior midline and progressed anteriorly to end precisely on the anterior midline. Though the number of bands described was variable, similar pigmented atrophic lesions or pigmented lines were present on the limbs of the same side in 3 out of the 5 cases. Due to the asymptomatic nature of the lesions, they caused only a cosmetic concern for the patients. They were stable and didn't show tendency to progress during follow up period of 2-30 years. Histopathology from five skin biopsies which were done on 3 patients showed unremarkable epidermis except hyperpigmentation of the basal layer. The dermis didn't reveal any pigmentary incontinence, inflammation, alteration of connective tissue including collagen and elastin. In one patient, perivascular lymphocytic infiltrate was present. They believed that this clinical atrophy was related to the loss of subcutaneous tissue; however, a deep biopsy from both the affected skin and contralateral sides to assess the thickness of subcutaneous tissue was originally not performed. Moulin *et al.* suggested the term "blaschkose" to differentiate it from the term "blaschkitis" that has an inflammatory and acquired nature [2].

Two years later, it was Bauman *et al.* in 1994, who reported a patient with a similar disease that was published in a German journal. He coined the term linear atrophoderma of Moulin. According to them, LAM belonged to the group of acquired linear dermatoses that follow BL and suggested that LAM was a variant of idiopathic atrophoderma of Pasini and Pierini (IAPP) [3]. However, the term LAM is a misnomer as there is no atrophoderma, the atrophy in LAM has been attributed to the thinning of subcutaneous tissue rather than the dermis. The use of ultrasound probes to determine skin thickness has revealed that there is thinning of the subcutaneous tissue underlying the lesions of LAM. Hence, the atrophy in the lesions of LAM is due to a decrease in the subcutaneous tissue [4].

EPIDEMIOLOGY

LAM is a rare disease. All the reported cases have been sporadic cases or short case series not exceeding five cases. Currently, there is not a single study available for LAM from which the author can describe its epidemiological parameters. Owing to the paucity of cases of LAM, the author has searched for the published cases of LAM since 1992 till the drafting of this chapter. Despite the meticulous search in, the author could find only 48 published cases of LAM (Table **16.1**).

Table 16.1. Forty eight published cases of linear atrophoderma of moulin.

Case No	Year of Publication	Authors	Reference	Age	sex	Sites	Histopathology	Other comments
1	1992	Moulin *et al.* 1st of 5	[2]	8	m	T	Basal Hyperpigmentation; perivascular lymphocytic infiltrate	-
2	1992	Moulin *et al.* 2nd of 5	[2]	7	f	T	Basal Hyperpigmentation	-
3	1992	Moulin *et al.* 3rd of 5	[2]	15	m	T	Basal Hyperpigmentation	-
4	1992	Moulin *et al.* 4th of 5	[2]	20	m	T	Skin Biopsy not done	-
5	1992	Moulin *et al.* 5th of 5	[2]	6	m	T/UL	Skin biopsy not done	-
6	1994	Baumann *et al.*	[3]	22	m	T/UL	Basal epidermal ballooning; perivascular lymphocytic infiltrate; increased dermal collagen.	-
7	1995	Larrègue *et al.*	[37]	15	m	T	Increased dermal collagen.	-
8	1996	Artola *et al.*	[38]	5	f	T	Acanthosis and basal hyperpigmentation; increased dermal collagen; perivascular lymphocytic infiltrate	Treatment with oral potassium aminobenzoate 12g/day stabilized lesions

(Table 16.1) cont.....

Case No	Year of Publication	Authors	Reference	Age	sex	Sites	Histopathology	Other comments
9	1996	Wollenberg *et al.*	[39]	5	f	UL	Atrophy in the epidermis; increased dermal collagen; perivascular lymphocytic infiltrate.	-
10	1997	Cecchi *et al.*	[17]	12	f	T/UL	Localized hyperpigmentation of basal epidermis	-
11	2000	Browne *et al.*	[13]	6	m	F/T/UL	Parakeratosis, acanthosis, hypogranulosis; perivascular lymphocytic infiltrate.	Face localization; preceding inflammatory phase
12	2000	Rompel *et al.*	[40]	12	f	T/L	Basal layer hyperpigmentation; focal vacuolar degeneration; perivascular lymphocytic infiltrate; thickened dermal collagen bundles.	Elevated serum IgE
13	2002	Martin *et al.*	[41]	9	m	T	Sclerotic reticular dermis; perivascular lymphocytes in the dermis.	-
14	2002	Miteva *et al.*	[42]	16	f	F/UL/LL	Psoriasiform epidermal hyperplasia with hyaline eosinophilic bodies; perivascular lymphocytic infiltrate; thickened dermal collagen bundles.	Face localization; Absence of band like lesions; association of hypopigmented atrophic lesions and telangiectatic macules
15	2003	Danarti *et al.* 1st of 4	[7]	13	f	T/UL	Perivascular lymphocytic infiltrate in the dermis	Penicillin G ineffective
16	2003	Danarti *et al.* 2nd of 4	[7]	24	f	T/UL	Skin biopsy not done	-

(Table 16.1) cont.....

Case No	Year of Publication	Authors	Reference	Age	sex	Sites	Histopathology	Other comments
17	2003	Danarti *et al.* 3rd of 4	[7]	36	f	LL	Unremarkable epidermis and dermis	-
18	2003	Danarti *et al.* 4th of 4	[7]	14	f	LL	Skin biopsy not done	-
19	2003	Utikal *et al.*	[8]	23	m	T/UL/LL	Unremarkable epidermis; perivascular lymphocytic infiltrate in the dermis; Dermal edema	Bilateral; telangiectatic skin lesions; penicillin G + PUVA caused satisfactory improvement
20	2003	Utikal *et al.*	[8]	2	f	T/UL/LL	Unremarkable epidermis; perivascular lymphocytic infiltrate in the dermis	Bilateral; telangiectatic macular lesions; Application of self-tanning cream caused homogenization of skin pigmentation
21	2005	Miteva *et al.*	[43]	9	m	T	Hyperpigmentation of basal epidermis; hyperkeratosis, irregular acanthosis; increased dermal collagen.	-
22	2005	Ang *et al.*	[5]	0	f	LL	Epidermal acanthosis with widening and blunting of rete ridges; decreased elastin fibres in dermis	Congenital case, hypopigmentation
23	2006	Atasoy *et al.*	[44]	16	m	T/UL	Epidermal atrophy; perivascular lymphocytic infiltrate; collagen fibers fragmented in dermis	Leukonychia; penicillin G ineffective
24	2008	Cecchi *et al.*	[19]	8	m	FN	Hyperpigmentation of basal epidermis; perivascular lymphocytic infiltrate	Neck localization.

(Table 16.1) cont.....

Case No	Year of Publication	Authors	Reference	Age	sex	Sites	Histopathology	Other comments
25	2008	Zampetti *et al.*	[9]	37	f	T/UL	Hyperpigmentation of basal epidermis; thickened dermal collagen bundles	Slight improvement with vitamin E + topical clobetasol propionate
26	2008	Lopez *et al.*	[15]	16	m	UL	Hyperpigmentation basal epidermis	-
27	2010	Ripert *et al.*	[45]	14	f	T	Hyperpigmentation basal epidermis; Civatte bodies; perivascular lymphocytic infiltrate; increased dermal collagen.	Elevated ANA
28	2010	Ozkaya *et al.*	[12]	19	f	T/LL	Acanthosis; hyperpigmentation of basal epidermis; elastic fibers slightly decreased in dermis	Bilateral; Twin spotting phenomenon-coexistence of lentiginosis form with classical LAM
29	2010	Schepis *et al.*	[46]	13	m	T	Hyperpigmentation of basal epidermis; perivascular lymphocytic infiltrate; Dermal edema	-
30	2011	Tukenmez *et al.*	[20]	17	f	FN	Hyperpigmentation of basal epidermis; perivascular lymphocytic infiltrate	Neck localization
31	2011	Norisugi *et al.*	[4]	25	m	T/LL	Hyperpigmentation of the lower epidermis; slight thickening of the collagen fibers in the reticular dermis; perivascular lymphocytes in the dermis	Evaluated skin atrophy in LAM by ultrasound probes.

(Table 16.1) cont.....

Case No	Year of Publication	Authors	Reference	Age	sex	Sites	Histopathology	Other comments
32	2012	Oiso *et al.*	[11]	12	m	T/UL/LL	Acanthosis; irregular, elongated rete ridges; different levels of melanin pigment synthesis; melanin present in hypopigmented streak	Hyper- and hypopigmented linear atrophoderma; segmental and spotty lentiginosis;
33	2012	Yucel *et al.*	[14]	NA	f	LL	Lentigo like lesion demonstrated a few melanophages and a slight perivascular lymphocytic infiltrate; hypopigmented plaque showed no abnormal findings.	Lentiginosis within plaques of hypopigmented LAM; Twin spotting phenomenon.
34	2012	Patsatsi *et al.*	[22]	17	f	T	Hyperpigmentation of basal epidermis; broad dermis with thickened collagen fibers; decreased subcutaneous fat tissue	Brownish atrophic plaques in a zosteriform distribution
35	2013	Villani *et al.* Ist of 4	[21]	8	m	LL	Hyperpigmentation of basal epidermis; perivascular Lymphocytic infiltrate; fragmented elastic fibres	Spontaneous improvement
36	2013	Villani *et al.* 2nd of 4	[21]	6	m	T/LL	Skin biopsy not done	-
37	2013	Villani *et al.* 3rd of 4	[21]	9	f	T	Skin biopsy not done	-
38	2013	Villani *et al.* 4th of 4	[21]	20	m	T/UL	Hyperpigmentation of the basal layer; perivascular lymphocytic infiltrate; thickened collagen in dermis	-
39	2013	Patrizi *et al.* ist of 2	[6]	28	m	T/UL/LL	Hyperpigmentation of the basal ; thickened collagen in dermis	-

(Table 16.1) cont.....

Case No	Year of Publication	Authors	Reference	Age	sex	Sites	Histopathology	Other comments
40	2013	Patrizi *et al.* 2nd of 2	[6]	70	f	T	Hyperpigmentation of the basal layer; superficial perivascular lymphocytic infiltrate; thickening of collagen bundles, decreased and fragmented elastin fibres	-
41	2013	Wongkietkachorn *et al.*	[28]	15	m	T/LL	Epidermal atrophy without any change in the dermis or collagen bundle or elastic tissue	Calcipotriol twice a day on abdominal lesions showed efficacy
42	2014	Golian *et al.*	[10]	10	m	T/UL/LL	Epidermis unremarkable; In mid dermis, thickened collagen bundles entrapping eccrine ducts; In deep dermis collagen is thickened and hyalinized; thicker elastin fibers in dermis	-
43	2014	Zaouak *et al.*	[29]	11	f	T/UL/LL	Hyperpigmentation of basal epidermis; perivascular lymphocytic infiltrate	Treatment with methotrexate 20 mg/week for 6 months improved skin pigmentation and atrophy

(Table 16.1) cont.....

Case No	Year of Publication	Authors	Reference	Age	sex	Sites	Histopathology	Other comments
44	2015	Niaki *et al.*	[27]	10	f	UL/LL	2 biopsies done 1.unremarkable epidermis with prominent melanin deposition in the basal layer; perivascular and focally interstitial lymphoid infiltrates without any obvious signs of sclerosis. 2. unremarkable mild dermal inflammatory changes with no evidence of dermal sclerosis or atrophic skin appendages	Topical steroids, vitamin D analogues, retinoid and hydroquinone treatments for 5 years were ineffective; Lesions coalesced together after 5 years of onset.
45	2016	Tan *et al.*	[47]	11	f	T/UL/LL	Slight upper dermal perivascular lymphocytic infiltrate. On comparing with the normal skin, the thickness of dermis was decreased and the collagen bundles in dermis were more compact.	Betamethasone, 0.1% cream twice a day for 6 months, proved ineffective; application of hydroquinone 4% cream for 2 years didn't help pigmentation
46	2016	Emre *et al.*	[48]	36	m	FN	Thinning of epidermis and flattening of the rete ridges; vacuolar degeneration in the basal layer of epidermis; perivascular mononuclear inflammatory infiltrates, slight edema, and diffuse melanophages in the papillary dermis	Face/neck localization.

(Table 16.1) cont.....

Case No	Year of Publication	Authors	Reference	Age	sex	Sites	Histopathology	Other comments
47	2017	Darung *et al.*	[49]	16	f	FN	Atrophic epidermis, melanin deposition in the basal layer; subcutaneous tissue apparently normal; Sparse periappendageal and perivascular infiltrates of lymphocytes with mild thickening of dermal collagen bundles.	Face localization
48	2018	Kharkar *et al.*	[30]	14	m	T	Acanthosis with slight hyperkeratosis, Significant melanin deposition in the basal layer of epidermis, Dense lymphocytic infiltrates with normal elastin and collagen in the dermis.	4 sessions of PRP caused reduction in the depth of the plaques; color and texture unaltered.

T: Trunk; UL: Upper limb; LL: Lower limb; FN: Face/neck; m: Male; f: Female; NA: Not available; PRP: Platelet rich plasma; LAM: Linear atrophoderma of Moulin.

Most of the published cases have shown the disease onset to be during childhood or adolescence. In the original case series by Moulin *et al.*, the age of onset ranged from 6-20 years [2]. Four-fifths of the cases of LAM have the age of onset less than or equal to 20 years, only one fifth of the cases had onset after 20 years of age. Rarely, LAM can involve extremes of ages which is explained by the appearance of LAM in a congenital case and development of lesions in a 70 year female (Range 0-70 years) [5, 6]. Some of the epidemiological parameters of these 48 published cases have been summarized in (Table **16.2**).

In the five cases reported by Moulin *et al.*, 4 were males. However, after the review of literature, it seems that the disease affects both males and females equally (male to female ratio of 1). The lesions usually affect the trunk and limbs. Out of the 5 cases described by Moulin *et al.*, first four cases had lesions localized to the trunk, only while the fifth case had the involvement of trunk as well as left arm [2]. This has been confirmed by subsequent reported cases. Table **16.2** shows that trunk has been the most affected part seen in 70.8% cases followed by upper limb (41.7%) and lower limb (39.6%) affected almost equally. In rare instances, it can involve face/neck (12.5%). Cases of LAM have been reported from different parts of the world and from different races. So, there is no racial predilection for LAM.

Table 16.2. Basic features of 48 published cases of LAM.

Total Cases Collected	48
Mean age of onset of disease	15.7 years (in one case age not specified)
Range	0-70 years
Males	24 (50%)
Females	24 (50%)
M/F ratio	1:1
Congenital cases	1 (2.1%)
Onset of disease before or at 20 years	39 (81.2%)
Onset of disease after 20 years	9 (18.8%)
Trunk involvement	34 (70.8%)
Upper limb involvement	20 (41.7%)
Lower limb involvement	19 (39.6%)
Face/neck involvement	6 (12.5%)

ETIOPATHOGENESIS

The etiopathogenesis of LAM has not been understood till date. All the reported cases so far have been sporadic. It is a well-known fact that dermatoses that follow BL are believed to be caused by a somatic mutation taking place early in embryogenesis resulting in a genotypic and phenotypic mosaicism. Some authors have proposed that LAM may reflect the action of an autosomal lethal gene surviving by mosaicism. Mosaicism is defined as the presence of two or more genetically distinct cell populations in an individual derived from a single zygote. A postzygotic mutation may cause a loss of the corresponding allele (wild type) at the locus of atrophoderma. This leads to a homozygous cell clone which later in the life becomes clinically manifested along the lines of Blaschko [7]. However, till date no gene responsible for LAM has been reported in the literature. Utikal *et al.* proposed that a secondary event (probably environmental factor) could affect these mutated cells, giving rise to the clinical manifestations of the disease [8]. There has been no triggering factor identified so far in the causation of LAM. Some authors have suspected the probable exposure of sun in collaboration with parasiticide substances and tomato plants as potential environmental factors causing the clinical manifestations of the disease [9].

CLINICAL PRESENTATION

LAM is characterized by hyperpigmented depressed plaques following the lines of Blaschko (Figs. **16.1, 16.2**).

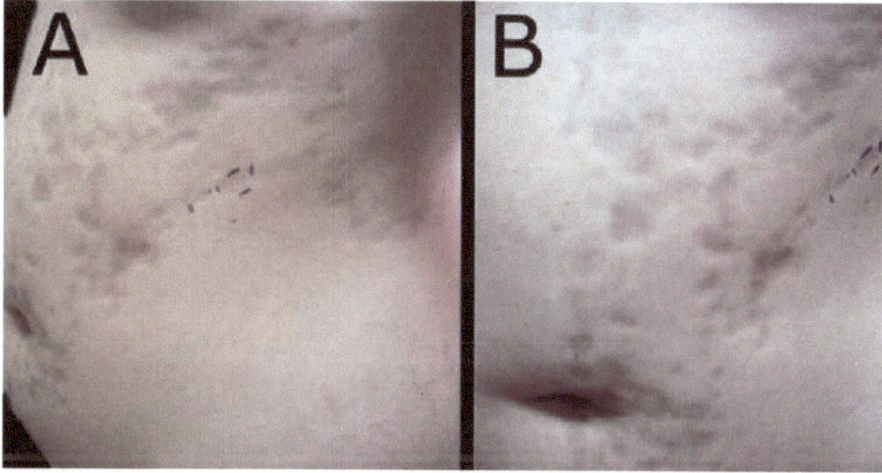

Fig. (16.1A & B). Depressed atrophic plaques on the left side of the trunk present along Blaschko lines. (Image credit: Patsatsi A, Kyriakou A, Chaidemenos G, Sotiriadis D. Linear atrophoderma of Moulin: a case report and review of the literature. Dermatol Pract Concept 2013: 3: 7–11. http://dx.doi.org/10.5826/dpc.0301a03.)

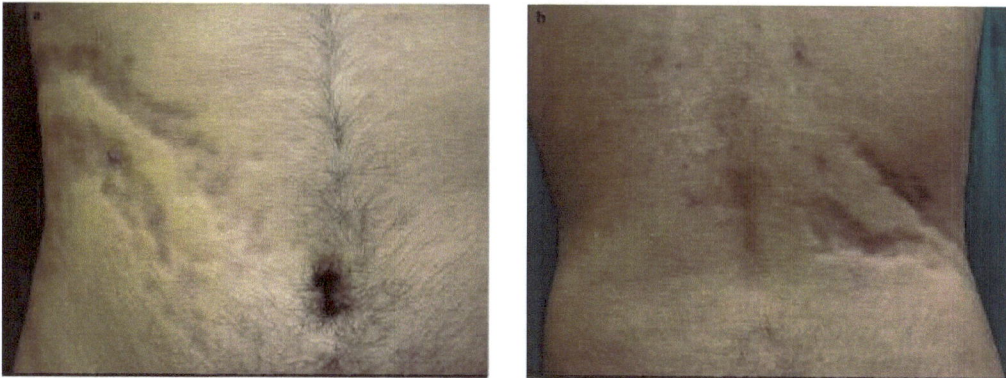

Fig. (16.2). (**a**) Two parallel bands of atrophic, linear hyperpigmented plaques along Blaschko's lines, extending from umbilicus to the right side of abdomen; (**b**) Two parallel bands of atrophic, linear hyperpigmented plaques along Blaschko's lines, extending from midline to the right side of the back. (Image credit: Kharkar VD, Abak BA, Mahajan SA. Linear atrophoderma of Moulin: A rare entity. Indian J Dermatol Venereol Leprol 2018;84:591-4.)

Around 80% of the cases have disease onset before or at 20 years of age. The lesions usually affect trunk and extremities without any evidence of long-term progression. These plaques are not associated with preceding inflammation, induration, or sclerosis. Trunk is the most common affected site followed by upper and lower limbs, which share almost equal frequencies. Rarely face/neck has been reported (Figs. **16.3**, **16.4**).

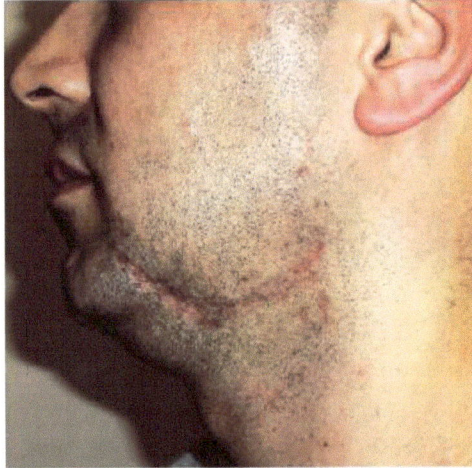

Fig. (16.3). The purplish brown, depressed lesion which followed the Blaschko lines on the chin and neck. (Image credit: Emre S, Metin A, Sungu N, Kilinc F, Demirseren DD. Linear atrophoderma of Moulin located on the face. Our Dermatol Online. 2016;7(2):204-206.)

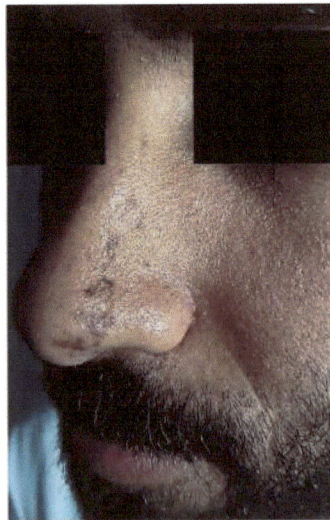

Fig. (16.4). Multiple hyperpigmented atrophic lesions present in a band like pattern over left side of nose following Blaschko lines. (Copyright: Arif T. Linear Atrophoderma of Moulin Localized to Face: An Exceedingly Rare Entity. J Skin Stem Cell. 2020 ; 7(2):e106255. doi: 10.5812/jssc.106255.)

LAM can rarely occur at the extremes of age. A congenital case and a woman at the age of 70 have been reported [5, 6]. Though, Moulin *et al.* presumed LAM to have unilateral localization, however, few bilateral cases have also been reported [8, 10 - 13]. Hyperpigmented bands are the most classical presentation of the disease; but less often hypopigmented variety has also been reported [11, 12, 14]. Several new clinical manifestations have been reported in LAM (Box **16.1**); whether they are atypical presentations of LAM or they represent a different dermatoses is questionable.

Box 16.1. New clinical findings reported in LAM.
Congenital presentation
Hypopigmented lesions
Preceding inflammation
Late onset of disease (70 years)
Facial/Neck localization
Elevated serum IgE
Associated telangiectasia
Bilateral presentation
Presence of leukonychia
Elevated ANA
Concomitant lentiginosis
Spontaneous improvement
Twin spotting
Disease activity even after five years of onset

Brown and Fisher have described a case of LAM having preceding inflammation. On that basis, they proposed that LAM has two variants, an inflammatory one, and the non-inflammatory type. They suggested that the initial inflammatory phase ultimately can lead to hyperpigmentation with atrophy [13]. Utikal *et al.* have reported two cases having linear atrophoderma with prominent telangiectatic erythema. They believed that these cases might present a novel variant of LAM or a separate disease entity [8].

HISTOPATHOLOGY

The histopathology of LAM has seen several modifications. In the original case series reported by Moulin *et al.*, in which skin biopsies were performed in three patients; there was only hyperpigmentation of the basal layer, whereas the rest of the epidermis and dermis was normal. In one of the three patients, perivascular lymphocytic infiltrate was present [2]. With subsequent reports of LAM being published, new histopathological findings have been reported by various authors. These include perivascular lymphocytic infiltrates, epidermal atrophy, decreased elastic tissue, altered dermal collagen, dermal atrophy, acanthosis, plasma cell infiltrate, dilated dermal blood vessels, *etc.* (Figs. **16.5-16.7**). [10].

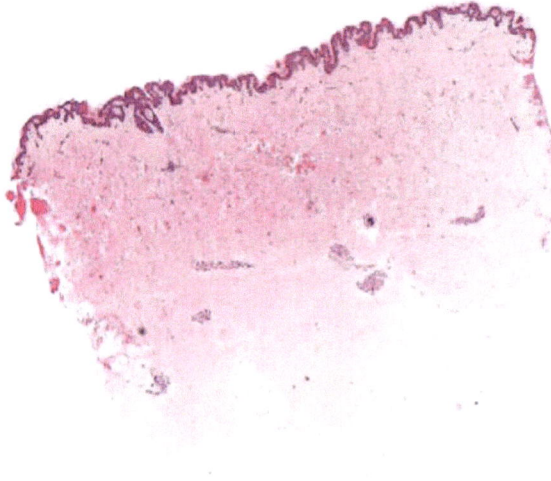

Fig. (16.5). Normal epidermis and broad dermis. (Image credit: Patsatsi A, Kyriakou A, Chaidemenos G, Sotiriadis D. Linear atrophoderma of Moulin: a case report and review of the literature. Dermatol Pract Concept 2013: 3: 7–11. http://dx.doi.org/10.5826/dpc.0301a03.)

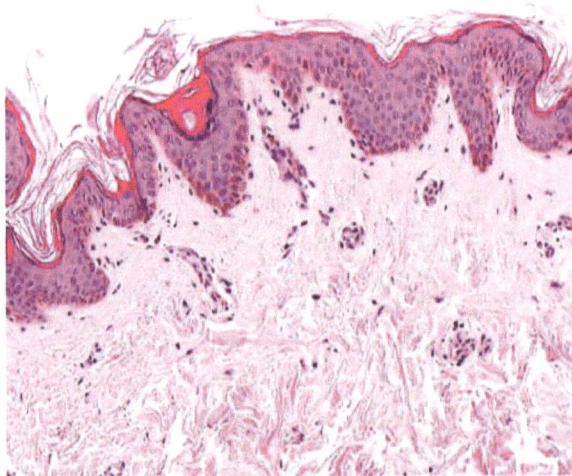

Fig. (16.6). Normal epidermis with hyperpigmented basal layer. (Image credit: Patsatsi A, Kyriakou A, Chaidemenos G, Sotiriadis D. Linear atrophoderma of Moulin: a case report and review of the literature. Dermatol Pract Concept 2013: 3: 7–11. http://dx.doi.org/10.5826/dpc.0301a03.)

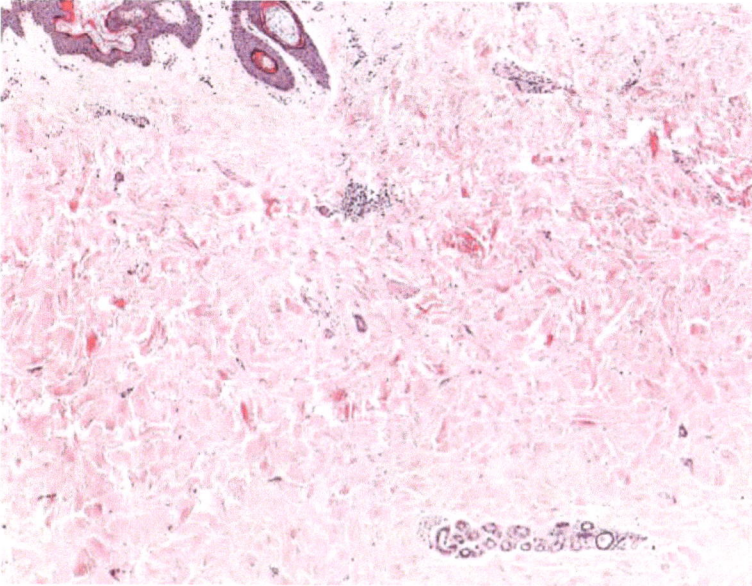

Fig. (16.7). Thickened collagen fibers in the dermis. (Image credit: Patsatsi A, Kyriakou A, Chaidemenos G, Sotiriadis D. Linear atrophoderma of Moulin: a case report and review of the literature. Dermatol Pract Concept 2013: 3: 7–11. http://dx.doi.org/10.5826/dpc.0301a03.)

Various histopathological findings that have been reported in LAM are summarized in Table **16.3**.

Table 16.3. Histopathological findings reported in LAM.

Basal layer hyperpigmentation	Hypogranulosis
Perivascular lymphocytic infiltrates	Parakeratosis
Altered dermal collagen	Psoriasiform epidermal hyperplasia with hyaline eosinophilic bodies
Decreased elastic tissue	Edema in the dermis
Acanthosis	Hyperkeratosis
Epidermal atrophy	Civatte bodies
Plasma cell infiltrate	Melanophages in the papillary dermis
Dilated dermal blood vessels	Periappendageal lymphocytic infiltrate
Dermal atrophy	Ballooning in basal epidermis

Perivascular lymphocytic inflammatory infiltrate in the dermis combined with abnormal collagen fibers has been the most common finding described in LAM [16]. Since, these cases presented sufficient clinical evidence to support a diagnosis of LAM, they suggested that LAM was not as limited in scope as has been described originally but probably comprised a wider set of clinical and histopathological features that fit rather within a spectrum of related disorders.

It is necessary to assess the subcutaneous tissue layer while making a diagnosis of LAM as the atrophy in LAM has been reported to be due to the loss of subcutaneous tissue. However, it is difficult to investigate the thickness of the subcutaneous tissue layer as it is easily missed in most of the routine punch skin biopsies. Thus, in order to assess the subcutaneous tissue, the skin biopsy, preferably an elliptical one has to be performed which is deep enough to reach the fascia so as to measure the entire thickness of subcutaneous tissue layer. In addition, a second skin biopsy from the contralateral side is advised to serve as a control. Hence, the correct way of taking a skin biopsy should consider the depth of biopsy specimen, somatic features of the patient (age, sex, skin color), stage of the disease, control biopsy from the contralateral normal skin, the dermatological history of the patient and follow up, and the area of the body from which skin biopsy has been taken. For instance, dermal collagen bundles in the back are normally thickened while thinned in the folds. Finally, an ultrasound assessment of the skin should also be done to look for the thickness of dermis and subcutaneous tissue layer [6, 16].

DIAGNOSIS

Diagnostic Criteria

LAM is a clinical diagnosis. However, histopathology and skin ultrasound may help in supporting its diagnosis. Classically, LAM is characterized by hyperpigmented depressed plaques following BL on the trunk and extremities without any evidence of long-term progression. These plaques are not associated with inflammation, induration, or sclerosis. Hyperpigmentation of basal layer with unremarkable changes in epidermal and dermal layers including collagen and elastin, was the characteristic histopathological finding reported in LAM by Moulin *et al.* [2]. Ultrasound probes to assess skin thickness have shown that there is thinning of the subcutaneous tissue underlying the lesions of LAM. Thus, the atrophy in LAM is due to a decrease in subcutaneous tissue rather than dermis. This explains why the term "atrophoderma" in LAM is a misnomer as there is no atrophy in the dermis. Based on initial case presentations of LAM, some diagnostic criteria were suggested for LAM summarized in Table **16.4** [1 - 3, 7, 16, 17].

Table 16.4. Diagnostic criteria for LAM [1 - 3, 7, 16, 17].

1.	Onset during childhood or adolescence.
2.	Development of hyperpigmented, slightly atrophic, unilateral lesions following Blaschko lines on the trunk or limbs.
3.	Absence of preceding inflammation and absence of subsequent induration or scleroderma.
4.	Stable, non-progressive clinical course without a pattern of remission.
5.	Histologic findings showing hyperpigmentation of the basal epidermis and a normal dermis with unaltered connective tissue and elastic fibres.

Diagnostic Insufficiency

Though the above diagnostic criteria apply to the classical cases of LAM as reported by Moulin *et al.* and other cases that are in their initial phase of disease progression. However, the subsequent published cases of LAM do not comply with these diagnostic criteria, yet they have been published by several reputed Journals under the term LAM. Since the first description of LAM by Moulin *et al.*, several authors throughout the world have reported cases with variable clinical and histopathological findings such as preceding inflammation, telangiectasias, collagen sclerosis, psoriasiform changes, *etc.* not fulfilling the diagnostic criteria of LAM and yet have been published under the umbrella term LAM. As a result of diversification in the cases of LAM, some researchers proposed the concept of atypical variants of LAM while others presumed that different disease entities were wrongly published as LAM [3, 5, 18]. Thus, the question arises whether all those cases represented classical LAM as described by Moulin *et al.* or they represented a related dermatosis; depends upon whether we confine to the diagnosis of LAM as described by Moulin *et al.*, or consider those cases that do not adhere to classical presentation as atypical variants of LAM, or consider LAM to be a diseases spectrum rather than a discrete entity where lesions may have varied clinical and histopathological findings. Thus, it is clear that the suggested diagnostic criteria of LAM are not sufficient because there are scores of cases that do not fulfil these criteria and still have been published under the name of LAM. Thus, it becomes imperative for us to revisit or update these diagnostic criteria [1]. The author has tried to explain why the existing diagnostic criteria of LAM are neither sufficient nor accurate in making the diagnosis of LAM by analysing each criterion and comparing them with the clinically published cases of LAM.

Onset During Childhood or Adolescence

Though this criterion holds good for most cases of LAM, but it is not exclusive. A congenital case of linear atrophoderma in a 9 month old Hispanic girl that had been present on her right leg since birth has been reported. On the contrary, LAM has been described in a 70 year old female [6]. Zampetti *et al.* described a 42-year-old Caucasian woman who presented with a 5-year history of atrophic brown macules on the left arm and trunk [9]. Similarly, in 2003, Danarti *et al.* reported four cases of LAM one of them was aged 38 years [7]. Hence it is clear that LAM can occur at any age and its onset cannot be limited to childhood or adolescence only.

Development of Hyperpigmented, Slightly Strophic, Unilateral Lesions Following Blaschko Lines on the Trunk or Limbs

By analysing this criterion, there are three parameters contained in it that include hyperpigmented lesions (color of lesions), unilateral localisation (unilateral vs bilateral) and presence of lesions on trunk or limbs (affected sites). There are cases of LAM where not only hyperpigmented but also hypopigmented lesions were described [11, 12, 14]. Regarding unilateral localization of lesions in LAM, the author has found five cases where the lesions were present bilaterally [8, 10 - 13]. Cases of LAM localised to neck have also been described [19, 20]. Hence, one can clearly understand that this criterion is not adequate for diagnosing LAM. This implies that lesions of LAM can be hyper/hypopigmented, unilateral/bilateral and can involve trunk/limbs/head/neck.

Absence of Preceding Inflammation and Absence of Subsequent Induration or Scleroderma

Moulin *et al* had proposed absence of preceding inflammation for diagnosing LAM [2]. However, a case of LAM with prior inflammation was reported by Brown and Fisher. Based on that case, they suggested that LAM consists of two variants viz., inflammatory and non-inflammatory types. They proposed that the initial inflammatory phase may later cause hyperpigmentation with atrophy [13]. Apart from this, there are dozens of reported cases of LAM in which histopathology has revealed increased and thickened collagen bundles in the dermis similar to morphea [6, 21, 22]. Though LAM is known for lacking an antecedent inflammatory phase unlike that of morphea, but in exceedingly rare cases, prior inflammation may be present.

Stable, Non-progressive Clinical Course Without a Pattern of Remission

The usual clinical course followed by LAM is a stable and non-progressive one. However, an interesting case with disease progression even after 5 years has been reported. Niaki *et al* have described a case of LAM who developed lesions similar to LAM at the age of 10 years and histopathology supported the diagnosis of

LAM. She was treated with long trials of topical steroids, retinoid, vitamin D analogues and hydroquinone for the next 5 years without any evidence of clinical improvement. At the age of 15 years, the existing lesions coalesced to form band like hyperpigmented atrophic plaques similar to LAM. The repeat biopsy was taken which ruled out morphea and they re-established the diagnosis of LAM [27]. This case suggests that LAM may not always follow a non-progressive course.

Histological Findings Showing Hyperpigmentation of the Basal Epidermis and a Normal Dermis with Unaltered Connective Tissue and Elastic Fibres

From the original case series by Moulin *et al.*, they reported only basal layer hyperpigmentation; and in one case, there were perivascular lymphocytic infiltrates; however the rest of the epidermis and dermis was unremarkable [2]. With subsequent cases of LAM being reported, several authors have described new histopathological findings in LAM. These include epidermal atrophy, perivascular lymphocytic infiltrates, altered dermal collagen, acanthosis, decreased elastic tissue, dilated dermal blood vessels and plasma cell infiltrate (Table **16.3**) [1, 13]. It is surprising that perivascular lymphocytic inflammatory infiltrate in the dermis in combination with abnormal collagen fibres has been found to be the most common histopathological finding described in LAM [5]. However, it needs to be understood these subsequent cases with new histopathological findings presented sufficient clinical evidence in favour of diagnosis of LAM. Hence, these authors proposed that LAM was not as limited in scope as has been described originally by Moulin *et al.* but probably comprised a wider set of clinical and histopathological features that fit rather within a spectrum of related disorders [13].

It is evident that all the five criteria of LAM are neither specific nor sufficient for diagnosing it. This implies to the fact that either those cases who are not complying with the original diagnostic criteria of LAM are referring to a different dermatoses; or they represent atypical or novel varieties of LAM; or we need to redefine this controversial entity and reframe its diagnostic criteria with a wider set of clinical and histopathological findings to account for the varied clinical and histopathological features reported in the cases of LAM. The author is of the opinion that LAM is not limited in scope in its clinical or histopathological findings as was proposed earlier but rather encompasses a disease spectrum where there are varied clinical and histopathological features. Another plausible explanation for the varied histopathological findings in LAM is that probably the histopathological examinations were done at different stages in the evolution of lesions of LAM. It is possible that initially there can be only basal hyperpigmentation in the lesions. As the disease progresses it involves dermis leading to other histopathological findings related to dermis like abnormal collagen, perivascular lymphocytic infiltrates, *etc.* Thus, it may be imperative to follow up the patient and repeat biopsies should be taken to make a final diagnosis [16]. In author's opinion, a global working group on LAM must be established to redefine LAM and its diagnostic criteria should be updated in order to prevent any confusion in diagnosing and treating this rare disease entity.

DIFFERENTIAL DIAGNOSIS

The differential diagnosis of LAM includes those disorders which have hyperpigmented lesions with a variable amount of atrophy following BL and histopathology showing basal hyperpigmentation with altered collagen in the dermis (Table 16.5).

IAPP is differentiated from LAM by the characteristic atrophic plaques with cliff drop borders, usually in a bilateral distribution. It rarely occurs along BL and the atrophy in IAPP has been attributed to the loss of dermal tissue [23, 24]. Morphea usually has an initial inflammatory phase and the lesions have lilac colored rings. Induration and sclerosis on histopathology is the hallmark of morphea. The prognosis of morphea is less favourable and can lead to complications in contrast to LAM [25]. Blaschkoid lichen planus can also be considered as differential when the clinical atrophy in LAM is not well established. However, pruritic nature of the lesions and the histopathology suggestive of LP easily differentiates it from LAM [16, 26]. Linear & whorled nevoid hypermelanosis can be differentiated by its early onset at birth or soon after birth and absence of atrophy in the lesions. Linear post-inflammatory hyperpigmentation can be ruled out by the history of preceding dermatosis. In addition, atrophy will be absent in that case.

Table 16.5. Differential diagnosis of LAM [16].

Parameter	LAM	IAPP	Linear Morphea	Blaschkoid LP	LWNHM
Age of onset	Childhood or adolescence	Adolescence or early adulthood	Childhood or later	Childhood	Soon after or at birth
Lesion morphology	Hyperpigmented atrophic linear lesions along BL.	Circumscribed hyperpigmented atrophic lesions with cliff-drop borders.	Hyperpigmented to ivory white lesions with lilac borders and with induration and sclerosis.	Pruritic, violaceous papules in a linear fashion along BL.	Hyperpigmented macules along BL with no atrophy or inflammation.
Lesion distribution	Trunk, extremities	Trunk, arms	Extremities, head and neck,	Extremities	Trunk, extremities

(Table 16.5) cont.....

Parameter	LAM	IAPP	Linear Morphea	Blaschkoid LP	LWNHM
Evolution	Stable after initial progression	Present for a long duration	Unpredictable	Progressive	Progresses for a few years before stabilizing.
Atrophy	Atrophy of subcutaneous tissue	Atrophy of the dermis.	Involvement of skin and subcutis and may extend into deeper structures including muscles and bone.	No atrophy	No atrophy.
Histo-pathology	Only basal cell pigmentation in classical cases. Newer findings include chronic lymphocytic infiltrate, altered dermal collagen, decreased elastin, *etc.*	Thickening and homogenization of dermal collagen with dermal edema and mononuclear infiltrate. Epidermis is normal.	Epidermal atrophy with thickening and homogenization in dermal collagen with entrapment of adenexa with prominent inflammation.	Hyperkeratosis, hypergranulosis, basal cell vacuolization, Civette bodies and band like infiltrate at the dermo-epidermal junction.	Basal layer pigmentation with prominence or vacuolization of melanocytes.
Prognosis	Good, non-progressive	Progressive with new lesions developing and enlarging variably over 10-20 years.	Poor prognosis, contractures and arrested growth of involved limb.	Self-limiting	Good prognosis
Treatment	IV penicillin, Weekly methotrexate, topical calcipotriol, *etc.*	Topical corticosteroids, PUVA, Doxycycline, antimalarials, *etc.*	Steroids, methotrexate and other immunosuppressives and phototherapy.	Topical steroids	No treatment

LAM: Linear atrophoderma of Moulin, BL: Blaschko lines, IAPP: Idiopathic atrophoderma of Pasini and Pierini, LWNHM: Linear & whorled nevoid hypermelanosis, LP:Lichen planus

TREATMENT

No definitive treatment for LAM has been established yet. Several treatment modalities have been tried for LAM, however results have been unsatisfactory so far (Box **16.2**). These include oral potassium aminobenzoate (12g/day), intravenous penicillin, topical corticosteroids, heparin, phototherapy, combination of PUVA and penicillin; association of high-dose vitamin E (400 IU/day) and topical clobetasol propionate [21, 27]. Some authors have reported moderate efficacy with calcipotriol [28].

Box 16.2. Treatments tried in LAM.
Oral potassium aminobenzoate
Topical corticosteroids
Heparin
Intravenous penicillin
Phototherapy
Combination of PUVA and penicillin
High-dose vitamin-E and topical clobetasol propionate
Calcipotriol
Methotrexate
Intralesional platelet rich plasma

Zaouak *et al.* have claimed improvement in skin pigmentation and atrophy with methotrexate 20 mg/week for 6 months in an 11 year female having extensive lesions of LAM [29]. Recently, Kharkar *et al.* have carried out four sessions of intralesional platelet rich plasma (PRP) injections for LAM. They reported partial response after 4 sessions. They reported a reduction in the depth of the plaques; however, the color and the texture of the skin remained unaltered. They speculated that the growth factors present in PRP may help in the atrophy of subcutaneous tissue which is characteristic of LAM [30]. Since, most of the times, the condition is mainly esthetic; some authors have advised a self-tanning cream to a 15-year-old girl that caused homogenization of the skin pigmentation [8].

PROGNOSIS

The prognosis of LAM is very good. Most often the lesions are asymptomatic. In the original case series described by Moulin *et al.,* the lesions remained stable and didn't show tendency to progress during a follow up period of 2-30 years [2]. This excellent prognosis and lack of complications differentiates it from linear morphea which can cause significant cosmetic and functional morbidity as a result of flexion contractures, limb and facial asymmetry, extracutaneous manifestations, eye and CNS involvement. Fortunately, lesions of LAM, unlike that of linear morphea, that are present over joints have not proved troublesome as they do not cause joint contractures which is due to the lack of sclerosis and subsequent tightening of overlying tissues. It is important to mention the absence of complications in LAM to the patient to assure him that this condition should be considered as a cosmetic concern only.

TWIN SPOTTING IN LAM

Twin spotting has been considered as a particular type of loss of heterozygosity. When two different recessive mutations occur on either of a pair of homologous chromosomes, there is the emergence of two different homozygous daughter cells that form the stem cells of two different mutant lesions. These paired mutant lesions may be present on the same or on either side of the body. They may or may not follow lines of Blaschko. Some dermatological conditions which can be explained on the basis of twin spotting include melanotic and achromic twin nevi, phacomatosis pigmentovascularis and phacomatosis pigmentokeratotica, vascular twin nevi, lesions of overgrowth and deficient growth in Proteus syndrome, etc [31]. Apart from these, twin spotting has been implicated in several other associations [32]. The phenomenon of twin spotting may offer a plausible explanation for a number of paired skin conditions.

Two cases of LAM have been reported and surprisingly both from Turkey separately by Ozkaya *et al.* and Yucel *et al.* in 2010 and 2012, respectively. They have described two cases having segmental and spotty lentiginosis present within the lesions of LAM [12, 14]. Segmental lentiginosis is a condition characterized by circumscribed group of small, pigmented macules which are distributed unilaterally and arranged in a segmental/zosteriform pattern. This condition usually appears during childhood [32]. Previously, it has been reported to be colocalized within the lesions of nevus depigmentosus, nevoid hypopigmentation, and genital lichen sclerosus [33 - 36]. The authors of these two cases suggested that the occurrence of segmental and spotty lentiginosis within the lesions of LAM could be a new example of twin spotting. Twin spotting may occur as a result of allelic or nonallelic mutations. Allelic mutations involve dichotomic functional abnormalities of the same tissue *e.g.*, achromic and melanotic twin naevi or vascular twin naevi (naevus anaemicus and naevus telangiectaticus). On the contrary, unusual paired mutant skin lesions *e.g.*, phacomatosis pigmentokeratotica and phacomatosis pigmentovascularis are suggestive of nonallelic mutations [31].They concluded that the coexistence of segmental lentiginosis within lesions of LAM might represent a type of nonallelic twin spotting [12]. Whether these two cases represented a true association or just coincidence is a question of debate. We have to wait for some more cases to get published to support or refute this association.

Box 16.3. Learning points.
• The atrophy in LAM is due to the loss of subcutaneous tissue rather than the dermis.
• LAM can occur at any age; can be hyperpigmented or hypopigmented and can occur unilaterally or bilaterally.

cont.....

• The prognosis of LAM is excellent. Most often the lesions are asymptomatic and rarely show tendency to progress. Lack of complications unlike that of linear morphea differentiates it from the later.
• Twin spotting has been described in two cases of LAM that needs to be studied further.
• LAM is not as limited in scope as has been described originally but probably comprises a wider set of clinical and histopathological features.
• There is a need to redefine LAM and update its diagnostic criteria which at present neither seem to be sufficient nor accurate.

ACKNOWLEDGEMENTS

I am highly thankful to: A) Worthy Indian Journal of Dermatology, venereology and Leprology (IJDVL) and Dr Saumya panda (Editor-in-Chief, IJDVL) for granting me permission to share (Fig. **16.2**). B) Patsatsi A, Kyriakou A, Chaidemenos G and Sotiriadis D for granting me permission to share (Figs. **16.1**, **16.5-16.7**). C) Prof Piotr Brzezinski (Editor-in-Chief) and Prof. Lorenzo Martini (Subject Editor) of worthy Our Dermatology Online journal for their support in getting permission for (Fig. **16.3**). D) The worthy Journal of skin and stem cell for providing me assistance to get permission to share the published figure of my own article (Fig. **16.4**).

REFERENCES

[1]   Arif T. Linear atrophoderma of Moulin: Do we need to redefine this controversial disease entity? J Pak Assoc Dermatol 2019; 29(1): 1-3.

[2]   Moulin G, Hill MP, Guillaud V, Barrut D, Chevallier J, Thomas L. Acquired atrophic pigmented band-like lesions following Blaschko's lines. Ann Dermatol Venereol 1992; 119(10): 729-36.
       [PMID: 1296472]

[3]   Baumann L, Happle R, Plewig G, Schirren CG. Atrophodermia linearis moulin. Hautarzt 1994; 45(4): 231-6.
       [http://dx.doi.org/10.1007/s001050050066] [PMID: 8014049]

[4]   Norisugi O, Makino T, Hara H, Matsui K, Furuichi M, Shimizu T. Evaluation of skin atrophy associated with linear atrophoderma of Moulin by ultrasound imaging. J Am Acad Dermatol 2011; 65(1): 232-3.
       [http://dx.doi.org/10.1016/j.jaad.2009.12.005] [PMID: 21679833]

[5]   Ang G, Hyde PM, Lee JB. Unilateral congenital linear atrophoderma of the leg. Pediatr Dermatol 2005; 22(4): 350-4.
       [http://dx.doi.org/10.1111/j.1525-1470.2005.22415.x] [PMID: 16060875]

[6]   Patrizi A, Venturi M, Neri I, Pazzaglia M, Passarini B. Atrophoderma following the lines of Blaschko: An interesting diagnostic dilemma. Linear Atrophoderma of Moulin, blaschkolinear Atrophoderma of pasini and pierini or linear morphea? Clin Dermatol 2013; 1(1): 29-36.

[7]   Danarti R, Bittar M, Happle R, König A. Linear atrophoderma of Moulin: Postulation of mosaicism for a predisposing gene. J Am Acad Dermatol 2003; 49(3): 492-8.
       [http://dx.doi.org/10.1067/S0190-9622(03)00895-8] [PMID: 12963915]

[8]   Utikal J, Keil D, Klemke CD, Bayerl C, Goerdt S. Predominant telangiectatic erythema in linear atrophoderma of Moulin: Novel variant or separate entity? Dermatology 2003; 207(3): 310-5.
       [http://dx.doi.org/10.1159/000073096] [PMID: 14571076]

[9]   Zampetti A, Antuzzi D, Caldarola G, Celleno L, Amerio P, Feliciani C. Linear atrophoderma of moulin. Eur J Dermatol 2008; 18(1): 79-80.
[PMID: 18086596]

[10]   de Golian E, Echols K, Pearl H, Davis L. Linear atrophoderma of Moulin: A distinct entity? Pediatr Dermatol 2014; 31(3): 373-7.
[http://dx.doi.org/10.1111/pde.12003] [PMID: 23046463]

[11]   Oiso N, Kimura M, Itoh T, Kawada A. Variant of linear atrophoderma of Moulin: Hyper and hypopigmented linear atrophoderma with aberrant area cutanea and lentiginosis following the lines of Blaschko. J Dermatol 2012; 39(12): 1097-9.
[http://dx.doi.org/10.1111/j.1346-8138.2012.01627.x] [PMID: 22803683]

[12]   Özkaya E, Yazganoğlu KD. Lentiginosis within plaques of linear atrophoderma of Moulin: A twin-spotting phenomenon? Br J Dermatol 2010; 163(5): 1138-40.
[http://dx.doi.org/10.1111/j.1365-2133.2010.09952.x] [PMID: 20649796]

[13]   Browne C, Fisher BK. Atrophoderma of Moulin with preceding inflammation. Int J Dermatol 2000; 39(11): 850-2.
[http://dx.doi.org/10.1046/j.1365-4362.2000.00095-2.x] [PMID: 11123448]

[14]   Yücel S, Özcan D, Seçkin D. Lentiginosis within plaques of hypopigmented linear atrophoderma of Moulin: Another example of twin spotting? Int J Dermatol 2013; 52(11): 1427-9.
[http://dx.doi.org/10.1111/j.1365-4632.2011.05147.x] [PMID: 22913771]

[15]   López N, Gallardo MA, Mendiola M, Bosch R, Herrera E. A case of linear atrophoderma of Moulin. Actas Dermosifiliogr 2008; 99(2): 165-7.
[PMID: 18346448]

[16]   Arif T, Adil M, Sami M, Saeed N. Hyperpigmented patches following blaschko lines: Two probable cases of linear atrophoderma of moulin with subtle atrophy and a critical review of the subject. Indian J Paediatr Dermatol 2019; 20(3): 261-6.
[http://dx.doi.org/10.4103/ijpd.IJPD_97_18]

[17]   Cecchi R, Giomi A. Linear atrophoderma of Moulin. Acta Derm Venereol 1997; 77(6): 485.
[PMID: 9394993]

[18]   Ang GC, Lee JB. Linear atrophoderma of Moulin: Is it a single disease? J Am Acad Dermatol 2005; 52(5): 923-4.
[http://dx.doi.org/10.1016/j.jaad.2004.09.043] [PMID: 15858498]

[19]   Cecchi R, Bartoli L, Brunetti L, Pavesi M. Linear atrophoderma of Moulin localized to the neck. Dermatol Online J 2008; 14(6): 12.
[http://dx.doi.org/10.5070/D31W2688C0] [PMID: 18713593]

[20]   Tukenmez Demirci G, Altunay IK, Mertoglu E, Kucukunal A, Sakiz D. Linear atrophoderma of Moulin on the neck. J Dermatol Case Rep 2011; 5(3): 47-9.
[http://dx.doi.org/10.3315/jdcr.2011.1074] [PMID: 22187579]

[21]   Villani AP, Amini-Adlé M, Wagschal D, Balme B, Thomas L. Linear atrophoderma of moulin: Report of 4 cases and 20th anniversary case review. Dermatology 2013; 227(1): 5-9.
[http://dx.doi.org/10.1159/000347110] [PMID: 23989408]

[22]   Patsatsi A, Kyriakou A, Chaidemenos G, Sotiriadis D, Patsatsi A. Linear atrophodrma of Moulin: A case report and review of the literature. Dermatol Pract Concept 2013; 3(1): 7-11.
[http://dx.doi.org/10.5826/dpc.0301a03] [PMID: 23785629]

[23]   Arif T. Zosteriform idiopathic atrophoderma of pasini and pierini. Indian J Paediatr Dermatol 2019; 20(1): 60-3.
[http://dx.doi.org/10.4103/ijpd.IJPD_85_18]

[24]   Arif T, Adil M, Amin SS, Ahmed M. Atrophoderma of Pasini and Pierini in a blaschkoid pattern. J

Dtsch Dermatol Ges 2017; 15(6): 663-4.
[http://dx.doi.org/10.1111/ddg.13198] [PMID: 28346752]

[25]   Arif T, Adil M, Amin SS, *et al.* Clinico-epidemiological study of morphea from a tertiary care hospital. Curr Rheumatol Rev 2018; 14(3): 251-4.
[http://dx.doi.org/10.2174/1573397114666180410115553] [PMID: 29637865]

[26]   Adil M, Amin SS, Arif T. Blaschkoid lichen planus: A rare presentation of a common disease. Nasza Dermatol Online 2016; 7(3): 349-50.
[http://dx.doi.org/10.7241/ourd.20163.95]

[27]   Zahedi niaki O, Sissons W, Nguyen VH, Zargham R, Jafarian F. Linear atrophoderma of Moulin: An underrecognized entity. Pediatr Rheumatol Online J 2015; 13(1): 39.
[http://dx.doi.org/10.1186/s12969-015-0036-6] [PMID: 26438123]

[28]   Wongkietkachorn K, Intarasupht J, Srisuttiyakorn C, Aunhachoke K, Nakakes A, Niumpradit N. Linear atrophoderma of moulin: A case report and review of the literature. Case Rep Dermatol 2013; 5(1): 11-4.
[http://dx.doi.org/10.1159/000346747] [PMID: 23466694]

[29]   Zaouak A, Hammami Ghorbel H, Benmously-Mlika R, *et al.* A case of linear atrophoderma of Moulin successfully treated with methotrexate. Dermatol Ther 2014; 27(3): 153-5.
[http://dx.doi.org/10.1111/dth.12099] [PMID: 24903472]

[30]   Abak BA, Kharkar VD, Mahajan S. Linear atrophoderma of Moulin: A rare entity. Indian J Dermatol Venereol Leprol 2018; 84(5): 591-4.
[http://dx.doi.org/10.4103/ijdvl.IJDVL_136_17] [PMID: 30106014]

[31]   Happle R. Loss of heterozygosity in human skin. J Am Acad Dermatol 1999; 41(2): 143-61.
[http://dx.doi.org/10.1016/S0190-9622(99)70042-3] [PMID: 10426882]

[32]   Baba M, Akcali C, Seçkin D, Happle R. Segmental lentiginosis with ipsilateral nevus depigmentosus: Another example of twin spotting? Eur J Dermatol 2002; 12(4): 319-21.
[PMID: 12095874]

[33]   In SI, Kang HY. Partial unilateral lentiginosis colocalized with naevus depigmentosus. Clin Exp Dermatol 2008; 33(3): 337-9.
[http://dx.doi.org/10.1111/j.1365-2230.2007.02586.x] [PMID: 18419609]

[34]   Bolognia JL, Lazova R, Watsky K. The development of lentigines within segmental achromic nevi. J Am Acad Dermatol 1998; 39(2): 330-3.
[http://dx.doi.org/10.1016/S0190-9622(98)70383-4] [PMID: 9703146]

[35]   Kanitakis J, Souillet AL, Butnaru C, Claudy A. Melanocyte stimulation in focal dermal hypoplasia with unusual pigmented skin lesions: A histologic and immunohistochemical study. Pediatr Dermatol 2003; 20(3): 249-53.
[http://dx.doi.org/10.1046/j.1525-1470.2003.20313.x] [PMID: 12787276]

[36]   El Shabrawi-Caelen L, Soyer HP, Schaeppi H, *et al.* Genital lentigines and melanocytic nevi with superimposed lichen sclerosus: A diagnostic challenge. J Am Acad Dermatol 2004; 50(5): 690-4.
[http://dx.doi.org/10.1016/j.jaad.2003.09.034] [PMID: 15097951]

[37]   Larrègue M, Vabres P, Rat JP, Auriol F, de Giacomoni P. Atrophodermie pigmentée linéaire de Moulin. Ann Dermatol Venereol 1995; 122: 73s-4s.

[38]   Igarza A, Conejo-Mir S, Llopis C, Barrios L, Andreu C, Ortega N. Linear atrophoderma of Moulin: Treatment with potaba. Dermatology 1996; 193(4): 345-7.
[http://dx.doi.org/10.1159/000246288] [PMID: 8993965]

[39]   Wollenberg A, Baumann L, Plewig G. Linear atrophoderma of Moulin: A disease which follows Blaschko's lines. Br J Dermatol 1996; 135(2): 277-9.
[http://dx.doi.org/10.1111/j.1365-2133.1996.tb01160.x] [PMID: 8881673]

[40]   Rompel R, Mischke AL, Langner C, Happle R. Linear atrophoderma of Moulin. Eur J Dermatol 2000; 10(8): 611-3.
[PMID: 11125323]

[41]   Martin L, Georgescu V, Nizard S, Happle R, Estève E. Atrophodermie unilatérale suivant les lignes de Blaschko [Unilateral atrophoderma following Blaschko's lines: blaschkolinear morphoea or Moulin's linear atrophoderma?]. Ann Dermatol Venereol 2002; 129(4 Pt 1): 431–432.
[PMID: 12055546]

[42]   Miteva L, Obreshkova E. An unusual manifestation of linear atrophoderma of Moulin. Acta Derm Venereol 2002; 82(6): 479-80.
[http://dx.doi.org/10.1080/000155502762064737] [PMID: 12575866]

[43]   Miteva L, Nikolova K, Obreshkova E. Linear atrophoderma of Moulin. Int J Dermatol 2005; 44(10): 867-9.
[http://dx.doi.org/10.1111/j.1365-4632.2004.02221.x] [PMID: 16207193]

[44]   Atasoy M, Aliagaoglu C, Sahin O, Ikbal M, Gursan N. Linear atrophoderma of Moulin together with leuconychia: A case report. J Eur Acad Dermatol Venereol 2006; 20(3): 337-40.
[http://dx.doi.org/10.1111/j.1468-3083.2006.01434.x] [PMID: 16503901]

[45]   Ripert C, Vabres P. Linear atrophoderma of moulin associated with antinuclear antibodies. J Eur Acad Dermatol Venereol 2010; 24(1): 108-9.
[http://dx.doi.org/10.1111/j.1468-3083.2009.03371.x] [PMID: 19614857]

[46]   Schepis C, Palazzo R, Lentini M. A teen-ager with linear atrophoderma of Moulin. Dermatol Online J 2010; 16(2): 7.
[http://dx.doi.org/10.5070/D386K1K785] [PMID: 20178703]

[47]   Tan SK, Tay YK. Linear atrophoderma of Moulin. JAAD Case Rep 2016; 2(1): 10-2.
[http://dx.doi.org/10.1016/j.jdcr.2015.10.005] [PMID: 27051814]

[48]   Emre S, Metin A, Sungu N, Kilinc F, Demirseren DD. Linear atrophoderma of Moulin located on the face. Nasza Dermatol Online 2016; 7(2): 204-6.
[http://dx.doi.org/10.7241/ourd.20162.56]

[49]   Darung I, Rudra O, Samanta A, Agarwal M, Ghosh A. Linear atrophoderma of moulin over face: An exceedingly rare entity. Indian J Dermatol 2017; 62(2): 214-5.
[http://dx.doi.org/10.4103/ijd.IJD_469_16] [PMID: 28400647]

CHAPTER 17

Parry-Romberg Syndrome

Tasleem Arif[1,2,*]

[1] *Department of Dermatology, STDs, Leprosy and Aesthetics, Dar As Sihha Medical center, Dammam, Saudi Arabia*

[2] *Ellahi Medicare Clinic, Srinagar, Kashmir, India*

Chapter synopsis.
• Parry-Romberg syndrome (PRS) is a rare disease characterized by progressive hemi-facial atrophy of the skin and soft tissue and later causes atrophy of muscles and the underlying osteocartilaginous structures with or without neurological and other complications.
• The etiopathogenesis of PRS has not been clear till date. Several theories have been postulated which include autoimmune theory, vascular dysfunction, sympathetic dysfunction, genetic predisposition, trauma, infections, neural crest migration disorder, *etc.*
• The onset of PRS usually occurs during the first and second decades of life. After a span of 2-20 years, the disease usually "burns out" before acquiring stabilization.
• Histopathological examination usually shows atrophic epidermis, dermis, subcutaneous fat, skin adnexa, vessels, and/ or hair follicles. Whether, clinically patients have cutaneous sclerosis or not, histopathology will show homogenized and thickened dermal collagen bundles.
• Neurological, ophthalmological, dental and maxillofacial complications are usually present. Neurological complications are the most common extracutaneous manifestations; seizures and headaches being the most common presentations.
• The diagnosis of PRS is mainly based on typical clinical presentation and further supported by other investigations like skin histopathology and imaging modalities to look for related complications.
• There is no standard medical treatment currently available for PRS. Immunosuppressive therapies like systemic corticosteroids, methotrexate, cyclosporine, mycophenolate mofetil, cyclophosphamide and other treatments like PUVA, hydroxychloroquine, plasmapheresis, *etc.* have yielded variable success.
• Surgical and aesthetic treatments include lipo-injection, fat grafting, soft tissue fillers, dermal fat grafts, bone paste cranioplasty, adipofascial flaps, bone grafts, biocompatible porous polyethylene implants. Nasal reconstruction, lip repair, eyebrow repair, eyebrow lifting, face-lift, lip augmentation, Z-plasty, and hair transplant have been carried out for a better aesthetic outcome.
• There is enough evidence to support that morphea en coup de sabre and PRS lie on the same spectrum of disease.

* Corresponding author Tasleem Arif: Department of Dermatology, STDs, Leprosy and Aesthetics, Dar As Sihha Medical center, Dammam, Saudi Arabia and Ellahi Medicare Clinic, Srinagar, Kashmir, India; E-mail: dr_tasleem_arif@yahoo.com

Keywords: Autoimmune theory, Baraquer-Simons syndrome, *Borrellia burgdorferi*, Burnt-out phase, Cervical sympathectomy, Channelopathy, Congenital hemiatrophy, Dermal fat grafts, Enophthalmos, Facial asymmetry, Facial hemiatrophy, Fat grafting, Galeal flaps, Hyperactivity of the brain stem, Idiopathic hemifacial atrophy, Linear morphea en coup de sabre, Maxillofacial complications, Lipodystrophy, Neural crest migration disorder, Neurological complications, Parry-Romberg syndrome, Photographical evaluation, Primary hemifacial hypertrophy, Progressive facial hemiatrophy, Progressive hemifacial atrophy, Rasmussen encephalitis, Romberg syndrome, Sunken hemiface, Sympathetic dysfunction, Vascular dysfunction.

INTRODUCTION

Parry-Romberg syndrome (PRS) is a rare disorder characterized by progressive hemiatrophy of the skin and soft tissue of the face and later causes atrophy of muscles, cartilage, and the underlying bony structures with or without neurological complications [1, 2]. It was initially described by Drs Caleb Hillier Parry in 1825 and Moritiz Heinrich Romberg in 1846 [3, 4]. However, its current name progressive hemifacial atrophy (PHA) was coined by Eulenberg in 1871 [5]. PRS usually presents initially in children and young adults and gradually progresses over a variable time course which may range from 2 to 20 years, finally reaching a "burnt-out phase" and stabilizing for no apparent reason [6 - 10]. The highly variable signs and symptoms of the disorder coupled with the peculiar disease course put obstacles in elucidating the underlying pathophysiology of the disorder. Though, a specific etiology has not been described till date, several theories have been postulated to account for its causation. These include infection, trauma, sympathetic nervous system dysfunction, vascular abnormalities, inflammatory conditions, and autoimmune disorders, etc [1, 11 - 14]. Most often, it is restricted to one half of the face, however it can involve the arm, trunk, and leg [2]. It usually starts in the first decade of life although a late onset has been described in some cases [1, 2, 15]. Female preponderance has been noted in PRS. Though, it is assumed to be a sporadic disorder, rarely familial cases have also been described [16 - 18].

HISTORICAL BACKGROUND

Regardless of the etiology of PRS, evidence has suggested that the history of this disorder dates back to more than 2000 years (Table **17.1**).

Table 17.1. Historical background of Parry-Romberg syndrome.

2001	The history of PRS dates back to more than 2000 years. Appenzeller *et al.* conducted a study titled "Neurology in ancient faces" of 200 mummy portraits painted in color at the beginning of the first millennium. Two of them were found to have PRS. The diagnosis was based on facial features suggesting localized atrophy of the skin and subcutaneous tissues.
2017	Charlier *et al.* retrospectively described PRS in a major French revolution leader Mirabeau (1791).
1825	Late Caleb Hillier Parry presented the first description of Parry–Romberg syndrome.
1846	Moritiz Heinrich Romberg described the disorder.
1871	Eulenberg proposed the term "progressive hemifacial atrophy".
2015	Tolkachjov *et al.* used the synonyms for Parry–Romberg syndrome: idiopathic hemifacial atrophy, progressive hemiatrophy and Romberg syndrome.
2015	Nomura *et al.* suggested that progressive hemifacial atrophy (PHA) can progress in lupus profundus, lipodystrophy, morphea, and Parry–Romberg syndrome.

Appenzeller *et al.* conducted a study of 200 mummy portraits painted in color in 2001. They found two mummies to have this disease [19]. The diagnosis was suggested based on facial features of localized atrophy of the skin and subcutaneous tissues. PRS has been described in a major French revolution leader Mirabeau (1791) retrospectively by Charlier *et al.* in 2017 [20]. The description of first case of PRS was presented by "Collections from the Unpublished Medical Writings of the Late Caleb Hillier Parry" (1825) [3]. Moritiz Heinrich Romberg described the disorder in 1846 [4]. In 1871, it was Eulenberg who introduced the current nomenclature for this disorder: Progressive hemifacial atrophy (PHA) [5]. Tolkachjov *et al.* suggested synonyms for Parry–Romberg syndrome which include idiopathic hemifacial atrophy, progressive hemiatrophy (PHA) and Romberg syndrome [21]. Nomura *et al.* suggested that PHA could progress in morphea, lipodystrophy, lupus profundus, and PRS [22]. The term PHA has been used synonymously with PRS.

EPIDEMIOLOGY

The true incidence and epidemiologic parameters of PRS are not well known due to several reasons which include lack of standardized diagnostic criteria for the disease, rare occurrence of the disease and the overlap of clinical manifestations between PRS and morphea en coup de sabre (ECDS) [2, 23]. PRS is more prevalent in the female sex, similar to morphea. Chiu *et al.* have described a study of 32 pediatric patients, 66% of them were females [24]. Rogers carried out a review of 772 cases having Progressive facial hemiatrophy and found the female to male ratio of 3:1 [25].

ETIOPATHOGENESIS

The etiopathogenesis of PRS has not been elucidated till date. However, it seems to be heterogeneous. Several theories have been postulated which are summarized in (Box **17.1**).

Box 17.1. Proposed Etiopathogenesis of PRS.
Autoimmune theory
Trauma
Vascular dysfunction
Infections
Sympathetic dysfunction
Neural crest migration disorder
Disturbance of fat metabolism
Genetic predisposition
Channelopathy
Hyperactivity of the brain stem center

Autoimmune Theory

Autoimmune theory is one of the leading theories proposed in the pathogenesis of PRS. This theory is supported by the presence of other autoimmune disorders in some cases of PRS. These include rheumatoid arthritis (RA), systemic lupus erythematosus (SLE), generalized myopathy, *etc.* [26,27.]. Stone carried out a global survey of 205 patients of PRS using the internet. He found the medical history of vitiligo and thyroid dysfunction in 17% and 10% of patients, respectively [9]. He also found other autoimmune conditions in these responders like SLE (2%), inflammatory bowel disease (5%), ankylosing spondylitis (2%) and RA (4%) [9]. This theory is further supported by serological presence of autoantibodies. Patients with PRS have been found to have several autoantibodies in their sera such as rheumatoid factor, antinuclear antibodies, anticentromere, antidouble-stranded DNA, anticardiolipin, and antihistone antibodies; and cerebrospinal fluid oligoclonal bands [1, 28 - 30].

Trauma

Several cases of PRS have been reported following trauma. This has led to a possible trauma-induced theory. Some studies regarding PRS and ECDS have found trauma as an etiological factor in a good percentage of their study population. In a large survey of 205 PRS patients, a childhood history of head injury was found in 27% of responders. However, according to the author, only 12% of patients had trauma that was relevant to the disorder [9]. Sommer *et al.* in a case series of 12 patients of PRS found 33% had a history of preceding injury [31]. Trauma has been suggested to be the reason for PRS in about 24-34% of cases. It can be operative traumas like dental avulsion or thyroidectomy, accidental traumas or in the form of obstetric traumas like vacuum maneuvers or forceps [32 - 36].

Vascular Dysfunction

Vascular dysfunction has been considered another theory in the etiopathogenesis of morphea-like disorders such as PRS. In systemic sclerosis (SSC) and morphea, vascular changes have been implicated to cause extracellular matrix proliferation and collagen production [37]. Similarly, neuro-vasculitis has been suggested in ECDS and PRS [38, 39]. Pensler *et al.* carried out a study of 41 PRS patients in which they studied light microscopy performed on 19 tissue specimens and ultrastructural analysis on 6 patients. They found that chronic cell mediated vascular injury and incomplete endothelial regeneration caused a lymphocytic neuro-vasculitis along the branches of the trigeminal nerve. They believed that this neuro-vasculitis was a main factor in causing PRS in those patients [17].

Infections

Some infections have been implicated in the pathogenesis of PRS though they have not been proven yet. Herpes zoster in the trigeminal distribution or Bell's palsy have been suggested to be related to PRS. But these findings have not been confirmed so far [40]. The association of Lyme infection and *Borrelia burgdorferi* antibodies with morphea has been reported from European patients. However, authors from the United States, United Kingdom, and Turkey have not found such an association in their studies [41 - 45]. Sommer *et al.* reviewed 12 cases of PRS from Germany. None among them had Borrelia antibodies [31]. A recent study from Mexico by Gutierrez-Gomez *et al.* comprising 21 PRS patients and 6 morphea ECDS patients didn't find any association between IgG *Borrelia* antibodies and PRS [46]. Several studies from North America also failed to confirm a direct association between morphea and *Borrelia* [47 - 51]. Apart from these, several other infections have also been noted which include dental infections, diphtheria, otitis, tuberculosis, syphilis and rubella [36, 42, 52]. However, a definite association with PRS to this time has not been established.

Sympathetic Dysfunction

Sympathetic dysfunction has been suggested as a potential cause of PRS [53]. Animal Experiments have been carried out by Resende *et al.* in cats, dogs, and rabbits. They ablated their superior cervical ganglion at the age of 30 days and followed them for one year. They found that the animals developed features similar to PRS which included enophthalmos, hemifacial atrophy, localized alopecia, ocular atrophy, strabismus, slight bone atrophy on the side of the sympathectomy, keratitis and corneal ulceration [52]. In 1960, Moss and Crikelair also induced PRS like features following cervical sympathectomy in rats [54]. These findings suggest that that there is a role of sympathetic dysfunction in PRS.

Neural Crest Migration Disorder

Pichiecchio *et al.* have described migraine and intracranial aneurysms in PRS. In addition, PRS has been described in association with benign tumors like hamartomas, orbital neuromas, and mandibular odontogenic fibromas. Cranial vessels, craniofacial bone and cartilage, frontonasal masses and smooth muscles take origin from neural crest. These findings have raised the possibility of a neural crest migration disorder in PRS [7, 36].

Disturbance of Fat Metabolism

Some authors have reported lipodystrophy and diencephalic tissue melting in addition to facial atrophy in PRS. They have suggested a probable metabolic disorder affecting the adipose tissues in such patients [55, 56].

Genetic Predisposition

Familial cases in PRS have been reported and thus point to a genetic predisposition [18, 55, 57 - 59]. In the global survey of 205 patients with PRS, six patients (3%) had a history of facial asymmetry in the family members [9]. Some authors have suggested autosomal dominant inheritance with incomplete penetrance in PRS [59]. However, at this point no robust evidence has been provided for this hypothesis.

Channelopathy

In 2009, Mrabet *et al.* described paroxysmal kinesigenic dyskinesia in PRS. Paroxysmal kinesigenic dyskinesia is a movement disorder which is believed to be the result of a channelopathy. Based on this coexistence, the authors hypothesized that channelopathy may be a common pathogenic mechanism involved in both the disorders [60].

Hyperactivity of the Brain Stem Center

Lonchampt *et al.* have suggested hyperactivity of the brain stem center as a cause of PRS [53].

To summarize, a distinct etiology of PRS is still not clear. It seems that a combination of sympathetic dysfunction, autoimmune and vascular theories may provide a likely etiopathogenetic mechanism in PRS.

CLINICAL PRESENTATION

Disease Onset and Course

The onset of PRS usually occurs during the first and second decades of life. However, late-onset of the disease has also been described [31, 35]. After the initial presentation, the disease usually progresses slowly but remains self-limited [2]. During a span of 2-20 years, it usually "burns out" before achieving stabilization [14, 61]. Though, halting of the facial atrophy has been seen in majority of PRS patients, in the electronic survey of 205 PRS patients, 26% of the affected patients reported acceleration of the disease. Of these, 68% were women and nine women reported worsening of hemiatrophy of the face during pregnancy while eight women reported same after childbirth. Stress (26%) and surgery (8%) were the likely possible triggering factors for the disease acceleration among those who had progressive disease [9].

Skin Manifestations

PRS commonly affects the dermatomes of one or multiple branches of the trigeminal nerve. Clinically, PRS is characterized by mostly unilateral facial atrophy of the skin, soft tissues, muscles, and underlying osteocartilaginous structures (Figs. **17.1 - 17.11**) [1, 2]. Skin changes like dyspigmentation and scarring may be present in the affected areas but involvement of the skin epidermis is minimal. Intraoral involvement affecting tongue, teeth, gingiva, and palate has been described [23, 25, 35]. Due to the progressive shrinking and deformation of one side of the face, an appearance of sunken hemiface is created with ipsilateral enophthalmos, and deviation of the nose and mouth towards the diseased side [2]. The ultimate magnitude of deformity depends upon the duration of the disease. The disease affects the functionality in addition to the aesthetics of the face.

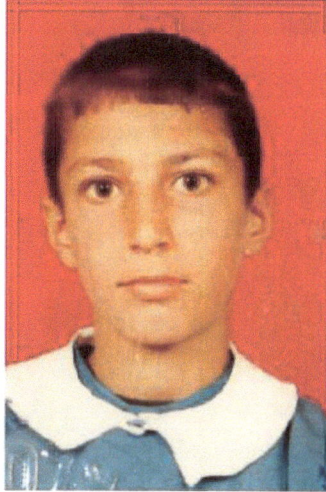

Fig. (17.1). At 8 years of age, very slight atrophy of the left side of the patient's face was apparent. [Image credit: Kaya M, Sel Yilmaz C, Kurtaran H, Gunduz M. Chronologic presentation of a severe case of progressive hemifacial atrophy (Parry–Romberg syndrome) with the loss of an eye. Case Rep Otolaryngol. 2014;2014:703017 Hindawi Limited/ CC BY 4.0]

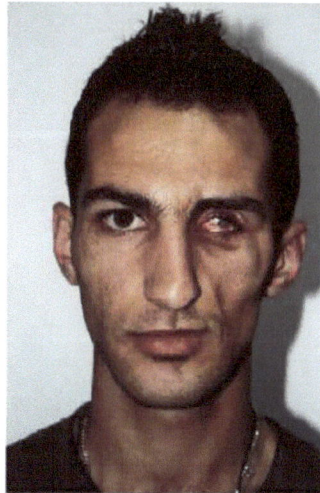

Fig. (17.2). Frontal view of the patient at 23 years of age, showing severe atrophy of fat and muscle tissue, and of the zygomatic arch on the left side, as well as shrinkage of the left eyeball and corneal atrophy. [Image credit: Kaya M, Sel Yilmaz C, Kurtaran H, Gunduz M. Chronologic presentation of a severe case of progressive hemifacial atrophy (Parry–Romberg syndrome) with the loss of an eye. Case Rep Otolaryngol. 2014;2014:703017/ Hindawi Limited/ CC BY 4.0]

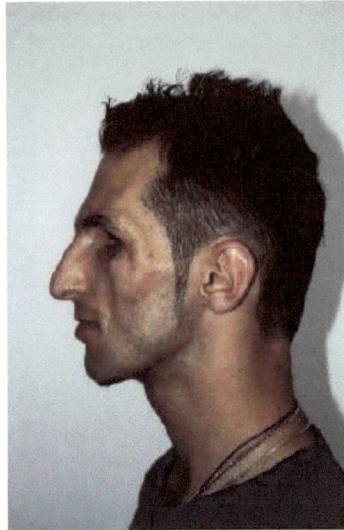

Fig. (17.3). Lateral view of left side of face. [Image credit: Kaya M, Sel Yilmaz C, Kurtaran H, Gunduz M. Chronologic presentation of a severe case of progressive hemifacial atrophy (Parry–Romberg syndrome) with the loss of an eye. Case Rep Otolaryngol. 2014;2014:703017 Hindawi Limited/ CC BY 4.0]

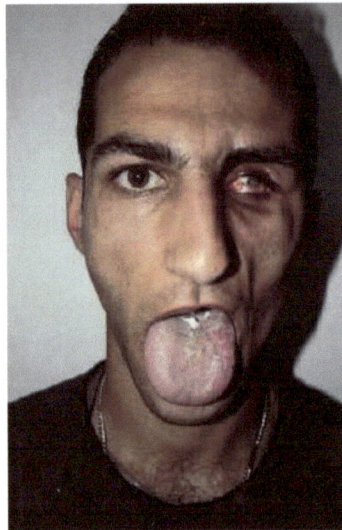

Fig. (17.4a). Atrophy and fissuring of the left hemi-glossus. [Image credit: Kaya M, Sel Yilmaz C, Kurtaran H, Gunduz M. Chronologic presentation of a severe case of progressive hemifacial atrophy (Parry–Romberg syndrome) with the loss of an eye. Case Rep Otolaryngol. 2014;2014:703017/ Hindawi Limited/ CC BY 4.0]

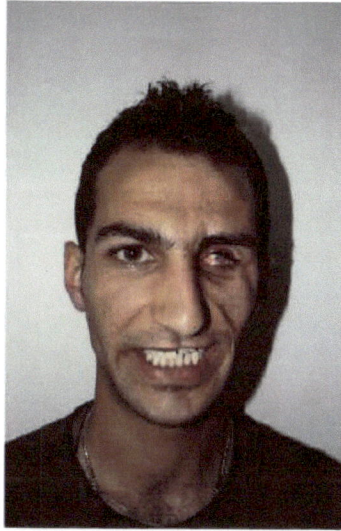

Fig. (17.4b). Maxillary atrophy has displaced the left upper teeth in an upward and backward Direction. [Image credit: Kaya M, Sel Yilmaz C, Kurtaran H, Gunduz M. Chronologic presentation of a severe case of progressive hemifacial atrophy (Parry–Romberg syndrome) with the loss of an eye. Case Rep Otolaryngol. 2014;2014:703017/ Hindawi Limited/ CC BY 4.0]

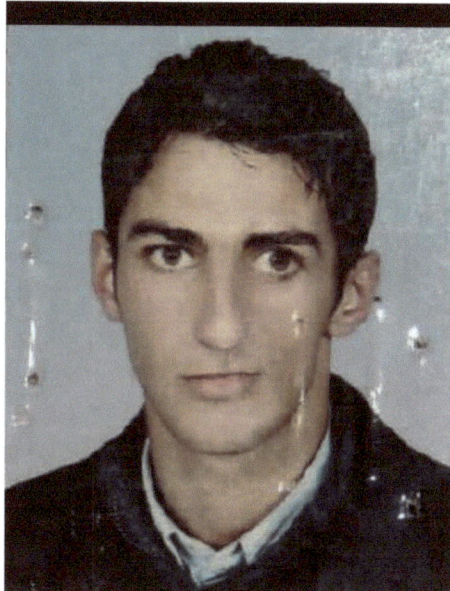

Fig. (17.5). The patient at 16 years of age, 1 year after the first autologous fat injection. [Image credit: Kaya M, Sel Yilmaz C, Kurtaran H, Gunduz M. Chronologic presentation of a severe case of progressive hemifacial atrophy (Parry–Romberg syndrome) with the loss of an eye. Case Rep Otolaryngol. 2014;2014:703017/Hindawi Limited/ CC BY 4.0]

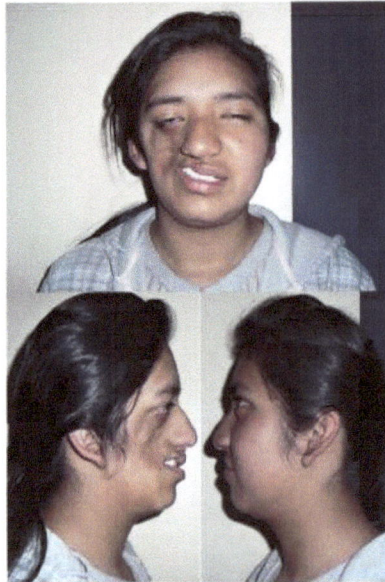

Fig. (17.6). A 17-year-old girl with Parry–Romberg syndrome. The subcutaneous tissue and underlying facial muscles on the right side of the face are severely atrophic, while the left side is unaffected. (Image credit: Desherinka-own work / Wikimedia Commons / CC BY-SA 3.0)

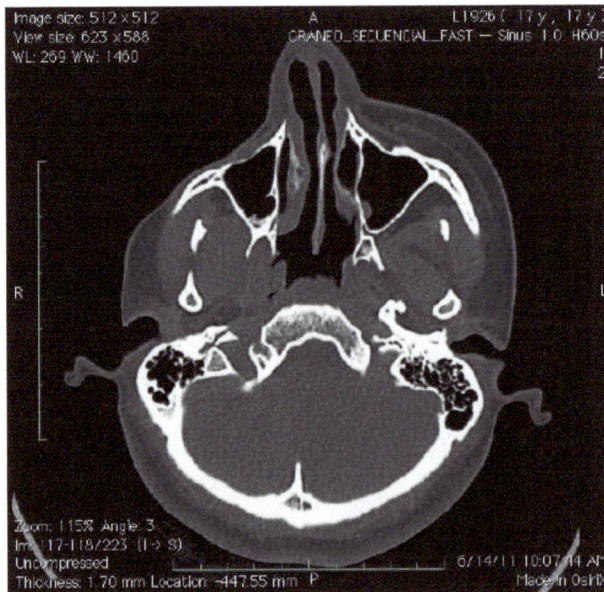

Fig. (17.7). An axial CT scan of a 17 year old girl with Parry Romberg syndrome, showing shrinkage and atrophy of the underlying subcutaneous tissue and underlying muscle, with no apparent involvement of the bone structure. (Image credit: Desherinka- own work/ Wikimedia Commons / CC BY-SA 3.0)

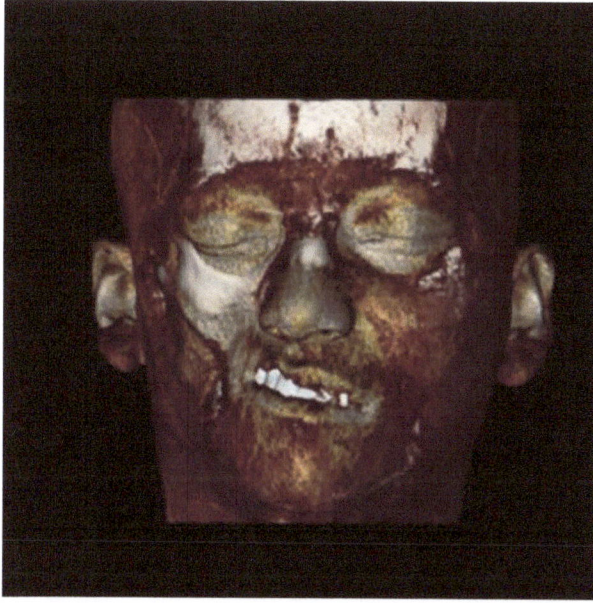

Fig. (17.8). A 3D, soft tissue reconstruction of a CT scan of a 17-year-old girl with Parry Romberg syndrome.(Image credit: Desherinka-own work / Wikimedia Commons / CC BY-SA 3.0)

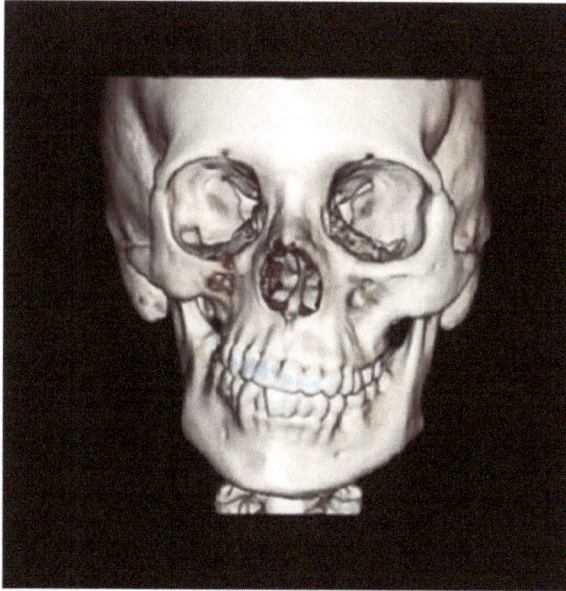

Fig. (17.9). A CT scan 3D bone reconstruction of a 17-year-old girl with Parry Romberg syndrome. (Image credit: Desherinka-own work / WIkimedia Commons / CC BY-SA 3.0)

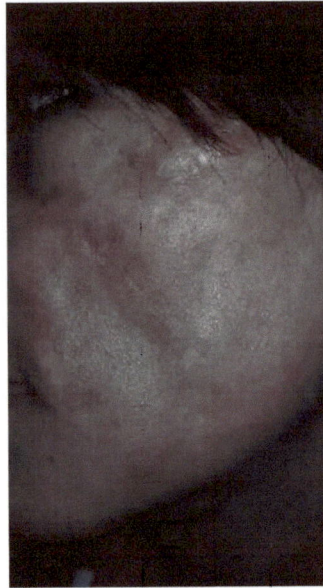

Fig. (17.10). Parry–Romberg syndrome in an adult female. There is atrophy of subcutaneous tissue and underlying facial muscles on the left side of the face. [Image credit: Dr Ömer Kutlu, Department of Dermatology and Venereology, Uşak University School of Medicine, Turkey]

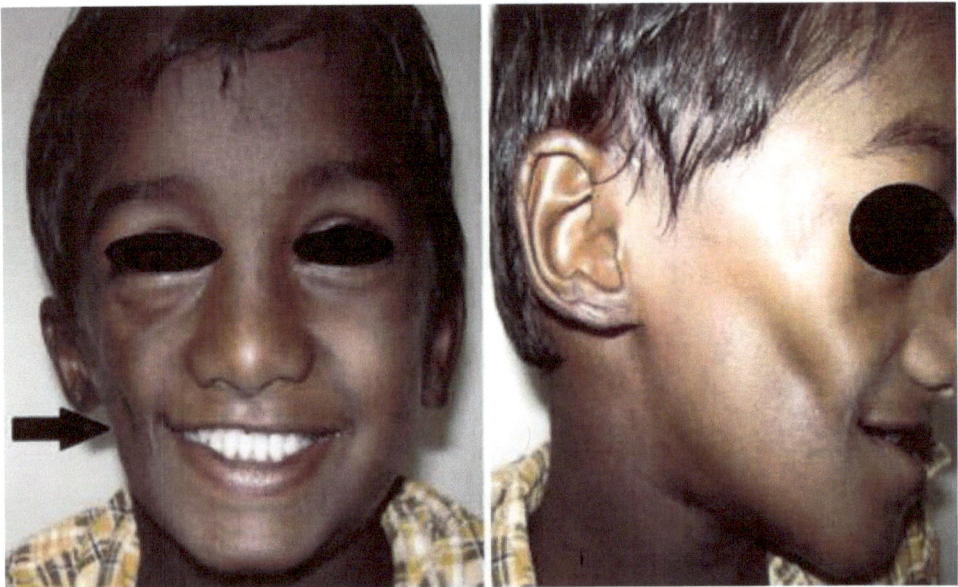

Fig. 17.11. Parry Romberg syndrome: Clinical photographs showing facial defects (a) Skewing of mouth, (b) Hollowing of cheek due to soft tissue atrophy. This patient also had circumscribed morphea over abdomen. [Copyright: Ramalingam A, Sreedevi A. A rare case of Parry Romberg syndrome with morphea. Our Dermatol Online. 2020;11(e):e133.1-e133.3. Courtesy: Dr Piotr Brzezinski, MD PhD]

Cutaneous Associations

PRS has been associated with several other dermatological conditions. These include segmental vitiligo, lupus profundus, hyperpigmentation, linear morphea ECDS, port-wine stain, Klippel-Trenaunay syndrome, etc [59, 61 - 77]. These have been summarized in (Box **17.2**).

Box 17.2. Dermatological conditions associated with PRS.
Segmental vitiligo
Port-wine stain
Klippel-Trenaunay syndrome
Linear morphea en coup de sabre
Lupus profundus
Morphea
Band-like alopecia
Raynaud's phenomenon

Among these, linear morphea ECDS forms a close differential of PRS and there has been a long debate whether ECDS and PRS are the same disorder or possess an overlap or they are the two manifestations of the same disease spectrum. This has been discussed separately at the end of the chapter.

Neurological Manifestations

Neurological complications are the most common extracutaneous manifestations seen in PRS patients. Among neurological manifestations, seizures and headaches are the most common presentations in such patients. Simple or complex partial seizures arising from the ipsilateral cerebral cortex are commonly seen in PRS. These may be resistant to treatment [31, 78]. Cranial neuropathies involving cranial nerves III, V, VI, and VII, have been reported in PRS patients [79, 80]. Trigeminal neuralgia has been described. Impingement of the nerve by the destruction of bony structures and vascular inflammation have been suggested for the neuralgia [81]. Aphasia or dysarthria has been reported due to disturbances in the speech [82]. Behavioral disorders and cognitive impairment have also been reported [24]. Due to the cranial tissue atrophy as well as alterations to intracranial vessels and tissue, several manifestations can occur like paresthesias, dysesthesias and hemiparesis [82, 83]. Vascular inflammation can cause hemorrhage, infarction and white matter hyper-density in these patients [73, 84]. Affected cerebellar areas in PRS patients have revealed dysplastic vessels. This may contribute to intracranial findings [85]. The constellation of dysplastic vessels, vascular damage and alteration in the vascular caliber may cause atrophy of cerebellum leading to neurological manifestations. Rarely, intracranial vascular malformations mostly in the form of dilation of intracranial blood vessels have been reported in these patients [39, 86, 87]. The various neurological manifestations in PRS patients have been mentioned in (Table **17.2**).

Table 17.2. Neurological manifestations of PRS.

Seizure	Headaches
Facial pain	Trigeminal neuralgia
Migraine	Brain atrophy
Hemiplegia	Cerebral microhemorrhage
Intracranial vascular malformations	Cerebellar syndrome
Paroxysmal kinesigenic dyskinesia	Syringomyelia
Hemianesthesia	Facial nerve palsy
Mental retardation	Aphasia
Oculomotor nerve palsy	Bilateral pyramidal tract involvement
Sympathetic hyperactivity	Torticollis
Agenesis of head of caudate nucleus	Vascular Aneurysm
Limb atrophy	Cystic leukoencephalopathy
Status migrainosus	Dura matter atrophy
Rasmussen syndrome	Trunk atrophy
Mandibular cramps	Alien hand syndrome
Subdural hygroma	chronic focal encephalitis
multiple intracranial cysts	complete agenesis of the corpus callosum
Cortical depression	Hyperactivity of brain stem center
CNS tumors	Fatal brain stem involvement

Ocular Manifestations

Ophthalmological manifestations have been described in PRS patients. These may range from mild visual impairment to complete blindness [88]. As a result of atrophy of deeper tissue, enophthalmos occurs in such patients. Dysfunction of the orbitalis muscle also ensues. The atrophy also affects eye ball, extraocular muscles and the eyelids. In some cases, the atrophy may be so severe to cause restrictive strabismus [89 - 91]. In few cases, retinal vasculitis has been reported in patients with PRS which supports the vascular etiopathogenesis. Other ophthalmological manifestations that have been reported in PRS include glaucoma, uveitis, neuroretinitis, cataracts, papillitis, heterochromia of iris, pigmentary changes of the retina and optical fundus [92 - 94]. Various Ophthalmological manifestations in PRS have been summarized in (Table **17.3**).

Table 17.3. Ocular manifestations of PRS.

Enophthalmos	Third Nerve Palsy
Eyelid atrophy	Glaucoma
Papillitis	Neuroretinitis
Uveitis	Amblyopia
Diplopia	Miosis
Restrictive strabismus	Iridocyclitis
Episcleritis	Bilateral vitreitis
Cataract	Retinal telangiectasis
Hypotropia	Exotropia
Extraocular muscle weakness	Upper eyelid retraction
Phthisis bulbi	Blepharoptosis
Orbital neurinomas	Esotropia
Retinal pigment changes	Decreased corneal sensitivity
Band keratopathy	Worsening of hyperopia
Severe ocular hypotony	Lagophthalmos
Loss of cilia	Pseudoptosis
Retinal vasculitis	Chorioretinal lesions
Eyeball Shrinkage	Blindness
Coat syndrome	Retinal detachment
Adie pupil	Duane retraction syndrome
Horner syndrome	Light staining of retina
Corneal exposure	Fuchs syndrome

Dental and maxillofacial manifestations

Dental and maxillofacial abnormalities are very common in PRS **(Box 17.3).**

Box 17.3. Maxillofacial and oro-dental manifestations in PRS.
Delayed teeth eruption
Odontogenic cyst

Box 17.3. Maxillofacial and oro-dental manifestations in PRS.
Mandibular odontogenous Fibroma
Dilaceration
Odontoma of mandible
Reduction in height and width of mandible on affected side
Root resorption
Dysphonia
Speech disorder.
Masticatory muscle spasm
Temporomandibular joint pain
Dental infections
Lingual atrophy
Locking of the jaw
Mandibular and maxillary bone hypoplasia

Mandible and masticatory muscles are frequently involved in patients with PRS. Some authors have suggested that teeth anomalies can help in identifying the age of onset in PRS patients [36]. Teeth abnormalities include crowding of teeth, short crowns and roots. Due to mandibular and maxillary hypoplasia, several functions become impaired like smiling, chewing, and speech impairment. However, hemi-facial atrophy and disturbances of other oro-glandular tissues such as the gingiva, lips, tongue and salivary glands can be responsible for the development of such symptoms. Dental infections are frequent in PRS patients. Temporomandibular joint pain, pain due to the masticatory muscle spasm, and locking of the jaw have been reported in these patients [95 - 98].

DIAGNOSIS

There are no universally acceptable diagnostic criteria available for PRS. The diagnosis of PRS is mainly based on typical clinical presentation that is further supported by other investigations like skin histopathology and imaging modalities. The characteristic clinical manifestations of PRS which aid in its diagnosis are the presence of unilateral idiopathic facial atrophy, typically involving the lower part of the face, without having significant involvement of skin epidermis. Deeper involvement in the form of subcutaneous fat, muscles and osteo-cartilaginous structures as well as other oro-dental structures like teeth, tongue and gingivae may also be present. The only differential which may pose a great challenge is the linear morphea ECDS. ECDS is considered when linear scleroderma presents in the fronto-parietal area of scalp involving medial or paramedian forehead. However, ECDS can also extend superiorly towards the scalp and inferiorly towards nasal sidewall, maxilla, chin and even neck [99 - 101].The cutaneous hyperpigmentation and sclerosis together with alopecia are the potential differentiating features of ECDS from PRS [23]. The relationship between ECDS and PRS has been discussed separately at the end of this chapter.

INVESTIGATIONS

Skin related investigations

Histopathological examination from the skin biopsy of PRS patients usually shows atrophic epidermis, dermis, subcutaneous fat, skin adnexa, vessels, and/ or hair follicles [17, 102]. Whether the patient has clinical findings of cutaneous sclerosis or not, histopathology will show homogenized and thickened dermal collagen bundles (Fig. **17.12**).

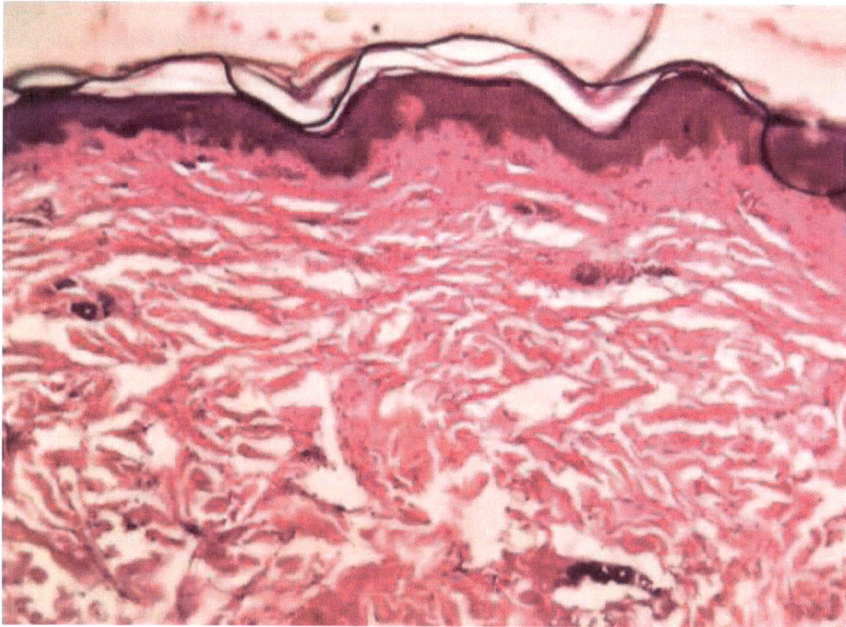

Fig. (17.12). Histopathology of Parry–Romberg syndrome (PRS) showing mild epidermal atrophy. Dense collagen bundles in the dermis with sparse inflammatory infiltrate. Findings similar to scleroderma (H&E 40×). (Image credit: Arif T, Fatima R, Sami M. Parry–Romberg syndrome: a mini review. Acta Dermatovenerol APA. 2020;29:193-199).

Cutaneous edema may be present. Dermal Inflammation in the form of lymphocytic infiltrates is variably present [82, 102]. A specific finding which can help in differentiating it from ECDS is the presence of degenerative changes of vascular endothelia [17, 76].

Skin ultrasound can be employed to measure the dermal thickness and echogenicity of the affected areas. This can give information about cutaneous sclerosis, help in monitoring of disease activity as well as assessing the treatment progress.

Photographical evaluation should be carried out by maintaining the serial photographs of the affected area and compared with subsequent follow up visits. Since, PRS progresses slowly and it may take a decade or two till stabilization, photographical records can help in disease evaluation.

Investigations for Neurological Complications

Neurological complications are frequently seen in PRS. Hence, in those patients who have neurologic symptoms, baseline imaging should be performed. Typical MRI findings include hyperintense white matter lesions on T2-weighted sequences. They are more prominently seen on the ipsilateral side. However, they are often seen bilaterally despite the lack of cutaneous involvement on the opposite side which means skin affliction is not necessary to manifest neurologically. It has been seen that these findings often do not progress irrespective of progressive skin and skeletal involvement. Cystic degeneration, encephalomalacia and cerebral atrophy have been reported on intracranial imaging of PRS patients [82]. Computed tomography (CT) scanning has also been used in evaluating PRS. However, it is less useful than MRI for evaluating lesions of brain parenchyma. Calcifications and alterations in the density of white matter are the typical changes seen on CT [78, 103]. In some cases, MRI findings may be seen in patients who lack clinical neurologic findings. Conversely, seizure activity may occur in patients before or in the absence of any abnormal MRI findings [78]. Similarly, cutaneous involvement does not correlate with CNS involvement [103]. Since, a direct correlation with cutaneous changes, clinical neurologic findings and MRI abnormalities is not always demonstrated; it becomes imperative to advise imaging of such patients, whether in the initial evaluation or in follow-up visits [78, 103].

In some patients silent white matter findings have been described [86]. However the significance of such findings is a difficult task to perform. Single-photo emission CT (SPECT) scan may be employed to study the regional blood flow in the affected area. It has been demonstrated that PRS patients having temporal lobe epilepsy were having hypoperfusion of the regional blood flow in the parieto-occipital area of their affected cerebral hemisphere [104]. Conversely, those PRS patients who had preserved cortical function and normal psychomotor development were having relatively increased regional cerebral blood flow of the affected cortical hemisphere on SPECT scan [105]. In some PRS patients demonstrating extensive white matter abnormalities on MRI, preserved cortical function can be demonstrated by SPECT scan, diffuse tensor imaging and proton MR spectroscopy [24]. In addition, those PRS patients having normal MRI report, SPECT scan may reveal abnormal findings [106]. Thus, the author concludes that while evaluation for neurological findings and an initial investigation with MRI is imperative, the additional evaluation of cerebral blood flow by SPECT can reveal more details of the CNS involvement and hence the prognosis in such patients.

In those patients who are suspected of having a seizure disorder, electroencephalography (EEG) should be advised. It has been demonstrated that those patients having abnormal EEG, findings are mainly on the ipsilateral side to the clinical involvement and most commonly have localized activity [78].

Investigations for Ocular Complications

Ophthalmological manifestations of PRS are common and can affect vision. Ophthalmology consultation should be advised for evaluation of vision, glaucoma, extra-ocular muscle weakness, restrictive strabismus, and inflammatory conditions of the eye associated with PRS [88, 89]. Retinal edema and optical disc swelling has been reported in some patients on ocular imaging which can lead to visual impairment and loss [107].

Investigations for Maxillofacial and Oro-dental Complications

Oro-dental involvement is common in PRS. This makes early evaluation necessary in order to reduce the deformity and complications related to mandible, teeth, maxilla, and other oral soft tissues. In order to monitor the disease progression, serial panoramic radiographs and photographs may be helpful. This can also help in planning for surgery and other orthodontic appliances [108]. Researchers have found that cone beam CT in combination with the mirror image of the normal unaffected side and superimposed on the diseased side is very helpful in making the assessment of the degree of asymmetry by clear linear, angular, and volumetric measurements. This has given orthodontists an additional insight to the therapeutic interventions in such patients [109].

DIFFERENTIAL DIAGNOSIS

The conditions which can mimic PRS have been mentioned in (Box **17.4**). Linear morphea ECDS at times becomes very difficult to be differentiated from PRS. Its relationship with PRS has been discussed at the end of this chapter.

Box 17.4. Differential diagnosis of PRS.
Linear morphea ECDS
Rasmussen encephalitis
Barraquer-Simons syndrome
Congenital hemiatrophy
Primary hemifacial hypertrophy

Rasmussen encephalitis (RE) or Rasmussen syndrome is characterized by unilateral cerebral hemispheric atrophy, abrupt onset of intractable motor seizures followed by hemiplegia and progressive neurologic deficits. It is a severe chronic inflammatory and immune-mediated disorder leading to brain damage. Histopathology from the affected cerebral tissue has shown chronic inflammation [110]. The unilateral localization, similar ages of onset, and presence of seizures has led to several reports of associations of PRS with RE thus making it difficult to differentiate the two entities [1, 8]. Some researchers have suggested that those cases of PRS that are complicated by epilepsy may have an overlap with RE [110]. However, patients with RE alone usually present with hemiparesis and severe intractable seizures [8]. On the other hand, the clinical hemiatrophy has only been described in PRS patients with coexisting ECDS or RE [1, 8]. In addition, brain biopsies of RE patients have shown distinct findings of reactive blood vessels, neuronal loss, and a pale background with chronic inflammatory cells and neutrophils [8]. Typically, brain biopsies are not done in PRS.

Baraquer-Simons syndrome is a type of acquired partial lipodystrophy affecting cephalothoracic region. It usually presents with an insidious onset of a bilaterally symmetrical subcutaneous fat atrophy involving face, neck, thorax, abdomen and upper extremities but sparing the lower limbs. Neurological manifestations include seizures, deafness, and intellectual impairment [111]. Systemic involvement in the form of the renal involvement and the bilateral nature of this disease can help in differentiating it from PRS. However, there are reports of associations of Baraquer-Simons syndrome and morphea [112].

Primary hemifacial hypertrophy (Hemifacial hypertrophy) is a rare disorder characterized by asymmetric enlargement of half of the head without hypertrophy of any other body part [113, 114]. It should be noted that in this disorder there is enlargement of one side of face while the other side is normal. This is in contrast to PRS where there is atrophy rather than hypertrophy.

TREATMENT

Medical Therapy

There is no standard treatment regimen currently available for PRS. The main aim of the treatment is to stop its progression in its early phase and improve patient's symptoms. Immunosuppressive therapy is justified in patients with CNS involvement. PRS being closely related to linear morphea ECDS, treatment modalities for scleroderma like immunosuppressive therapies, ranging from topical corticosteroids to systemic corticosteroids, immunomodulators, and plasmapheresis have also been used in PRS with varying degrees of success.

Methotrexate has been a standard drug for the treatment during active stage of the disease. Though its dosage has not been standardized, a dose ranging from 0.3-1 milligrams per kilogram of body weight per week (mg/kg/wk) either as an oral formulation or injectable form has been suggested. However, the maximum dose of methotrexate should not exceed 25mg/week. Methotrexate has been often combined with oral steroids in the form of prednisone over the first three months of the therapy. Combining the two is based on the fact that methotrexate has a delayed effect on inflammation and fibrosis. Most authors recommend two months of prednisone therapy at a dose of 1mg/kg/ day and then taper during the third month. Pulses of high doses of intra-venous methylprednisone using 1000 mg per day for three days a month for 6 months has been also used. The aim of this supra-pharmacological doses of steroid is to achieve the therapeutic effects of corticosteroids and to minimize the undesirable side effects. Generally, a long treatment course is needed as relapses are frequently reported after shorter treatment courses. The length of treatment course to induce remission and to reduce relapse is unknown and is believed to vary from case to case. Currently, a treatment course of 12-24 months with methotrexate is considered effective in inducing prolonged remission [61, 115 - 120].

Some patients who have failed to show beneficial response to methotrexate have shown variable success with other immunosuppressive agents such as cyclosporine, mycophenolate mofetil, and cyclophosphamide (Box **17.5**) [119, 121, 122]. In few cases, antimalarial drug (hydroxychloroquine) has also showed some efficacy [61]. Psoralens in collaboration with UVA-light (PUVA) has been reported to arrest disease activity in some PRS patients [43, 123].

Box 17.5. Medical treatment of PRS.
Methotrexate
Oral corticosteroids
Intra-venous methylprednisone pulse therapy
Cyclosporine
Mycophenolate mofetil
Cyclophosphamide
Hydroxychloroquine
PUVA

Surgical Treatment

Surgical management of PRS often requires a multidisciplinary approach. It may need repeated procedures, depending on the severity of the disease. The objective of surgical intervention in PRS patients is to correct the anatomy and function of affected facial structures and thus to decrease psychosocial effects [108, 124 - 126]. However, the timing of surgical intervention is a topic of debate. Most authors suggest that procedural treatment should be delayed until disease progression has stopped or stabilized. This approach avoids multiple surgeries as the defects progress. In addition, it also provides a stable skeletal foundation for the treating surgeon [127 - 129]. On the other hand, some researchers recommend earlier interventions despite active disease due to several reasons like psychosocial problems being faced by such patients, promotion of normal development of facial structures, and because of the fact that most patients will require multiple surgical interventions [126, 130]. Lack of confidence, low self-esteem due to the defective appearance, and bullying are the primary concerns forcing them to undergo surgical interventions [130]. Slack *et al.* in their study showed that early surgical intervention resulted in higher patient satisfaction scores [126]. It should be remembered that the timing of surgical intervention must be evaluated on an individual basis.

In cases where surgical intervention is delayed till disease stabilization has occurred, proper development of mandibles and symmetry of facial planes can be achieved with guided orthodontic appliances [124, 131]. Lipo-injection, fat grafting and other soft tissue fillers can be used for mild facial atrophy [126, 132 - 134]. In order to correct large volume atrophy, combined soft tissue and skeletal tissue approach is recommended which includes autologous fat infections, dermal fat grafts, bone paste cranioplasty and adipofascial flaps [135]. For correction of skeletal deformity, bone grafts and biocompatible porous polyethylene implants can be used [134, 135]. In addition, several procedures like nasal reconstruction, lip repair, eyebrow repair, eyebrow lifting, face-lift, lip augmentation, Z-plasty, and hair transplant can be employed in order to create a better aesthetic outcome [126, 130, 135].

Grading of Facial Atrophy and its Treatment

In order to provide the most effective treatment for facial atrophy in PRS, it is important to first grade the severity of tissue atrophy and then decide the treatment strategy. Accordingly, Guerrerosantos *et al.* divided 95 patients with clinical facial atrophy into four groups according to the severity of tissue atrophy and then decided treatment based on their classification system [136].

Type 1 Tissue Depression

Type 1 atrophy is very mild. There is thinning of the facial soft tissues. It is seen during acute phase of PRS usually between 10-20 years. The facial deformity is noticeable to the patient and to his family and friends but almost imperceptible to strangers.

Type 2 Tissue Depression

Type 2 atrophy is characterized by thinning of the soft tissues. However, there is no effect on cartilage or bone. The atrophy and loss of volume is more visible than type 1 deformity. Anyone looking at the patient can recognize it.

Type 3 Tissue Depression

In this facial atrophy, the soft tissues are thinner than in type 2. There is atrophy of cartilaginous and bony tissues. The deformity is clearly evident.

Type 4 Tissue Depression

It is the most severe type of facial tissue atrophy. The soft tissue atrophy is so severe that the skin is nearly attached to the underlying bones. The atrophy in cartilages and bone is more severe than type 3. These patients tend to have severe functional problems, especially those of nose and the lips apart from aesthetic deformities.

Treatment Protocol

For type 1 and 2 tissue depressions, they found successful results with lipo-injections and grafting into the muscle and periosteum or under the submucosal aponeurotic system because of the good vascularization. Patients with type 3 tissue depressions, received a combined treatment including lipo-injection sessions, dermis-fat grafts, galeal flaps, and bone and cartilage grafts. In patients with type 4 tissue depressions, the treatment remains similar to type 3. However, the thickness of the flaps and grafts is thicker than in type 3 [136].

RELATIONSHIP BETWEEN PRS AND LINEAR MORPHEA ECDS

Linear morphea ECDS is a type of linear morphea involving face and head [101, 137, 138]. It presents as an area of hyperpigmented (sometimes hypopigmented as well) indurated skin overlying the fronto-parietal area mainly unilateral (rarely bilateral), usually restricted to the forehead, and associated with a paramedian forehead scar separating normal skin from the atrophic one, however it can extend downwards as well. Induration of the skin is the characteristic finding [73, 99 - 101, 138]. Cicatricial alopecia is usually present on the affected side [139, 140].This type of linear morphea usually presents in the childhood and predominantly affects females, though late onset has also been described [100, 101, 141]. The clinical course of the disease is slow and progresses over a span of 2 to 20 years, after which stabilization is achieved. However, regaining of clinical activity after being quiescent for years, has also been described [99, 137]. Neurologic and ophthalmologic manifestations have also been reported similar to PRS, though less frequent [142 - 144]. The cause of linear morphea ECDS is not clear. Several factors have been proposed which include immune dysfunction, trauma, altered peripheral sympathetic nervous system, early cerebral inflammation and disturbed trigeminal nerve [53, 100, 138, 140, 145, 146].

Differentiating linear morphea ECDS from PRS has been very difficult [2].The two disease entities share several features. Both the diseases have relatively a similar age of onset (average age of onset of 11 years), predominantly affecting females, and clinically the lesions at presentation progress slowly over time till they acquire stabilization after several years ranging from 2-20 [2]. Neurological and ocular complications of the two are comparable [141]. Treatment response to immunosuppressive drugs may be seen in both [116, 119]. In some cases, features of the two diseases may overlap [61, 74, 147]. PRS and linear morphea ECDS have been found to coexist in many patients (Fig. **17.13**) [23, 106, 148, 149].

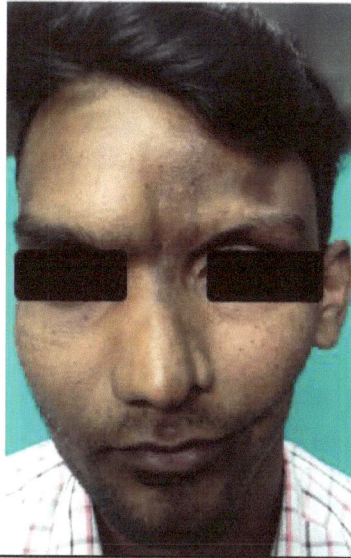

Fig. (17.13). ECDS and PRS in the same patient on the same side. This patient also had scarring alopecia in a linear pattern on the frontal scalp as a result of ECDS. There was visible atrophy on the left side of face behind the angle of mouth that was associated with atrophy of left side of the tongue consistent with PRS. [Image credit: a) Swetank; MLB Medical College, Jhansi, Uttar Pradesh, b) Mohammad Adil; Jawaharlal Nehru Medical College, Aligarh Muslim University, Aligarh, India, c) Arif T, Fatima R, Sami M. Parry–Romberg syndrome: a mini review. Acta Dermatovenerol APA. 2020;29:193-199.]

Furthermore, some researchers have described patients where ECDS converted into PRS with time [23, 106]. The prevalence of PRS in conjunction with ECDS has been reported in the range of 36.6% to 53.6% [61, 31].

Several studies have been carried out to differentiate PRS from ECDS on the basis of clinical and histopathological characteristics [23, 106, 150]. In 1992, Thomas Lehman stressed on two clinical features to differentiate between the two entities: a) In PRS, there is paramedian atrophy without significant induration of the overlying skin and, b) associated atrophy usually extends down the side of the face with tongue and mandibular involvement. According to him, ECDS should be considered when there is associated cutaneous induration in the area of the scalp and does not extend below the forehead [71]. However, there are several cases where ECDS has extended below the forehead and reached mandible and even neck. The author and his colleagues have reported two cases of ECDS where the lesions extended up to chin and neck [99, 101, 151]. In addition, there are several authors who have shown that the two diseases are closely related to each other and lie on the same spectrum of the disease [150, 152].

Orozco-Covarrubias *et al.* (2002) carried out a retrospective study to differentiate PRS and ECDS on the basis of clinical and histopathological criteria. In their series comprising 9 cases of PRS and 13 cases of ECDS, they found that the key differentiating clinical feature between the two entities was cutaneous sclerosis (present in 8 cases of ECDS and none in PRS). Hyperpigmentation and scarring alopecia were the characteristic features in ECDS while PRS was characterized by total hemi-facial involvement and ocular manifestations. On histopathological examination, a significant overlap existed. Connective tissue fibrosis was present in all ECDS cases and two cases of PRS. Adnexal atrophy was present in 11 cases of ECDS and three cases of PRS. Similarly, all ECDS cases demonstrated mononuclear cell infiltrates while the same was present in 6 cases of PRS [23]. Jablonska and Blaszczyk followed 71 cases of ECDS and PRS over a period of 20 years. They found that the clinical appearance of the two diseases changed progressively to the extent that the two often became indistinguishable [152]. These studies favor the concept that these two entities are closely related to each other and may lie on the same disease spectrum.

Duymaz *et al.* (2009) proposed some clinical guidelines to distinguish between the two diseases. The diagnosis of PRS was suggested if the patient presents with a unilateral facial atrophy involving the entire side of the face, usually deeper with absent or minimal preceding signs of inflammation or induration. The overlying skin is usually thin and soft, with normal hair and sclerosis is absent. Involvement of the underlying bone, skull, and other oro-dental structures like tongue, gingival, and palate is usually present. Morphea ECDS was considered if there is presence of a unilateral band-like sclerotic scar with hyperpigmentation on the frontoparietal area, restricted to the area above the eyebrow and without extension inferiorly, and most often preceded by induration of the skin. Cutaneous sclerosis in the form of hyperpigmented, hard, shiny, depressed and hairless skin is usually present. Progressive softening may occur in due course of time. However, they didn't study histopathologic findings [2].

It has been observed that in several cases, clinical findings of both the diseases are present in the same individual [31, 61, 71, 84, 153]. Co-existing morphea ECDS and PRS has been reported in some 28 to 42% of patients [31, 61, 153]. Christianson *et al.* performed a review of 235 patients with morphea, where facial hemi-atrophy was observed in 41.3% of the 29 morphea cases involving the facial, frontal and fronto-parietal areas [154]. Rogers carried out a review of 772 cases of PRS and mentioned that morphea ECDS as a potential initial presentation in some cases [25]. Blaszczyk and Jablonska evaluated 58 cases of ECDS. Features of PRS developed in 20 cases [150]. In addition, conversion of ECDS into PRS at the same physical location has been described in few cases [150, 152].

Tollefson and Witman studied a retrospective review of 54 patients of morphea ECDS and PRS. They concluded that their findings support the view that these two entities fall on the same spectrum of disease. Of the 28 patients having PRS, 71.4% had facial sclerosis, and 53.6% had lesions of ECDS. Conversely, of the 41 patients having morphea ECDS, they found that 36.6% also had PRS. Surprisingly, on histopathological examination, those PRS patients who did not have cutaneous sclerosis on clinical presentation, showed findings consistent with morphea [61]. Similar results have been reported by other studies [31, 148]. In conclusion, though ECDS and PRS may be distinguished by some clinical features; however, clinical and histopathological characteristics of the two often overlap in the same patient. Thus, it seems plausible to state that ECDS and PRS fall on the same spectrum of disease.

Proposed classification for linear morphea ECDS-PRS disease spectrum: Based on the ongoing discussion, the author believes that ECDS and PRS lie on the same spectrum of disease. Where there can be pure clinical forms of ECDS and PRS on one side, on the other, there can be variable overlap between the two or the two may coexist together or ECDS may transform into PRS in due course of time. With such a notion, the author has proposed a classification system for the ECDS-PRS disease spectrum (Table **17.4**).

Table 17.4. Proposed classification of linear morphea ECDS-PRS disease spectrum.

Type of Disease	Terminology	Description
Type-1	ECDS only	Linear morphea, unilateral or bilateral, restricted to the forehead but may extend superiorly to fronto-parietal scalp or more. Skin is hyper/hypo-pigmented, indurated associated with paramedian forehead scar. Cutaneous sclerosis and scarring alopecia present. Neurological, ocular, maxillofacial and oro-dental complications may or may not be present. Histopathological findings consistent with cutaneous sclerosis.
Type-2	ECDS with downward extension	Type-1 disease with downward extension to orbit/ nose/maxilla/lips/oral cavity/chin/neck or lower.
Type-3	ECDS-PRS overlap	When features of both ECDS and PRS are present simultaneously in the same patient and at the same site. It can be of two types: Type-3a: ECDS-PRS overlap ECDS predominant: when the features of ECDS predominate over PRS Type-3b: ECDS-PRS overlap PRS predominant: when the features of PRS predominate over ECDS.
Type-4	PRS only	De-novo hemifacial atrophy (or rarely bilateral) of the skin inferior to the forehead and involving dermatomes of one or more branches of the trigeminal nerve. The atrophy involves subcutaneous tissue, fat, muscle, and osteocartilaginous structures. Preceding signs of skin inflammation, induration, and cutaneous sclerosis are characteristically absent or minimal. Neurological, ocular, maxillofacial and oro-dental complications are usually present.

(Table 17.4) cont.....

Type of Disease	Terminology	Description
Type-5	Coexistent ECDS and PRS	When both ECDS and PRS are present in the same patient at two different sites whether simultaneously or not. *e.g.*, on one side, there is PRS and on the other side, there is ECDS; however, the two are present in their pure clinical forms without overlap features. Also, a patient who has ECDS on one side and after several years, develops PRS on the other side (and vice versa) but the original ECDS maintained its form.
Type-6	PRS with trunk and/or extremity involvement	Type-4 disease with trunk and/or extremity involvement.
Type-7	ECDS converting to PRS	These are the cases who start clinically and histopathologically as ECDS. After a variable time of follow up, severity of disease increases as well as complications while the skin becomes atrophic, losing induration and becoming soft and disease acquires features consistent with diagnosis of PRS.

ECDS: En coup de sabre; **PRS:** Parry-Romberg syndrome.

This classification will help in classifying the disease spectrum, identifying diseases with overlap or coexistence or conversion. It can be beneficial for epidemiological research purpose. It can also help in deciding a specific treatment protocol for the different classes of the disease spectrum.

Box 17.6. Learning points.
• PRS is mostly restricted to one half of the face, however it can involve trunk and limbs.
• Other dermatological conditions like segmental vitiligo, lupus profundus, morphea, band-like alopecia, hyperpigmentation, linear morphea en coup de sabre, port-wine stain and Klippel-Trenaunay syndrome may be associated with it.
• A specific finding which can help in differentiating PRS from ECDS is the presence of degenerative changes of vascular endothelia on histopathology.
• Skin ultrasound can help in measuring the dermal thickness and echogenicity of the affected areas. This can help in detecting cutaneous sclerosis, monitoring of disease activity as well as assessing the treatment progress.
• A direct correlation between cutaneous changes, clinical neurologic findings and MRI abnormalities is not always present in PRS. Hence, imaging should be advised in such patients, whether in the initial work up or in follow-up visits.
• ECDS and PRS share several disease characteristics. Both have relatively a similar age of onset, predominantly affecting females, have comparable neurological and ocular complications, response to immunosuppressive drugs seen in both and clinically lesions progresses slowly over time until stabilization attained after several years.
• ECDS and PRS seem to lie on the same disease spectrum. Though there can be pure clinical forms of ECDS and PRS, there can be a variable overlap between the two or the two may coexist or ECDS may transform into PRS in due course of time.

REFERENCES

[1]   Longo D, Paonessa A, Specchio N, *et al.* Parry-Romberg syndrome and Rasmussen encephalitis: Possible association; clinical and neuroimaging features. J Neuroimaging 2009; 20: 1-6.
        [PMID: 19555404]

[2]   Duymaz A, Karabekmez FE, Keskin M, Tosun Z. Parry-Romberg Syndrome. Ann Plast Surg 2009; 63(4): 457-61.
        [http://dx.doi.org/10.1097/SAP.0b013e31818bed6d] [PMID: 19745718]

[3]   Parry CH. Collections from the unpublished medical writings of the late Caleb Hillier Parry. London: Underwoods 1825; pp. 478-80.

[4]   Romberg HM. Krankheiten des nervensystems (IV: Trophoneurosen) (in German). Klinische Ergebnisse. Berlin: Forrtner; 1846; 75-81.

[5]   Eulenberg A. Hemiatrophia facialis progressiva (in German). Lehrbuch der functionellen nervenkrankheiten auf physiologischer basis. Berlin: Verlag von August Hirschwald; 1871; 712-26.

[6]   Aynaci FM, Şen Y, Erdöl H, Ahmetoğlu A, Elmas R. Parry-Romberg syndrome associated with Adie's pupil and radiologic findings. Pediatr Neurol 2001; 25(5): 416-8.
        [http://dx.doi.org/10.1016/S0887-8994(01)00333-2] [PMID: 11744320]

[7]   Pichiecchio A, Uggetti C, Grazia Egitto M, Zappoli F. Parry-Romberg syndrome with migraine and intracranial aneurysm. Neurology 2002; 59(4): 606-8.
        [http://dx.doi.org/10.1212/WNL.59.4.606] [PMID: 12196658]

[8]   Shah JR, Juhász C, Kupsky WJ, *et al.* Rasmussen encephalitis associated with Parry–Romberg syndrome. Neurology 2003; 61(3): 395-7.
        [http://dx.doi.org/10.1212/WNL.61.3.395] [PMID: 12913207]

[9]   Stone J. Parry–Romberg syndrome. Neurology 2003; 61(5): 674-6.
        [http://dx.doi.org/10.1212/WNL.61.5.674] [PMID: 12963760]

[10]   Moko SB, Mistry Y, Blandin de Chalain TM. Parry–Romberg syndrome: Intracranial MRI appearances. J Craniomaxillofac Surg 2003; 31(5): 321-4.
        [http://dx.doi.org/10.1016/S1010-5182(03)00028-3] [PMID: 14563334]

[11]   Blitstein MK, Vecchione MJ, Tung GA. Parry-Romberg syndrome. Appl Radiol 2011; 40: 34-6.
        [http://dx.doi.org/10.37549/AR1797]

[12]   Sharma M, Bharatha A, Antonyshyn OM, Aviv RI, Symons SP. Case 178: Parry-Romberg Syndrome. Radiology 2012; 262(2): 721-5.
        [http://dx.doi.org/10.1148/radiol.11092104] [PMID: 22282187]

[13]   Jayanandan M, Adhavan UR, Gopalakrishnan S, Mahendra L, Madasamy R. Parry Romberg syndrome: A case report and discussion. J Oral Maxillofac Pathol 2012; 16(3): 406-10.
        [http://dx.doi.org/10.4103/0973-029X.102498] [PMID: 23248475]

[14]   El-Kehdy J, Abbas O, Rubeiz N. A review of Parry-Romberg syndrome. J Am Acad Dermatol 2012; 67(4): 769-84.
        [http://dx.doi.org/10.1016/j.jaad.2012.01.019] [PMID: 22405645]

[15]   Mendonca J, Viana SL, Freitas F, Lima G. Late-onset progressive facial hemiatrophy (Parry-Romberg syndrome). J Postgrad Med 2005; 51(2): 135-6.
        [PMID: 16006711]

[16]   Jurkiewicz MJ, Nahai F, Jurkiewicz MJ. The use of free revascularized grafts in the amelioration of hemifacial atrophy. Plast Reconstr Surg 1985; 76(1): 44-54.
        [http://dx.doi.org/10.1097/00006534-198507000-00007] [PMID: 4011779]

[17]   Pensler JM, Murphy GF, Mulliken JB. Clinical and ultrastructural studies of Romberg's hemifacial

atrophy. Plast Reconstr Surg 1990; 85(5): 669-74.
[http://dx.doi.org/10.1097/00006534-199005000-00001] [PMID: 2326349]

[18]   Anderson PJ, Molony D, Haan E, David DJ. Familial Parry–Romberg disease. Int J Pediatr Otorhinolaryngol 2005; 69(5): 705-8.
[http://dx.doi.org/10.1016/j.ijporl.2004.12.004] [PMID: 15850693]

[19]   Appenzeller O, Stevens JM, Kruszynski R, Walker S. Neurology in ancient faces. J Neurol Neurosurg Psychiatry 2001; 70(4): 524-9.
[http://dx.doi.org/10.1136/jnnp.70.4.524] [PMID: 11254781]

[20]   Charlier P, Froesch P, Tollefson M. Parry-Romberg syndrome on a major French revolution leader: Mirabeau, 1791. J Craniofac Surg 2017; 28(2): 582.
[http://dx.doi.org/10.1097/SCS.0000000000003091] [PMID: 27617816]

[21]   Tolkachjov SN, Patel NG, Tollefson MM. Progressive hemifacial atrophy: A review. Orphanet J Rare Dis 2015; 10(1): 39.
[http://dx.doi.org/10.1186/s13023-015-0250-9] [PMID: 25881068]

[22]   Nomura H, Egami S, Yokoyama T, Sugiura M. Case of rapid progression of hemiatrophy on the face: a new clinical entity? Case Rep Dermatol Med 2015; 2015: 1-2.
[http://dx.doi.org/10.1155/2015/478640] [PMID: 26380125]

[23]   Orozco-Covarrubias L, Guzmán-Meza A, Ridaura-Sanz C, Carrasco Daza D, Sosa-De-Martinez C, Ruiz-Maldonado R. Scleroderma 'en coup de sabre' and progressive facial hemiatrophy. Is it possible to differentiate them? J Eur Acad Dermatol Venereol 2002; 16(4): 361-6.
[http://dx.doi.org/10.1046/j.1468-3083.2002.00442.x] [PMID: 12224693]

[24]   Chiu YE, Vora S, Kwon EKM, Maheshwari M. A significant proportion of children with morphea en coup de sabre and Parry-Romberg syndrome have neuroimaging findings. Pediatr Dermatol 2012; 29(6): 738-48.
[http://dx.doi.org/10.1111/pde.12001] [PMID: 23106674]

[25]   Rogers BO. Progressive facial hemiatrophy: Romberg's disease: A review of 772 cases. Third International Congress Plastic Surgery. 681.

[26]   Poniecki A, Bernacka K, Hryszko S. Romberg-type hemiatrophy in a case of severe rheumatoid arthritis. Wiad Lek 1971; 24(13): 1313-5.
[PMID: 5094453]

[27]   Kleiner-Baumgarten A, Sukenik S, Horowitz J. Linear scleroderma, hemiatrophy and systemic lupus erythematosus. J Rheumatol 1989; 16(8): 1141-3.
[PMID: 2585414]

[28]   Kayanuma K, Oguchi K. A case of progressive hemifacial atrophy associated with immunological abnormalities. Rinsho Shinkeigaku 1994; 34(10): 1058-60.
[PMID: 7834954]

[29]   Garcia-de la Torre I, Castello-Sendra J, Esgleyes-Ribot T, Martinez-Bonilla G, Guerrerosantos J, Fritzler MJ. Autoantibodies in Parry-Romberg syndrome: A serologic study of 14 patients. J Rheumatol 1995; 22(1): 73-7.
[PMID: 7699686]

[30]   Gonul M, Dogan B, Izci Y, Varol G. Parry-Romberg syndrome in association with anti-dsDNA antibodies: A case report. J Eur Acad Dermatol Venereol 2005; 19(6): 740-2.
[http://dx.doi.org/10.1111/j.1468-3083.2005.01290.x] [PMID: 16268883]

[31]   Sommer A, Gambichler T, Bacharach-Buhles M, von Rothenburg T, Altmeyer P, Kreuter A. Clinical and serological characteristics of progressive facial hemiatrophy: A case series of 12 patients. J Am Acad Dermatol 2006; 54(2): 227-33.
[http://dx.doi.org/10.1016/j.jaad.2005.10.020] [PMID: 16443052]

[32]   Asher SW, Berg BO. Progressive hemifacial atrophy: report of three cases, including one observed

over 43 years, and computed tomographic findings. Arch Neurol 1982; 39(1): 44-6.
[http://dx.doi.org/10.1001/archneur.1982.00510130046011] [PMID: 7055447]

[33] Delaire J, Lumineau JP, Mercier J, Plenier V. Romberg's syndrome. Progressive facial hemiatrophy. Rev Stomatol Chir Maxillofac 1983; 84(6): 313-21.
[PMID: 6367008]

[34] Claudy AL, Segault D, Rousset H, Moulin G. Facial hemiatrophy, homolateral cervical linear scleroderma and thyroid disease. Ann Dermatol Venereol 1992; 119(8): 543-5.
[PMID: 1485755]

[35] Archambault LS, Fromm NK. Progressive facial hemiatrophy; report of three cases. Arch Neurol Psychiatry 1932; 27(3): 529-84.
[http://dx.doi.org/10.1001/archneurpsyc.1932.02230150045004]

[36] Ruhin B, Bennaceur S, Verecke F, Louafi S, Seddiki B, Ferri J. Progressive hemifacial atrophy in the young patient: Physiopathologic hypotheses, diagnosis and therapy. Rev Stomatol Chir Maxillofac 2000; 101(6): 287-97.
[PMID: 11242767]

[37] Sartori-Valinotti JC, Tollefson MM, Reed AM. Updates on morphea: Role of vascular injury and advances in treatment. Autoimmune Dis 2013; 2013: 1-8.
[http://dx.doi.org/10.1155/2013/467808] [PMID: 24319593]

[38] Miedziak AI, Stefanyszyn M, Flanagan J, Eagle RC Jr. Parry-Romberg syndrome associated with intracranial vascular malformations. Arch Ophthalmol 1998; 116(9): 1235-7.
[http://dx.doi.org/10.1001/archopht.116.9.1235] [PMID: 9747688]

[39] Bosman T, Van Beijnum J, Van Walderveen MAA, Brouwer PA. Giant intracranial aneurysm in a ten-year-old boy with parry romberg syndrome. A case report and literature review. Interv Neuroradiol 2009; 15(2): 165-73.
[http://dx.doi.org/10.1177/159101990901500205] [PMID: 20465894]

[40] Wolf SM, Verity MA. Neurological complications of progressive facial hemiatrophy. J Neurol Neurosurg Psychiatry 1974; 37(9): 997-1004.
[http://dx.doi.org/10.1136/jnnp.37.9.997]

[41] Abele DC, Bedingfield RB, Chandler FW, Given KS. Progressive facial hemiatrophy (Parry-Romberg syndrome) and borreliosis. J Am Acad Dermatol 1990; 22(3): 531-3.
[http://dx.doi.org/10.1016/S0190-9622(08)80402-1] [PMID: 2107220]

[42] Stern HS, Elliott LF, Beegle PH Jr. Progressive hemifacial atrophy associated with Lyme disease. Plast Reconstr Surg 1992; 90(3): 479-83.
[http://dx.doi.org/10.1097/00006534-199209000-00020] [PMID: 1513894]

[43] Baskan EB, Kaçar SD, Turan A, Saricaoglu H, Tunali S, Adim SB. Parry–Romberg syndrome associated with borreliosis: Could photochemotherapy halt the progression of the disease? Photodermatol Photoimmunol Photomed 2006; 22(5): 259-61.
[http://dx.doi.org/10.1111/j.1600-0781.2006.00238.x] [PMID: 16948828]

[44] Sahin MT, Bariş S, Karaman A. Parry-Romberg syndrome: A possible association with borreliosis. J Eur Acad Dermatol Venereol 2004; 18(2): 204-7.
[http://dx.doi.org/10.1111/j.1468-3083.2004.00862.x] [PMID: 15009307]

[45] Goodlad JR, Davidson MM, Gordon P, Billington R, Ho-Yen DO. Morphoea and Borrelia burgdorferi: Results from the Scottish Highlands in the context of the world literature. Mol Pathol 2002; 55(6): 374-8.
[http://dx.doi.org/10.1136/mp.55.6.374] [PMID: 12456775]

[46] Gutiérrez-Gómez C, Godínez-Hana AL, García-Hernández M, *et al.* Lack of IgG antibody seropositivity to *Borrelia burgdorferi* in patients with Parry-Romberg syndrome and linear morphea *en coup de sabre* in Mexico. Int J Dermatol 2014; 53(8): 947-51.

[http://dx.doi.org/10.1111/ijd.12105] [PMID: 24527729]

[47] Daoud MS, Daniel Su WP, Leiferman KM, Perniciaro C. Bullous morphea: Clinical, pathologic, and immunopathologic evaluation of thirteen cases. J Am Acad Dermatol 1994; 30(6): 937-43.
[http://dx.doi.org/10.1016/S0190-9622(94)70113-X] [PMID: 8188883]

[48] Payne DA, Payne DA, Tyring SK, Sánchez RL. Borrelia burgdorferi DNA and Borrelia hermsii DNA are not associated with morphea or lichen sclerosus et atrophicus in the southwestern United States. Arch Dermatol 1997; 133(9): 1174.
[http://dx.doi.org/10.1001/archderm.1997.03890450126024] [PMID: 9301604]

[49] Fan W, Leonardi CL, Penneys NS. Absence of Borrelia burgdorferi in patients with localized scleroderma (morphea). J Am Acad Dermatol 1995; 33(4): 682-4.
[http://dx.doi.org/10.1016/0190-9622(95)91311-4] [PMID: 7673508]

[50] Dillon WI, Saed GM, Fivenson DP. Borrelia burgdorferi DNA is undetectable by polymerase chain reaction in skin lesions of morphea, scleroderma, or lichen sclerosus et atrophicus of patients from North America. J Am Acad Dermatol 1995; 33(4): 617-20.
[http://dx.doi.org/10.1016/0190-9622(95)91281-9] [PMID: 7673495]

[51] DeVito JR, Merogi AJ, Vo T, *et al.* Role of Borrelia burgdorferi in the pathogenesis of morphea/scleroderma and lichen sclerosus et atrophicus: A PCR study of thirty-five cases. J Cutan Pathol 1996; 23(4): 350-8.
[http://dx.doi.org/10.1111/j.1600-0560.1996.tb01309.x] [PMID: 8864923]

[52] Resende LA, Dal Pai V, Alves A. Experimental study of progressive facial hemiatrophy: effects of cervical sympathectomy in animals. Rev Neurol 1991; 147(8-9): 609-11.
[PMID: 1962072]

[53] Lonchampt P, Emile J, Pélier-Cady MC, Cadou B, Barthelaix A. Central sympathetic dysregulation and immunological abnormalities in a case of progressive facial hemiatrophy (Parry-Romberg disease). Clin Auton Res 1995; 5(4): 199-204.
[http://dx.doi.org/10.1007/BF01824007] [PMID: 8520214]

[54] Moss ML, Crikelair GF. Progressive facial hemiatrophy following cervical sympathectomy in the rat. Arch Oral Biol 1960; 1(3): 254-IN14.
[http://dx.doi.org/10.1016/0003-9969(60)90052-2] [PMID: 14424619]

[55] Wartenberg R. Progressive facial hemiatrophy. Arch Neurol Psychiatry 1945; 54(2): 75-96.
[http://dx.doi.org/10.1001/archneurpsyc.1945.02300080003001]

[56] Decourt J, Aubry M, Blanchard J. Hemiatrophie faciale lingual et velopalatine et maladie de Basedow associee. Rev Neurol 1941; 34: 135-40.

[57] Ignatowicz R, Michałowicz R, Kmieć T, Jóźwiak S. Familial form of Parry-Romberg syndrome. Pol Tyg Lek 1985; 40(2): 47-9.
[PMID: 3975172]

[58] Leão M, da Silva ML. Progressive hemifacial atrophy with agenesis of the head of the caudate nucleus. J Med Genet 1994; 31(12): 969-71.
[http://dx.doi.org/10.1136/jmg.31.12.969] [PMID: 7891383]

[59] Lewkonia RM, Lowry RB, Opitz JM. Progressive hemifacial atrophy (Parry-Romberg syndrome) report with review of genetics and nosology. Am J Med Genet 1983; 14(2): 385-90.
[http://dx.doi.org/10.1002/ajmg.1320140220] [PMID: 6601461]

[60] Mrabet Khiari H, Masmoudi S, Mrabet A. [Association of Parry-Romberg syndrome and paroxymal kinesigenic dyskinesia]. Rev Neurol 2009; 165(5): 489-92.
[http://dx.doi.org/10.1016/j.neurol.2008.08.003] [PMID: 18930510]

[61] Tollefson MM, Witman PM. En coup de sabre morphea and Parry-Romberg syndrome: A retrospective review of 54 patients. J Am Acad Dermatol 2007; 56(2): 257-63.
[http://dx.doi.org/10.1016/j.jaad.2006.10.959] [PMID: 17147965]

[62]   Thapa R, Ghosh A, Dhar S. Parry-Romberg syndrome with band-like alopecia. Indian J Pediatr 2009; 76(7): 760.
[http://dx.doi.org/10.1007/s12098-009-0167-1] [PMID: 19693456]

[63]   Creus L, Sanchez-Regaña M, Salleras M, Chaussade V, Umbert P. Parry-Romberg syndrome associated with homolateral segmental vitiligo. Ann Dermatol Venereol 1994; 121(10): 710-1.
[PMID: 7793760]

[64]   Moseley BD, Burrus TM, Mason TG, Shin C. Contralateral cutaneous and MRI findings in a patient with Parry-Romberg syndrome. J Neurol Neurosurg Psychiatry 2010; 81(12): 1400-1.
[http://dx.doi.org/10.1136/jnnp.2009.202044] [PMID: 20802222]

[65]   Grossberg E, Scherschun L, Fivenson DP. Lupus profundus: Not a benign disease. Lupus 2001; 10(7): 514-6.
[http://dx.doi.org/10.1191/096120301678416105] [PMID: 11480852]

[66]   Lane TK, Cheung J, Schaffer JV. Parry-Romberg syndrome with coexistent morphea. Dermatol Online J 2008; 14(10): 21.
[http://dx.doi.org/10.5070/D38DK1B0FW] [PMID: 19061620]

[67]   Rischebieth RH. Progressive facial hemiatrophy (Parry-Romberg syndrome). Proc Aust Assoc Neurol 1976; 13: 109-12.
[PMID: 1028996]

[68]   Al-Khenaizan S, Al-Watban L. Parry-Romberg syndrome. Overlap with linear morphea. Saudi Med J 2005; 26(2): 317-9.
[PMID: 15770315]

[69]   Klene C, Massicot P, Ferrière-Fontan I, Sarlangue J, Fontan D, Guillard JM. Saber-cut scleroderma and Parry-Romberg facial hemiatrophy. Nosologic problems. Neurologic complications. Ann Pediatr 1989; 36(2): 123-5.
[PMID: 2930126]

[70]   Wakhlu A, Agarwal V, Aggarwal A, Misra R. Parry Romberg syndrome: A close differential diagnosis of linear scleroderma en coup de sabre. J Assoc Physicians India 2003; 51: 980.
[PMID: 14719588]

[71]   Lehman TJ. The Parry Romberg syndrome of progressive facial hemiatrophy and linear scleroderma en coup de sabre. Mistaken diagnosis or overlapping conditions? J Rheumatol 1992; 19(6): 844-5.
[PMID: 1404118]

[72]   Auvinet C, Glacet-Bernard A, Coscas G, Cornelis P, Cadot M, Meyringnac C. Parry-Romberg progressive facial hemiatrophy and localized scleroderma. Nosologic and pathogenic problems. J Fr Ophtalmol 1989; 12(3): 169-73. [in French].
[PMID: 2695557]

[73]   Paprocka J, Jamroz E, Adamek D, Marszal E, Mandera M. Difficulties in differentiation of Parry–Romberg syndrome, unilateral facial sclerodermia, and Rasmussen syndrome. Childs Nerv Syst 2006; 22(4): 409-15.
[http://dx.doi.org/10.1007/s00381-005-1262-x] [PMID: 16247619]

[74]   Slimani S, Hounas F, Ladjouze-Rezig A. Multiple linear sclerodermas with a diffuse Parry–Romberg syndrome. Joint Bone Spine 2009; 76(1): 114-6.
[http://dx.doi.org/10.1016/j.jbspin.2008.07.009] [PMID: 18993106]

[75]   Maletic J, Tsirka V, Ioannides P, Karacostas D, Taskos N. Parry-Romberg syndrome associated with localized scleroderma. Case Rep Neurol 2010; 2(2): 57-62.
[http://dx.doi.org/10.1159/000314927] [PMID: 20671858]

[76]   Pinheiro TP, Silva CC, Silveira CS, Botelho PC, Pinheiro Md, Pinheiro JdeJ. Progressive Hemifacial Atrophy case report. Med Oral Patol Oral Cir Bucal 2006; 11(2): E112-4.
[PMID: 16505785]

[77]   Gambichler T, Kreuter A, Hoffmann K, Bechara FG, Altmeyer P, Jansen T. Bilateral linear scleroderma "en coup de sabre" associated with facial atrophy and neurological complications. BMC Dermatol 2001; 1(1): 9.
[http://dx.doi.org/10.1186/1471-5945-1-9] [PMID: 11741509]

[78]   Yano T, Sawaishi Y, Toyono M, Takaku I, Takada G. Progressive facial hemiatrophy after epileptic seizures. Pediatr Neurol 2000; 23(2): 164-6.
[http://dx.doi.org/10.1016/S0887-8994(00)00168-5] [PMID: 11020643]

[79]   Sathornsumetee S, Schanberg L, Rabinovich E, Lewis D Jr, Weisleder P. Parry-Romberg syndrome with fatal brain stem involvement. J Pediatr 2005; 146(3): 429-31.
[http://dx.doi.org/10.1016/j.jpeds.2004.10.026] [PMID: 15756237]

[80]   Viana M, Glastonbury CM, Sprenger T, Goadsby PJ. Trigeminal neuropathic pain in a patient with progressive facial hemiatrophy (parry-romberg syndrome). Arch Neurol 2011; 68(7): 938-43.
[http://dx.doi.org/10.1001/archneurol.2011.126] [PMID: 21747035]

[81]   Dalla Costa G, Colombo B, Dalla Libera D, Martinelli V, Comi G. Parry Romberg Syndrome associated with chronic facial pain. J Clin Neurosci 2013; 20(9): 1320-2.
[http://dx.doi.org/10.1016/j.jocn.2012.08.020] [PMID: 23528409]

[82]   Cory RC, Clayman DA, Faillace WJ, McKee SW, Gama CH. Clinical and radiologic findings in progressive facial hemiatrophy (Parry-Romberg syndrome). AJNR Am J Neuroradiol 1997; 18(4): 751-7.
[PMID: 9127045]

[83]   Strenge H, Cordes P, Sticherling M, Brossmann J. Hemifacial atrophy: A neurocutaneous disorder with coup de sabre deformity, telangiectatic naevus, aneurysmatic malformation of the internal carotid artery and crossed hemiatrophy. J Neurol 1996; 243(9): 658-60.
[http://dx.doi.org/10.1007/BF00878663] [PMID: 8892068]

[84]   Menni S, Marzano AV, Passoni E. Neurologic abnormalities in two patients with facial hemiatrophy and sclerosis coexisting with morphea. Pediatr Dermatol 1997; 14(2): 113-6.
[http://dx.doi.org/10.1111/j.1525-1470.1997.tb00216.x] [PMID: 9144696]

[85]   Chbicheb M, Gelot A, Rivier F, *et al.* Parry-Romberg's syndrome and epilepsy. Rev Neurol 2005; 161(1): 92-7.
[http://dx.doi.org/10.1016/S0035-3787(05)84980-X] [PMID: 15678008]

[86]   Aoki T, Tashiro Y, Fujita K, Kajiwara M. Parry-Romberg syndrome with a giant internal carotid artery aneurysm. Surg Neurol 2006; 65(2): 170-3.
[http://dx.doi.org/10.1016/j.surneu.2005.05.006] [PMID: 16427416]

[87]   Catala M. Progressive intracranial aneurysmal disease in a child with progressive hemifacial atrophy (Parry-Romberg disease): Case report. Neurosurgery 1998; 42(5): 1195-6.
[http://dx.doi.org/10.1097/00006123-199805000-00161] [PMID: 9588570]

[88]   Miller MT, Sloane H, Goldberg MF, Grisolano J, Frenkel M, Mafee MF. Progressive hemifacial atrophy (Parry-Romberg disease). J Pediatr Ophthalmol Strabismus 1987; 24(1): 27-36.
[http://dx.doi.org/10.3928/0191-3913-19870101-07] [PMID: 3559850]

[89]   Dawczynski J, Thorwarth M, Koenigsdoerffer E, Schultze-Mosgau S. Interdisciplinary treatment and ophthalmological findings in Parry-Romberg syndrome. J Craniofac Surg 2006; 17(6): 1175-6.
[http://dx.doi.org/10.1097/01.scs.0000236440.20592.be] [PMID: 17119425]

[90]   Balan P, Gogineni SB, Shetty SR, D'souza D. Three-dimensional imaging of progressive facial hemiatrophy (Parry-Romberg syndrome) with unusual conjunctival findings. Imaging Sci Dent 2011; 41(4): 183-7.
[http://dx.doi.org/10.5624/isd.2011.41.4.183] [PMID: 22232729]

[91]   Khan AO. Restrictive strabismus in Parry-Romberg syndrome. J Pediatr Ophthalmol Strabismus 2007; 44(1): 51-2.

[http://dx.doi.org/10.3928/01913913-20070101-09] [PMID: 17274338]

[92]   Bellusci C, Liguori R, Pazzaglia A, Badiali L, Schiavi C, Campos EC. Bilateral Parry-Romberg syndrome associated with retinal vasculitis. Eur J Ophthalmol 2003; 13(9-10): 803-6.
[http://dx.doi.org/10.1177/1120672103013009-1014] [PMID: 14700105]

[93]   Cohen JS. Congenital nonprogressive facial hemiatrophy with ipsilateral eye abnormalities and juvenile glaucoma. Ann Ophthalmol 1979; 11(3): 413-6.
[PMID: 110207]

[94]   Yildirim Ö, Dinç E, Öz Ö. Parry-Romberg syndrome associated with anterior uveitis and retinal vasculitis. Can J Ophthalmol 2010; 45(3): 289-90.
[http://dx.doi.org/10.3129/i09-241] [PMID: 20379281]

[95]   Talacko AA, Reade PC. Hemifacial atrophy and temporomandibular joint pain-dysfunction syndrome. Int J Oral Maxillofac Surg 1988; 17(4): 224-6.
[http://dx.doi.org/10.1016/S0901-5027(88)80044-4] [PMID: 3139790]

[96]   Kaufman MD. Masticatory spasm in facial hemiatrophy. Ann Neurol 1980; 7(6): 585-7.
[http://dx.doi.org/10.1002/ana.410070614] [PMID: 7436363]

[97]   Fayad S, Steffensen B. Root resorptions in a patient with hemifacial atrophy. J Endod 1994; 20(6): 299-303.
[http://dx.doi.org/10.1016/S0099-2399(06)80821-6] [PMID: 7931029]

[98]   Tsuda N, Yamamoto K, Fukusako T, Morimatsu M. A case of unilateral lingual atrophy and ipsilateral muscular atrophy supplied by trigeminal nerve in relation to progressive facial hemiatrophy. Rinsho Shinkeigaku 1991; 31(9): 1007-9.
[PMID: 1769148]

[99]   Arif T, Majid I. Can lesions of 'en coup de sabre' progress after being quiescent for a decade? Iran J Dermatol 2015; 18: 77-9.

[100]   Arif T, Majid I, Ishtiyaq Haji ML. Late onset 'en coup de sabre' following trauma: Rare presentation of a rare disease. Nasza Dermatol Online 2015; 6(1): 49-51.
[http://dx.doi.org/10.7241/ourd.20151.12]

[101]   Arif T, Sami M. En coup de sabre' extending from scalp to neck: An extremely rare presentation. J Pak Assoc Dermatol 2018; 28(3): 381-3.

[102]   Bergler-Czop B, Lis-Swiety A. Brzezi_nska-Wcislo L. Scleroderma linearis: Hemiatrophia faciei progressiva (Parry-Romberg syndrome) without any changes in CNS and linear scleroderma "en coup de sabre" with CNS tumor. BMC Neurol 2009; 9: 39.
[http://dx.doi.org/10.1186/1471-2377-9-39] [PMID: 19635150]

[103]   Doolittle DA, Lehman VT, Schwartz KM, Wong-Kisiel LC, Lehman JS, Tollefson MM. CNS imaging findings associated with Parry–Romberg syndrome and en coup de sabre: correlation to dermatologic and neurologic abnormalities. Neuroradiology 2015; 57(1): 21-34.
[http://dx.doi.org/10.1007/s00234-014-1448-6] [PMID: 25304124]

[104]   DeFelipe J, Segura T, Arellano JI, et al. Neuropathological findings in a patient with epilepsy and the Parry-Romberg syndrome. Epilepsia 2001; 42(9): 1198-203.
[http://dx.doi.org/10.1046/j.1528-1157.2001.45800.x] [PMID: 11580770]

[105]   Okumura A, Ikuta T, Tsuji T, et al. Parry-Romberg syndrome with a clinically silent white matter lesion. AJNR Am J Neuroradiol 2006; 27(8): 1729-31.
[PMID: 16971623]

[106]   Blaszczyk M, Królicki L, Krasu M, Glinska O, Jablonska S. Progressive facial hemiatrophy: Central nervous system involvement and relationship with scleroderma en coup de sabre. J Rheumatol 2003; 30(9): 1997-2004.
[PMID: 12966605]

[107]   Raina UK, Seth A, Gupta R, Goel N, Gupta A, Ghosh B. Parry-Romberg syndrome studied by spectral-domain optical coherence tomography. Ophtha Surg Las Imag Ret 2014; 45: 1-4.
[http://dx.doi.org/10.3928/23258160-20140115-01]

[108]   You KH, Baik HS. Orthopedic and orthodontic treatment of Parry-Romberg syndrome. J Craniofac Surg 2011; 22(3): 970-3.
[http://dx.doi.org/10.1097/SCS.0b013e31820fe339] [PMID: 21558909]

[109]   Oosterkamp BC, Damstra J, Jansma J. Facial asymmetry: the benefits of cone beam computerized tomography. Ned Tijdschr Tandheelkd 2010; 117(5): 269-73.
[http://dx.doi.org/10.5177/ntvt2010.05.09150] [PMID: 20506903]

[110]   Carreño M, Donaire A, Barceló MI, *et al.* Parry Romberg syndrome and linear scleroderma in coup de sabre mimicking Rasmussen encephalitis. Neurology 2007; 68(16): 1308-10.
[http://dx.doi.org/10.1212/01.wnl.0000259523.09001.7a] [PMID: 17438222]

[111]   Simsek-Kiper PO, Roach E, Utine GE, Boduroglu K. Barraquer-Simons syndrome: A rare clinical entity. Am J Med Genet A 2014; 164(7): 1756-60.
[http://dx.doi.org/10.1002/ajmg.a.36491] [PMID: 24788242]

[112]   Payapvipapong K, Niumpradit N, Nakakes A, Buranawuti K. A rare case of acquired partial lipodystrophy *(Barraquer-Simons syndrome)* with localized scleroderma. Int J Dermatol 2014; 53(1): 82-4.
[http://dx.doi.org/10.1111/j.1365-4632.2011.05435.x] [PMID: 23675994]

[113]   Bergman JA. Primary hemifacial hypertrophy. Review and report of a case. Arch Otolaryngol Head Neck Surg 1973; 97(6): 490-4.
[http://dx.doi.org/10.1001/archotol.1973.00780010504015] [PMID: 4704449]

[114]   Gorlin RJ, Meskin LH. Congenital hemihypertrophy. J Pediatr 1962; 61(6): 870-9.
[http://dx.doi.org/10.1016/S0022-3476(62)80198-X] [PMID: 13949299]

[115]   Zulian F, Cuffaro G, Sperotto F. Scleroderma in children. Curr Opin Rheumatol 2013; 25(5): 643-50.
[http://dx.doi.org/10.1097/BOR.0b013e3283641f61] [PMID: 23912318]

[116]   Kreuter A, Gambichler T, Breuckmann F, *et al.* Pulsed high-dose corticosteroids combined with low-dose methotrexate in severe localized scleroderma. Arch Dermatol 2005; 141(7): 847-52.
[http://dx.doi.org/10.1001/archderm.141.7.847] [PMID: 16027298]

[117]   Zulian F, Vallongo C, Patrizi A, *et al.* A long-term follow-up study of methotrexate in juvenile localized scleroderma (morphea). J Am Acad Dermatol 2012; 67(6): 1151-6.
[http://dx.doi.org/10.1016/j.jaad.2012.03.036] [PMID: 22657157]

[118]   Goldberg-Stern H, deGrauw T, Passo M, Ball WS Jr. Parry-Romberg syndrome: Follow-up imaging during suppressive therapy. Neuroradiology 1997; 39(12): 873-6.
[http://dx.doi.org/10.1007/s002340050525] [PMID: 9457714]

[119]   Korkmaz C, Adapinar B, Uysal S. Beneficial effect of immunosuppressive drugs on Parry-Romberg syndrome: A case report and review of the literature. South Med J 2005; 98(9): 939-41.
[http://dx.doi.org/10.1097/01.smj.0000177355.43001.ff] [PMID: 16217992]

[120]   Hashkes PJ, Becker ML, Cabral DA, *et al.* Methotrexate: New uses for an old drug. J Pediatr 2014; 164(2): 231-6.
[http://dx.doi.org/10.1016/j.jpeds.2013.10.029] [PMID: 24286573]

[121]   Martini G, Ramanan AV, Falcini F, Girschick H, Goldsmith DP, Zulian F. Successful treatment of severe or methotrexate-resistant juvenile localized scleroderma with mycophenolate mofetil. Rheumatology 2009; 48(11): 1410-3.
[http://dx.doi.org/10.1093/rheumatology/kep244] [PMID: 19713439]

[122]   Bergler-Czop B, Lis-Swiety A, Brzezinska-Wcislo L. Scleroderma linearis: Hemiatrophia faciei progressiva (Parry-Romberg syndrom) without any changes in CNS and linear scleroderma "en coup

de sabre" with CNS tumor. BMC Neurol 2009; 9: 39.
[http://dx.doi.org/10.1186/1471-2377-9-39]

[123] Gambichler T, Kreuter A, Rotterdam S, Altmeyer P, Hoffmann K. Linear scleroderma 'en coup de sabre' treated with topical calcipotriol and cream psoralen plus ultraviolet A. J Eur Acad Dermatol Venereol 2003; 17(5): 601-2.
[http://dx.doi.org/10.1046/j.1468-3083.2003.00626.x] [PMID: 12941109]

[124] De Vasconcelos Carvalho M, Do Nascimento GJF, Andrade E, Andrade M, Sobral APV. Association of aesthetic and orthodontic treatment in Parry-Romberg syndrome. J Craniofac Surg 2010; 21(2): 436-9.
[http://dx.doi.org/10.1097/SCS.0b013e3181cfe917] [PMID: 20216455]

[125] Grippaudo C, Deli R, Grippaudo FR, Di Cuia T, Paradisi M. Management of craniofacial development in the Parry-Romberg syndrome: Report of two patients. Cleft Palate Craniofac J 2004; 41(1): 95-104.
[http://dx.doi.org/10.1597/02-066] [PMID: 14697063]

[126] Slack GC, Tabit CJ, Allam KA, Kawamoto HK, Bradley JP. Parry-Romberg Reconstruction. J Craniofac Surg 2012; 23(7) (1): S27-31.
[http://dx.doi.org/10.1097/SCS.0b013e318258bd11] [PMID: 23154357]

[127] Siebert JW, Longaker MT. Secondary craniofacial management following skeletal correction in facial asymmetry. Application of microsurgical techniques. Clin Plast Surg 1997; 24(3): 447-58.
[http://dx.doi.org/10.1016/S0094-1298(20)31038-5] [PMID: 9246512]

[128] Siebert JW, Anson G, Longaker MT. Microsurgical correction of facial asymmetry in 60 consecutive cases. Plast Reconstr Surg 1996; 97(2): 354-63.
[http://dx.doi.org/10.1097/00006534-199602000-00013] [PMID: 8559818]

[129] Roddi R, Riggio E, Gilbert PM, Hovius SER, Michiel Vaandrager J, van der Meulen JCH. Clinical evaluation of techniques used in the surgical treatment of progressive hemifacial atrophy. J Craniomaxillofac Surg 1994; 22(1): 23-32.
[http://dx.doi.org/10.1016/S1010-5182(05)80292-6] [PMID: 8175994]

[130] Palmero MLH, Uziel Y, Laxer RM, Forrest CR, Pope E. En coup de sabre scleroderma and Parry-Romberg syndrome in adolescents: Surgical options and patient-related outcomes. J Rheumatol 2010; 37(10): 2174-9.
[http://dx.doi.org/10.3899/jrheum.100062] [PMID: 20843909]

[131] Al-Aizari NA, Azzeghaiby SN, Al-Shamiri HM, Darwish S, Tarakji B. Oral manifestations of Parry-Romberg syndrome: A review of literature. Avicenna J Med 2015; 5(2): 25-8.
[http://dx.doi.org/10.4103/2231-0770.154193] [PMID: 25878963]

[132] Grimaldi M, Gentile P, Labardi L, Silvi E, Trimarco A, Cervelli V. Lipostructure technique in Romberg syndrome. J Craniofac Surg 2008; 19(4): 1089-91.
[http://dx.doi.org/10.1097/SCS.0b013e318176354a] [PMID: 18650738]

[133] Slack GC, Tabit CJ, Allam KA, Kawamoto HK, Bradley JP. Parry-romberg reconstruction. Ann Plast Surg 2014; 73(3): 307-10.
[http://dx.doi.org/10.1097/SAP.0b013e31827aeb0d] [PMID: 23676519]

[134] Hu J, Yin L, Tang X, Gui L, Zhang Z. Combined skeletal and soft tissue reconstruction for severe Parry-Romberg syndrome. J Craniofac Surg 2011; 22(3): 937-41.
[http://dx.doi.org/10.1097/SCS.0b013e31820fe27d] [PMID: 21558914]

[135] Yu-Feng L, Lai G, Zhi-Yong Z. Combined treatments of facial contour deformities resulting from Parry-Romberg syndrome. J Reconstr Microsurg 2008; 24(5): 333-42.
[http://dx.doi.org/10.1055/s-2008-1080536] [PMID: 18597216]

[136] Guerrerosantos J, Guerrerosantos F, Orozco J. Classification and treatment of facial tissue atrophy in Parry-Romberg disease. Aesthetic Plast Surg 2007; 31(5): 424-34.
[http://dx.doi.org/10.1007/s00266-006-0215-4] [PMID: 17700981]

[137] Arif T, Adil M, Amin SS, Sami M, Raj D. Concomitant en coup de sabre and plaque type morphea in the same patient: A rare occurrence. Przegl Dermatol 2017; 5: 570-4.
[http://dx.doi.org/10.5114/dr.2017.71222]

[138] Arif T, Adil M, Amin SS, *et al.* Clinico-epidemiological study of morphea from a tertiary care hospital. Curr Rheumatol Rev 2018; 14(3): 251-4.
[http://dx.doi.org/10.2174/1573397114666180410115553] [PMID: 29637865]

[139] Menascu S, Padeh S, Hoffman C, Ben-Zeev B. Parry-Romberg syndrome presenting as status migrainosus. Pediatr Neurol 2009; 40(4): 321-3.
[http://dx.doi.org/10.1016/j.pediatrneurol.2008.11.007] [PMID: 19302950]

[140] Arif T, Adil M, Suhail Amin S, Alam M. Morphea «En Coup De Sabre» at the site of healed herpes zoster ophthalmicus. Actas Dermosifiliogr 2019; 110(7): 617-9.
[http://dx.doi.org/10.1016/j.ad.2018.03.022] [PMID: 30201544]

[141] Kister I, Inglese M, Laxer RM, Herbert J. Neurologic manifestations of localized scleroderma: A case report and literature review. Neurology 2008; 71(19): 1538-45.
[http://dx.doi.org/10.1212/01.wnl.0000334474.88923.e3] [PMID: 18981376]

[142] Hickman JW, Sheils WS. Progressive facial hemiatrophy: Report of a case with marked homolateral involvement. Arch Intern Med 1964; 113(5): 716-20.
[http://dx.doi.org/10.1001/archinte.1964.00280110096019] [PMID: 14120599]

[143] Donley DE. Facial hemiatrophy associated with epilepsy: Report of a case. J Nerv Ment Dis 1935; 82(1): 33-9.
[http://dx.doi.org/10.1097/00005053-193507000-00004]

[144] Obermoser G, Pfausler BE, Linder DM, Sepp NT. Scleroderma en coup de sabre with central nervous system and ophthalmologic involvement: Treatment of ocular symptoms with interferon gamma. J Am Acad Dermatol 2003; 49(3): 543-6.
[http://dx.doi.org/10.1067/S0190-9622(03)00901-0] [PMID: 12963929]

[145] Marzano AV, Menni S, Parodi A, *et al.* Localized scleroderma in adults and children. Clinical and laboratory investigations on 239 cases. Eur J Dermatol 2003; 13(2): 171-6.
[PMID: 12695134]

[146] Fry JA, Alvarellos A, Fink CW, Blaw ME, Roach ES. Intracranial findings in progressive facial hemiatrophy. J Rheumatol 1992; 19(6): 956-8.
[PMID: 1404134]

[147] Arif T, Fatima R, Sami M. Parry-Romberg syndrome: A mini review. Acta Dermatovenerol Alp Panonica Adriat 2020; 29(4): 193-9.
[PMID: 33348939]

[148] Falanga V, Medsger TA Jr, Reichlin M, Rodnan GP. Linear Scleroderma. Ann Intern Med 1986; 104(6): 849-57.
[http://dx.doi.org/10.7326/0003-4819-104-6-849] [PMID: 3486617]

[149] Jablonska S, Blaszczyk M, Rosinka D. Progressive facial hemiatrophy and scleroderma en coup de sabre: Clinical presentation and course as related to the onset in early childhood and young adults. Arch Argent Dermatol 2007; 56: 257-63.

[150] Blaszczyk M, Jablonska S. Linear scleroderma en Coup de Sabre. Relationship with progressive facial hemiatrophy (PFH). Adv Exp Med Biol 1999; 455: 101-4.
[http://dx.doi.org/10.1007/978-1-4615-4857-7_14] [PMID: 10599329]

[151] Davis WC, Saunders TS. Scleroderma of the face involving the gingiva. Arch Derm Syphilol 1946; 54(2): 133-5.
[http://dx.doi.org/10.1001/archderm.1946.01510370017002] [PMID: 20995032]

[152] Jablonska S, Blaszczyk M. Long-lasting follow-up favours a close relationship between progressive

facial hemiatrophy and scleroderma en coup de sabre. J Eur Acad Dermatol Venereol 2005; 19(4): 403-4.
[http://dx.doi.org/10.1111/j.1468-3083.2005.00979.x] [PMID: 15987282]

[153] Jun JH, Kim HY, Jung HJ, *et al.* Parry-romberg syndrome with en coup de sabre. Ann Dermatol 2011; 23(3): 342-7.
[http://dx.doi.org/10.5021/ad.2011.23.3.342] [PMID: 21909205]

[154] Christianson HB, Dorsey CS, O'Leary PA, Kierland RR. Localized scleroderma. AMA Arch Derm 1956; 74(6): 629-39.
[http://dx.doi.org/10.1001/archderm.1956.01550120049012]

CHAPTER 18

Lichen Sclerosus

Muazzez Cigdem Oba[1], **Defne Ozkoca**[2] and **Tugba Kevser Uzuncakmak**[3,*]

[1] *Department of Dermatology and Venereology, Sancaktepe Sehit Prof. Dr. Ilhan Varank Research and Training Hospital, Istanbul, Turkey*

[2] *Department of Dermatology and Venereology, Cerrahpasa Medical Faculty, Istanbul University-Cerrahpasa, Istanbul, Turkey*

[3] *Memorial Health Group, Sisli Hospital, Istanbul, Turkey*

Chapter synopsis.
• Lichen sclerosus (LS) is a chronic mucocutaneous inflammatory disease, which involves genital and extragenital skin.
• The etiology of the disease is unknown but several factors including genetic factors, autoimmunity, hormonal factors, infections, and drugs have been suspected.
• The disease has a predilection for females, with the ratio ranging between 3:1 and 10:1. For extragenital involvement, male to female ratio is 1:1.
• Extragenital LS presents with polygonal porcelain-white papules and plaques accompanied by follicular delling and ecchymosis. The condition is most commonly located on the buttocks, thighs, breasts, submammary area, neck, back, chest, shoulders, axillae, and the flexural surface of the wrists.
• Histopathology reveals an atrophic epidermis with the basal vacuolar change, papillary dermal edema, homogenized collagen, and lymphocytic infiltrate beneath the edema.
• Diagnosis depends on clinical examination and is confirmed by histopathology.
• Treatment modalities include topical steroids, topical tacrolimus, phototherapy, antibiotics, and methotrexate among others.

Keywords: Atrophy, Autoimmunity, Corticosteroids, Chrysalis structures, Dermoscopy, Diagnosis, Differential diagnosis, Extragenital, Genital, Histopathology, Inflammation, Inflammoscopy, Lichen sclerosus, Lichenoid inflammation, Keratotic plugs, Malignancy, Methotrexate, Morphea, Phototherapy, Tacrolimus, Sclerosis.

---

* **Corresponding author Tugba Kevser Uzuncakmak:** Memorial Health Group, Sisli Hospital, Istanbul, Turkey; E-mail: tkevserustunbas@gmail.com

Tasleem Arif (Ed.)

INTRODUCTION

Lichen sclerosus (LS) is a chronic inflammatory mucocutaneous disease of genital and extragenital skin. Etiology is poorly understood, however, the role of genetics, autoimmunity and infections, among others, is postulated. The disease commonly involves the anogenital region, where it is usually a scarring condition with a chronic progressive course. Thus, it may cause significant functional (dyspareunia, dysuria) and cosmetic problems (changing the appearance of genitalia). There is a risk of malignant transformation in approximately 5% of genital LS cases [1]. Extragenital LS is thought to affect 15-20% of all patients with LS [2]. Cutaneous LS most commonly involves the upper trunk and does not have a premalignant potential. However, it may cause diagnostic difficulties by simulating various dermatologic conditions including morphea, and is more treatment-resistant [1]. While there are numerous studies about female and male genital LS, studies focusing on extragenital form of the disease are scarce. Thus, this chapter will primarily focus on extragenital LS along with a discussion on genital LS when necessary, in order to define similarities and contrasts between the two forms.

HISTORICAL BACKGROUND

In 1887, the description of a patient with lichenification and pruritus of the vulva along with coalescent papules on the trunk and forearms, by Hallopeau, is usually considered to be the first clinical description of LS [3]. However, in 1875, Weir's report of a case presenting with oral and vulvar "ichthyosis" was possibly the first LS patient described [4, 5]. From his first case until 1898, Hallopeau continued to describe three new cases of LS, which he considered to be an atrophic form of lichen planus due to oral mucosal involvement [6]. From late 1800s to early 1900s, various independent scientists presented the same disease, under different names [3, 4, 7 - 14]. The synonyms used in dermatologic literature to designate LS are listed in (Table **18.1**). Of note, as can be seen in the (Table **18.1**), Breisky's definition of "kraurosis vulvae" in gynecologic literature had preceded Hallopeau's definition in dermatologic literature [7]. Kraurosis vulvae was not linked to LS until 1920 [5]. Similarly, urologic literature referred LS as "balanitis xerotica obliterans" by Stühmer's definition, which was only linked to LS in 1941 [5, 14]. Darier published the classical histopathological features of LS in 1892 [8]. As atrophy is not always present in LS lesions, International Society for the Study of Vulvar Disease proposed the term "lichen sclerosus" in 1976, and since then, this nomination has widely gained acceptance [15].

Table 18.1. Various synonyms of lichen sclerosus.

Synonym	Author/Year/Reference
Oral and vulvar ichthyosis	Weir, 1875 [4]
Kraurosis vulvae	Breisky, 1885 [7]
Atrophic lichen planus ("lichen plan atrophique")	Hallopeau, 1887 [3]
Sclerotic lichen planus ("lichen plan sclereux")	Darier, 1892 [8]
Playing card scleroderma ("kartenblattförmige sklerodermie")	Unna, 1894 [9]
White spot disease	Westberg, 1901 [10]
Lichen albus	Von Zumbusch, 1906 [11]
Lichen planus sclerosus et atrophicus	Montgomery and Ormsby, 1907 [12]
Dermatitis lichenoides chronica atrophicans	Csillag, 1909 [13]
Balanitis xerotica Obliterans	Stühmer, 1928 [14]

EPIDEMIOLOGY

Lichen sclerosus may affect patients of all ages and both sexes. However, there is a bimodal distribution of the age of onset. Women are mostly affected in premenarchal and postmenopausal periods [1]. In men, the first peak occurs during childhood while the second peak affects adult men in the late fourth decade [1, 16]. The disease has a predilection for females, with the ratio ranging between 3:1 and 10:1 [17]. For extragenital involvement, this ratio was reported as 1:1, while for extragenital bullous disease, it is similar to that of genital LS [18, 19]. Although reported in various ethnic groups, the condition is seemingly more common in Caucasians [20]. The prevalence of the disorder is difficult to determine owing to the fact that the patients may apply to various specialties, that not all physicians are conversant with LS, and that patients may not present to physicians because of embarrassment or because the disease does not cause any symptoms [1]. An estimated prevalence is between 1:300 and 1:1000 [20]. Extragenital LS affects about 15-20% of all patients with LS [18]. Isolated extragenital LS constitutes only 6% of LS [1]. Extragenital lesions occur more frequently in women, affecting 11% and 13% of women in different series [21 - 23], whereas extragenital disease is rare or absent in men [16, 24].

ETIOPATHOGENESIS

Etiopathogenetic factors involved in the development of LS are summarized in (Box **18.1**).

Box 18.1. Etiopathogenetic factors involved in the development of LS.
• Genetic factors (Positive family history, HLA associations)
• Autoimmunity (See Box 18.2)
• Hormonal factors
• Trauma and chronic irritation
• Infections (HPV, Borrelia, EBV, HCV)
• Drugs

Genetic Factors

A genetic predisposition presumably contributes to the development of LS. An observational cohort study conducted in a UK vulvar diseases clinic including 1052 females (children and adults) with genital LS revealed a positive family history in 12% of the patients [25]. Although not statistically significant, patients with a family history of LS had more commonly associated autoimmune disease compared to patients with sporadic LS [25]. In a Scottish population based case-control study, 8.7% of women with genital LS had a relative affected by genital LS while there was no familial history of genital LS in the control group [26]. A very similar result of 8.6% positive family history of LS was reported in a Dutch cohort study involving 117 LS patients (114 females, 2 males, and one patient who was not willing to state gender) between 8 and 73 years [27].

Associations between several human leukocyte antigen (HLA) class II antigens and LS were reported, the most important being HLA DQ7. Studies have shown that HLA DQ7 occurred in 50% of women and 45% of men with LS [28, 29]. An even stronger association was reported between pediatric vulvar LS and the presence of HLA DQ7 in 66% of cases. The authors suggested a role of HLA DQ7 in the early onset of disease [30]. However, another study involving 187 women with LS and 354 healthy controls, did not establish any association between the time of onset of the disease and HLA DQ and DR antigens. The latter study demonstrated an increased frequency of DRB1*12 (DR12) which appears to be involved in the susceptibility to the disease, and a decreased frequency of DRB1*0301/04 (DR17) which appears to be involved in the protection from the disease [31]. Other HLA markers that have been reported in familial cases of LS include HLA B*08, B*18, B*15, B*57, CW*03, CW*07, CW*18, DRB1*04, DRB1*07, DRB4* [32, 33].

Autoimmunity

There is evidence to suggest that autoimmune mechanisms may play a role in the etiopathogenesis of LS, as listed in (Box **18.2**).

Box 18.2. Factors suggesting an autoimmune etiology for LS.
• Female preponderance
• Association with autoimmune disorders
• Family history of autoimmune diseases
• Presence of circulating auto-antibodies (organ specific and skin specific)
• Presence of autoreactive T cells
• Impaired immune tolerance
• HLA-subtype susceptibility

Similar to various autoimmune diseases, LS is more common in women [1]. In a study involving 350 women with histopathologically proven LS, 21.5% had at least one autoimmune disease, 21% had a positive family history of autoimmune diseases and 42% had circulating auto-antibodies [34]. In this cohort, the most common autoimmune comorbidities were thyroid disease, alopecia areata, vitiligo and pernicious anemia. In a study involving 26 LS patients and 443 controls, organ specific autoantibodies against thyroid and gastric parietal cells were demonstrated in 40% and 44% of LS patients, respectively, which was significantly more common than controls [35]. A strikingly high prevalence of thyroid disease reaching 30% was reported in 211 women with histopathologically confirmed LS [36]. Another study involving 202 vulvar LS patients found the presence of thyroid disease in 19% of cases [23]. In a large case-control study, autoimmune diseases were also shown to be significantly more prevalent in women with LS (28%), as compared with controls (9%) [37]. However, the latter study did not find a difference in the prevalence of circulating antibodies between patients and controls. A higher incidence of autoimmune diseases, in patients and their relatives, was also found in men with LS, in some studies [38, 39].

Humoral autoimmunity to several specific skin proteins was reported in LS patients. Whether these antibodies are pathogenic or represent an epiphenomenon is not known [40, 41]. IgG autoantibodies against extracellular matrix protein 1 (ECM1) were identified in 67% of the sera of women with LS [40]. Significantly higher serum levels of anti-ECM1 antibodies were also found in men with LS, compared to controls [41]. Several studies have shown the presence of antibodies against the basement membrane zone (BMZ) proteins in patients with LS.

Howard *et al.* reported BMZ antibodies in 30% of 90 adult female LS patients by serum indirect immunofluorescence. Immunoblotting was performed in seven patients and revealed antibodies to BP180 in six patients and BP230 in one patient [42]. However, despite these findings, authors reported a doubtful role for the BMZ antibodies in the pathogenesis of LS. In fact, the antibodies were of low-titer and direct immunofluorescence did not show in vivo deposition of autoantibodies [42]. Baldo *et al.* demonstrated circulating autoreactive T cells targeting the non-collagenous (NC)16A domain of BP180 as well as autoantibodies to BP180 [43]. Autoantibodies targeting BP180 were also detected in four of nine children with vulvar LS [44]. However, Gambichler and co-workers did not find a significant difference in the frequency of anti-BMZ antibodies, especially those targeting the disease-relevant NC16A domain, between 147 LS patients and 36 healthy controls [45].

Loss of immune tolerance is possibly another autoimmune mechanism triggering LS development. Terlou *et al.* observed a strong T helper1 (Th1) response and increased expression of microRNA (miR)-155 in LS lesions. As a key regulator of immune response, miR-155 has been shown to result in alterations in T-regulatory cell (Treg) phenotype and thus in the reduction of their suppressive functions [46]. Confirming the results of the latter study, a study comprising 31 biopsies from male and female genital LS patients, demonstrated a lesional increase of forkhead box protein (FOXP) 3-positive T-regs and low interleukin (IL)-10 expression. This pattern, lacking the expected positive correlation between Tregs and IL-10, is also thought to represent the reduced suppressive functions of Tregs in LS [47].

However, the pathogenetic role of autoimmune factors has been questioned in recent studies [16, 26, 48]. In their population based study, Higgins *et al.* reported no difference in the rate of concomitant autoimmune diseases between women with and without LS [26]. The association with autoimmune diseases is shown to be significantly more common (odds ratio: 4.3) in women as compared to men [49]. Authors hypothesized that pathogenetic mechanisms underling the development of LS may differ between men and women [49]. Edmonds *et al.* found that only 7% of 329 males with genital LS had associated autoimmune diseases, and Kantere *et al.* reported that the prevalence of autoimmune diseases and autoantibodies was not increased in 100 male patients with LS as compared to general population [16, 48]. Using whole genome microarrays, Edmonds *et al.* did not detect any autoimmunity-associated gene expression pattern in male genital LS [50].

Hormonal Factors

A hormonal pathogenesis was suggested in LS due to higher incidence observed in post-menopausal women [17]. In women with genital LS, significantly decreased circulating levels of dihydrotestosterone, free testosterone and androstenedione were reported [51]. Immunohistochemical studies have shown the loss of androgen receptors genital and extragenital LS lesions [52, 53]. A case-control study including 40 premenopausal patients with LS and 110 healthy control subjects demonstrated an odds ratio of 2.5 for the development of LS for patients using oral contraceptives with anti-androgenic activity [54]. In addition, estrogen receptor beta was highly expressed in LS, in contrast to its absence in normal tissues, while estrogen receptor alpha expression was shown to be decreased or absent [53, 55].

Trauma and Chronic Irritation

Mechanical trauma is a well-recognized trigger to the development of LS lesions, also known as isomorphic (Koebner) phenomenon [56]. Typical lesions of LS were reported to occur at the sites of injections [57 - 60], jellyfish sting [61], surgical scars [62, 63], thermal burn scar [64], skin graft scar [65], irradiated [66 - 69] and sunburnt areas of the skin [70], areas under pressure of tight clothings [56, 71] and peristomal sites [72, 73], striae distensae [74] and varicose veins [75]. In addition, cases of childhood LS associated with sexual abuse were reported [76]. Koebnerization of genital LS due to trauma might possibly explain this coexistence [76, 77]. In a case of vulvar LS, recurrence of LS was reported on pudendal thigh skin flap, which was performed for the treatment of vulvar squamous cell carcinoma [78]. Hypotheses that may explain the development of disease on transferred tissue include tissue inherent positional information as well as local factors such as urine, sweat, friction or microbiome. Koebnerization in LS is further discussed under subsection Dermoscopy.

Infections

The role of infections in the pathogenesis of LS is controversial. Infectious agents incriminated in triggering LS are discussed below.

Human Papilloma Virus Infection

Drut *et al.* detected koilocyte-like changes in the epidermis of prepuce samples in prepubertal boys with LS, and HPV was isolated in 70% of samples [79]. In addition, HPV reactivation was detected following application of topical immunosuppressive therapies such as potent steroids and tacrolimus [80, 81]. The therapeutic benefit of imiquimod in LS also suggests a potential causative role of HPV in genital LS [82]. In a recent review, the prevalence of HPV infection was reported to range between 0% and 80%, with a median prevalence of 8% and 29%, in women and men, respectively [83]. However, considering that HPV infection is very frequent in general population, these associations may be co-incidental and do not establish a pathogenetic role of HPV in LS [16, 83].

Borrelia Infection

Results of the studies regarding the etiological role of Borrelia infection are controversial. Studies from the U.S.A and U.K. have refuted any association [84 - 86]. Some studies from Europe suggest a possible link between Borrelia species and the development of LS [85, 87 - 89]. However, other studies from Europe have failed to demonstrate any significant association [90, 91].

Ebstein-Barr Virus Infection

Ebstein-Barr virus (EBV) is another viral agent implicated in the etiology of LS. In a preliminary study involving 34 women with genital LS and 17 controls, EBV was isolated in 26.5% and 0% of patients and controls, respectively [92]. Another study demonstrated a higher EBV infection rate in 47 male LS patients compared to 30 healthy men [93]. However, the role of EBV needs to be further investigated [93].

Hepatitis C Infection

Few case reports have suggested a possible relationship between hepatitis C (HCV) infection and LS [94, 95]. However, a study including 61 men with genital LS revealed that all patients were HCV seronegative [96].

Drugs

There are anecdotal reports of LS triggered by the use of drugs, such as carbamazepine and imatinib [97, 98]. An inverse association was found between use of beta-blockers and angiotensin-converting-enzyme (ACE) inhibitors and presence of vulvar LS [99]. The anti-inflammatory effects of ACE inhibitors may possibly underlie their protective role. Beta-blockers might prevent LS development by increasing keratinocyte proliferation and lymphocyte motility, and decreasing lymphocyte differentiation through blocking of cyclic AMP [99].

CLINICAL PRESENTATION

Although pruritus is occasionally present, the extragenital lesions of LS are most commonly asymptomatic [5]. The extent of the disease may vary from a single small lesion to widespread involvement [100]. The condition is most commonly located on the buttocks, thighs, breasts, submammary area, neck, back, chest, shoulders, axillae, and flexural surface of the wrists [1, 5, 101, 102]. Less common sites of involvement include the face [103, 104], scalp [105, 106], and palmoplantar region [107, 108]. Sites involved by extragenital LS are summarized in (Box **18.3**).

Box 18.3. Sites involved by extragenital LS.
• Buttocks
• Thighs
• Breasts
• Submammary area
• Neck
• Back
• Chest
• Shoulders
• Axillae
• Extremities
• Face
• Scalp
• Palmoplantar region
• Oral mucosa
• Nails

Classical clinical features of extragenital LS resemble those of genital LS with polygonal porcelain white papules and plaques accompanied by follicular delling and ecchymosis. Clinical photograph of a case of extragenital LS on the breast can be seen in Fig. (**18.1**).

Long-lasting cutaneous lesions become atrophic [109, 110]. Several atypical forms of extragenital LS exist, including bullous [111 - 114], Blaschkoid [115 - 117], and keratotic variants [101, 110]. Oral mucosal involvement is a rare feature of extragenital LS [109]. In a recent systematic review, demographic and clinical characteristics of 41 histologically proven oral LS cases were reported [118]. Mean age of the patients was 34 years and 66% of the patients were female.

Majority of the lesions consisted of asymptomatic white, homogenous plaques, which were most commonly located on labial and buccal mucosa and the lips. Other sites of involvement were the gingiva and the tongue. Of note, base of the mouth was spared in all patients. Malignant transformation of oral LS has not been reported. A more rare feature in extragenital LS is the nail involvement. Case reports of nail disease due to LS exist [119, 120]. Extragenital LS of the nails may lead to atrophic nails and irreversible loss of the nail plate [119, 120].

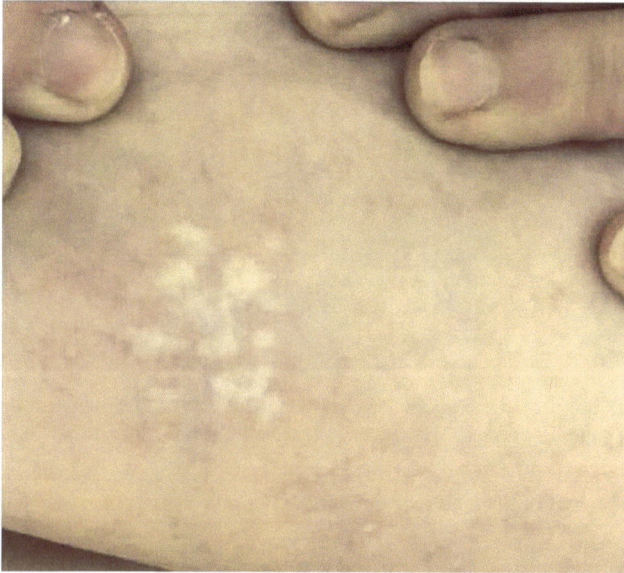

Fig. (18.1). White shiny grouped papules can be seen on the breast. [Image credit: Özkoca D, Üstünbaş Uzuncakmak TK, Kutlubay Z. PRP-induced lichen scleroatrophicus. Cerrahpasa Med J, accepted for publication].

HISTOPATHOLOGY

Histologically, LS is characterized by alterations both in the epidermis and the dermis. The histopathological findings vary according to the duration of the disease. In early lesions, atrophic epidermis with loss of rete ridges, lichenoid inflammatory pattern including band-like lymphocytic infiltrate in dermoepidermal junction, edema in papillary dermis and a compact orthokeratotic hyperkeratosis, vacuolar degeneration of the basal layer, hyalinization of subepithelial collagen, decreased elastic fibers in the upper dermis and dilated blood vessels under the basement membrane may be seen (Fig. **18.2**). The vacuolar interface dermatitis and dermal sclerosis have been mentioned as the minimum diagnostic criteria for LS. However, early lesions may lack dermal sclerosis. In older lesions, histology shows a reduced number of mononuclear cells and superficial sclerosing pattern with dispersed patchy islands of mononuclear cells within the hyalinized dermis [121]. List of histopathologic findings of extragenital LS can be found in (Box **18.4**). Recently, a case report of acrosyringeal variant of extragenital LS was published with typical features of LS confined to acrosyringium [122].

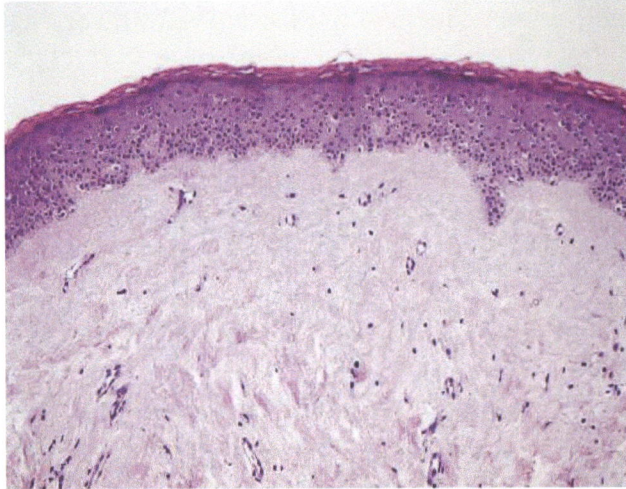

Fig. (18.2). Histopathology of lichen sclerosus showing epidermal atrophy, loss of rete ridges, dermal sclerosis and edema in papilary dermis. (Hematoxylin and eosin, original magnification x10).

Box 18.4. Histopathological findings of extragenital lichen sclerosus [123, 124].
• Atrophy of the epidermis
• Hyperkeratosis
• Follicular plugging
• Lichenoid inflammatory infiltrate (in very early lesions near basal layer, later in mid-dermis)
• Papillary dermal edema
• Vacuolar degeneration of the basal layer
• Hyalinization of subepithelial collagen
• Vascular dilatation
• Loss of elastic fibers in upper dermis

DIAGNOSIS

The diagnosis of LS is mainly based on patient history and clinical findings. The presence of the autoimmune diseases in the patient and family, examination of the mucosae, extragenital skin and completed by a gynecological/urological examination should be noted. A biopsy can be performed in cases who have atypical clinical presentation, non-healing ulceration and no response to recommended treatment choices. Imaging tests are not initially necessary if there is no urinary obstruction secondary to severe stenosing genital involvement.

Japanese guidelines have established diagnostic criteria for LS (Table **18.2**) [102]. Diagnosis of LS can be made if both clinical and histopathologic criteria are fulfilled and four diseases are excluded.

Table 18.2. Criteria for diagnosis of lichen sclerosus.

1. Clinical	Presence of white sclerotic plaques with well-circumscribed atrophy.
2. Histopathologic	Hyperkeratosis, epidermal atrophy, liquefactive degeneration, intradermal edema, lymphocytic infiltration and hyaline homogenization of collagen fibers
Exclude	Localized scleroderma, chronic eczema, vitiligo vulgaris, lichen planus.

Dermoscopy

Dermoscopy is helpful in the diagnosis and follow-up of LS. Larre Borges *et al.* studied the dermoscopic features of 29 histologically diagnosed LS lesions (14 genital, 15 extragenital) [123]. Later, Errichetti *et al.* analyzed dermoscopic features of 35 cutaneous LS and 51 morphea lesions [124]. Accordingly; patchy white-yellowish structureless areas are the most common finding in extragenital LS lesions reflecting the atrophy (Fig. **18.3**) [123, 124]. Keratotic plugs are the other important pattern, which are seen as round to oval, white to yellow circles similar to comedo-like openings, especially seen in extragenital LS (Fig. **18.4**). Keratotic plugs are only present in early extragenital LS lesions with duration of less than 1.5 years [123]. Chrysalis structures that are white intersecting lines, can be seen in polarized dermoscopy of extragenital LS. In contrast to keratotic plugs, they are more prevalent in lesions with duration longer than 1.5 years. Histologically, chrysalis structures correspond to increased amount of collagen bundles in fibrotic tissue. Erythematous areas, as a sign of inflammation, and hemorrhagic spots, as a sign of erythrocyte extravasation, can be observed in cutaneous LS (Fig. **18.5**) [124]. Surface scales, corresponding to hyperkeratosis, are also common dermoscopic findings in extragenital LS. Though much less common than in genital LS, linear and dotted vessels may also be seen in dermoscopic examination of extragenital LS [123]. List of dermoscopic findings of extragenital LS can be found in (Box **18.5**). Dermoscopy can also aid clinician in patient follow-up. Disappearance of white structureless areas in dermoscopy is a clue to therapeutic response [125].

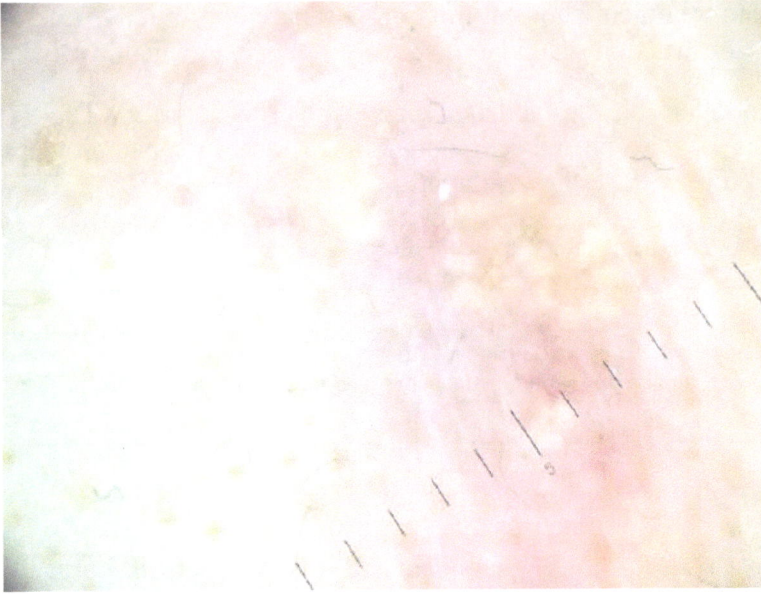

Fig. (18.3). Dermoscopy of extragenital LS revealing white- yellowish structureless areas, erythematous areas and linear vessels.

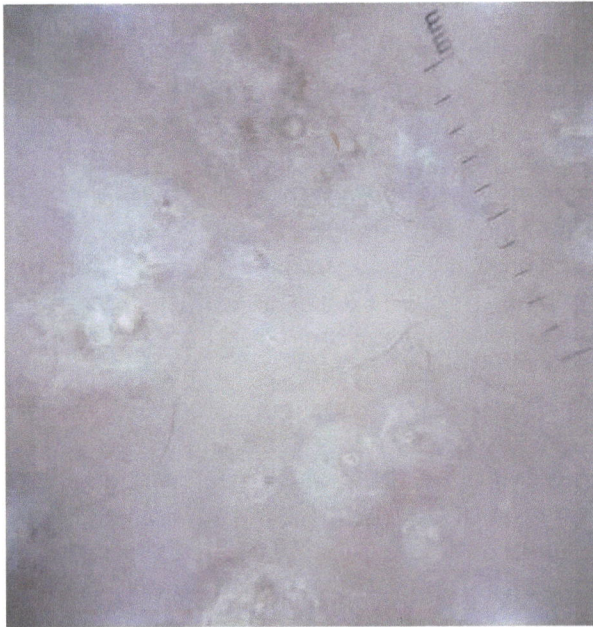

Fig. (18.4). Dermoscopy of extragenital LS revealing white structureless areas and keratotic plugs.

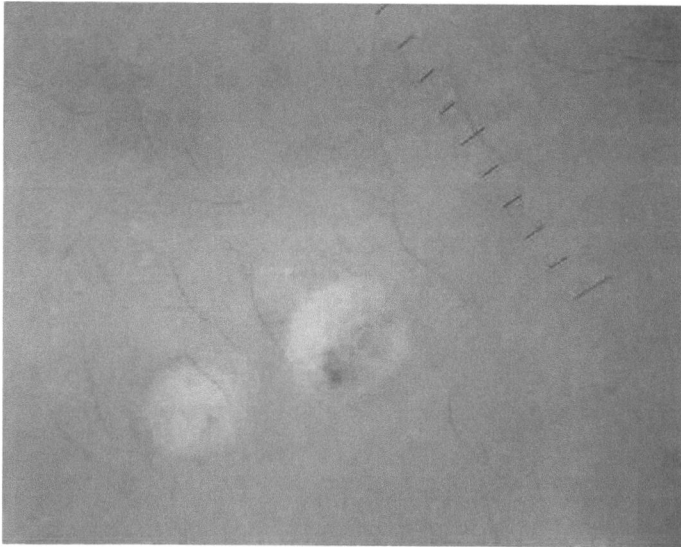

Fig. (18.5). Dermoscopy of extragenital LS revealing white structureless areas and hemorrhagic spots.

Box 18.5. Dermoscopic findings of extragenital lichen sclerosus [123, 124].
• White- yellowish structureless areas (most common finding)
• Erythematous areas
• Scales
• Keratotic plugs (in early lesions)
• Chrysalis structures (long-lasting lesions)
• Hemorrhagic spots
• Linear vessels
• Dotted vessels
• Gray dots
• Brown lines
• Erosion

Reflectance Confocal Microscopy

In vivo reflectance confocal microscopy can be used in the diagnosis of inflammatory skin diseases. However, data is scarce about extragenital LS consisting of a case report and a case series of 7 patients [126, 127]. At epidermal level, the most striking finding is round dark structures containing bright amorphous material, which correspond to follicular plugs [126, 127]. In some patients, tortuous horizontalized acrosyringium can be seen [127]. In addition atrophic epidermis and hyperkeratosis are observed [126]. In the upper dermis, scattered bright inflammatory cells and coarse collagen structures in bundles may be seen [126, 127].

KOEBNER'S PHENOMENON IN LICHEN SCLEROSUS

Koebnerization is a well-recognized feature of LS, especially common at extragenital sites [109]. According to the classification of Boyd and Neldner, LS is under category III, with lesions that occasionally localize to areas of trauma [128]. Main reports on Koebnerization at extragenital sites and their putative stimuli are summarized in Table **18.3**.

Table 18.3. Koebner response in extragenital lichen sclerosus.

Putative Stimulus for Koebner Response	Site/Trigger for Koebner Response
Radiation induced cytokine release, skin trauma due to irradiation.	Radiotherapy [66 - 69]
Skin trauma	Injection/vaccination site [57 - 60], jellyfish sting [61], thermal burn scar [64], severe sunburn [70], skin graft scar [65], striae distensae [74]
Mechanical trauma, occlusion, irritation.	Peristomal sites [72, 73]
Chronic pressure, friction.	Tight clothing [56, 71]
Lymphatic pressure due to impaired drainage	Old surgery scar [62, 63]
Venous pressure	Varicose veins [75]

In clinical practice, the occurrence of LS in Koebnerized sites may be a clue to detect the primary focus of the disease, which might have gone unnoticed [71]. Symptomatic relief can be obtained by avoidance of the stimuli that cause Koebner's phenomenon [56]. Moreover, Koebnerization should be kept in mind during the surgical treatment of genital LS. In patients undergoing circumcision, topical steroids should be continued if there is ongoing disease activity at the time of surgery, in order to prevent Koebnerization [109].

LICHEN SCLEROSUS AND MORPHEA: WHAT IS THE RELATIONSHIP?

Lichen sclerosus and morphea (localized scleroderma) are both connective tissue diseases that affect the skin [129]. They are chronic inflammatory skin diseases characterized clinically by sclerotic skin plaques and histopathologically by dermal inflammatory infiltrate and dermal fibrosis [130]. Although there are many similarities between the two conditions, their exact relationship is controversial

[130]. In the landmark article published by Peterson *et al.* in 1995, LS was classified as a subtype of plaque morphea as they considered LS a superficial variant of morphea [131]. However, their prognoses are different [132]. It is controversial to include LS under the entity of morphea, many authors consider them as two different entities [130, 133].

A significantly higher prevalence of genital LS was reported in patients with morphea [130, 134]. Coexistence of extragenital LS and morphea in the same patient at different sites has been reported [135 - 139]. Concomitant LS and morphea in monozygotic twins was reported [140]. Furthermore, LS and morphea can even be encountered in the same lesion [60, 141, 142]. These observations favor a common pathogenetic background of two diseases. Lutz *et al.* hypothesized LS to be the genital manifestation of morphea [130]. However, LS and morphea can be differentiated by several important aspects (Table **18.4**). According to current data, LS and morphea are different entities but they are both included in sclerodermoid skin conditions [143].

Table 18.4. Differences between morphea and lichen sclerosus.

Parameter	Lichen Sclerosus	Morphea
Epidemiology [17, 133]	Female:Male: 3:1-10:1	Female:Male: 2.4:1-4.2:1
Etiology [20, 133]	Autoimmunity	Vascular injury triggers increased fibroblastic activity
Clinical features [121]	Atrophic, polygonal white papules or thin plaques Affects genitals, upper trunk	Indurated plaques with peripheral violaceous hue, and ivory center. Affects trunk, extremities, and scalp.
Dermoscopy [124]	White-yellow structureless areas, keratotic plugs, hemorrhagic spots	White fibrotic beams.
Histopathology [121]	Atrophic epidermis, basal vacuolar change Loss of elastic fibers	Reticular dermal fibrosis. Preservation of elastic fibers.
Antibodies [121, 133]	Against extracellular matrix protein-1 (ECM-1)	Antinuclear antibody (ANA) Anti-single strand DNA (ssDNA) Antihistone antibodies (AHA).
Prognosis [20, 132]	Malignant transformation risk of about 5% in genital LS cases	Rare malignant transformation, only 16 cases reported since 1952.

DIFFERENTIAL DIAGNOSIS

In the differential diagnosis of LS, many diseases can be counted according to the age of the patient, the location of the lesions and the duration of the lesion (Box **18.6**).

Box 18.6. Differential diagnosis of lichen sclerosus.
• Lichen planus
• Lichen nitidus
• Vitiligo
• Idiopathic guttate hypomelanosis
• Morphea
• Scleroderma
• Immunobullous disorders
• Squamous cell carcinoma
• Contact dermatitis
• Mycosis fungoides
• Psoriasis
• Graft-versus-host disease
• Discoid lupus erythematosus
• Porokeratosis
• Sarcoidosis

Lichen Planus

Lichen planus shares several clinical and pathologic features with LS, such as clinical involvement of both skin and mucosa, erosions of mucosa and lymphocytic infiltration at dermoepidermal junction [144]. Clinically, symmetrical distribution of the lesions and post inflammatory hyperpigmentation favors diagnosis of lichen planus [145]. In addition, LS has distinguishing histopathological features including basal cell degeneration, civatte bodies and focal hypergranulosis [144]. Histopathology also helps in differentiation of keratotic variant of LS and hypertrophic lichen planus [101].

Lichen Nitidus

Lichen nitidus is considered in the differential diagnosis of extragenital LS, especially when the latter presents clinically with small, pinhead sized lesions [122]. Shiny papules of lichen nitidus typically involve genitalia, upper extremities and trunk, are usually asymptomatic and may show Koebner's phenomenon. Despite these clinical similarities, histopathology of lichen nitidus shows well-circumscribed, granulomatous, lymphohistiocytic infiltrates, which are embraced by elongated rete ridges [146].

Vitiligo

Vitiligo can simulate both genital and extragenital lichen sclerosus lesions with milky-white lesions [147]. The term "vitiligoid lichen sclerosus" defines lesions with clinical appearance of vitiligo, which were correctly diagnosed only after histopathological examination. Clinically vitiligoid LS cases were reported as isolated oral, isolated genital and orogenital involvements, which are also common locations for vitiligo vulgaris. Wood's lamp examination may help in the differential diagnosis of LS with vitiligo as the latter shows white accentuation [122]. Dermal sclerosis and lichenoid or vacuolar interface dermatitis points to the definite diagnosis of LS [147, 148]. It should also be kept in mind that vitiligo can also occur concomitantly with extragenital LS [149, 150].

Idiopathic guttate hypomelanosis

Idiopathic guttate hypomelanosis (IGH) is characterized by asymptomatic, well-circumscribed, polygonal, white macules. They may clinically resemble extragenital LS. However, IGH mostly involves extensor surface of the forearms and anterior aspect of legs in a symmetrical fashion [151]. In addition, Wood's lamp examination of IGH lesions demonstrate white accentuation [122, 151]. Dermoscopically, IGH shows porcelain-white macules and cloudy-sky pattern, which is defined as hyperpigmented networks within or surrounding the lesions [152].

Morphea

Morphea can have close resemblance to extragenital LS. Dermoscopy, confocal microscopy and histopathology help in their differential diagnosis [126]. In a study comparing dermoscopic features of morphea and cutaneous LS, white fibrotic beams were 100% specific for morphea, while white-yellow structureless areas, keratotic plugs and hemorrhagic spots were 100% specific for cutaneous LS [124]. Of note, white-yellowish structureless areas of LS are brighter and often have sharper margins due to fibrosis in superficial dermis. On the other hand, fibrotic beams of morphea are more opaque and have less defined margins as fibrosis affects the lower reticular dermis [124]. Definite distinction between morphea and LS can be made by histopathological findings. While LS is characterized by atrophic epidermis, basal vacuolar change and loss of elastic fibers, morphea shows reticular dermal fibrosis and preserved elastic fibers [121]. A rare case of linear LS involving the forehead and scalp, closely resembling linear morphea clinically, was correctly diagnosed by the typical histopathologic features [153]. Morphea as a differential diagnosis of LS, is also discussed under subsection Reflectance Confocal Microscopy and differences are outlined in (Table **18.4**).

Systemic Sclerosis

Systemic sclerosis can mimic clinical and pathologic findings of LS and two diseases may occur concomitantly [154, 155]. Differing from LS, cutaneous lesions of scleroderma has associated skin thickening [122]. Although cutaneous findings may be similar in two diseases, accompanying clinical features of systemic sclerosis such as Raynaud's phenomenon, acral sclerosis, lung disease and circulating autoantibodies make their clinical differentiation [155].

Immunobullous disorders

Immunobullous disorders including mucous membrane pemphigoid (MMP) should be taken into account in differential diagnosis of both genital and extragenital LS [1]. In genitalia, blistering, erosions and scarring caused by MMP may closely mimic LS [156]. Furthermore, extragenital bullous LS presents with flaccid bullae and erosions on the trunk and extremities, which are clinically indistinguishable from MMP [19, 157]. Direct immunofluorescence findings with linear C3 deposition along dermoepidermal junction and indirect immunofluorescence studies on salt-split skin are gold standard for correct diagnosis of MMP [156]. Apart from MMP, a differential diagnosis list for extragenital bullous LS is provided in (Table **18.5**) [157 - 164].

Table 18.5. Differential diagnosis of extragenital bullous LS.

Disease	Clues Differentiating from LS
Bullous pemphigoid [159]	Pruritus is common. Linear deposits of IgG and C3 along the dermoepidermal junction, by DIF.
Pemphigus vulgaris [159]	Flaccid bullae that break easily to leave erosions and bulla remnants . Histopathologically suprabasilar blister formation.
Senile purpura [160]	Occurs on sun exposed skin. Histopathologically, vascular ectasia with extravasated erythrocytes.
Bullous arthropod reaction [161]	Severe itching. History of insect bite.
Bullous morphea [138]	Histopathologically reticular dermal fibrosis, atrophy of skin appendages.

(Table 18.5) cont.....

Disease	Clues Differentiating from LS
Bullous lichen planus [162]	Bullae over typical lichen planus papules. Histologically basal cell degeneration, civatte bodies.
Bullous lupus erythematosus [163]	Clinical features of SLE. Linear or granular deposition of IgG and/or IgM and often IgA at the basement membrane zone by DIF.
Circumscribed lymphangioma [164]	Grouped vesicles Dermoscopically hypopion-like lacunes Histopathologically, lymphatic ducts with thin walls in the papillary dermis.

Squamous Cell Carcinoma

Squamous cell carcinoma (SCC) can develop as an ulcer and/or hyperkeratotic plaque upon anogenital LS lesions [165]. Extragenital LS lesions practically do not transform into malignancy. However, inflammatory, well-demarcated lesions of extragenital LS may clinically resemble Bowen's disease. Histopathologic examination is necessary for definitive diagnosis [166].

Contact Dermatitis

Contact dermatitis may mimic LS lesions. On the other hand, in a case report, Tammaro *et al.* postulated a possible association between nickel allergy and extragenital LS [167]. In suspected cases, history of contact with sensitizing agents should be taken and if necessary patch-testing should be done using appropriate standard series along with patch-testing of any product that come in contact with the lesions in order to rule out allergic contact dermatitis [63, 72].

Mycosis Fungoides

Mycosis fungoides (MF), may be a clinical and histopathological simulator of LS [168, 169]. Hypopigmented patches and plaques of MF showing atrophy might clinically mimic LS. Clinical examination for typical MF lesions elsewhere should be performed [168]. Furthermore, MF has distinctive dermoscopic features including fine short linear vessels, spermatozoa-like vessels and orange-yellowish patchy areas [170]. Histopathology of early LS may lack dermal sclerosis and may show lichenoid reaction along with basilar epidermotropism that may be confused with MF. Immunohistochemistry might be helpful as presence of CD4-positive and CD8-positive T cells favor diagnosis of MF and LS, respectively. However, there are CD8-positive MF cases, especially in hypopigmented variant. Repeat biopsy is crucial for diagnostic confirmation [169].

Psoriasis

Psoriasis may present with well-demarcated, scaly lesions that can be considered in differential diagnosis of both genital and extragenital LS [17, 166]. Blaschkoid extragenital LS can mimic other dermatoses that follow Blaschko lines such as linear psoriasis [117]. In studies with vulvar LS patients, it was shown that LS patients had an increased prevalence of psoriasis [23, 171]. Both diseases can occur at sites of trauma as they show Koebner's phenomenon. Questioning a positive family history for psoriasis can be helpful. Histopathological examination is needed to make the definite diagnosis [17].

Graft-versus-host Disease

Graft-versus-host disease (GVHD) is a common immunological reaction that results from hematopoietic stem cell transplantation, less frequently from solid organ transplantations and blood transfusions [172]. Clinical spectrum of chronic GVHD is classified as lichenoid and sclerodermoid. Chronic GVHD can present with LS like lesions that show atrophy, scaling and follicular plugging and is considered the most superficial variant of sclerodermoid GVHD. Lesions favor the neck and upper trunk. Clinically, history of stem cell transplantation and associated findings of chronic GVHD such as ulcers, xerosis, ichthyosis, poikiloderma etc. help in their differentiation. Histopathologically, both diseases share similar features [173].

Discoid Lupus Erythematosus

Discoid lupus erythematosus (DLE) needs to be differentiated from extragenital LS, as the latter may occasionally involve face and scalp [174]. Facial lesions of LS was termed as "annular atrophic plaques of the face" in several cases in literature, with inconsistent histopathologic findings some showing features of DLE, others LS [175]. On the scalp, atrophy, sclerosis and hyperkeratosis caused by LS mimics DLE [105, 106]. A negative direct immunofluorescence study rules out the diagnosis of DLE [106, 176].

Porokeratosis

Porokeratosis is considered among differential diagnoses of LS. The disease presents with asymptomatic plaques that have atrophy in the center, hyperkeratosis at the periphery. Sites of involvement include hands and feet, neck, shoulders and genitalia, which are similar to that of extragenital LS. The presence of cornoid lamella in histopathology of porokeratosis allows diagnostic confirmation [177].

Sarcoidosis

Sarcoidosis lesions may resemble extragenital LS. Micropapular or lichenoid perifollicular sarcoidosis may be indistinguishable from LS [178]. As other granulomatous diseases, dermoscopy of sarcoidal lesions display orange-yellow structureless areas along with focused linear branching vessels [179]. Typical histologic findings of sarcoidosis with epitheloid giant cells and macrophages forming non-caseating granulomas help confirm diagnosis [178].

Differential Diagnosis of Oral LS

Oral LS lesions need special consideration as they occur mostly as isolated lesions. Differential diagnosis of the most common white plaque-like lesions that may be confused with oral LS are listed in (Table **18.6**) [118, 180, 181].

Table 18.6. Oral lesions mimicking oral lichen sclerosus [118, 180, 181].

Disease	Clues Differentiating from LS
Oral lichen planus	Symmetrical involvement May include reticular areas More often symptomatic Histologically no dermal hyalinization
Leukoplakia	Older patients Smoking, alcohol consumption history Histologically hyperkeratosis, dysplasia
Frictional keratosis	Chronic cheek or lip biting, poor-fitting dentures Histologically hyperkeratosis and acanthosis
Chronic hyperplastic candidiasis (candidal leukoplakia)	Verrucous plaques Most commonly involves anterior buccal mucosa Smear shows pseudohyphae
Vitiligo	LS involving the lip major diagnostic challenge Histopathologically absent/decreased melanin Loss of melanocytes by immunohistochemistry
Oral submucosal fibrosis	Affects most parts of oral cavity Reduction of mouth opening
Tobacco pouch keratosis	Velvety texture Restricted to the area in contact with the snuff Histologically acanthosis, orthokeratosis, marked parakeratosis

(Table 18.6) cont.....

Disease	Clues Differentiating from LS
Morphea	Very rare Associated mostly with linear morphea Typically involves lip, gingiva, alveolar bone

TREATMENT

Options for the treatment of extragenital LS and their levels of evidence/grades of recommendation are listed in (Table **18.7**) [17, 182].

Table 18.7. Evidence based treatment of extragenital LS [17, 182].

Treatment	Level of Evidence/Grade of Recommendation
Topical ultrapotent steroids	Level of evidence 3/grade of recommendation D
Topical tacrolimus 0.1% ointment	Level of evidence 3/grade of recommendation D
Topical calcipotriol	Level of evidence 3/grade of recommendation D
UVA1 phototherapy for ten weeks	Level of evidence 1 +/grade of recommendation B
Systemic steroids/methotrexate	Level of evidence 3/grade of recommendation D
Sulphasalazine (salazopyrine) 1–2 g/day	Level of evidence 3/grade of recommendation D
Potassium para-aminobenzoate	Level of evidence 1 +/grade of recommendation B
Oral vitamin D	Level of evidence 3/grade of recommendation D

Topical Steroids

Potent topical steroids (*e.g.*, clobetasol propionate 0.05%) are the first line in the treatment of extragenital lichen sclerosus, though not as effective as in genital LS [183]. Despite their regular use for extragenital LS, there are no randomized controlled trials or case series about the use of topical corticosteroids in this indication [1].

The possible adverse effects of long-term potent corticosteroid use are atrophy, striae and telangiectasia formation, systemic absorption, rebound lesions upon treatment cessation, fungal infections, bacterial infections, herpes simplex virus or human papilloma virus activation [1].

Topical Calcineurin Inhibitors

Topical calcineurin inhibitors have both anti-inflammatory and immunomodulatory actions by inhibiting calcineurin phosphatase and reducing T-cell activation and cytokine production. The two topical calcineurin inhibitors that are widely used are tacrolimus and pimecrolimus. They are approved to be used in patients older than 2 years of age. Topical calcineurin inhibitors are commonly used in many dermatological disorders due to their steroid-sparing effects [184]. The most common side effects of topical calcineurin inhibitor use are burning sensation and itching, which may last for 14 days [185].

Although commonly used for genital LS, topical calcineurin inhibitors have less evidence as treatment options of extragenital LS [109]. In fact, in a comparative study involving 10 anogenital and six extragenital LS patients were treated with tacrolimus ointment twice daily. Only one patient with extragenital LS responded partially to tacrolimus, whereas nine of 10 patients with anogenital LS responded to therapy [186]. Combined treatment of tacrolimus and psoralen plus UVA (PUVA) therapy was used in case report to increase efficacy of tacrolimus ointment [187]. Lastly, in a case report, topical 1% pimecrolimus was unsuccessful in treating extragenital LS [188].

Topical Calcipotriol

There is one case report on successful treatment of extragenital LS with topical calcipotriol under occlusion, twice daily application for 12 weeks [189].

Phototherapy

Phototherapy is also a treatment alternative in treatment resistance LS cases, especially in extragenital localization [1]. Ultraviolet-A1 (UVA1) therapy has been used in the treatment of morphea and scleroderma successfully, which have pathophysiological similarities to LS. In a clinical trial, ten patients with extragenital LS were treated with low dose UVA1 phototherapy four times weekly with single UVA1 doses of 20 J/cm^2. Forty sessions were administered and low dose UVA1 therapy was shown to be an effective treatment option both clinically and regarding ultrasonic improvement of skin thickness [190]. As LS involves epidermis and superficial dermis, narrow-band UVB (NB-UVB) was also considered among treatment options of extragenital LS. To date, there are at least six cases of extragenital LS that were successfully treated with NB-UVB. Colbert *et al.* reported a case of extragenital LS that was successfully treated with narrow band ultraviolet-B, in only three sessions. Treatment was continued three sessions a week for three months [191]. Kreueter *et al.* reported successful treatment of several extragenital LS patients with NB-UVB. Authors recommended application of at least 30 sessions to obtain significant clinical effects. They also showed that immunohistochemical staining with matrix metalloproteinases was increased in an extragenital LS patient following phototherapy [192]. Uzuncakmak *et al.* reported complete resolution of folliculocentric hyperkeratotic LS in a 7-year-old child following 20 sessions of NB-UVB [110]. Likewise, Montegi *et al.* observed a significant improvement of widespread extragenital LS lesions after five weeks of NB-UVB given thrice weekly [193]. Herz-Ruelas *et al.* reported a case of acral bullous lichen sclerosus improved with narrow-band UVB, which did not tolerate UVA-1 treatment due to pain, in a total of 27 sessions of low dose narrow-band UVB treatment [194]. NB-UVB was also successfully used in the treatment of a case of blaschkoid LS along with topical steroids and calcineurin inhibitors [117]. As for PUVA therapy, there are two case reports showing complete remission of extragenital LS in a 66-yea--old woman and a 10 year-old-girl after total UVA doses of 61 J/cm^2 and 31.7 J/cm^2 [195, 196].

Methotrexate

Current guidelines recommend methotrexate among treatment options of extragenital LS [109, 182]. As methotrexate is a successful treatment option of morphea, it was also used for the treatment of extragenital LS in two case reports. Both patients had therapy-resistant disease, which was resolved by 10 and 15 mg weekly methotrexate [197, 198]. Low dose methotrexate combined with pulsed high dose corticosteroids was retrospectively evaluated for severe refractory extragenital LS in seven patients. Authors reported significant clinical benefit and no recurrence for at least three months [199]. A recent study involving 28 LS patients with 24 extragenital involvement, an initial response of 75% and sustained improvement of 50% were reported [200].

Sulphasalazine

Oral sulphasalazine (salazopyrine) was reported to be effective in a case of extragenital LS, with sustained remission for 10 years [201].

Antibiotics

Penicillin and cephalosporins can be tried in genital LS patients that are resistant to topical steroids [182]. Shelly *et al.* treated 15 LS patients with antibiotics, among them four patients with extragenital LS. Three patients had favorable improvement and one had great improvement. Authors recommended ceftriaxone 1 g intramuscular injections every two weeks for three times, followed by treatment on a need basis once a month. Alternatively penicillin G benzathine suspension 2.4 million units intramuscular injections every two weeks for three times, followed by treatment on a need basis once a month can be used. A case of extensive bullous LS was also successfully treated with ceftriaxone and systemic steroids [202]. A similar case with extensive bullous LS reported by Madan and Cox responded to doxycycline [203].

Potassium Para-aminobenzoate

Potassium para-aminobenzoate, in doses ranging from 4 g to 24 g daily, was reported to improve cutaneous LS in a case series of five patients [204]. However, a double blind placebo controlled trial failed to establish any difference between potassium para-aminobenzoate 12 mg daily and placebo [205].

Oral vitamin D

Considering beneficial effects of oral calcitriol in morphea, Ronger *et al.* administered oral calcitriol in a generalized cutaneous LS patient and they reported dramatic response [206].

Others

Cyclosporine

There is a case-series of 5 refractory vulvar LS patients successfully treated with oral cyclosporine [207]. However, there are no studies investigating the role of cyclosporine in extragenital LS.

Hydroxyurea (hydroxycarbamide)

Hydroxyurea 1 g daily was shown to be effective in the treatment of one case of vulvar LS [208]. However, there is no evidence for its use for extragenital disease.

Laser

Laser therapy can be considered in localized lesions of extragenital LS [209]. Pulsed dye laser completely resolved extragenital LS lesions after 4 sessions in an adolescent patient [210]. Combined pulsed dye laser and photodynamic therapy using 5-aminolevulinic acid were shown to be more effective in treating extragenital LS lesions than laser therapy alone, in two case reports [209, 211]. However, it should be kept in mind that combined therapy is more expensive and more painful [209]. A case report of extragenital LS describes successful result with ablative erbium:YAG laser [63].

Topical and Systemic Retinoids

Topical retinoids can be used as alternate therapy along with topical steroids for the treatment of extragenital LS [183, 196]. Oral acitretin was shown to be effective in the treatment of male and female genital LS in clinical trials [212, 213]. For extragenital LS, there are several case reports [113, 214, 215].

Hydroxychloroquine

Oral hydroxychloroquine 200 mg daily was shown to halt extragenital bullous disease progression in a case report. However, a spontaneous remission cannot be ruled out due to short history [216]. García-Doval *et al.* reported a bullous LS case that failed to respond to hydroxychloroquine [217]. Current guidelines do not recommend hydroxychloroquine treatment in LS [182].

PROGNOSIS

Malignant transformation of extragenital LS is extremely rare, as compared to anogenital LS which predisposes to the development of squamous cell carcinoma in 5% of cases [218]. To date, only two patients were reported in literature who developed three squamous cell carcinomas on extragenital LS lesions [218, 219]. It is postulated that chronic inflammation of LS has triggered the malignant transformation. However, previous phototherapy and immunosuppressive treatments may have played a role [218]. Patients with extragenital LS do not need follow-up for the disease itself. In case of treatment with a systemic agent or phototherapy, appropriate visits should be performed for drug monitoring and assessment of efficacy [109].

Box 18.7. Learning points.
• Although they share common pathogenetic mechanisms, LS and morphea are different entities but they are both included in sclerodermoid skin conditions.
• Dermoscopy is a helpful adjunct in the diagnosis and follow-up of LS. It reveals patchy white yellowish structureless areas, keratotic plugs in early lesions and chrysalis structures in late lesions.
• Many inflammatory disorders such as lichen planus, morphea, vitiligo, contact dermatitis, and malignant mucocutaneous disorders such as mycosis fungoides and squamous cell carcinoma can mimic extragenital LS.
• Ultrapotent or potent topical corticosteroids are the first line therapeutic agents in LS. For widespread lesions, UVA1 phototherapy is preferred, with a level of evidence 1+.
• Systemic treatment options in recalcitrant cases include methotrexate, sulphasalazine, antibiotics and potassium para-aminobenzoate.
• Malignant transformation of extragenital LS is practically non-existent.

REFERENCES

[1]   Fistarol SK, Itin PH. Diagnosis and treatment of lichen sclerosus: an update. Am J Clin Dermatol 2013; 14(1): 27-47.
[http://dx.doi.org/10.1007/s40257-012-0006-4] [PMID: 23329078]

[2]   Powell JJ, Wojnarowska F. Lichen sclerosus. Lancet 1999; 353(9166): 1777-83.
[http://dx.doi.org/10.1016/S0140-6736(98)08228-2] [PMID: 10348006]

[3]   Hallopeau H. Leçons cliniques sur les maladies cutanées et syphiliques. Union Med 1887; 43: 742-7.

[4]   Weir RF. Icthyosis of the tongue and vulva. N Y State J Med 1875; 246.

[5]   Meffert JJ, Davis BM, Grimwood RE. Lichen sclerosus. J Am Acad Dermatol 1995; 32(3): 393-416.
[http://dx.doi.org/10.1016/0190-9622(95)90060-8] [PMID: 7868709]

[6]   Gahan E. Hallopeau's communications on lichen sclerosus et atrophicus. Arch Dermatol 1954; 69(4): 435-7.
[http://dx.doi.org/10.1001/archderm.1954.01540160037006] [PMID: 13147546]

[7]   Breisky A. Uber Kraurosis vulvae. Z Heilkr 1885; 6: 69.

[8]   Darier J. Lichen plan sclereux. Ann Dermatol Syph 1892; 3: 833-7.

[9]   Unna P. Kartenblattförmige sklerodermie. Lehrbuch der speziellen path Anatomie 1894; 112.

[10]   Westberg F. Ein Fall von mit weissen Flecken einhergehender, bisher nicht bekannter Dermatose. Monatschr Prakt Dermatol 1901; 33: 355-61.

[11]   Von Zumbusch LR. Über Lichen albus, eine bisher unbeschriebene Erkrankung. Arch Dermatol Res 1906; 82(3): 339-50.
[http://dx.doi.org/10.1007/BF01823927]

[12]   Montgomery F, Ormsby O. White spot disease. morphea guttata and lichen planus sclerosus et atrophicus. J Cutan Dis 1907; 25: 1-16.

[13]   Csillag J. Dermatitis lichenoides chronica atrophicans. Ikonographia Dermatol 1909; 4: 147.

[14]   Stühmer A. Balanitis xerotica obliterans *(post operationem)* und ihre Beziehungen zur Kraurosis glandis et praeputii penis. Arch Dermatol Res 1928; 156(3): 613-23.
[http://dx.doi.org/10.1007/BF01828558]

[15]   Kaufman RH, DiPaola GR, Friedrich EG, Hewitt J, Woodruff JD. New nomenclature for vulvar disease. J Cutan Pathol 1976; 3(3): 159-61.
[http://dx.doi.org/10.1111/j.1600-0560.1976.tb01105.x] [PMID: 1002872]

[16]   Edmonds EVJ, Hunt S, Hawkins D, Dinneen M, Francis N, Bunker CB. Clinical parameters in male genital lichen sclerosus: A case series of 329 patients. J Eur Acad Dermatol Venereol 2012; 26(6): 730-7.
[http://dx.doi.org/10.1111/j.1468-3083.2011.04155.x] [PMID: 21707769]

[17]   Kirtschig G. Lichen sclerosus-presentation, diagnosis and management. Dtsch Arztebl Int 2016; 113(19): 337-43.
[PMID: 27232363]

[18]   Knio Z, Kurban M, Abbas O. Lichen sclerosis: Clinicopathological study of 60 cases from Lebanon. Int J Dermatol 2016; 55(10): 1076-81.
[http://dx.doi.org/10.1111/ijd.13336] [PMID: 27229659]

[19]   Sauder MB, Linzon-Smith J, Beecker J. Extragenital bullous lichen sclerosus. J Am Acad Dermatol 2014; 71(5): 981-4.
[http://dx.doi.org/10.1016/j.jaad.2014.06.037] [PMID: 25088813]

[20]   Tasker GL, Wojnarowska F. Lichen sclerosus. Clin Exp Dermatol 2003; 28(2): 128-33.
[http://dx.doi.org/10.1046/j.1365-2230.2003.01211.x] [PMID: 12653695]

[21]   Meyrick Thomas RH, Ridley CM, McGibbon DH, Black MM. Anogenital lichen sclerosus in women. J R Soc Med 1996; 89(12): 694-8.
[http://dx.doi.org/10.1177/014107689608901210] [PMID: 9014881]

[22]   Cooper SM, Gao XH, Powell JJ, Wojnarowska F. Does treatment of vulvar lichen sclerosus influence its prognosis? Arch Dermatol 2004; 140(6): 702-6.
[http://dx.doi.org/10.1001/archderm.140.6.702] [PMID: 15210461]

[23]   Simpkin S, Oakley A. Clinical review of 202 patients with vulval lichen sclerosus: A possible association with psoriasis. Australas J Dermatol 2007; 48(1): 28-31.
[http://dx.doi.org/10.1111/j.1440-0960.2007.00322.x] [PMID: 17222298]

[24]   Riddell L, Edwards A, Sherrard J. Clinical features of lichen sclerosus in men attending a department of genitourinary medicine. Sex Transm Infect 2000; 76(4): 311-3.
[http://dx.doi.org/10.1136/sti.76.4.311] [PMID: 11026891]

[25]   Sherman V, McPherson T, Baldo M, Salim A, Gao XH, Wojnarowska F. The high rate of familial lichen sclerosus suggests a genetic contribution: An observational cohort study. J Eur Acad Dermatol Venereol 2010; 24(9): 1031-4.
[http://dx.doi.org/10.1111/j.1468-3083.2010.03572.x] [PMID: 20202060]

[26]   Higgins CA, Cruickshank ME. A population-based case–control study of aetiological factors associated with vulval lichen sclerosus. J Obstet Gynaecol 2012; 32(3): 271-5.
[http://dx.doi.org/10.3109/01443615.2011.649320] [PMID: 22369403]

[27]   Kirtschig G, Kuik D. A dutch cohort study confirms familial occurrence of anogenital lichen sclerosus. J Womens Health Care 2014; 3: 209.

[28]   Marren P, Jell J, Charnock FM, Bunce M, Welsh K, Wojnarowska F. The association between lichen sclerosus and antigens of the HLA system. Br J Dermatol 1995; 132(2): 197-203.
[http://dx.doi.org/10.1111/j.1365-2133.1995.tb05013.x] [PMID: 7888355]

[29]   Azurdia RM, Luzzi GA, Byren I, *et al.* Lichen sclerosus in adult men: A study of HLA associations and susceptibility to autoimmune disease. Br J Dermatol 1999; 140(1): 79-83.
[http://dx.doi.org/10.1046/j.1365-2133.1999.02611.x] [PMID: 10215772]

[30]   Powell J, Wojnarowska F, Winsey S, Marren P, Welsh K. Lichen sclerosus premenarche: Autoimmunity and immunogenetics. Br J Dermatol 2000; 142(3): 481-4.
[http://dx.doi.org/10.1046/j.1365-2133.2000.03360.x] [PMID: 10735954]

[31]   Gao XH, Barnardo MCMN, Winsey S, *et al.* The association between HLA DR, DQ antigens, and vulval lichen sclerosus in the UK: HLA DRB1*12 and its associated DRB1*12/DQB1*0301/04/09/010 haplotype confers susceptibility to vulval lichen sclerosus, and HLA DRB1*0301/04 and its associated DRB1*0301/. J Invest Dermatol 2005; 125(5): 895-9.
[http://dx.doi.org/10.1111/j.0022-202X.2005.23905.x] [PMID: 16297186]

[32]   Şentürk N, Aydın F, Birinci A, *et al.* Coexistence of HLA-B*08 and HLA-B*18 in four siblings with Lichen sclerosus. Dermatology 2004; 208(1): 64-6.
[http://dx.doi.org/10.1159/000075049] [PMID: 14730240]

[33]   Aslanian FMNP, Marques MTQ, Matos HJ, *et al.* HLA markers in familial Lichen sclerosus. JDDG - J Ger Soc Dermatology 2006; 4: 842-7.
[http://dx.doi.org/10.1111/j.1610-0387.2006.06087.x]

[34]   Meyrick Thomas RH, Ridley CM, McGibbon DH, Black MM. Lichen sclerosus et atrophicus and autoimmunity—a study of 350 women. Br J Dermatol 1988; 118(1): 41-6.
[http://dx.doi.org/10.1111/j.1365-2133.1988.tb01748.x] [PMID: 3342175]

[35]   Goolamali SK, Barnes EW, Irvine WJ, Shuster S. Organ-specific antibodies in patients with lichen sclerosus. BMJ 1974; 4(5936): 78-9.
[http://dx.doi.org/10.1136/bmj.4.5936.78] [PMID: 4414943]

[36]   Birenbaum DL, Young RC. High prevalence of thyroid disease in patients with lichen sclerosus. J Reprod Med 2007; 52(1): 28-30.
[PMID: 17286064]

[37]   Cooper SM, Ali I, Baldo M, Wojnarowska F. The association of lichen sclerosus and erosive lichen planus of the vulva with autoimmune disease: A case-control study. Arch Dermatol 2008; 144(11): 1432-5.
[http://dx.doi.org/10.1001/archderm.144.11.1432] [PMID: 19015417]

[38]   Meyrick Thomas RH, Ridley CM, Black MM. The association of lichen sclerosus et atrophicus and autoimmune-related disease in males. Br J Dermatol 1983; 109(6): 661-4.
[http://dx.doi.org/10.1111/j.1365-2133.1983.tb00546.x] [PMID: 6652042]

[39]   Bjekić M, Šipetić S, Marinković J. Risk factors for genital lichen sclerosus in men. Br J Dermatol 2011; 164(2): 325-9.
[http://dx.doi.org/10.1111/j.1365-2133.2010.10091.x] [PMID: 20973765]

[40]   Oyama N, Chan I, Neill SM, et al. Autoantibodies to extracellular matrix protein 1 in lichen sclerosus. Lancet 2003; 362(9378): 118-23.
[http://dx.doi.org/10.1016/S0140-6736(03)13863-9] [PMID: 12867112]

[41]   Edmonds EVJ, Oyama N, Chan I, Francis N, McGrath JA, Bunker CB. Extracellular matrix protein 1 autoantibodies in male genital lichen sclerosus. Br J Dermatol 2011; 165(1): 218-9.
[http://dx.doi.org/10.1111/j.1365-2133.2011.10326.x] [PMID: 21428972]

[42]   Howard A, Dean D, Cooper S, Kirtshig G, Wojnarowska F. Circulating basement membrane zone antibodies are found in lichen sclerosus of the vulva. Australas J Dermatol 2004; 45(1): 12-5.
[http://dx.doi.org/10.1111/j.1440-0960.2004.00026.x] [PMID: 14961902]

[43]   Baldo M, Bailey A, Bhogal B, Groves RW, Ogg G, Wojnarowska F. T cells reactive with the NC16A domain of BP180 are present in vulval lichen sclerosus and lichen planus. J Eur Acad Dermatol Venereol 2010; 24(2): 186-90.
[http://dx.doi.org/10.1111/j.1468-3083.2009.03375.x] [PMID: 19686329]

[44]   Baldo M, Bhogal B, Groves RW, Powell J, Wojnarowska F. Childhood vulval lichen sclerosus: autoimmunity to the basement membrane zone protein BP180 and its relationship to autoimmunity. Clin Exp Dermatol 2010; 35(5): 543-5.
[http://dx.doi.org/10.1111/j.1365-2230.2010.03827.x] [PMID: 20456392]

[45]   Gambichler T, Höxtermann S, Skrygan M, et al. Occurrence of circulating anti-bullous pemphigoid antibodies in patients with lichen sclerosus. J Eur Acad Dermatol Venereol 2011; 25(3): 369-70.
[http://dx.doi.org/10.1111/j.1468-3083.2010.03739.x] [PMID: 20524944]

[46]   Terlou A, Santegoets LAM, van der Meijden WI, et al. An autoimmune phenotype in vulvar lichen sclerosus and lichen planus: A Th1 response and high levels of microRNA-155. J Invest Dermatol 2012; 132(3): 658-66.
[http://dx.doi.org/10.1038/jid.2011.369] [PMID: 22113482]

[47]   Gambichler T, Belz D, Terras S, Kreuter A. Humoral and cell-mediated autoimmunity in lichen sclerosus. Br J Dermatol 2013; 169(1): 183-4.
[http://dx.doi.org/10.1111/bjd.12220] [PMID: 23301780]

[48]   Kantere D, Alvergren G, Gillstedt M, Pujol-Calderón F, Tunbäck P. Clinical features, complications and autoimmunity in male lichen sclerosus. Acta Derm Venereol 2017; 97(3): 365-9.
[http://dx.doi.org/10.2340/00015555-2537] [PMID: 27671756]

[49]   Kreuter A, Kryvosheyeva Y, Terras S, et al. Association of autoimmune diseases with lichen sclerosus in 532 male and female patients. Acta Derm Venereol 2013; 93(2): 238-41.
[http://dx.doi.org/10.2340/00015555-1512] [PMID: 23224274]

[50]   Edmonds E, Barton G, Buisson S, et al. Gene expression profiling in male genital lichen sclerosus. Int J Exp Pathol 2011; 92(5): 320-5.

[http://dx.doi.org/10.1111/j.1365-2613.2011.00779.x] [PMID: 21718371]

[51]   Friedrich EG Jr, Kalra PS. Serum levels of sex hormones in vulvar lichen sclerosus, and the effect of topical testosterone. N Engl J Med 1984; 310(8): 488-91.
[http://dx.doi.org/10.1056/NEJM198402233100803] [PMID: 6537989]

[52]   Clifton MM, Bayer Garner IB, Kohler S, Smoller BR. Immunohistochemical evaluation of androgen receptors in genital and extragenital lichen sclerosus: Evidence for loss of androgen receptors in lesional epidermis. J Am Acad Dermatol 1999; 41(1): 43-6.
[http://dx.doi.org/10.1016/S0190-9622(99)70404-4] [PMID: 10411409]

[53]   Taylor AH, Guzail M, Al-Azzawi F. Differential expression of oestrogen receptor isoforms and androgen receptor in the normal vulva and vagina compared with vulval lichen sclerosus and chronic vaginitis. Br J Dermatol 2008; 158(2): 319-28.
[http://dx.doi.org/10.1111/j.1365-2133.2007.08371.x] [PMID: 18076706]

[54]   Günthert AR, Faber M, Knappe G, Hellriegel S, Emons G. Early onset vulvar Lichen Sclerosus in premenopausal women and oral contraceptives. Eur J Obstet Gynecol Reprod Biol 2008; 137(1): 56-60.
[http://dx.doi.org/10.1016/j.ejogrb.2007.10.005] [PMID: 18055095]

[55]   Lagerstedt M, Huotari-Orava R, Nyberg R, Mäenpää JU, Snellman E, Laasanen SL. Reduction in ERRα is associated with lichen sclerosus and vulvar squamous cell carcinoma. Gynecol Oncol 2015; 139(3): 536-40.
[http://dx.doi.org/10.1016/j.ygyno.2015.10.016] [PMID: 26499936]

[56]   Todd P, Halpern S, Kirby J, Pembroke A. Lichen sclerosus and the Kobner phenomenon. Clin Exp Dermatol 1994; 19(3): 262-3.
[http://dx.doi.org/10.1111/j.1365-2230.1994.tb01183.x] [PMID: 8033394]

[57]   Anderton RL, Abele DC. Lichen sclerosus et atrophicus in a vaccination site. Arch Dermatol 1976; 112(12): 1787.
[http://dx.doi.org/10.1001/archderm.1976.01630370067015] [PMID: 1008571]

[58]   Monteagudo B, Cabanillas M, Bellido D, Suárez-Amor Ó, Ramírez-Santos A, de la Cruz A. Lichen sclerosus atrophicus at an insulin injection site: an unusual koebner phenomenon. Actas Dermo-Sifiliográficas 2010; 101(6): 563-5.
[http://dx.doi.org/10.1016/S1578-2190(10)70849-0] [PMID: 20738983]

[59]   Vishwanath T, Ghate S, Shinde G, Lahoria V, Binny B, Sonwane A. Koebnerization of lichen sclerosus et atrophicus at insulin injection sites. A rare case with dermoscopic features. Indian J Dermatol 2021; 66(2): 224.
[http://dx.doi.org/10.4103/ijd.IJD_634_18] [PMID: 34188297]

[60]   Arif T, Adil M, Amin SS, Mahtab A. Concomitant morphea and lichen sclerosus et atrophicus in the same plaque at the site of intramuscular drug injection: an interesting case presentation. Acta Dermatovenerol Alp Panonica Adriat 2018; 27(2): 111-3.
[http://dx.doi.org/10.15570/actaapa.2018.23] [PMID: 29945269]

[61]   Pérez-López I, Garrido-Colmenero C, Blasco-Morente G, Tercedor-Sánchez J. Koebner phenomenon in a patient with lichen sclerosus following a jellyfish sting: An exceptional morphology. Actas Dermo-Sifiliográficas 2015; 106(3): 238-9.
[http://dx.doi.org/10.1016/j.adengl.2015.01.013] [PMID: 25597413]

[62]   Pock L. Koebner Phenomenon in Lichen sclerosus et atrophicus. Dermatology 1990; 181(1): 76-7.
[http://dx.doi.org/10.1159/000247872] [PMID: 2394311]

[63]   Mendieta-Eckert M, Ocerin-Guerra I, Landa-Gundin N. Lichen sclerosus et atrophicus in a surgical scar treated with fractional laser. J Cosmet Laser Ther 2017; 19(2): 106-8.
[http://dx.doi.org/10.1080/14764172.2016.1262955] [PMID: 27911123]

[64]   Meffert JJ, Grimwood RE. Lichen sclerosus et atrophicus appearing in an old burn scar. J Am Acad

Dermatol 1994; 31(4): 671-3.
[http://dx.doi.org/10.1016/S0190-9622(08)81738-0] [PMID: 8089298]

[65] Glaser KS, Glaser EN, Piliang M, Anthony J. Extragenital lichen sclerosus et atrophicus within a skin graft scar. JAAD Case Rep 2018; 4(9): 938-40.
[http://dx.doi.org/10.1016/j.jdcr.2018.09.007] [PMID: 30320200]

[66] Yates VM, King CM, Dave VK. Lichen sclerosus et atrophicus following radiation therapy. Arch Dermatol 1985; 121(8): 1044-7.
[http://dx.doi.org/10.1001/archderm.1985.01660080098024] [PMID: 4026344]

[67] Vujovic O. Lichen sclerosus in a radiated breast. CMAJ 2010; 182(18): E860.
[http://dx.doi.org/10.1503/cmaj.091800] [PMID: 20974722]

[68] Nemer KM, Anadkat MJ. Postirradiation lichen sclerosus et atrophicus. JAMA Dermatol 2017; 153(10): 1067-9.
[http://dx.doi.org/10.1001/jamadermatol.2017.0823] [PMID: 28538963]

[69] Bonfill-Ortí M, Martínez-Molina L, Penín RM, Marcoval J. Extragenital lichen sclerosus induced by radiotherapy. Actas Dermosifiliogr 2019; 110(1): 69-71.
[http://dx.doi.org/10.1016/j.ad.2017.09.024] [PMID: 29566881]

[70] Milligan A, Graham-Brown RA, Burns DA. Lichen sclerosus et atrophicus following sunburn. Clin Exp Dermatol 1988; 13(1): 36-7.
[PMID: 3208439]

[71] Ronnen M, Suster S, Kahana M, Schewach-Millet M. Bilateral Koebner phenomenon in lichen sclerosus et atrophicus. Int J Dermatol 1987; 26(2): 117-8.
[http://dx.doi.org/10.1111/j.1365-4362.1987.tb00539.x] [PMID: 3570583]

[72] Ah-Weng A, Charles-Holmes R. Peristomal lichen sclerosus affecting colostomy sites. Br J Dermatol 2000; 142(1): 177-8.
[http://dx.doi.org/10.1046/j.1365-2133.2000.03265.x] [PMID: 10819544]

[73] Al-Niaimi F, Lyon C. Peristomal lichen sclerosus: The role of occlusion and urine exposure? Br J Dermatol 2013; 168(3): 643-6.
[http://dx.doi.org/10.1111/bjd.12014] [PMID: 22913573]

[74] Baykal C, Kobaner GB, Copur S, Buyukbabani N. Lichen sclerosus on the sites of striae distensae and a surgical scar in a patient with coexistent morphea. Acta Dermatovenerol Croat 2019; 27(1): 44-6.
[PMID: 31032793]

[75] Noakes RR, Spelman L. Kobnerization in a woman with generalized lichen sclerosus. Australas J Dermatol 2004; 45(2): 144-5.
[http://dx.doi.org/10.1111/j.1440-0960.2004.00063.x] [PMID: 15068467]

[76] Warrington SA, de San Lazaro C. Lichen sclerosus et atrophicus and sexual abuse. Arch Dis Child 1996; 75(6): 512-6.
[http://dx.doi.org/10.1136/adc.75.6.512] [PMID: 9014605]

[77] Ridley CM. Genital lichen sclerosus (lichen sclerosus et atrophicus) in childhood and adolescence. J R Soc Med 1993; 86(2): 69-75.
[PMID: 8433310]

[78] Wolf B, Horn LC, Höckel M. Anogenital lichen sclerosus: Change of tissue position as pathogenetic factor. Gynecol Oncol Rep 2017; 20: 73-4.
[http://dx.doi.org/10.1016/j.gore.2017.03.003] [PMID: 28349117]

[79] Drut RM, Gómez MA, Drut R, Lojo MM. Human papillomavirus is present in some cases of childhood penile lichen sclerosus: An in situ hybridization and SP-PCR study. Pediatr Dermatol 1998; 15(2): 85-90.
[http://dx.doi.org/10.1046/j.1525-1470.1998.1998015085.x] [PMID: 9572688]

[80]   von Krogh G, Dahlman-Ghozlan K, Syrjänen S. Potential human papillomavirus reactivation following topical corticosteroid therapy of genital lichen sclerosus and erosive lichen planus. J Eur Acad Dermatol Venereol 2002; 16(2): 130-3.
[http://dx.doi.org/10.1046/j.1468-3083.2002.00420.x] [PMID: 12046814]

[81]   Bilenchi R, Poggiali S, De Padova LA, Pisani C, De Paola M, Fimiani M. Human papillomavirus reactivation following topical tacrolimus therapy of anogenital lichen sclerosus. Br J Dermatol 2007; 156(2): 405-6.
[http://dx.doi.org/10.1111/j.1365-2133.2006.07662.x] [PMID: 17223903]

[82]   Vignale Peirano R, Acosta Dibarraz G, Paciel Vaz J, González Domínguez V. Presencia del virus del papiloma humano en lesiones de liquen escleroso y atrófico vulvar. Estudio por inmunohistoquímica e hibridización in situ. Actas Dermosifiliogr 2002; 93(6): 389-92.
[http://dx.doi.org/10.1016/S0001-7310(02)76596-4]

[83]   Hald AK, Blaakaer J. The possible role of human papillomavirus infection in the development of lichen sclerosus. Int J Dermatol 2018; 57(2): 139-46.
[http://dx.doi.org/10.1111/ijd.13697] [PMID: 28737238]

[84]   DeVito JR, Merogi AJ, Vo T, *et al.* Role of Borrelia burgdorferi in the pathogenesis of morphea/scleroderma and lichen sclerosus et atrophicus: a PCR study of thirty-five cases. J Cutan Pathol 1996; 23(4): 350-8.
[http://dx.doi.org/10.1111/j.1600-0560.1996.tb01309.x] [PMID: 8864923]

[85]   Fujiwara H, Fujiwara K, Hashimoto K, *et al.* Detection of Borrelia burgdorferi DNA (B garinii or B afzelii) in morphea and lichen sclerosus et atrophicus tissues of German and Japanese but not of US patients. Arch Dermatol 1997; 133(1): 41-4.
[http://dx.doi.org/10.1001/archderm.1997.03890370047008] [PMID: 9006371]

[86]   Edmonds E, Mavin S, Francis N, Ho-Yen D, Bunker C. *Borrelia burgdorferi* is not associated with genital lichen sclerosus in men. Br J Dermatol 2009; 160(2): 459-60.
[http://dx.doi.org/10.1111/j.1365-2133.2008.08969.x] [PMID: 19077073]

[87]   Schempp C, Bocklage H, Lange R, Kölmel HW, Orfanos CE, Gollnick H. Further evidence for Borrelia burgdorferi infection in morphea and lichen sclerosus et atrophicus confirmed by DNA amplification. J Invest Dermatol 1993; 100(5): 717-20.
[http://dx.doi.org/10.1111/1523-1747.ep12472369] [PMID: 8491994]

[88]   Özkan S, Atabey N, Fetil E, Erkizan V, Güneş AT. Evidence for Borrelia burgdorferi in morphea and lichen sclerosus. Int J Dermatol 2000; 39(4): 278-83.
[http://dx.doi.org/10.1046/j.1365-4362.2000.00912.x] [PMID: 10809977]

[89]   Eisendle K, Grabner T, Kutzner H, Zelger B. Possible role of Borrelia burgdorferi sensu lato infection in lichen sclerosus. Arch Dermatol 2008; 144(5): 591-8.
[http://dx.doi.org/10.1001/archderm.144.5.591] [PMID: 18490585]

[90]   Alonso-Llamazares J, Persing DH, Anda P, Gibson LE, Rutledge BJ, Iglesias L. No evidence for Borrelia burgdorferi infection in lesions of morphea and lichen sclerosus et atrophicus in Spain. A prospective study and literature review. Acta Derm Venereol 1997; 77(4): 299-304.
[PMID: 9228224]

[91]   Zollinger T, Mertz KD, Schmid M, Schmitt A, Pfaltz M, Kempf W. *Borrelia* in granuloma annulare, morphea and lichen sclerosus: a PCR-based study and review of the literature. J Cutan Pathol 2010; 37(5): 571-7.
[http://dx.doi.org/10.1111/j.1600-0560.2009.01493.x] [PMID: 20015188]

[92]   Aidé S, Lattario FR, Almeida G, do Val IC, da Costa Carvalho M. Epstein-Barr virus and human papillomavirus infection in vulvar lichen sclerosus. J Low Genit Tract Dis 2010; 14(4): 319-22.
[http://dx.doi.org/10.1097/LGT.0b013e3181d734f1] [PMID: 20885159]

[93]   Zhang Y, Fu Q, Zhang X. The presence of human papillomavirus and Epstein-Barr virus in male

Chinese lichen sclerosus patients: A single center study. Asian J Androl 2016; 18(4): 650-3.
[PMID: 26289401]

[94] Boulinguez S, Bernard P, Lacour JP, *et al.* Bullous lichen sclerosus with chronic hepatitis C virus infection. Br J Dermatol 1997; 137(3): 474-6.
[http://dx.doi.org/10.1111/j.1365-2133.1997.tb03767.x] [PMID: 9349358]

[95] Yashar S, Han KF, Haley JC. Lichen sclerosus-lichen planus overlap in a patient with hepatitis C virus infection. Br J Dermatol 2004; 150(1): 168-9.
[http://dx.doi.org/10.1111/j.1365-2133.2004.05707.x] [PMID: 14746647]

[96] Shim TN, Bunker CB. Male genital lichen sclerosus and hepatitis C. Br J Dermatol 2012; 167(6): 1398-9.
[http://dx.doi.org/10.1111/j.1365-2133.2012.11065.x] [PMID: 22612734]

[97] Pranteda G, Muscianese M, Grimaldi M, *et al.* Lichen sclerosus et atrophicus induced by carbamazepine: A case report. Int J Immunopathol Pharmacol 2013; 26(3): 791-4.
[http://dx.doi.org/10.1177/039463201302600326] [PMID: 24067479]

[98] Skupsky H, Abuav R, High W, Pass C, Goldenberg G. Development of lichen sclerosus et atrophicus while receiving a therapeutic dose of imatinib mesylate for chronic myelogenous leukemia. J Cutan Pathol 2010; 37(8): 877-80.
[http://dx.doi.org/10.1111/j.1600-0560.2009.01398.x] [PMID: 19703239]

[99] Baldo M, Ali I, Wojnarowska F. The contribution of drugs to lichen sclerosus. Clin Exp Dermatol 2014; 39(2): 234.
[http://dx.doi.org/10.1111/ced.12264] [PMID: 24450847]

[100] Kawamura E, Kanekura T, Mera Y, Uchimiya H, Kanzaki T. Generalized lichen sclerosus et atrophicus: Report of a case. J Dermatol 2005; 32(12): 1048-50.
[http://dx.doi.org/10.1111/j.1346-8138.2005.tb00900.x] [PMID: 16471476]

[101] Criado PR, Lima FHSD, Miguel DS, Valente NYS, Vasconcellos C, Sittart JAS. Lichen sclerosus: A keratotic variant. J Eur Acad Dermatol Venereol 2002; 16(5): 504-5.
[http://dx.doi.org/10.1046/j.1468-3083.2002.00542.x] [PMID: 12428848]

[102] Hasegawa M, Ishikawa O, Asano Y, *et al.* Diagnostic criteria, severity classification and guidelines of lichen sclerosus et atrophicus. J Dermatol 2018; 45(8): 891-7.
[http://dx.doi.org/10.1111/1346-8138.14171] [PMID: 29265410]

[103] Jee MS, Kim HH, Chang SE, *et al.* Lichen sclerosus et atrophicus of the face. Korean J Dermatol 2002; 40: 1434-6.

[104] Feng S, Yu L, Li Z. Lichen sclerosus of face: A case report and review of literature. Indian J Dermatol 2016; 61(1): 120.
[http://dx.doi.org/10.4103/0019-5154.174096] [PMID: 26955133]

[105] Foulds IS. Lichen sclerosus et atrophicus of the scalp. Br J Dermatol 1980; 103(2): 197-200.
[http://dx.doi.org/10.1111/j.1365-2133.1980.tb06591.x] [PMID: 7426417]

[106] Kawakami Y, Oyama N, Hanami Y, Kimura T, Kishimoto K, Yamamoto T. A case of lichen sclerosus of the scalp associated with autoantibodies to extracellular matrix protein 1. Arch Dermatol 2009; 145(12): 1458-60.
[http://dx.doi.org/10.1001/archdermatol.2009.313] [PMID: 20026864]

[107] Purres J, Krull EA. Lichen sclerosus et atrophicus involving the palms. Arch Dermatol 1971; 104(1): 68-9.
[http://dx.doi.org/10.1001/archderm.1971.04000190070010] [PMID: 5120165]

[108] Petrozzi JW, Wood MG, Tisa V. Palmar-plantar lichen sclerosus et atrophicus. Arch Dermatol 1979; 115(7): 884.
[http://dx.doi.org/10.1001/archderm.1979.04010070060028] [PMID: 453905]

[109] Lewis FM, Tatnall FM, Velangi SS, *et al.* British Association of Dermatologists guidelines for the management of lichen sclerosus. Br J Dermatol 2018; 178(4): 839-53.
[http://dx.doi.org/10.1111/bjd.16241] [PMID: 29313888]

[110] Uzuncakmak TK, Akdeniz N, Suslu H, Zemheri E, Karadag AS. Folliculocentric hyperkeratotic lichen sclerosus in a 7-year-old child successfully treated with narrowband ultraviolet B phototherapy. Clin Exp Dermatol 2018; 43(1): 91-3.
[http://dx.doi.org/10.1111/ced.13216] [PMID: 28940561]

[111] Ballester I, Bañuls J, Pérez-Crespo M, Lucas A. Extragenital bullous lichen sclerosus atrophicus. Dermatol Online J 2009; 15(1): 6.
[http://dx.doi.org/10.5070/D357M4H6NW] [PMID: 19281711]

[112] Khatu S, Vasani R. Isolated, localised extragenital bullous Lichen sclerosus et atrophicus: A rare entity. Indian J Dermatol 2013; 58(5): 409.
[http://dx.doi.org/10.4103/0019-5154.117351] [PMID: 24082218]

[113] Parr K, Trinh T-VT, Butler D. Disseminated extragenital bullous lichen sclerosus. Indian Dermatol Online J 2014; 5(1): 66-8.
[http://dx.doi.org/10.4103/2229-5178.126037] [PMID: 24616861]

[114] Quatrano NA, Shvartsbeyn M, Meehan SA, Pomerantz R, Pomeranz MK. Extragenital bullous lichen sclerosus. Dermatol Online J 2015; 21: 13030/qt1rc0z3n8.
[http://dx.doi.org/10.5070/D32112029533]

[115] Libow LF, Coots NV. Lichen sclerosus following the lines of Blaschko. J Am Acad Dermatol 1998; 38(5): 831-3.
[http://dx.doi.org/10.1016/S0190-9622(98)70468-2] [PMID: 9591796]

[116] Choi SW, Yang JE, Park HJ, Kim CW. A case of extragenital lichen sclerosus following Blaschko's lines. J Am Acad Dermatol 2000; 43(5): 903-4.
[http://dx.doi.org/10.1067/mjd.2000.101876] [PMID: 11044817]

[117] Nair PA, Diwan NG. Extragenital lichen sclerosus et atrophicus along the lines of Blaschko. Indian Dermatol Online J 2015; 6(5): 342-4.
[http://dx.doi.org/10.4103/2229-5178.164486] [PMID: 26500867]

[118] Kakko T, Salo T, Siponen MK. Oral lichen sclerosus: A systematic review of reported cases and two new cases. Int J Dermatol 2018; 57(5): 521-8.
[http://dx.doi.org/10.1111/ijd.13870] [PMID: 29313955]

[119] Kossard S, Cornish N. Localized lichen sclerosus with nail loss. Australas J Dermatol 1998; 39(2): 119-20.
[http://dx.doi.org/10.1111/j.1440-0960.1998.tb01263.x] [PMID: 9611385]

[120] Ramrakha-Jones VS, Paul M, McHenry P, Burden AD. Nail dystrophy due to lichen sclerosus? Clin Exp Dermatol 2001; 26(6): 507-9.
[http://dx.doi.org/10.1046/j.1365-2230.2001.00878.x] [PMID: 11678877]

[121] Dalal V, Kaur M, Rai C, Singh A, Ramesh V. Histopathological spectrum of lichen sclerosus Et atrophicus. Ind J Dermat Diagn Dermat 2017; 4(1): 8.
[http://dx.doi.org/10.4103/ijdpdd.ijdpdd_66_16]

[122] Lee SB, Heo JH, Yoon HS, *et al.* Acrosyringeal variant of extragenital lichen sclerosus et atrophicus. J Cutan Pathol 2020; 47(11): 1039-41.
[http://dx.doi.org/10.1111/cup.13776] [PMID: 32533734]

[123] Larre Borges A, Tiodorovic-Zivkovic D, Lallas A, *et al.* Clinical, dermoscopic and histopathologic features of genital and extragenital lichen sclerosus. J Eur Acad Dermatol Venereol 2013; 27(11): 1433-9.
[http://dx.doi.org/10.1111/j.1468-3083.2012.04595.x] [PMID: 22646723]

[124] Errichetti E, Lallas A, Apalla Z, Di Stefani A, Stinco G. Dermoscopy of morphea and cutaneous lichen sclerosus: Clinicopathological correlation study and comparative analysis. Dermatology 2017; 233(6): 462-70.
[http://dx.doi.org/10.1159/000484947] [PMID: 29237158]

[125] Behera B, Palit A, Mitra S, Sethy M. Dermoscopy as a tool for assessing the therapeutic response in a case of extra-genital lichen sclerosus et atrophicus. Indian Dermatol Online J 2021; 12(1): 169-71.
[http://dx.doi.org/10.4103/idoj.IDOJ_182_20] [PMID: 33768045]

[126] Lacarrubba F, Pellacani G, Verzì AE, Pippione M, Micali G. Extragenital lichen sclerosus: Clinical, dermoscopic, confocal microscopy and histologic correlations. J Am Acad Dermatol 2015; 72(1) (Suppl.): S50-2.
[http://dx.doi.org/10.1016/j.jaad.2014.07.008] [PMID: 25500042]

[127] Jacquemus J, Debarbieux S, Depaepe L, Amini M, Balme B, Thomas L. Reflectance confocal microscopy of extra-genital lichen sclerosus atrophicus. Skin Res Technol 2016; 22(2): 255-8.
[http://dx.doi.org/10.1111/srt.12246] [PMID: 26058682]

[128] Boyd AS, Neldner KH. The isomorphic response of Koebner. Int J Dermatol 1990; 29(6): 401-10.
[http://dx.doi.org/10.1111/j.1365-4362.1990.tb03821.x] [PMID: 2204607]

[129] Laga AC, Larson A, Granter SR. Histopathologic spectrum of connective tissue diseases commonly affecting the skin. Surg Pathol Clin 2017; 10(2): 477-503.
[http://dx.doi.org/10.1016/j.path.2017.01.012] [PMID: 28477892]

[130] Lutz V, Francès C, Bessis D, et al. High frequency of genital lichen sclerosus in a prospective series of 76 patients with morphea: Toward a better understanding of the spectrum of morphea. Arch Dermatol 2012; 148(1): 24-8.
[http://dx.doi.org/10.1001/archdermatol.2011.305] [PMID: 22004877]

[131] Peterson LS, Nelson AM, Su WPD. Classification of morphea (localized scleroderma). Mayo Clin Proc 1995; 70(11): 1068-76.
[http://dx.doi.org/10.4065/70.11.1068] [PMID: 7475336]

[132] Heck J, Olk J, Kneitz H, Hamm H, Goebeler M. Long-standing morphea and the risk of squamous cell carcinoma of the skin. (JDDG) J Ger Soc Dermatology 2020; 18: 669-73.
[http://dx.doi.org/10.1111/ddg.14096]

[133] Fett N, Werth VP. Update on morphea. J Am Acad Dermatol 2011; 64(2): 217-28.
[http://dx.doi.org/10.1016/j.jaad.2010.05.045] [PMID: 21238823]

[134] Kreuter A, Wischnewski J, Terras S, Altmeyer P, Stücker M, Gambichler T. Coexistence of lichen sclerosus and morphea: A retrospective analysis of 472 patients with localized scleroderma from a German tertiary referral center. J Am Acad Dermatol 2012; 67(6): 1157-62.
[http://dx.doi.org/10.1016/j.jaad.2012.04.003] [PMID: 22533994]

[135] Tremaine R, Adam JE, Orizaga M. Morphea coexisting with lichen sclerosus et atrophicus. Int J Dermatol 1990; 29(7): 486-9.
[http://dx.doi.org/10.1111/j.1365-4362.1990.tb04840.x] [PMID: 2228375]

[136] Blaya B, Gardeazabal J. Martínez de Lagrán Z, Díaz-Pérez JL. Patient with generalized guttate morphea and lichen sclerosus et atrophicus. Actas Dermosifiliogr 2008; 99(10): 808-11.
[http://dx.doi.org/10.1016/S0001-7310(08)74962-7] [PMID: 19091221]

[137] Kim DH, Lee KR, Kim TY, Yoon MS. Coexistence of lichen sclerosus with morphoea showing bilateral symmetry. Clin Exp Dermatol 2009; 34(7): e416-8.
[http://dx.doi.org/10.1111/j.1365-2230.2009.03396.x] [PMID: 19754732]

[138] Yasar S, Mumcuoglu CT, Serdar ZA, Gunes P. A case of lichen sclerosus et atrophicus accompanying bullous morphea. Ann Dermatol 2011; 23 (Suppl. 3): S354-9.
[http://dx.doi.org/10.5021/ad.2011.23.S3.S354] [PMID: 22346277]

[139] Requena López S, Hidalgo García Y, Gómez Díez S, Vivanco Allende B. Morphea and Extragenital Lichen Sclerosus et Atrophicus After Influenza Vaccination. Actas Dermo-Sifiliográficas 2018; 109(1): 86-8.
[http://dx.doi.org/10.1016/j.adengl.2017.11.018] [PMID: 29025691]

[140] Lis-Święty A, Mierzwińska K, Wodok-Wieczorek K, Widuchowska M, Brzezińska-Wcisło L. Co-existence of lichen sclerosus and localized scleroderma in female monozygotic twins. J Pediatr Adolesc Gynecol 2014; 27(6): e133-6.
[http://dx.doi.org/10.1016/j.jpag.2013.11.010] [PMID: 24841519]

[141] Rongioletti F, Caratti F, Rebora A. Concomitance of lichen sclerosus et atrophicus and morphea in the same lesions. J Eur Acad Dermatol Venereol 1994; 3(3): 407-10.
[http://dx.doi.org/10.1111/j.1468-3083.1994.tb00386.x]

[142] Das A, Gupta S, Singh S, Pant L. Coexisting morphea with lichen sclerosus et atrophicus in a single lesion. A rare case report. Bangladesh J Med Sci 2016; 15(1): 145-7.
[http://dx.doi.org/10.3329/bjms.v15i1.20483]

[143] Gloster HM, Gebauer LE, Mistur RL. Scleroderma and Sclerodermoid Skin Conditions. Absolute Dermatology Review. Cham: Springer 2016; pp. 119-27.
[http://dx.doi.org/10.1007/978-3-319-03218-4_35]

[144] Patel B, Gupta R, Vora VR. Extra genital lichen sclerosus et atrophicus with cutaneous distribution and morphology simulating lichen planus. Indian J Dermatol 2015; 60(1): 105.
[http://dx.doi.org/10.4103/0019-5154.147873] [PMID: 25657434]

[145] Corbalán-Vélez R, Pérez-Ferriols A, Jiménez JR. Lichen sclerosus et atrophicus affecting the wrists and left ankle and clinically simulating lichen planus. Cutis 2001; 67(5): 417-9.
[PMID: 11381860]

[146] Arizaga AT, Gaughan MD, Bang RH. Generalized lichen nitidus. Clin Exp Dermatol 2002; 27(2): 115-7.
[http://dx.doi.org/10.1046/j.1365-2230.2002.00971.x] [PMID: 11952701]

[147] Carlson JA, Grabowski R, Mu XC, Del Rosario A, Malfetano J, Slominski A. Possible mechanisms of hypopigmentation in lichen sclerosus. Am J Dermatopathol 2002; 24(2): 97-107.
[http://dx.doi.org/10.1097/00000372-200204000-00001] [PMID: 11979069]

[148] Attili V, Attili S. Vitiligoid lichen sclerosus: A reappraisal. Indian J Dermatol Venereol Leprol 2008; 74(2): 118-21.
[http://dx.doi.org/10.4103/0378-6323.39693] [PMID: 18388368]

[149] Lee H, Kim YJ, Oh SH. Segmental vitiligo and extragenital lichen sclerosus et atrophicus simultaneously occurring on the opposite sides of the abdomen. Ann Dermatol 2014; 26(6): 764-5.
[http://dx.doi.org/10.5021/ad.2014.26.6.764] [PMID: 25473235]

[150] Kwon IH, Kye H, Seo SH, Ahn HH, Kye YC, Choi JE. Synchronous onset of symmetrically associated extragenital lichen sclerosus and vitiligo on both breasts and the vulva. Ann Dermatol 2015; 27(4): 456-7.
[http://dx.doi.org/10.5021/ad.2015.27.4.456] [PMID: 26273168]

[151] Bulat V, Šitum M, Maričić G, *et al.* Idiopathic Guttate Hypomelanosis: A Comprehensive Overview. J Pigment Disord 2014; 01: 1-4.

[152] Al-Refu K. Dermoscopy is a new diagnostic tool in diagnosis of common hypopigmented macular disease: A descriptive study. Dermatol Rep 2018; 11(1): 7916.
[http://dx.doi.org/10.4081/dr.2018.7916] [PMID: 31119026]

[153] Ganesan L, Parmar H, Das J, Gangopadhyay A. Extragenital lichen sclerosus et atrophicus. Indian J Dermatol 2015; 60(4): 420.
[http://dx.doi.org/10.4103/0019-5154.160516] [PMID: 26288432]

[154] Marfatia Y, Surani A, Baxi R. Genital lichen sclerosus et atrophicus in females: An update. Indian J Sex Transm Dis AIDS 2019; 40(1): 6-12.
[http://dx.doi.org/10.4103/ijstd.IJSTD_23_19] [PMID: 31143853]

[155] Farrell AM, Marren PM, Wojnarowska F. Genital lichen sclerosus associated with morphoea or systemic sclerosis: clinical and HLA characteristics. Br J Dermatol 2000; 143(3): 598-603.
[http://dx.doi.org/10.1111/j.1365-2133.2000.03717.x] [PMID: 10971336]

[156] Marren P, Walkden V, Mallon E, Wojnarowska F. Vulval cicatricial pemphigoid may mimic lichen sclerosus. Br J Dermatol 1996; 134(3): 522-4.
[http://dx.doi.org/10.1046/j.1365-2133.1996.43766.x] [PMID: 8731681]

[157] Arnold N, Manway M, Stephenson S, Lipkin H. Extragenital bullous lichen sclerosus on the anterior lower extremities: Report of a case and literature review. Dermatol Online J. 2017;2 3: 0-4.

[158] Phan M, Sou E, Al Sannaa G, Erwin M, Sanchez R. Dermal Hemorrhage: A Clue to Lichen Sclerosus et Atrophicus. Cureus 2020; 12(7): e9343.
[http://dx.doi.org/10.7759/cureus.9343] [PMID: 32850217]

[159] Kershenovich R, Hodak E, Mimouni D. Diagnosis and classification of pemphigus and bullous pemphigoid. Autoimmun Rev 2014; 13(4-5): 477-81.
[http://dx.doi.org/10.1016/j.autrev.2014.01.011] [PMID: 24424192]

[160] Piccolo D, Soyer HP, Schaeppi H, Chimenti S. Morphologic stages of senile purpura. G Ital Dermatol Venereol 1999; 134: 553-6.

[161] Collins P, Sepede J. Bullous arthropod bite reaction. BMJ Case Rep 2018; 11(1): e228079.
[http://dx.doi.org/10.1136/bcr-2018-228079] [PMID: 30567148]

[162] Verma R, Vasudevan B, Kinra P, Vijendran P, Badad A, Singh V. Bullous lichen planus. Indian J Dermatol Venereol Leprol 2014; 80(3): 279.
[http://dx.doi.org/10.4103/0378-6323.132275] [PMID: 24823424]

[163] Harris-Stith R, Erickson QL, Elston DM, David-Bajar K. Bullous eruption: A manifestation of lupus erythematosus. Cutis 2003; 72(1): 31-7.
[PMID: 12889712]

[164] Gomides MDA, Costa LD, Berbert ALCV, Janones RS. Cutaneous lymphangioma circumscriptum: The relevance of clinical, dermoscopic, radiological, and histological assessments. Clin Case Rep 2019; 7(4): 612-5.
[http://dx.doi.org/10.1002/ccr3.2007] [PMID: 30997047]

[165] Funaro D. Lichen sclerosus: A review and practical approach. Dermatol Ther 2004; 17(1): 28-37.
[http://dx.doi.org/10.1111/j.1396-0296.2004.04004.x] [PMID: 14756888]

[166] Rotsztejn H, Trznadel-Grodzka E, Krawczyk T. Lichen sclerosus mimicking Bowen's disease. Adv Dermat Allerg 2012; 4: 321-3.
[http://dx.doi.org/10.5114/pdia.2012.30474]

[167] Tammaro A, Magri F, Iacovino C, Zollo V, Parisella FR, Persechino S. Lichen sclerosus et atrophicus and allergic contact dermatitis: A significant association. J Cosmet Dermatol 2019; 18(6): 1935-7.
[http://dx.doi.org/10.1111/jocd.12915] [PMID: 30864217]

[168] Parera E, Toll A, Gallardo F, Bellosillo B, Pujol RM, Martí R. Lichen sclerosus et atrophicus-like lesions in mycosis fungoides. Br J Dermatol 2007; 157(2): 411-3.
[http://dx.doi.org/10.1111/j.1365-2133.2007.08024.x] [PMID: 17573868]

[169] Suchak R, Verdolini R, Robson A, Stefanato CM. Extragenital lichen sclerosus et atrophicus mimicking cutaneous T-cell lymphoma: Report of a case. J Cutan Pathol 2010; 37(9): 982-6.
[http://dx.doi.org/10.1111/j.1600-0560.2009.01452.x] [PMID: 19903217]

[170] Lallas A, Apalla Z, Lefaki I, *et al.* Dermoscopy of early stage mycosis fungoides. J Eur Acad Dermatol Venereol 2013; 27(5): 617-21.

[http://dx.doi.org/10.1111/j.1468-3083.2012.04499.x] [PMID: 22404051]

[171] Eberz B, Berghold A, Regauer S. High prevalence of concomitant anogenital lichen sclerosus and extragenital psoriasis in adult women. Obstet Gynecol 2008; 111(5): 1143-7.
[http://dx.doi.org/10.1097/AOG.0b013e31816fdcdf] [PMID: 18448747]

[172] Weinberg JL, Rosenbach M, Kim EJ, Kovarik CL. Lichen sclerosus et atrophicus-like graft versus host disease post stem cell transplant. Dermatol Online J 2009; 15(9): 4-7.
[http://dx.doi.org/10.5070/D36J26J40D] [PMID: 19930991]

[173] Schaffer JV, McNiff JM, Seropian S, Cooper DL, Bolognia JL. Lichen sclerosus and eosinophilic fasciitis as manifestations of chronic graft-versus-host disease: Expanding the sclerodermoid spectrum. J Am Acad Dermatol 2005; 53(4): 591-601.
[http://dx.doi.org/10.1016/j.jaad.2005.06.015] [PMID: 16198778]

[174] Yesudian PD, Sugunendran H, Bates CM, O'Mahony C. Lichen sclerosus. Int J STD AIDS 2005; 16(7): 465-474, 474.
[http://dx.doi.org/10.1258/0956462054308440] [PMID: 16004624]

[175] Adams BB, Mutasim DF. Annular lichen sclerosus et atrophicus. Cutis 2001; 67(3): 249-50.
[PMID: 11270301]

[176] Marren P, Berker D, Millard P, Wojnarowska F. Bullous and haemorrhagic lichen sclerosus with scalp involvement. Clin Exp Dermatol 1992; 17(5): 354-6.
[http://dx.doi.org/10.1111/j.1365-2230.1992.tb00231.x] [PMID: 1458645]

[177] Ferreira FR, Santos LDN, Tagliarini FANM, Lira MLA. Porokeratosis of Mibelli literature review and a case report. An Bras Dermatol 2013; 88(6 suppl 1): 179-82.
[http://dx.doi.org/10.1590/abd1806-4841.20132721] [PMID: 24346913]

[178] Levine EG, Osztreicher P, Heymann WR. Sarcoidosis mimicking lichen sclerosus. Int J Dermatol 2005; 44(3): 238-9.
[http://dx.doi.org/10.1111/j.1365-4632.2004.02041.x] [PMID: 15807735]

[179] Errichetti E, Stinco G. Dermoscopy in General Dermatology: A Practical Overview. Dermatol Ther 2016; 6(4): 471-507.
[http://dx.doi.org/10.1007/s13555-016-0141-6] [PMID: 27613297]

[180] Brown AR, Dunlap CL, Bussard DA, Lask JT. Lichen sclerosus et atrophicus of the oral cavity. Oral Surg Oral Med Oral Pathol Oral Radiol Endod 1997; 84(2): 165-70.
[http://dx.doi.org/10.1016/S1079-2104(97)90064-0] [PMID: 9269018]

[181] Messadi DV, Waibel JS, Mirowski GW. White lesions of the oral cavity. Dermatol Clin 2003; 21(1): 63-78, vi.
[http://dx.doi.org/10.1016/S0733-8635(02)00069-4] [PMID: 12622269]

[182] Kirtschig G, Becker K, Günthert A, et al. Evidence-based (S3) Guideline on (anogenital) Lichen sclerosus. J Eur Acad Dermatol Venereol 2015; 29(10): e1-e43.
[http://dx.doi.org/10.1111/jdv.13136] [PMID: 26202852]

[183] Guerriero C, Manco S, Paradisi A, Capizzi R, Fossati B, Fabrizi G. Extragenital lichen sclerosus and atrophicus treated with topical steroids and retinoids in a child with vitiligo. Int J Immunopathol Pharmacol 2008; 21(3): 757-9.
[http://dx.doi.org/10.1177/039463200802100333] [PMID: 18831946]

[184] Guenther L, Lynde C, Poulin Y. Off-label use of topical calcineurin inhibitors in dermatologic disorders. J Cutan Med Surg 2019; 23(4_suppl): 27S-34S.
[http://dx.doi.org/10.1177/1203475419857668] [PMID: 31476936]

[185] Jablonowska O, Wozniacka A, Zebrowska A. Lichen sclerosus. Przegl Dermatol. 2021; 108:126–36.

[186] Kim GW, Park HJ, Kim HS, et al. Topical tacrolimus ointment for the treatment of lichen sclerosus, comparing genital and extragenital involvement. J Dermatol 2012; 39(2): 145-50.

[http://dx.doi.org/10.1111/j.1346-8138.2011.01384.x] [PMID: 22044240]

[187] Valdivielso-Ramos M, Bueno C, Hernanz JM. Significant improvement in extensive lichen sclerosus with tacrolimus ointment and PUVA. Am J Clin Dermatol 2008; 9(3): 175-9.
[http://dx.doi.org/10.2165/00128071-200809030-00006] [PMID: 18429647]

[188] Arican O, Ciralik H, Sasmaz S. Unsuccessful treatment of extragenital lichen sclerosus with topical 1% pimecrolimus cream. J Dermatol 2004; 31(12): 1014-7.
[http://dx.doi.org/10.1111/j.1346-8138.2004.tb00646.x] [PMID: 15801267]

[189] Kreuter A, Gambichler T, Sauermann K, Jansen T, Altmeyer P, Hoffmann K. Extragenital lichen sclerosus successfully treated with topical calcipotriol: evaluation by in vivo confocal laser scanning microscopy. Br J Dermatol 2002; 146(2): 332-3.
[http://dx.doi.org/10.1046/j.1365-2133.2002.4653_3.x] [PMID: 11903254]

[190] Kreuter A, Gambichler T, Avermaete A, et al. Low-dose ultraviolet A1 phototherapy for extragenital lichen sclerosus: Results of a preliminary study. J Am Acad Dermatol 2002; 46(2): 251-5.
[http://dx.doi.org/10.1067/mjd.2002.118552] [PMID: 11807437]

[191] Colbert RL, Chiang MP, Carlin CS, Fleming M. Progressive extragenital lichen sclerosus successfully treated with narrowband UV-B phototherapy. Arch Dermatol 2007; 143(1): 19-20.
[http://dx.doi.org/10.1001/archderm.143.1.19] [PMID: 17224537]

[192] Kreuter A, Gambichler T. Narrowband UV-B phototherapy for extragenital lichen sclerosus. Arch Dermatol 2007; 143(9): 1209.
[http://dx.doi.org/10.1001/archderm.143.9.1213-a] [PMID: 17875895]

[193] Motegi SI, Sekiguchi A, Fujiwara C, Yamazaki S, Ishikawa O. Extragenital lichen sclerosus successfully treated with narrowband-UVB phototherapy. Eur J Dermatol 2018; 28(5): 710-1.
[PMID: 30325310]

[194] Herz-Ruelas ME, Barboza-Quintana O, Cuéllar-Barboza A, Cárdenas-de la Garza JA, Gómez-Flores M. Acral bullous lichen sclerosus intolerant to UVA□1 successfully treated with narrowband ultraviolet B phototherapy. Photodermatol Photoimmunol Photomed 2019; 35(5): 378-80.
[http://dx.doi.org/10.1111/phpp.12478] [PMID: 31062884]

[195] von Kobyletzki G, Freitag M, Hoffmann K, Altmeyer P, Kerscher M. Balneophotochemotherapie mit 8-Methoxypsoralen bei Lichen sclerosus et atrophicus. Hautarzt 1997; 48(7): 488-91.
[http://dx.doi.org/10.1007/s001050050615] [PMID: 9333629]

[196] Dalmau J, Baselga E, Roé E, Alomar A. Psoralen-UVA treatment for generalized prepubertal extragenital lichen sclerosus et atrophicus. J Am Acad Dermatol. 2006; 55(2 Suppl): S56-8.

[197] Nayeemuddin F, Yates VM. Lichen sclerosus et atrophicus responding to methotrexate. Clin Exp Dermatol 2008; 33(5): 651-2.
[http://dx.doi.org/10.1111/j.1365-2230.2008.02721.x] [PMID: 18507666]

[198] Ürün M, Gürsel Ürün Y, Sarıkaya Solak S. A case of extragenital linear lichen sclerosus along the lines of Blaschko responding to methotrexate. Acta Dermatovenerol Alp Panonica Adriat 2020; 29(3): 149-51.
[PMID: 32975302]

[199] Kreuter A, Tigges C, Gaifullina R, Kirschke J, Altmeyer P, Gambichler T. Pulsed high-dose corticosteroids combined with low-dose methotrexate treatment in patients with refractory generalized extragenital lichen sclerosus. Arch Dermatol 2009; 145(11): 1303-8.
[http://dx.doi.org/10.1001/archdermatol.2009.235] [PMID: 19917961]

[200] Cuellar-Barboza A, Bashyam AM, Ghamrawi RI, Aickara D, Feldman SR, Pichardo RO. Methotrexate for the treatment of recalcitrant genital and extragenital lichen sclerosus: A retrospective series. Dermatol Ther 2020; 33(4): e13473.
[http://dx.doi.org/10.1111/dth.13473] [PMID: 32347617]

[201] Taveira M, Selores M, Costa V, Massa A. Generalized morphea and lichen sclerosus et atrophicus

successfully treated with sulphasalazine. J Eur Acad Dermatol Venereol 1999; 12(3): 283-4.
[http://dx.doi.org/10.1111/j.1468-3083.1999.tb01053.x] [PMID: 10461662]

[202] Breier F, Khanakah G, Stanek G, *et al.* Isolation and polymerase chain reaction typing of Borrelia afzelii from a skin lesion in a seronegative patient with generalized ulcerating bullous lichen sclerosus et atrophicus. Br J Dermatol 2001; 144(2): 387-92.
[http://dx.doi.org/10.1046/j.1365-2133.2001.04034.x] [PMID: 11251580]

[203] Madan V, Cox NH. Extensive bullous lichen sclerosus with scarring alopecia. Clin Exp Dermatol 2009; 34(3): 360-2.
[http://dx.doi.org/10.1111/j.1365-2230.2008.02919.x] [PMID: 19018788]

[204] Penneys NS. Treatment of lichen sclerosus with potassium para-aminobenzoate. J Am Acad Dermatol 1984; 10(6): 1039-42.
[http://dx.doi.org/10.1016/S0190-9622(84)80332-1] [PMID: 6736322]

[205] Buxton PK, Priestley GC. Para-aminobenzoate in lichen sclerosus et atrophicus. J Dermatolog Treat 1990; 1(5): 255-6.
[http://dx.doi.org/10.3109/09546639009086746]

[206] Ronger S, Viallard AM, Meunier-Mure F, Chouvet B, Balme B, Thomas L. Oral calcitriol: a new therapeutic agent in cutaneous lichen sclerosis. J Drugs Dermatol 2003; 2(1): 23-8.
[PMID: 12852377]

[207] Bulbul Baskan E, Turan H, Tunali S, Toker SC, Saricaoglu H. Open-label trial of cyclosporine for vulvar lichen sclerosus. J Am Acad Dermatol 2007; 57(2): 276-8.
[http://dx.doi.org/10.1016/j.jaad.2007.03.006] [PMID: 17442452]

[208] Tomson N, Sterling JC. Hydroxycarbamide: a treatment for lichen sclerosus? Br J Dermatol 2007; 157(3): 622.
[http://dx.doi.org/10.1111/j.1365-2133.2007.07991.x] [PMID: 17553032]

[209] Passeron T, Lacour JP, Ortonne JP. Comparative treatment of extragenital lichen sclerosus with methylaminolevulinic Acid pulsed dye laser-mediated photodynamic therapy or pulsed dye laser alone. Dermatol Surg 2009; 35(5): 878-80.
[http://dx.doi.org/10.1111/j.1524-4725.2009.01148.x] [PMID: 19389089]

[210] Greve B, Hartschuh W, Raulin C. Extragenitaler Lichen sclerosus et atrophicus. Behandlung durch gepulsten Farbstofflaser. Hautarzt 1999; 50(11): 805-8.
[http://dx.doi.org/10.1007/s001050050988] [PMID: 10591791]

[211] Alexiades-Armenakas M. Laser-mediated photodynamic therapy of lichen sclerosus. J Drugs Dermatol 2004; 3(6) (Suppl.): S25-7.
[PMID: 15624739]

[212] Ioannides D, Lazaridou E, Apalla Z, Sotiriou E, Gregoriou S, Rigopoulos D. Acitretin for severe lichen sclerosus of male genitalia: A randomized, placebo controlled study. J Urol 2010; 183(4): 1395-9.
[http://dx.doi.org/10.1016/j.juro.2009.12.057] [PMID: 20171665]

[213] Bousema MT, Romppanen U, Geiger J-M, *et al.* Acitretin in the treatment of severe lichen sclerosus et atrophicus of the vulva: A double-blind, placebo-controlled study. J Am Acad Dermatol 1994; 30(2): 225-31.
[http://dx.doi.org/10.1016/S0190-9622(94)70021-4] [PMID: 8288782]

[214] Basak PY, Basak K. Lichen sclerosus et atrophicus of the scalp: Satisfactory response to acitretin. J Eur Acad Dermatol Venereol 2002; 16(2): 183-5.
[http://dx.doi.org/10.1046/j.1468-3083.2002.00392_10.x] [PMID: 12046836]

[215] Formiga AdeA, Torres IdeS, Rocha BdeO, *et al.* Disseminated extragenital lichen sclerosus et atrophicus treated with acitretin. Skinmed 2014; 12(1): 62-3.
[PMID: 24720089]

[216] Wakelin SH, James MP. Extensive lichen sclerosus et atrophicus with bullae and ulceration-improvement with hydroxychloroquine. Clin Exp Dermatol 1994; 19(4): 332-4.
[http://dx.doi.org/10.1111/j.1365-2230.1994.tb01208.x] [PMID: 7955478]

[217] García-Doval I, Peteiro C, Sánchez-Aguilar D, Toribio J. Extensive bullous lichen sclerosus et atrophicus unresponsive to hydroxychloroquine. Clin Exp Dermatol 1996; 21(3): 247.
[http://dx.doi.org/10.1111/j.1365-2230.1996.tb00081.x] [PMID: 8914380]

[218] Sergeant A, Vernall N, Mackintosh LJ, McHenry P, Leman JA. Squamous cell carcinoma arising in extragenital lichen sclerosus. Clin Exp Dermatol 2009; 34(7): e278-9.
[http://dx.doi.org/10.1111/j.1365-2230.2008.03195.x] [PMID: 19438563]

[219] Sotillo Gago I, Martínez Sahuquillo A, Matilla A, García Pérez A. Epitelioma espinocelular sobre liquen escleroatrófico cutáneo. Spinocellular epithelioma following scleroatrophic autoaneous licher. Actas Dermosifiliogr 1977; 68(3-4): 219-20.
[PMID: 868604]

Pediatric Morphea

Katarzyna Wolska-Gawron[1] and **Dorota Krasowska**[1,*]

[1] *Department of Dermatology, Venereology and Pediatric Dermatology, Medical University of Lublin, Lublin, Poland*

Chapter synopsis.
• Morphea is a rare autoimmune disease characterized by inflammation and limited sclerosis of the skin and underlying tissues.
• Pediatric morphea represents about 15% of all morphea cases and most frequently affects children aged 7-10 years, especially girls.
• The etiopathogenesis of morphea has not been fully revealed. However, it is assumed that genetic and environmental factors as well as immunological and vascular disorders are involved.
• Pediatric morphea is divided into five clinical types: linear, circumscribed, mixed, generalized, and disabling pansclerotic.
• The clinical course of the disease includes three stages: early inflammation, progressive sclerosis and atrophy.
• Management of morphea is based on the clinical type of the disease, its severity and activity, the extent of skin lesions, and the patient's age.

Keywords: Childhood morphea, Clinical types, Circumscribed morphea, Classification, Diagnosis, Deep morphea, Differential diagnosis, En coup de sabre, Extracutaneous manifestations, Generalized morphea, Lilac ring, Linear morphea, Juvenile localized scleroderma, Mixed morphea, Morphea in children, Monitoring, Morbidity, Management, Parry-Romberg syndrome, Pediatric morphea.

INTRODUCTION

Morphea is a rare autoimmune disease characterized by inflammation and limited sclerosis of the skin and underlying tissues (subcutaneous tissue, fascia, muscles, and bones). Morphea is most common among women (2,6-6 times more often), with the peak incidence among 40-50 years [1].

---

* **Corresponding author Dorota Krasowska:** Department of Dermatology, Venereology and Pediatric Dermatology, Medical University of Lublin, Lublin, Poland; E-mail: dor.krasowska@gmail.com

Pediatric morphea represents about 15% of all morphea cases and most frequently affects children aged 7-10 years, especially girls [2, 3]. Nonetheless, rare cases of congenital morphea have been described (about 0.8% of all morphea cases) [4]. The estimated prevalence of pediatric morphea is 0.34-2.7 cases/100,000/year, however, the real incidence can be higher due to differential difficulties [5]. The clinical manifestation of pediatric morphea is varied based on the disease activity and the extent of tissue involvement [1]. The clinical course of the disease includes three stages: early inflammation, progressive sclerosis and atrophy [3, 6]. The most common clinical type of pediatric morphea (linear morphea) requires prompt immunosuppressive therapy, otherwise it may lead to irreversible orthopedic sequelae [2].The disease is typically diagnosed on the basis of its clinical picture, however, in case of any doubts, a histopathological examination should be performed [7].

ETIOPATHOGENESIS

The etiopathogenesis of morphea has not been fully elucidated. However, it is assumed that genetic and environmental factors as well as immunological and vascular disorders are involved (Fig. **19.1**) [8, 9]. Latest reports have shown human leucocyte antigens such as HLA-B*37, HLA-DR5, HLA-DR8, HLA-DR11; individual and/or a family history of autoimmune diseases predispose to the development of morphea [8, 9]. Moreover, epigenetic factors (*i.e.* decreased DNA methylation and histone acetylation, changed expression of individual miRNA molecules, *e.g.* miRNA-181b-5p, miRNA-223-3p, miRNA-210-3p, let 7i-5p, miRNA-21-5p) are no less important [10]. A number of external factors contribute to morphea onset in susceptible patients – *i.e.* injuries (surgery, injection, tooth extraction, vaccination, insect bites), repeated friction (especially along waistline, groins) and drug use (bisoprolol, bleomycin, D-penicillamine, TNF-α inhibitors) [9]. The above mentioned factors can activate keratinocytes for inflammatory mediators release, which then stimulate immune cells, including lymphocytes, endothelial cells and fibroblasts [9]. Consequently, the production of extracellular matrix increases, what clinically manifests as skin fibrosis and sclerosis [9].

CLINICAL PRESENTATION

According to Pediatric Rheumatology European Society, pediatric morphea is divided into five clinical types: linear, circumscribed, mixed, generalized, and disabling pansclerotic (Table **19.1**) [2, 11]. The differences between morphea in children and adults are presented in (Table **19.2**) [12].

Predisposing factors (genetic)

- HLA (DRB1*04:04, B*37)
- Mosaicism
- Autoimmune medical history (patient/family)

External factors

Epigenetic factors
- miRNA, *e.g.* ↓ miR-7, miR-196a
- Decreased DNA methylation and histone acetylation

Generating factors
- Injury/surgical procedure
- Injections/vaccinations
- Insect bites
- Radiation therapy
- Drugs

FGF receptor 1,2

Epidermis

TLR-4

Keratinocyte
TGF-β, IL-I, IL-6, TNF-α, PDGF, FGF, CCL-2, SI00A9, endothelin, fibrillin-I, α-melanotropin, FLII

Dermis

Dermis-epidermis signal paths
(Wnt jagged Notch)

Endothelial cell

VCAM-I, ICAM-I, E-selectin, t-PA, PAI- I

Damage/activation of the endothelium

Fibroblast

PDGF, CTGF, TGF-β, FGF

IL-1, IL-2, IL-4, IL-6, IL-13, IL-17B, IL-22, TNF-α, TGF-β

Lymphocyte

Production of extracellular matrix
(type I and type III collagen)

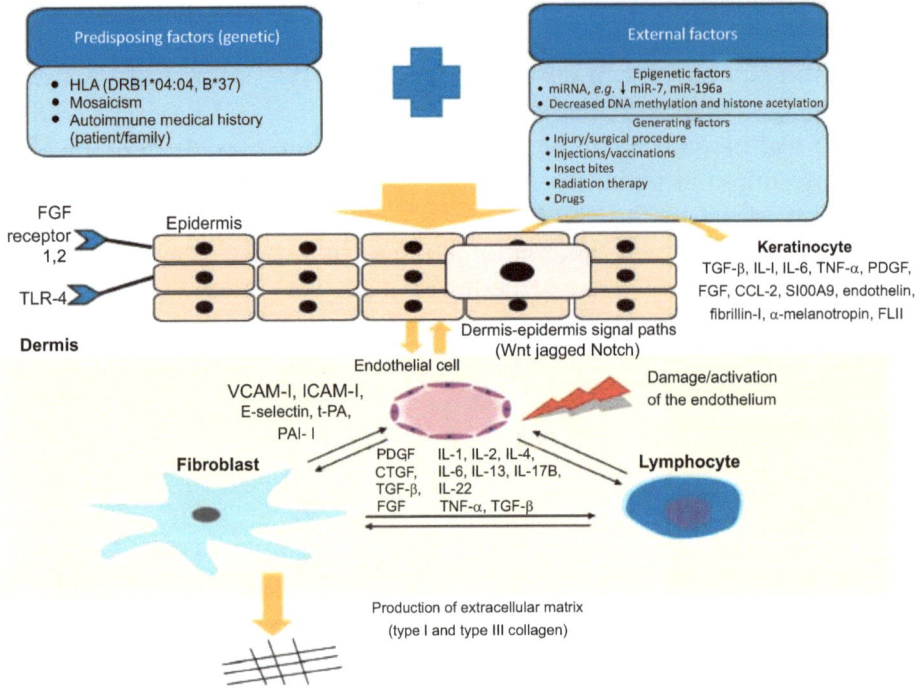

Fig. (19.1). The etiopathogenesis of morphea [8].

Table 19.1. Classification of pediatric morphea published by Pediatric Rheumatology European Society [2, 11].

Type of Morphea	Subtype of Morphea		Description	
Linear	Of extremities		linear, band-like sclerotic lesions occurring along Blaschko's lines	
	Of head and neck	En coup de sabre		
		Progressive facial hemiatrophy/		
Circumscribed	Superficial		Oval/round lesions of >1 cm in diameter, occurring in 1 or 2 different anatomical locations	Involving epidermis and dermis
	Deep			Involving deep layers of the skin, subcutaneous tissue, muscle
Mixed			linear + circumscribed linear + generalized	
Generalized			≥ 4 areas of skin induration, ≥ 3 cm in diameter, in ≥ 2 anatomic sites.	
Pansclerotic			Circumferential involvement of limb(s) affecting the epidermis, dermis, subcutaneous tissue, muscle and bone.	

Table 19.2. Differentiation between morphea in children and adults [12].

Clinical Feature	Children	Adults
Age of onset	7-10 years	20-40 years
Most common clinical type of morphea	Linear	Plaque
Prognosis	Poorer	Better
Orthopedic sequelae	More frequent	Less frequent
Extracutaneous manifestations	More frequent	Less frequent

Linear Morphea

It is the most common type of pediatric morphea representing about 50% of all cases [2]. It manifests with at least one band of sclerosis following Blaschko lines, usually distributed unilaterally, affecting extremities, head and neck. Linear pediatric morphea has severe course and may lead to irreversible sequelae, unless immunosuppressive treatment is introduced at time [3, 11].

Linear Pediatric Morphea Involving Extremities

Linear pediatric morphea involving extremities most commonly affects lower limbs, however upper extremities may also be involved (Fig. **19.2**). The risk of orthopedic complications (joint mobility restrictions, contractures, limb asymmetry, limb atrophy, growth disorders) is estimated at 30-50%, especially when morphea lesions are distributed near the joints [3, 13, 14]. Articular symptoms do not always correlate with the distribution of skin lesions [12].

Linear Pediatric Morphea of Head and Neck

Linear pediatric morphea of head and neck manifests as en coup de sabre (ECDS) or Parry-Romberg syndrome (PRS) / progressive hemifacial atrophy (PHA). Most consider these subtypes as the same spectrum of the disease due to frequent coexistence (24-48% of cases) [2]. Both ECDS and PRS were commonly acknowledged self-limiting, with the active disease stage persisting 2-10 years prior to "burnout", although latest studies have revealed that its recurrence is alike to other autoimmune disorders [15].

En Coup De Sabre

En coup de sabre usually presents as a linear, unilateral depression on the frontoparietal scalp or paramedian forehead, resembling "stroke from a sword" (Fig. **19.3**) [16]. It advances through the stages of inflammation, sclerosis, and atrophy, frequently ranging from the eyebrow to the scalp, with cicatricial alopecia development (Fig. **19.4**) [16, 17]. Nonetheless, cases of ECDS spreading below the eyebrows with the involvement of the eyelids, eyelashes or the skin of the nose have been reported [17]. In rare cases, double lines may occur [18].

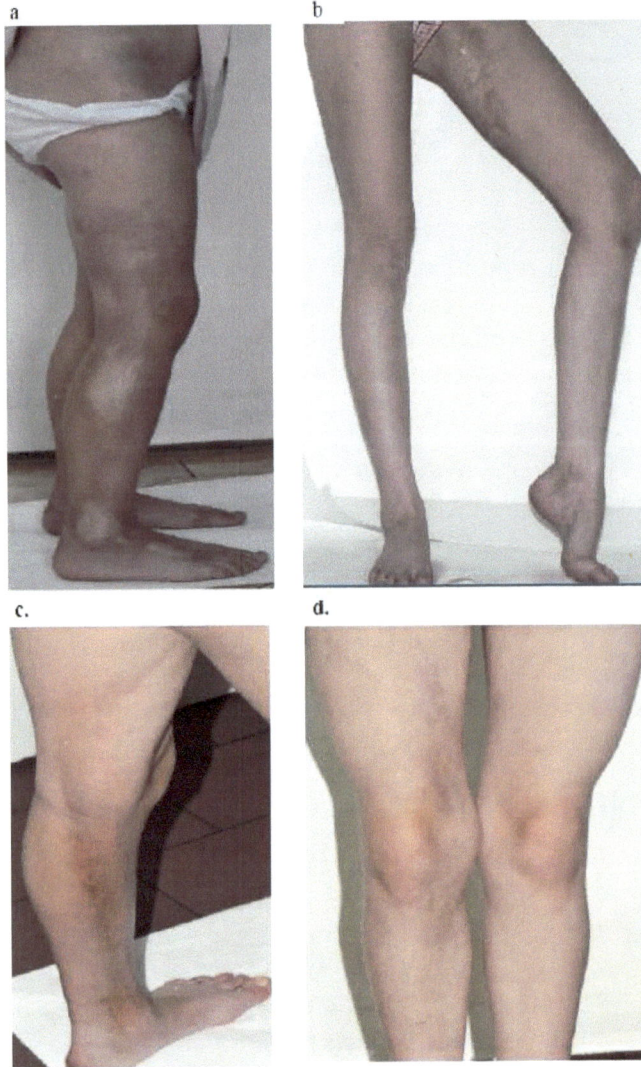

Fig. (19.2). Children with linear morphea of extremities. **a**) Linear sclerotic band with hyperpigmentation extending from the right hip to the foot. **b**) Linear sclerotic plaque with associated hyperpigmentation and atrophy on the inner left thigh and the medial malleolus. **c**) Linear sclerotic plaque distributed on the medial part of the left lower leg. d) Dermal atrophy on the right lower extremity with sclerotic plaques above and below the knee.

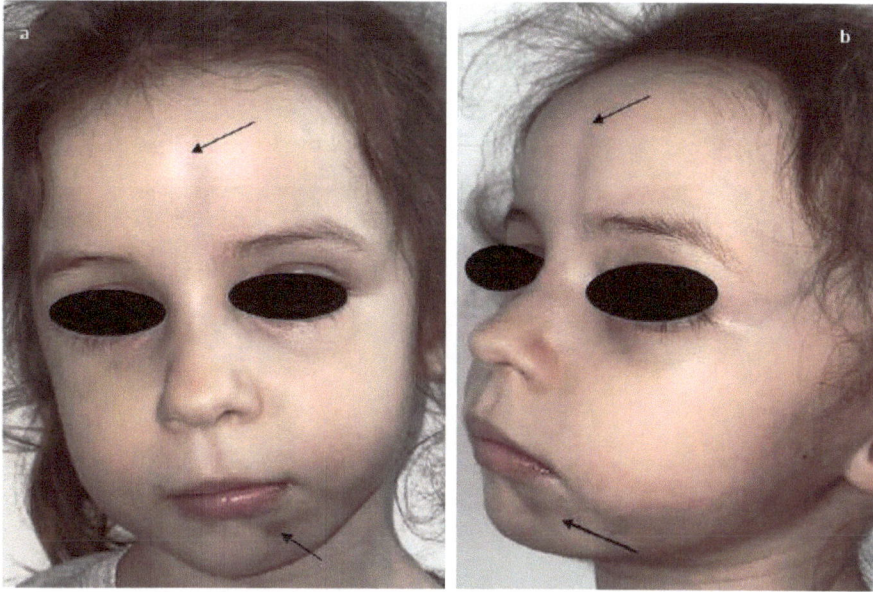

Fig. (19.3). En coup de sabre. Unilateral depression on paramedian forehead and visible atrophy on left side of chin **a)** frontal view; **b)** lateral view.

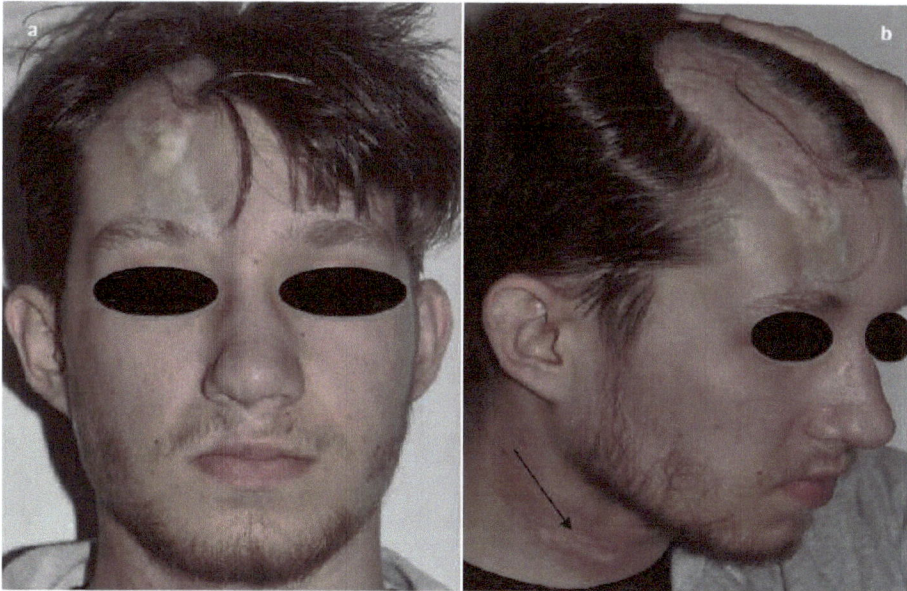

Fig. (19.4). En coup de sabre with associated circumscribed plaque morphea. **a)** Sclerosis and atrophy extending from the right eyebrow to the scalp with associated cicatricial alopecia of the scalp. **b)** Circumscribed plaque morphea on neck characterized by ivory white sclerosis.

Parry-Romberg Syndrome

Parry-romberg syndrome is characterized by progressive unilateral atrophy of the skin, soft tissues of the face and bones (Figs. **19.5** and **19.6**). Generally, PRS is restricted to one half of the face but in 20% of patients may broaden to other parts of the body including ipsilateral or contralateral trunk, upper and lower extremities [19, 20]. The disease usually progresses slowly and the defect becomes more pronounced over years [16]. PRS has been described in detail in chapter 17.

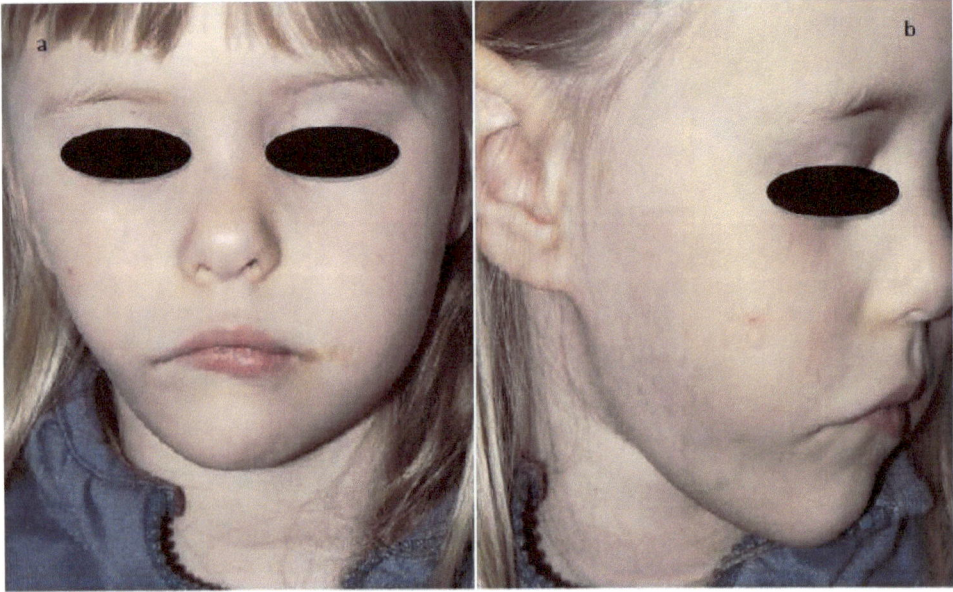

Fig. (19.5). Parry Romberg syndrome. Unilateral atrophy of skin and soft tissues involving the right cheek and chin. **a**) Frontal view, **b**) lateral view

Most authors claim that cutaneous sclerosis, hyperpigmentation and alopecia usually develop in the ECDS, while PRS does not show skin thickening at any stage [21]. Both patients with ECDS and PRS are at risk of developing neurologic (seizures, headache, migraine, hemiparesis, stroke, cognitive decline, intracranial vessel anomalies, dysarthria, aphasia, learning disabilities, behavioral disorders), ocular (enophthalmos, uveitis, white uveitis, episcleritis, strabismus, orbital cavity defects, lid atrophy, diplopia, Horner's syndrome, mydriasis, blindness) and odontostomatologic complications (unilateral tongue atrophy, jaw hypoplasia, short roots on affected side, unilateral cross bite, deficiency of soft and hard palate, wasting of masticatory muscles) [15, 22 - 29]. In 70-75% of cases, ocular and neurological symptoms correlate with the distribution of skin lesions [12]. However, in some cases, extracutaneous manifestations may anticipate prominent cutaneous development setting up challenge to dermatologists. The differentiation between en coup de sabre and PRS is presented in (Table **19.3**) [16, 30].

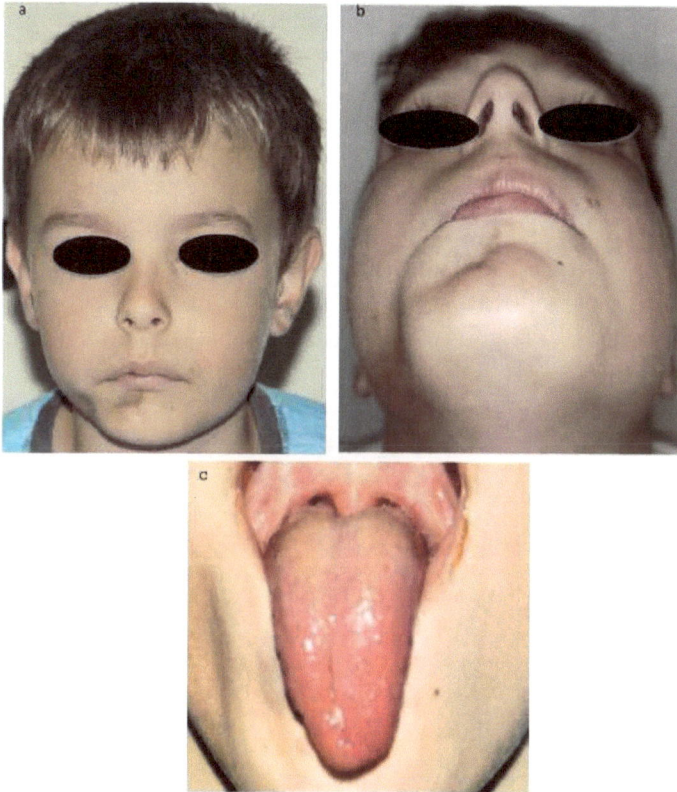

Fig. (19.6). Progressive facial hemiatrophy involving right side of the face (**a**, **b**). Right hemi-glossal atrophy (**c**).

Table 19.3. Differentiation between en coup de sabre and PRS [16, 30].

Clinical Feature	En Coup De Sabre	Progressive Facial Hemiatrophy
Characteristics of skin lesions	Sclerosis Hyperpigmentation	Atrophy
Typical distribution of lesions	Forehead, scalp	Nose, cheek
Alopecia	Present	Absent
Neurological involvement	Present	Present
Ocular involvement	Present	Present
Oral cavity involvement	Present	Present

Circumscribed Morphea

involves about 26–37% of patients and is characterized by the presence of multiple oval/round lesions with the diameter > 1 cm, restricting to the dermis (superficial subtype) or affecting deeper tissues (deep subtype) [2, 31]. At the beginning of the disease, lesions present as erythematous macules with porcelain-yellow sclerosis in the middle part, sometimes surrounded by inflammatory border (lilac rings) (Fig. **19.7**) [2, 31]. Over time, they become atrophic and dyspigmented (hyper-/hypopigmented), accompanied by telangiectasia in some cases (Fig. **19.8**) [2, 32]. The typical distribution of circumscribed morphea lesions include the skin of the trunk, groins and lower back [3].Deep morphea is characterized by the presence of sclerosis found within the deep layers of the skin, subcutaneous tissue, fasciae and muscles; usually distributed symmetrically on the extremities (Fig. **19.9**).

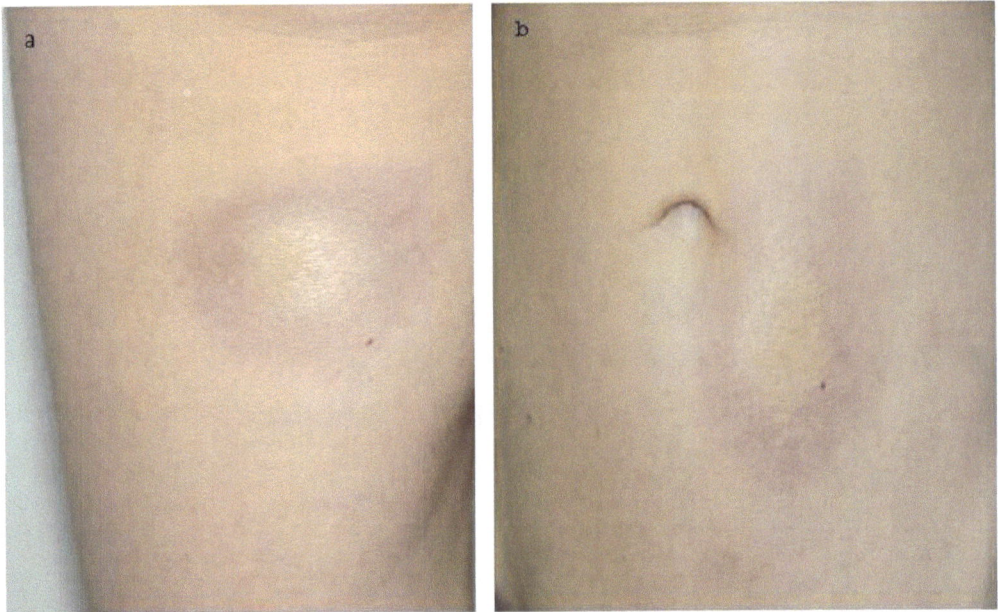

Fig. (19.7). Erythematous plaque with porcelain-yellow sclerosis in the center, surrounded by lilac ring localized on the thigh (**a**) and the abdomen (**b**).

Mixed Morphea

in children represents about 15% of all pediatric morphea cases. It manifests by a combination of clinical features typical for at least two subtypes of morphea (principally linear morphea and circumscribed morphea) [33, 34] (Fig. **19.10**).

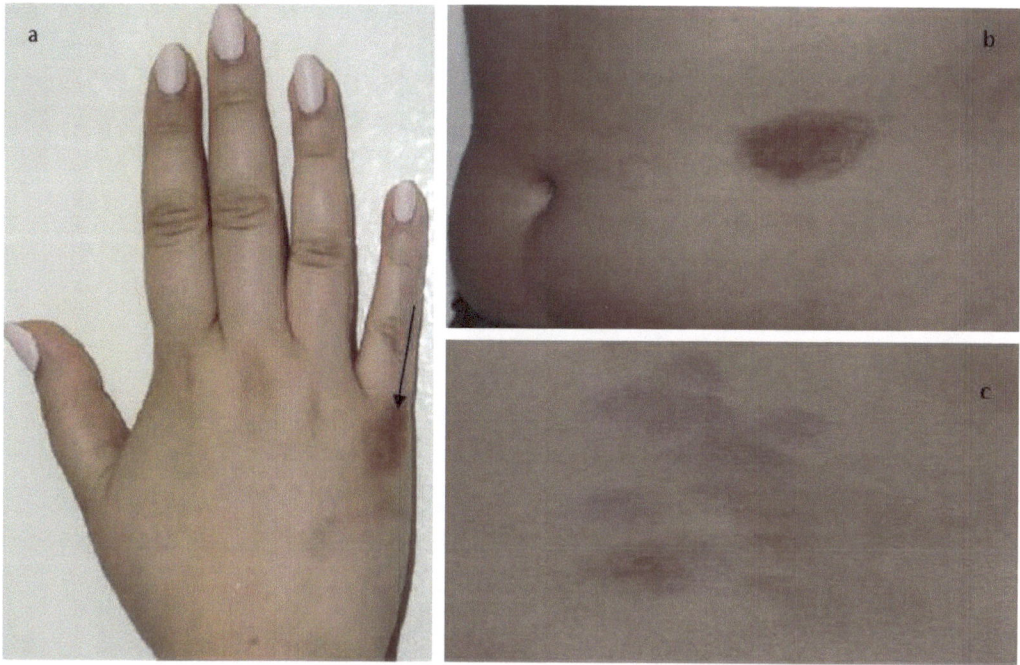

Fig. (19.8). Hyperpigmented indurated plaques in the course of circumscribed morphea localized on the right hand (**a**), abdomen (**b**) and back (**c**).

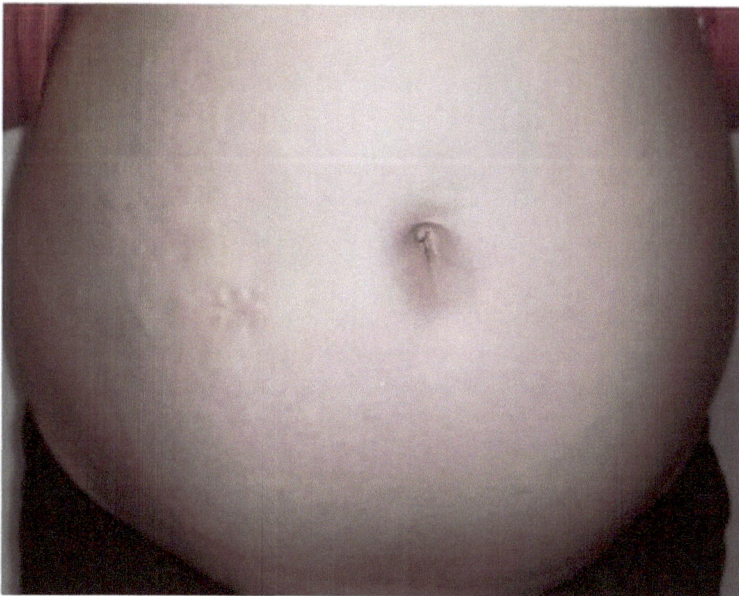

Fig. (19.9). Deep morphea involving abdomen. Sclerosis was found within the deep layers of the skin and subcutaneous tissue

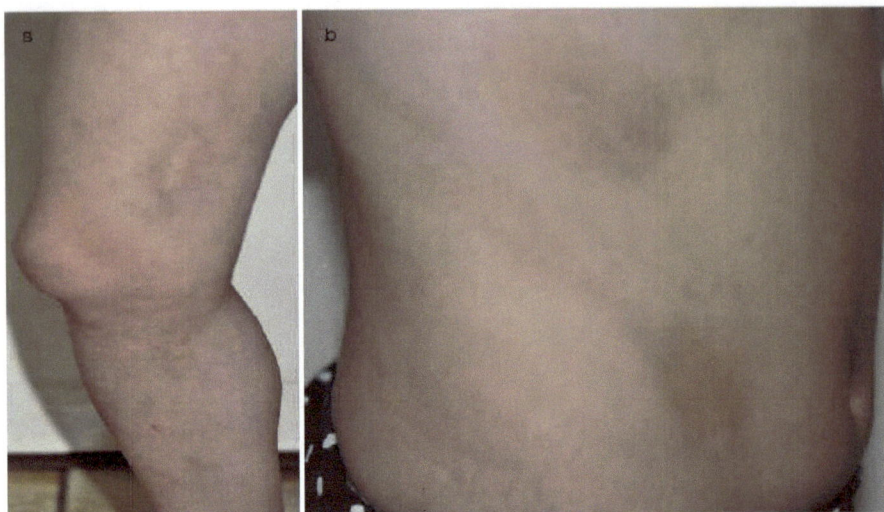

Fig. (19.10). Mixed morphea having Coexisting linear (**a**) and circumscribed (**b**) morphea in the same patient

Generalized Morphea

is rare in children (7–8% of cases) and manifests with the presence of ≥4 sclerotic areas with a diameter of ≥3 cm that affects ≥2/7 anatomical areas (head and neck, front trunk, back trunk, right upper limb, left upper limb, right lower limb, left lower limb) (Figs. **19.11** and **19.12**) [5]. Some authors set a threshold for the involvement of at least 30% of body surface [2]. Generalized morphea frequently involves the trunk and limbs, sparing the face, palms and feet [24]. Skin lesions may be accompanied by the systemic symptoms such as fatigue, muscle or joint pain.

Disabling Pansclerotic Scleroderma

is a rare (1–2% of cases) and very severe type of morphea, which mainly affects pediatric patients [1, 2]. It manifests with circumferential, full-thickness involvement of the skin, subcutaneous tissues, muscles and bones, affecting the trunk, limbs, head, without palms and soles [2]. Extensive sclerotic areas may drive to contractures and progress to disability [2, 3]. Children with disabling pansclerotic scleroderma have impaired wound healing response, they suffer more often from ulcers, what makes them predisposed to develop squamous cell carcinoma (SCC) [3, 6].

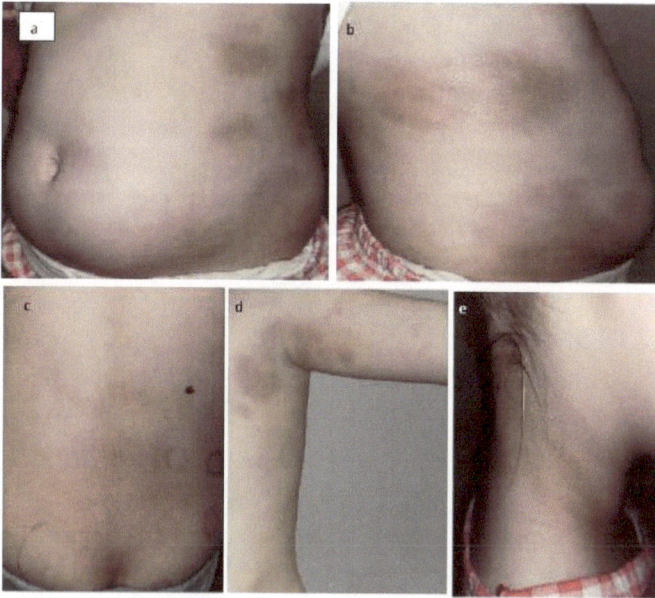

Fig. (19.11). Generalized morphea in a patient with disseminated erythematous and indurated plaques involving abdomen, chest, back, arm and neck (**a**, **b**, **c**, **d**, **e**). Some plaques have central ivory white sclerosis.

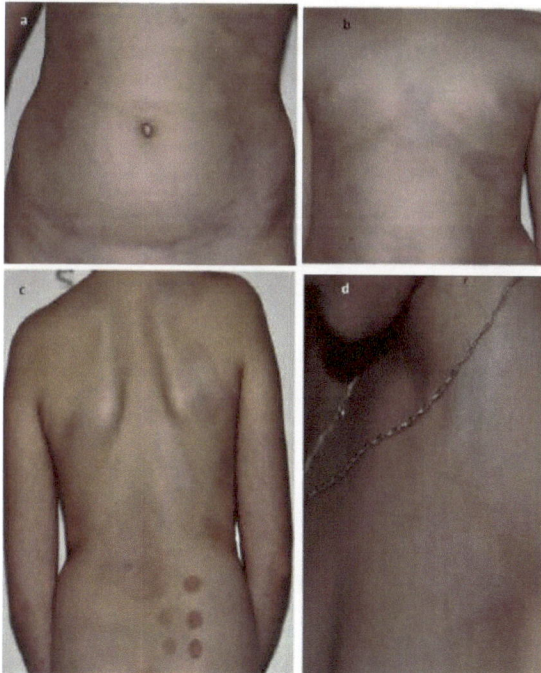

Fig. (19.12). Disseminated erythematous plaques with central sclerosis, surrounded by lilac rings distributed on the abdomen (**a**), chest (**b**), back (**c**) and neck (**d**).

European Dermatology Forum distinguishes idiopathic atrophoderma of Pasini and Pierini (IAPP)–a subtype of limited morphea which is a bit more common in children than adults [3, 34]. It manifests with a mild course and the development of oval, sharply demarcated, greyish brown lesions, either flat or slightly depressed, without accompanying skin induration (Fig. **19.13**) [6].They often arise symmetrically on the proximal parts of extremities and trunk, mainly affecting buttocks and lower back [1]. IAPP has been discussed in detail in chapter 15.

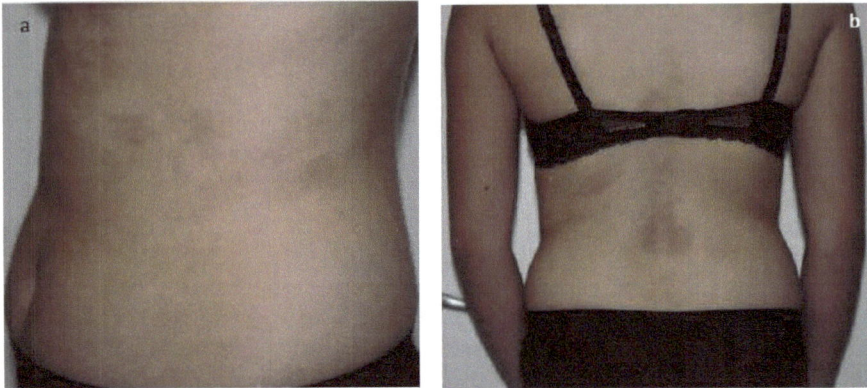

Fig. (19.13). Greyish brown flat lesions without accompanying skin induration distributed over the skin of the abdomen (**a**) and back (**b**).

EXTRACUTANEOUS MANIFESTATIONS.

Extracutaneous symptoms affect about 20-40% of children with morphea (Table **19.4**) [2, 15, 35]. Musculoskeletal manifestations are the most frequent among patients with linear, generalized and pansclerotic morphea, whereas eye and neurological involvement prevails in ECDS and PRS [2, 15, 35].

Table 19.4. Extracutaneous manifestations of pediatric morphea [2, 7, 15].

Organ/System	Frequency	Symptoms
Musculoskeletal system	19%	Joint pain, arthritis, contractures, limb asymmetry, scoliosis, odonto-stomatologic abnormalities
Nervous system	5%	Seizures, headaches, neuropathies, difficulties with concentration, learning disabilities, behavioral disorders
Eyes	3,2%	Uveitis, episcleritis, strabismus, enophthalmia, orbital cavity defects, lid atrophy
Gastrointestinal tract	<2%	
Respiratory tract	<2%	
Kidneys	<2%	

LABORATORY TESTS

Routine laboratory tests (Box **19.1**) in children with morphea include complete blood count, erythrocyte sedimentation rate (ESR) and C-reactive protein (CRP). Elevation of acute phase reactants is recognized during the early, inflammatory phase of the disease, especially in the course of linear and deep types [2, 7]. Peripheral blood eosinophilia is seen in up to 62% of patients with generalized, deep and linear morphea [1, 2]. Children presenting with muscle and joint symptoms, particularly along with the course of linear, generalized and deep morphea, as well as disabling pansclerotic morphea, may demonstrate elevated rheumatoid factor, aldolase, creatinine kinase and lactate dehydrogenase [2, 32, 34]. Evaluation of anti-unclear autoantibodies (ANA) and serological testing for Borrelia infection are no longer routinely recommended, as they are not disease-specific and do not correlate with the course of morphea [1, 7].

Box 19.1. Laboratory tests [2, 7].
• Complete blood count, CRP, ESR – routine laboratory tests.
• Rheumatoid factor, aldolase, creatinine kinase, lactate dehydrogenase –recommended in case of muscle and joint symptoms.
• Anti-unclear autoantibodies, serological testing for Borrelia infection - no longer routinely recommended.

MONITORING OF THE DISEASE

Based on current knowledge, it is not recommended to perform routine diagnostic tests for internal organ involvement in every child with morphea [1, 7]. Pediatric patients with the most severe morphea types (linear and generalized morphea, disabling pansclerotic scleroderma), revealing manifestations of systemic organ involvement, should undergo appropriate imaging deemed by the clinician. Children with linear morphea of extremities require regular rheumatologic assessment of the risk of developing bone and joint sequelae [7]. The involvement of the head and neck in the course of progressive facial hemiatrophy and en coup de sabre demand assessment of the central nervous system (CNS), eyes, temporomandibular joints (TMJ) and teeth based on the pattern presented in Table **19.5** [7, 15, 35]. "White uveitis" is the inflammation without prominent symptoms of eye involvement, diagnosed in about 3.2–8.3% of the patients with Juvenile localized scleroderma JLS [7]. Choroid assessment in the slit lamp is recommended every 6 months (ECDS, PRS) or every 12 months (other types of JLS sparing head) for the first 4 years of the disease [7].

Table 19.5. Monitoring the course of pediatric morphea [7, 15, 35].

Clinical type of JLS	Extracutaneous Manifestations	Imaging/Consultations	Frequency
Linear JLS of the head and neck	CNS	Neurological assessment with MRI	At the time of diagnosis and repeated upon appearance of neurologic symptoms.
	Eyes	Ophthalmic assessment with choroid examination in the slit lamp.	Every 6 months for the first 4 years of the disease.
	TMJ and teeth	Dental evaluation with panoramic radiograph and rheumatologic assessment (if applicable with MRI).	Every 6 months.
Linear JLS of the limbs	Joints	Rheumatologic assessment MRI.	When the lesion crosses the joint.
Others	Eyes	Choroid examination in the slit lamp.	Every 12 months for the first 4 years of the disease.

JLS: Juvenile localized scleroderma; TMJ: Temporomandibular joint.

DIAGNOSIS

The diagnosis of pediatric morphea is based on its typical clinical appearance and exclusion of other diseases manifesting with a similar clinical picture [7]. In case of any doubts, a histopathological examination of a skin biopsy should be performed [7].

DIFFERENTIAL DIAGNOSIS

The differential diagnosis of the pediatric morphea based on the type of JLS and its clinical stage is presented in Table **19.6** [3, 34].

Table 19.6. Differential diagnosis of the pediatric morphea [3, 34].

Type of Pediatric Morphea		Differential Diagnosis
Linear		Panniculitis, progressive lipodystrophy, localized lipodystrophy, steroid atrophy, lupus erythematosus profundus.
Circumscribed	Erythematous plaques with lilac ring.	Erythema migrans, fixed erythema, hemangioma, granuloma annulare, cutaneous mastocytosis.
	Skin thickening.	Lichen sclerosus, necrobiosis lipoidica.
	Dyspigmentation.	Vitiligo, café au lait spots, post-inflammatory hyperpigmentation, lichen planus actinicus.
	Atrophy.	Scarring, acrodermatitis chronic atrophicans, lichen sclerosus.

(Table 19.6) cont.....

Type of Pediatric Morphea	Differential Diagnosis
Generalized	Graft versus host disease, systemic sclerosis, mixed connective tissue, nephrogenic systemic fibrosis, scleromyxedema, pseudoscleroderma.
Pansclerotic	Systemic sclerosis.

TREATMENT

The evaluation of disease activity and severity is pivotal in children with morphea to introduce the convenient treatment regimen [1]. Moreover, assessing the disease activity is crucial to evaluate the response to therapy. Management of morphea is based on the clinical type of the disease, its severity and activity, the extent of skin lesions and patient's age [36].

Pediatric Morphea with a Mild Course

Circumscribed superficial morphea and atrophoderma of Pasini and Pierini are generally of cosmetic concern [35]. Pediatric patients with limited skin involvement respond well to the topical therapy (Box **19.2**) [7]. Topical corticosteroids (TC) are efficient in the therapy of active, inflammatory lesions, however, the potency of TC should be adjusted to the age of the child. Some experts emphasize that the use of TC ought to be limited for the risk of skin atrophy [7].Calcineurin inhibitors and calcipotriol, applied in monotherapy or combination twice daily for 3 months (preferably under occlusion), are the treatment of choice [1, 36]. Topical imiquimod may be used to reduce skin thickening of circumscribed morphea [35]. Localized, small and non-progressive lesions without crossing a joint, can be managed by UVA-1 phototherapy or narrowband UVB. This treatment option is available for children above the age of 12. PUVA-therapy is not recommended in pediatric morphea due to its probable carcinogenic effect.

Box 19.2. Treatment of pediatric morphea with a mild course [7, 35].
• Topical corticosteroids
• Topical calcineurin inhibitors
• Topical calcipotriol
• Topical imiquimod
• Phototherapy (UVA-1 or UVB narrowband)

Pediatric Morphea with a Severe Course

Severe cases of JLS with expanded tissue involvement (linear morphea of the extremities, en coup se sabre, Parry-Romberg syndrome, generalized morphea, disabling pansclerotic scleroderma) require immunosuppressive therapy (Box **19.3**) upon diagnosis, before markers of tissue damage appear (hyperpigmentation, atrophy of the skin and subcutaneous tissue) [35, 36]. According to current recommendations, patients with JLS which involve significant cosmetic defects or sclerotic patches distributed over the skin of the joins, demand prompt introduction of methotrexate (MTX) [7, 35, 37]. MTX should be used in monotherapy or in combination with corticosteroids taken orally or intravenously. A recommended MTX dose in pediatric patients is 15 mg/m^2/week (max. 25 mg/week), given orally or subcutaneously for at least 1 year [3, 7, 34]. The dose of corticosteroids ought to be adjusted to the route of administration and a patient's body weight – prednisone administered orally at the dose of 0.5–2 mg/kg/day in 2–3 divided doses (max 60 mg/day) for 2–4 weeks with consecutive stepwise dose reduction; intravenous pulses of methylprednisolone at the dose of 30 mg/kg/day (max 1g) in concordance with one out of two regimens (for 3 following days along 3–6 months or 1 dose/week for 12 months [7]. In the absence of clinical response after 3 months therapy or presence of disease activity markers (appearance of new lesions or enlargement of existing lesions, lilac ring, skin induration) after 6 months, a modification in the treatment regimen should be introduced [7]. The second-line treatment for severe JLS include mycophenolate mofetil (MMF). In agreement with CARRA recommendations, the drug dose should be customized to a patient's body weight: <40 kg - 600 mg/m^2 twice a day; 40-50 kg– 750 mg/m^2 twice a day; >50 kg/m^2 - 1,000 mg/m^2 twice a day [36, 38].

Box 19.3. Treatment of pediatric morphea with a severe course [35, 36].
• Methotrexate
• Corticosteroids
• Mycophenolate mofetil
• Surgical management

Surgical management is devoted for children with severe types of JLS, complicated by limb asymmetry, joint contractures or cosmetic defects induced by atrophic lesions [3, 34]. Surgical procedures should be performed in non-active phases of JLS (after at least 6 months with no disease activity markers) due to the lowest risk of relapse. Otherwise, introduction of immunosuppressive drug after the surgical procedure is necessary. The literature presents cases of limb asymmetry successfully corrected by Achilles tendon shortening or epiphysiodesis [39, 40]. Furthermore, patients with linear morphea of the head successfully treated with autologous fat transplants, synthetic tissue fillers (such as hyaluronic acid, poly-L lactic acid) and orbital implants were described [41 - 43].

Box 19.4. Learning points.
• Morphea is an autoimmune disease manifested by inflammation and limited sclerosis of the skin and underlying tissues.
• Morphea is typically diagnosed on the basis of its clinical picture, however, in case of any doubts, a histopathological examination should be performed.
• The most common clinical type of pediatric morphea is linear morphea.
• Children with limited skin involvement (circumscribed superficial morphea, atrophoderma of Pasini and Pierini) respond well to the topical therapy.
• Severe cases of pediatric morphea with expanded tissue involvement (linear morphea of the extremities, en coup se sabre, Parry-Romberg syndrome, generalized morphea, disabling pansclerotic scleroderma) require prompt immunosuppressive therapy.

REFERENCES

[1] Krasowska D, Rudnicka L, Dańczak-Pazdrowska A, *et al.* Localized scleroderma (morphea). Diagnostic and therapeutic recommendations of the polish dermatological society. Przegl Dermatol 2019; 106(4): 333-53.
[http://dx.doi.org/10.5114/dr.2019.88252]

[2] Aranegui B, Jiménez-Reyes J. Morphea in Childhood: An Update. Actas Dermo-Sifiliográficas 2018; 109: pp. 312-22.

[3] Kreuter A, Krieg T, Worm M, *et al.* German guidelines for the diagnosis and therapy of localized scleroderma. J Dtsch Dermatol Ges 2016; 14(2): 199-216.
[http://dx.doi.org/10.1111/ddg.12724] [PMID: 26819124]

[4] Zulian F, Vallongo C, de Oliveira SKF, *et al.* Congenital localized scleroderma. J Pediatr 2006; 149(2): 248-51.
[http://dx.doi.org/10.1016/j.jpeds.2006.04.052] [PMID: 16887444]

[5] Li SC. Scleroderma in children and adolescents. Pediatr Clin North Am 2018; 65(4): 757-81.
[http://dx.doi.org/10.1016/j.pcl.2018.04.002] [PMID: 30031497]

[6] Wolska-Gawron K, Krasowska D. Localized scleroderma classification and tools used for the evaluation of tissue damage and disease activity/severity. Przegl Dermatol 2017; 3: 269-89.
[http://dx.doi.org/10.5114/dr.2017.68775]

[7] Constantin T, Foeldvari I, Pain CE, *et al.* Development of minimum standards of care for juvenile localized scleroderma. Eur J Pediatr 2018; 177(7): 961-77.
[http://dx.doi.org/10.1007/s00431-018-3144-8] [PMID: 29728839]

[8] Wolska-Gawron K, Bartosińska J, Krasowska D. MicroRNA in localized scleroderma: A review of literature. Arch Dermatol Res 2020; 312(5): 317-24.
[http://dx.doi.org/10.1007/s00403-019-01991-0] [PMID: 31637470]

[9] Saracino AM, Denton CP, Orteu CH. The molecular pathogenesis of morphoea: From genetics to future treatment targets. Br J Dermatol 2017; 177(1): 34-46.
[http://dx.doi.org/10.1111/bjd.15001] [PMID: 27553363]

[10] Wolska-Gawron K, Bartosińska J, Rusek M, Kowal M, Raczkiewicz D, Krasowska D. Circulating miRNA-181b-5p, miRNA-223-3p, miRNA-210-3p, let 7i-5p, miRNA-21-5p and miRNA-29a-3p in

patients with localized scleroderma as potential biomarkers. Sci Rep 2020; 10(1): 20218.
[http://dx.doi.org/10.1038/s41598-020-76995-2] [PMID: 33214624]

[11]   Laxer RM, Zulian F. Localized scleroderma. Curr Opin Rheumatol 2006; 18(6): 606-13.
[http://dx.doi.org/10.1097/01.bor.0000245727.40630.c3] [PMID: 17053506]

[12]   Timpane S, Brandling-Bennett H, Kristjansson AK. Autoimmune collagen vascular diseases: Kids are not just little people. Clin Dermatol 2016; 34(6): 678-89.
[http://dx.doi.org/10.1016/j.clindermatol.2016.07.002] [PMID: 27968927]

[13]   Schoch JJ, Schoch BS, Werthel JD, McIntosh AL, Davis DMR. Orthopedic complications of linear morphea: Implications for early interdisciplinary care. Pediatr Dermatol 2018; 35(1): 43-6.
[http://dx.doi.org/10.1111/pde.13336] [PMID: 29119592]

[14]   Torok KS. Pediatric scleroderma: Systemic or localized forms. Pediatr Clin North Am 2012; 59(2): 381-405.
[http://dx.doi.org/10.1016/j.pcl.2012.03.011] [PMID: 22560576]

[15]   Glaser DH, Schutt C, VonVille HM, Schollaert-Fitch K, Torok K. Linear Scleroderma of the Head. Updates in management of Parry Romberg Syndrome and En coup de sabre: A rapid scoping review across subspecialties. Eur J Rheumatol 2020; 7 (1): S48-57.
[http://dx.doi.org/10.5152/eurjrheum.2019.19183] [PMID: 35929860]

[16]   Khamaganova I. Progressive hemifacial atrophy and linear scleroderma en coup de sabre: A spectrum of the same disease? Front Med 2018; 4: 258.
[http://dx.doi.org/10.3389/fmed.2017.00258] [PMID: 29445726]

[17]   Mears KA, Servat JJ, Black EH. Linear scleroderma en coup de sabre affecting the upper eyelid and lashes. Graefes Arch Clin Exp Ophthalmol 2012; 250(7): 1097-9.
[http://dx.doi.org/10.1007/s00417-011-1911-6] [PMID: 22249315]

[18]   Kreuter A, Mitrakos G, Hofmann S, *et al.* Localized scleroderma of the head and face area: A retrospective cross-sectional study of 96 patients from 5 german tertiary referral centres. Acta Derm Venereol 2018; 98(6): 603-5.
[http://dx.doi.org/10.2340/00015555-2920] [PMID: 29507998]

[19]   Jain RS, Kumar S, Srivastava T. Lower limb onset Parry–Romberg syndrome: An unusual presentation of a rare disease. Oxf Med Case Rep 2016; 2016(8): omw031.
[http://dx.doi.org/10.1093/omcr/omw031] [PMID: 29497540]

[20]   Panda A, Pathi J, Mishra P, Kumar H. Parry–Romberg syndrome affecting one half of the body. J Int Soc Prev Commun Dent 2016; 6(4): 387-90.
[http://dx.doi.org/10.4103/2231-0762.186792] [PMID: 27583230]

[21]   Jun JH, Kim HY, Jung HJ, *et al.* Parry-romberg syndrome with en coup de sabre. Ann Dermatol 2011; 23(3): 342-7.
[http://dx.doi.org/10.5021/ad.2011.23.3.342] [PMID: 21909205]

[22]   Chiu YE, Vora S, Kwon EKM, Maheshwari M. A significant proportion of children with morphea en coup de sabre and Parry-Romberg syndrome have neuroimaging findings. Pediatr Dermatol 2012; 29(6): 738-48.
[http://dx.doi.org/10.1111/pde.12001] [PMID: 23106674]

[23]   Zannin ME, Martini G, Athreya BH, *et al.* Juvenile scleroderma working group of the pediatric rheumatology european society (PRES). Ocular involvement in children with localised scleroderma: A multi-centre study. Br J Ophthalmol 2007; 91(10): 1311-4.
[http://dx.doi.org/10.1136/bjo.2007.116038] [PMID: 17475707]

[24]   Fledelius HC, Danielsen PL, Ullman S. Ophthalmic findings in linear scleroderma manifesting as facial en coup de sabre. Eye 2018; 32(11): 1688-96.
[http://dx.doi.org/10.1038/s41433-018-0137-9] [PMID: 29973692]

[25]   Vafa A, Gevorgyan O, De D, Hassan S. Retinal vasculitis the first clue in the diagnosis of progressive

hemifacial atrophy. Eur J Rheumatol 2019; 6(4): 219-22.
[http://dx.doi.org/10.5152/eurjrheum.2019.18100] [PMID: 31329538]

[26] Kapoor A, Kumar S, Bhagyalakshmi N. Localized scleroderma causing enophthalmos: A rare entity. Indian J Ophthalmol 2018; 66(11): 1611-2.
[http://dx.doi.org/10.4103/ijo.IJO_303_18] [PMID: 30355873]

[27] Fea AM, Aragno V, Briamonte C, Franzone M, Putignano D, Grignolo FM. Parry romberg syndrome with a wide range of ocular manifestations: A case report. BMC Ophthalmol 2015; 15(1): 119.
[http://dx.doi.org/10.1186/s12886-015-0093-0] [PMID: 26340917]

[28] Niklander S, Marín C, Martínez R, Esguep A. Morphea en coup de sabre: An unusual oral presentation. J Clin Exp Dent 2017; 9(2): 0.
[http://dx.doi.org/10.4317/jced.53151] [PMID: 28210455]

[29] Al-Aizari NA, Azzeghaiby SN, Al-Shamiri HM, Darwish S, Tarakji B. Oral manifestations of Parry-Romberg syndrome: A review of literature. Avicenna J Med 2015; 5(2): 25-8.
[http://dx.doi.org/10.4103/2231-0770.154193] [PMID: 25878963]

[30] Amaral TN, Marques Neto JF, Lapa AT, Peres FA, Guirau CR, Appenzeller S. Neurologic involvement in scleroderma en coup de sabre. Autoimmune Dis 2012; 2012: 1-6.
[http://dx.doi.org/10.1155/2012/719685] [PMID: 22319646]

[31] Browning JC. Pediatric Morphea. Dermatol Clin 2013; 31(2): 229-37.
[http://dx.doi.org/10.1016/j.det.2012.12.002] [PMID: 23557652]

[32] Florez-Pollack S, Kunzler E, Jacobe HT. Morphea: Current concepts. Clin Dermatol 2018; 36(4): 475-86.
[http://dx.doi.org/10.1016/j.clindermatol.2018.04.005] [PMID: 30047431]

[33] Asano Y, Fujimoto M, Ishikawa O, *et al.* Diagnostic criteria, severity classification and guidelines of localized scleroderma. J Dermatol 2018; 45(7): 755-80.
[http://dx.doi.org/10.1111/1346-8138.14161] [PMID: 29687475]

[34] Knobler R, Moinzadeh P, Hunzelmann N, *et al.* European Dermatology Forum S1-guideline on the diagnosis and treatment of sclerosing diseases of the skin, Part 1: Localized scleroderma, systemic sclerosis and overlap syndromes. J Eur Acad Dermatol Venereol 2017; 31(9): 1401-24.
[http://dx.doi.org/10.1111/jdv.14458] [PMID: 28792092]

[35] Zulian F, Culpo R, Sperotto F, *et al.* Consensus-based recommendations for the management of juvenile localised scleroderma. Ann Rheum Dis 2019; 78(8): 1019-24.
[http://dx.doi.org/10.1136/annrheumdis-2018-214697] [PMID: 30826775]

[36] Wolska-Gawron K, Michalska-Jakubus M, Krasowska D. Localized scleroderma. Current treatment options. Przegl Dermatol 2017; 104(6): 606-18.
[http://dx.doi.org/10.5114/dr.2017.71833]

[37] Foeldvari I. New developments in juvenile systemic and localized scleroderma. Rheum Dis Clin North Am 2013; 39(4): 905-20.
[http://dx.doi.org/10.1016/j.rdc.2013.05.003] [PMID: 24182860]

[38] Li SC, Torok KS, Pope E, *et al.* Childhood arthritis and rheumatology research alliance (CARRA) localized scleroderma workgroup. development of consensus treatment plans for juvenile localized scleroderma: A roadmap toward comparative effectiveness studies in juvenile localized scleroderma. Arthr Care Res 2012; 64(8): 1175-85.
[PMID: 22505322]

[39] Handler MZ, Wulkan AJ, Stricker SJ, Schachner LA. Linear morphea and leg length discrepancy: Treatment with a leg-lengthening procedure. Pediatr Dermatol 2013; 30(5): 616-8.
[http://dx.doi.org/10.1111/pde.12169] [PMID: 23756319]

[40] Lehman AM, Patel MS. Childhood-onset hemiatrophy caused by unilateral morphea. Clin Dysmorphol 2009; 18(4): 213-4.

[http://dx.doi.org/10.1097/MCD.0b013e32832a9e0c] [PMID: 19543082]

[41] Thareja SK, Sadhwani D, Alan Fenske N. En coup de sabre morphea treated with hyaluronic acid filler. Report of a case and review of the literature. Int J Dermatol 2015; 54(7): 823-6.
[http://dx.doi.org/10.1111/ijd.12108] [PMID: 24168261]

[42] Dinulos JGH. Cosmetic procedures in children. Curr Opin Pediatr 2011; 23(4): 395-8.
[http://dx.doi.org/10.1097/MOP.0b013e328348112d] [PMID: 21670683]

[43] Marangoni RG, Lu TT. The roles of dermal white adipose tissue loss in scleroderma skin fibrosis. Curr Opin Rheumatol 2017; 29(6): 585-90.
[http://dx.doi.org/10.1097/BOR.0000000000000437] [PMID: 28800024]

CHAPTER 20

Eosinophilic Fasciitis

Sueli Carneiro[1,*], Renata Cavalcante[1] and Marcia Ramos-e-Silva[1]

[1] *Sector of Dermatology and Post-Graduation Course in Dermatology, University Hospital and School of Medicine, Federal University of Rio de Janeiro, Rio de Janeiro, Brazil*

Chapter synopsis.
• Eosinophilic fasciitis (EF) is a rare disease of sudden onset, characterized by edema, erythema, and rigidity of the limbs, in addition to thickening of the muscle fascia. It is characterized by the absence of sclerodactyly, Raynaud's phenomenon, and capillary changes in the nail folds.
• It was first reported by Shulman in 1974 with scleroderma-like changes associated with peripheral eosinophilia, hypergammaglobulinemia, and increased erythrocyte sedimentation rate.
• About 30 to 46% of patients of EF have a history of intense or unusual physical exercise or a history of trauma. Several drugs, including hemodialysis, radiotherapy, and graft-versus-host disease have also been implicated in its etiology.
• Diagnosis is primarily based on a well-taken history and good clinical examination. Clinically, there is symmetrical and woody edema associated with painful erythema of sudden origin, sparing face, hands, fingers, and feet.
• Histologically, thickening of the muscle fascia is observed, in addition to an infiltrate of lymphocytes, plasma cells, histiocytes, and eosinophils.
• Early diagnosis and treatment are extremely important for clinical response and complete regression of the condition. Spontaneous improvement can occur; however, most cases require drug treatment.

Keywords: *Borrelia burgdorferi*, Chronic synovitis, Eosinophilia, Eosinophilic fasciitis, Erythrocyte sedimentation rate, Fasciitis, Fibrosis, Groove sign, Hypergammaglobulinemia, Joint contractures, Localized scleroderma, Magnetic resonance imaging, Morphea, Peripheral eosinophilia, Scleroderma, Shulman syndrome, Stiffness, Tenosynovitis, Thickening of fascia, Valley sign.

INTRODUCTION AND HISTORICAL BACKGROUND

Eosinophilic fasciitis (EF) is a rare disease, characterized by a sudden onset of edema, erythema and stiffness of the limbs (thickening of the subcutaneous tissue,

* **Corresponding author Sueli Carneiro:** Sector of Dermatology and Post-Graduation Course in Dermatology, University Hospital and School of Medicine, Federal University of Rio de Janeiro, Rio de Janeiro, Brazil; E-mail: sueli@hucff.ufrj.br

Tasleem Arif (Ed.)

fascia and muscle) [1]. Also called as, Shulman syndrome, its first case was reported in 1974 by Shulman with scleroderma-like changes associated with peripheral eosinophilia, hypergammaglobulinemia, and increased erythrocyte sedimentation rate (ESR) [2]. The relationship between EF and systemic sclerosis (SSC), a disorder with similar clinical and histopathological features, is still not clear; and, although both have symmetrical hardening of the limbs, EF is characterized by the absence of sclerodactyly, Raynaud's phenomenon and capillary changes in the nail folds [3].

Shulman described two patients who presented with peripheral eosinophilia, swelling of the extremities, induration of the skin and soft tissues accompanied by joint contractures in the limbs [2]. In 1975, Rodnan *et al.* reported seven patients with similar signs and symptoms seen by Shulman the year before [4]. They found a large number of inflamed cells in the muscle, fascia and subcutaneous tissue in addition to the peripheral eosinophilia, which was 30% or more of leukocytes [5]. Barnes *et al.*, in 1979, published a study of 20 cases of EF, showing that the common histopathological alterations were thickening of fascia and perivascular inflammatory infiltrate [5].

EPIDEMIOLOGY

EF is a rare connective tissue disease, with fewer than 300 cases reported in the literature [1]. It affects men and women between 37 and 50 years of age and its etiology is not fully understood [5].

Yamamoto *et al.*, in 2020, examined 31 Japanese patients with EF. These authors observed a ratio of male: female of 2.3:1 and a mean age of 47.7 years. They also found some triggering factors associated with EF like muscle training, sports, walking or sitting for a long time, physical work, insect bite and drugs. They observed co-occurrence of morphea in 9 cases (29%), and malignancies in 3 [6]. Several characteristics of various published cases of EF have been summarized in (Tables **20.1** and **20.2**) [1, 5, 7 - 69].

Table 20.1. Some published cases of Eosinophilic Fasciitis [1,5,7 - 69].

Publication Number	Year of Publication	Authors	Refs.	Age	No of Patients	Sex	Sites	Histopathology	Other Comments
1	1976	Atherton *et al.*	7	49	1	M	T; UL	Normal epidermis with an increase of normal fibrous tissue.	-

(Table 20.1) cont.....

Publication Number	Year of Publication	Authors	Refs.	Age	No of Patients	Sex	Sites	Histopathology	Other Comments
2	1977	Krauser *et al.*	9	22	1	F	UL	Severe thickening of the deep fascia associated with lymphocytes and plasma cell infiltrate.	-
3	1978	Weinstein *et al.*	8	55	1	F	UL	Inflammation and thickening of fascia.	Associated with eosinophilia. Good response to treatment with steroids
4	1979	Lupton *et al.*	10	53/59	2	f/m	UL/LL	On histopathology, the fascia was four times thicker than the dermis and epidermis. In addition to an infiltrate composed of lymphocytes, plasma cells, histiocytes and eosinophils	Report of two cases of patients between 50-60 years of age with edema, erythema and hardening of limbs; started by physical exercise
5	1979	Barnes *et al.*	5	20-68	20	f/m	LL/UL	Thickening of muscular fascia with edema and inflammation. Lymphocyte infiltration is observed.	Of the patients evaluated, only 5 had an early diagnosis. All 20 individuals had biopsies showing the characteristic morphological changes of EF. The biopsies were taken from areas of active disease.
6	1979	Jarret *et al*	11	59	1	F	UL	The biopsy showed a thick sclerotic fascia with strong lymphocyte infiltrate, plasma cells, occasional histiocytes and some eosinophils.	Report of a case with clinical and histological characteristic of EF but with progression as scleroderma.
7	1979	Nassonova *et al*	12	26-52	6	m/f	LL/UL	The fascia was thickened in all cases. Inflammatory changes in the fascia of the perimysial tissue were observed in the muscle. Eosinophils were found in the fascia. Most cells were lymphocytes with a variable number of plasma cells. In most cases, the inflammatory infiltrates had a perivascular distribution.	-

(Table 20.1) cont.....

Publication Number	Year of Publication	Authors	Refs.	Age	No of Patients	Sex	Sites	Histopathology	Other Comments
8	1979	Haim *et al*	13	63	1	F	A, UL; LL ; A;C	The biopsy showed some lymphocytes in the dermis, with little eosinophilic infiltrate, mainly seen around blood vessels and sebaceous glands. An inflammatory infiltrate composed of lymphocytes, plasma cells, histiocytes and eosinophils was observed, an infiltrate that extended to the subcutaneous tissue and fascia.	-
9	1979	Abeles *et al.*	14	69	1	M	LL/ UL	Thickened fascia with the infiltrate of lymphocytes, eosinophils and neutrophils.	EF has a benign course and does not involve internal organs.
10	1979	Chalmers *et al.*	15	22	1	F	LL/ UL	Fascia with inflammatory infiltrate; an increase of dermal collagen.	A rare condition with good prognosis due to the good response to steroids.
11	1979	Robinson	16	32-61	2	F	LL; UL	Perivascular infiltrate of lymphocytes and histiocytes.	-
12	1979	Thivolet *et al.*	17	53	1	M	LL/ UL/ T	Infiltrates of plasma cells, histiocytes, eosinophils. Plasma cells in fascia and muscular septa.	High eosinophilia, immune complexes, hiperimmunoglobulinemia.
13	1980	Moore *et al.*	18	38	1	F	LL/ UL/T/F	Infiltrates of lymphocytes and plasma cells.	-
14	1981	Janin-Mercier *et al.*	19	55	1	F	LL/ UL	Infiltrates of lymphocytes and plasma cells in epimysium; sclerosis in some areas of fascia.	Electronic microscopy showing alterations in the biopsy of the patient with EF.
15	1982	Solomon *et al.*	20	53	1	M	LL/UL	Deep biopsies showed marked thickening of the fascia between muscle and fat, in addition to infiltration with plasma cells, lymphocytes and rare eosinophils	Improvement of symptoms of EF after treatment with cimetidine.

(Table 20.1) cont.....

Publication Number	Year of Publication	Authors	Refs.	Age	No of Patients	Sex	Sites	Histopathology	Other Comments
16	1982	Kennedy *et al.*	21	64	1	M	LL/ UL	Infiltrates of lymphocytes, plasma cells, and eosinophils.	Association of EF with erosive arthritis.
17	1983	Naguwa *et al.*	22	55	1	F	LL/ UL	Infiltrate of inflammatory cells; thickening of fascia.	Report of six patients with EF treated with steroids.
18	1984	Allen	23	58	1	F	LL/ UL	Thickening of fascia, with infiltrates of plasma cells, and lymphocytes.	The patient with EF treated with hydroxychloroquine.
19	1985	Silverman *et al.*	24	1	27	F	LL	Thickened fascia, muscles and fat, with infiltrates of inflammatory cells.	-
20	1985	Piette *et al.*	25	17	1	F	UL	Biopsy revealed thickened fibrotic fascia containing inflammatory cells. Polymorphic infiltrate seen in the fascia.	EF in a child, associated with neurologic involvement.
21	1986	Jones *et al.*	26	30-52	6	F/M	UL	Thickened fascia up to eight times more than normal, with infiltrates of lymphocytes and plasma cells.	Report of six patients with EF who evolved to carpal tunnel syndrome.
22	1988	Narayanan *et al.*	27	51	1	F	A/ LL/ UL	Edema and inflammation of the dermis.	Eosinophilia found is secondary to aplastic anemia.
23	1988	Valentini *et al.*	28	33-52	2	M	LL / UL	The biopsy revealed thickening of the fascia with an infiltrate of inflammatory cells. The muscle also contained lymphohistiocytic infiltrates.	-
24	1989	Grisanti *et al.*	29	4	1	M	LL	Histiocytes, eosinophils and mononuclear cells in fascia.	-
25	1989	Thomson *et al.*	30	33-38	2	F/ m	UL/ LL	Dermal collagen and septal thickening, and lymphocytic infiltrate.	Two siblings developed EF in a period of six months. Both with identical HLA-A, B, DR and DQ antigens, leading to the possibility of genetic influence.
26	1990	Cotsarelis *et al.*	31	59	1	F	LL/ UL	Sclerosis and infiltration of lymphocytes in the fascia.	L-tryptophan as a trigger factor for EF.

(Table 20.1) cont.....

Publication Number	Year of Publication	Authors	Refs.	Age	No of Patients	Sex	Sites	Histopathology	Other Comments
27	1990	Magaro *et al.*	32	45	1	M	LL; UL	Histopathologically, dermal sclerosis was observed which extended to subcutaneous tissues. Lymphocytic and eosinophilic perivascular infiltrate was also seen. In the fascia, there was a significant inflammatory infiltrate composed of lymphocytes, plasma cells and eosinophils.	-
28	1991	Hamilton	33	62	1	F	T/UL	Thickening of fascia and septae, lymphocytic infiltrate.	-
29	1991	Ching *et al.*	34	13	1	M	UL/ LL	Thickened fascia with infiltrate including eosinophils.	-
30	1991	Chalker *et al.*	35	71	1	M	UL	The thickened reticular dermis, with greater deposition of collagen. Inflammatory cells in the thickened fascia.	-
31	1992	Ishikawa *et al.*	36	24	1	F	UL LL	Inflammation of fascia with histiocytes and eosinophils.	Case report of a young woman who developed eosinophilia-myalgia syndrome associated with the ingestion of L-tryptophan, present in fitness protein tablets.
32	1992	Ching *et al.*	37	30	1	M	LL/ UL	Dermal thickening; inflammatory infiltrate with histiocytes, plasma cells, lymphocytes and rare eosinophils.	Patient with EF and good response to the use of prednisone associated with ketotifen.

(Table 20.1) cont.....

Publication Number	Year of Publication	Authors	Refs.	Age	No of Patients	Sex	Sites	Histopathology	Other Comments
33	1993	Wong *et al.*	38	26	1	M	LL/ UL	The skin biopsy showed in the deep dermis and subcutaneous tissue a moderate chronic inflammatory cell infiltrate containing numerous plasma cells and neutrophils.	Typical presentation of EF with ulcers similar to vasculitis.
34	1993	Gaffney *et al.*	39	52	1	M	LL	Infiltration of fascia and septum fibers with mononuclear inflammatory infiltrate.	-
35	1994	Juncá *et al.*	40	69	1	M	UL	Inflammatory infiltrate with thickening of fibrous septa. Thickened fascia and muscles with infiltrate of inflammatory cells.	EF associated to non-Hodgkin lymphoma.
36	1994	O'Laughlin *et al.*	41	21	1	M	UL	Thickening of fascia and inflammatory cell infiltrate.	Importance of the association of physiotherapy for rehabilitation of patients with EF.
37	1995	Baffoni *et al.*	42	52	1	F	UL/LL	A deep biopsy showed sclerosis of subcutaneous tissue and deep fascia. A perivascular inflammatory infiltrate composed of mononuclear cells, neutrophils and nuclear debris were present, apparently creating a pattern of leukocytoclastic vasculitis.	Patient with lupus associated to EF.
38	1996	Hashimoto *et al.*	43	49	1	M	UL/ LL	Accumulation of collagen in the dermis, thickened fascia. Inflammatory infiltrate with lymphocytes, histiocytes and eosinophils.	First report of an EF patient with specific *Borrelia burgdorferi* DNA in a skin sample.
39	1997	Achura *et al.*	44	21	1	F	UL/LL	Hard fibrosis with infiltrate of lymphocytes and eosinophils.	-

(Table 20.1) cont.....

Publication Number	Year of Publication	Authors	Refs.	Age	No of Patients	Sex	Sites	Histopathology	Other Comments
40	1998	Smith *et al.*	45	50	1	F	UL	Skin biopsy not done.	Probable lansoprazole induced EF
41	1999	Bachmeyer *et al.*	46	53	1	M	UL/ LL	Thickened collagen bundles, with an inflammatory infiltrate of lymphocytes and eosinophils, affecting fascia, subcutaneous tissue and muscle.	Association of autoimmune disease with EF.
42	2000	Hayashi *et al.*	47	50	1	M	LL/UL	Infiltrate of inflammatory cells, and eosinophils in the dermis.	Good response to the use of cyclosporine.
43	2001	Vannucci *et al.*	48	40	1	F	T/UL	Thickening and inflammatory infiltrate of fascia.	EF associated with epilepsy.
44	2002	Quintero-Ofl-Rio *et al.*	49	1-13	3	F	LL/UL	Fascia with dense infiltrate of cells including lymphocytes and eosinophils. Stromal fibrosis, hyalinization, and degenerative alterations.	Involvement of EF in infancy.
45	2003	Jacob *et al.*	50	60	1	F	LL/UL	Thickened fascia with infiltrate of plasma cells, lymphocytes and rare eosinophils.	EF associated with polycythemia vera.
46	2004	Owens *et al.*	51	46	1	F	UL	Abundant mononuclear cells.	-
47	2005	Carneiro *et al.*	52	35	1	M	UL/LL	Infiltrate of lymphocytes, plasma cells and eosinophils around dermal vessels.	-
48	2006	Pillen *et al.*	53	14	1	M	UL/LL	The biopsy revealed lymphocyte infiltrate, plasma cells, histiocytes and some eosinophilic granulocytes.	EF as differential diagnosis in infancy
49	2007	Endo *et al.*	54	29/ 68	2	F	UL /LL	Fibrosis and infiltrate of inflammatory cells	-
50	2008	Jaimes-Hernández *et al.*	55	42-50	3	M/F	LL/ UL/ A	Thickening of fascia.	Good response to cyclosporine
51	2009	Ronneberg *et al.*	56	35/ 68	2	F/M	LL/ UL	Unspecified fibrotic alterations of fascia	MR has an important role in the diagnosis of EF; can substitute the block biopsy.

(Table 20.1) cont.....

Publication Number	Year of Publication	Authors	Refs.	Age	No of Patients	Sex	Sites	Histopathology	Other Comments
52	2010	Servy *et al.*	57	49	1	M	UL/ LL	Sclerosis of fascia; infiltrate of plasma cells, lymphocytes and eosinophils.	-
53	2011	Chun *et al.*	58	36 / 52	2	m/ f	UL	Infiltrate of plasma cells, lymphocytes and histiocytes	-
54	2012	Manzini *et al.*	59	45/ 60	3	M/F	UL/ LL/ T	Inflammatory infiltrate of plasma cells, histiocytes and eosinophils. Thickening of fascia.	D-penicillamine as steroid saver.
55	2013	Lese *et al.*	60	16	1	M	UL	Infiltrate with plasma cells, lymphocytes, histiocytes and eosinophils.	-
56	2014	Alonso-Castro *et al.*	61	66	1	M	UL/ C	Infiltrate of inflammatory cells, thickened collagen bundles in the reticular dermis.	Good response to azathioprine.
57	2015	Espinoza *et al.*	62	43	1	M	UL	Fasciitis with lymphocytes and eosinophils. Perivascular infiltrate.	Response to tocilizumab, regression of the clinical picture of EF and of the articular involvement.
58	2016	Lamback *et al.*	1	44	1	M	LL/ UL/ A	Interstitial edema and inflammatory infiltrate.	-
59	2017	Whitlock *et al.*	63	43	1	F	LL	Thickened fascia, with perivascular infiltrate.	-
60	2018	Sato *et al.*	64	75	1	M	UL/ LL/ T	Thickened collagen bundles.	-
61	2019	El-Jammal *et al.*	65	61	1	M	UL	Fascia with lymphocytic inflammatory infiltrate.	-
62	2020	Mastrantonio *et al.*	66	53	1	M	UL	Lichen sclerosis associated with morphea.	EF associated with aplastic anemia.
63	2021	Jimenez- Garcia; *et al*	67	34	1	F	UL/ LL	Thickening of the collagen fibers of the dermis and an inflammatory infiltrate	EF in pregnancy. Treatment with infliximab.
64	2021	Asaoka *et al.*	68	66	1	F	UL/ LL	Thickening of fascia with inflammatory cell infiltrate.	-

(Table 20.1) cont.....

Publication Number	Year of Publication	Authors	Refs.	Age	No of Patients	Sex	Sites	Histopathology	Other Comments
65	2021	Daniels P, *et al*	69	61	1	F	UL/ LL/ C	Muscle biopsy revealed endomysial and perimysial inflammation that was accompanied by mild perifascicular atrophy. The fibroadipose tissue showed inflammation with T lymphocytes and predominant macrophages and the presence of few B lymphocytes and plasma cells.	-

T: Trunk; UL: Upper limb; LL: Lower limb; C: Chest; A: Abdomen FN: Face/neck; m: Male; f: Female; NA: Not available; EF: Eosinophilic fasciitis

Table 20.2. Basic features of published cases of EF [1, 5, 7-69].

Total cases collected	107
Mean age of onset of disease	41.3 years
Range	1-71 years
Males	51
Females	56
M/F ratio	0,910
Onset of disease before or at 20 years	8
Onset of disease after 20 years	99
Trunk involvement	7
Upper limb involvement	98
Lower limb involvement	82
Face/chest/ neck/ abdomen involvement	8

ETIOPATHOGENESIS

The pathophysiology of EF remains unclear. It is suspected that there is a triggering factor. Jinnin *et al.*, in 2018, established diagnostic criteria, severity classification and treatment guidelines for EF. They concluded that 30 to 46% of individuals with EF had a history of intense or unusual physical exercise or a history of trauma with the formation of hematomas. However, they recognized that this evidence is level D [3]. They also observed positive cases for the

Borrelia burgdorferi antibody, which would favor the hypothesis of infection by Borrelia [3]. Some authors believe that inflammation of the injured fascia stimulates an autoimmune response against antigens released into the tissue [5].

Drugs such as phenytoin, statins, ramipril, and heparin have been implicated, in addition to hemodialysis, radiotherapy, and graft-versus-host disease [3].

There are reports that dermal fibroblasts from EF patients have a higher expression of type I collagen and fibronectin. In EF, fibrogenesis is the result of increased levels of tissue inhibitors of metalloproteinase-1 (TIMP-1) in the tissue while there are decreased serum levels of matrix metalloproteinase-1 (MMP-1) [70].

It is postulated that mast cells may release mediators, such as histamine, which stimulate fibroblast proliferation [71]. Increased levels of several chemokines like interleukin-5 (IL-5), interleukin-2 (IL-2), increased interferon-gamma (IFN-γ), and leukemia inhibitory factor by peripheral blood mononuclear cells may contribute to the onset of EF [71]. There is increased expression of the growth factor beta messenger RNA in muscle fascia-derived fibroblasts [71].

CLINICAL PRESENTATION

EF is a sclerodermiform syndrome with painful and progressive edema, which results in the hardening of the muscle, fascia (Figs. **20.1** and **20.2**) and subcutaneous tissue, resulting in muscle contracture and shortening of the tendons [72].

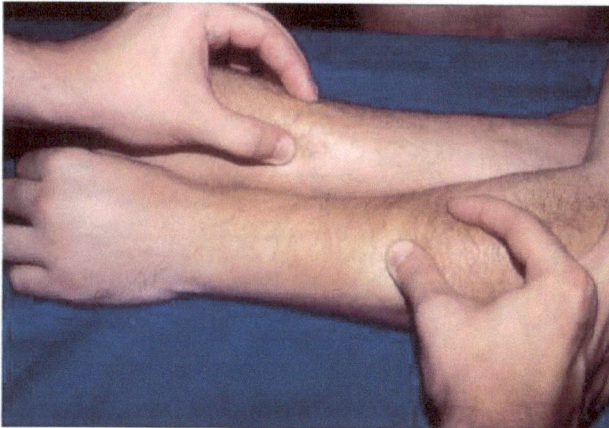

Fig. (20.1). Infiltrated areas in both forearms. (From Carneiro S, Brotas A, Lamy F, *et al*. Eosinophilic Fasciitis. Cutis 2005;75(4):228-32. With permission).

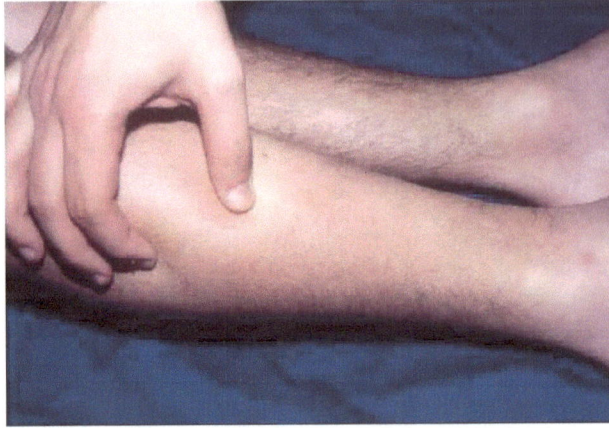

Fig. (20.2). Infiltrated area in the right leg, sclerosis of skin, and sparse hair in the affected area. (From Carneiro S, Brotas A, Lamy F, *et al*. Eosinophilic Fasciitis. Cutis 2005;75(4):228-32. With permission).

Diagnosis is primarily based on a well-taken clinical history and accurate physical examination. Clinically, there is symmetrical and woody edema associated with painful erythema of sudden origin, sparing face, hands, fingers and feet [74].

The regions usually affected are the forearms, arms, legs, thighs, and trunk. Sometimes skin presents with a "peau d'orange" appearance, which is characterized by the presence of irregularities and prominent hair follicles [70]. When the affected region is elevated, one or more grooves are observed in the paths of the superficial veins, visible along the inner surface of the limbs, sparing hands, and trunk, known as the 'valley sign or groove sign' (Fig. **20.3**) [3].

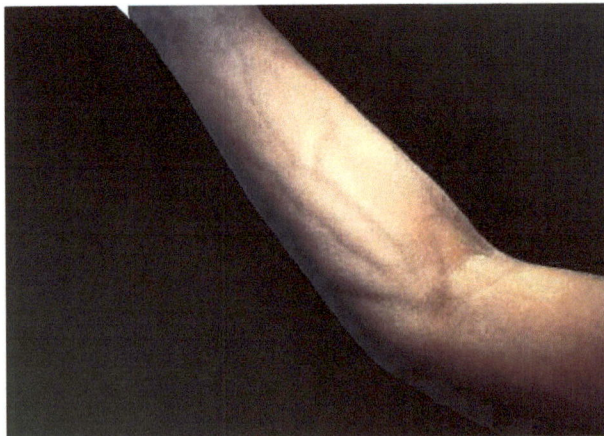

Fig. (20.3). Groove sign in eosinophilic fasciitis. Image credit Dr. Mayara Ferro Barbosa, Dermatologist.

In contrast, morphea is characterized by violaceous erythematous skin lesions. As the disease progresses, the plaques become hardened, and may present a violet halo, called a 'lilac ring'. In some patients, there is the onset of hyperpigmentation associated with the plaques [74].

Trunk thickening can result in refractory fibrosis and therefore restrictive lung disease [72].

Extracutaneous involvement is characterized by chronic synovitis and tenosynovitis [72]; secondary to stiffening of the limb, resulting in flexion contracture of the fingers [70]. Median nerve compression can lead to carpal tunnel syndrome [70]. Some patients may have systemic symptoms (Box **20.1**), such as weight loss, asthenia, and myalgia [73].

Box 20.1. Clinical findings reported in EF [3, 70-74].
Symmetrical involvement of extremities (sparing hands)
Hard, erythematous, painful lesions with "peau d'orange" appearance.
Previous triggering factors (extreme physical exercise, use of some drugs).
Affects middle age people.
Located on the limbs.
Peripheral eosinophilia.
Hypergammaglobulinemia.
Increased ESR and aldolase.
May have systemic symptoms.
May have spontaneous resolution.

Jinnin *et al.*, in 2018, considered joint contracture or limited movement of each limb as severity criteria. The deterioration of skin symptoms would also add one point to the criteria list and two points or more are considered markers of disease severity [3].

HISTOPATHOLOGY

Diagnostic confirmation is made by the histopathological examination (Table **20.3**). The biopsy should be deep enough to include the muscle so that the biopsy sample must comprise the tissue from the skin to the fascia [3, 72, 74, 75].

Table 20.3. Histopathological findings reported in EF [3, 72, 74, 75].

Thickening of fascia	Normal dermis (in the majority of cases)
Inflammatory infiltrate	Presence of eosinophils (not present sometimes)
Sclerosis	Accumulation of lymphocytes, plasmacytes, and histiocytes in the fibrous septum and fascia
Deposition of neo collagen in fascia and fibrous septum	Loss of dermal appendages and atrophy of the dermis

The epidermis is rarely affected. The dermis can be fibrotic and lymphohistiocytic and plasma cell infiltrate (Figs. **20.4** and **20.5**) can be observed in the dermis [74, 75].

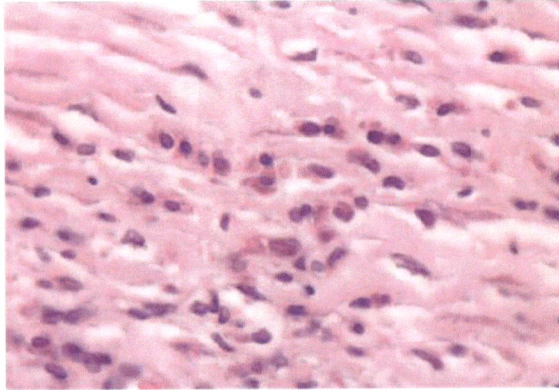

Fig. (20.4). Inflammatory cells at the muscular fascia and adjacent adipose tissue (HE X 200). (From Carneiro S, Brotas A, Lamy F, *et al*. Eosinophilic Fasciitis. Cutis 2005;75(4):228-32. With permission).

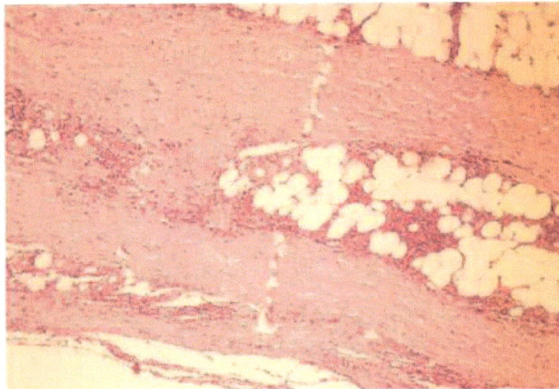

Fig. (20.5). Numerous eosinophils among inflammatory cells (400X HE). (From Carneiro S, Brotas A, Lamy F, *et al*. Eosinophilic Fasciitis. Cutis 2005;75(4):228-32. With permission).

The fascia is thickened two to fifteen times its normal size with focal or diffuse perivascular lymphocytic infiltrate with increased eosinophils [3, 72, 74, 75]. Eosinophils infiltrate primarily the deep epimysium and perimysium [72, 74, 75]. The absence of eosinophils does not exclude the diagnosis.

Barnes *et al.*, in 1979, studying 20 biopsies of EF, observed a yellow-whitish, sclerotic fascia, adherent to the subjacent skeletal muscle, and 2 to 15 times thicker than normal [5].

At the beginning of the disease there is an infiltrate of inflammatory cells: lymphocytes, plasmacytes, histiocytes, and eosinophils [5]. In later phases, the structures become thickened and sclerotic [76].

The biopsy should be deep enough to include fascia and muscle, and should be performed before initiating the treatment, since steroids and immunosuppressants can disguise the diagnosis [5, 76].

DIAGNOSIS

The diagnostic criteria for EF have been mentioned in (Boxes **20.2** and **20.3**) [3, 76].

Mazori *et al.* [76] drew attention to the similarities and differences between EF and SSC (Box **20.2**) and, although both have symmetrical hardening of the extremities, they have different prognoses and treatments. On the one hand, systemic corticosteroids, which are the treatment of choice for SSC, should be avoided or used in small doses for EF. Also in EF, extracutaneous involvement is limited to joint contractures and/or hematological alterations, not requiring systemic investigation.

Box 20.2. Diagnostic criteria of EF (modified from Mazori *et al.*) [76].
Major criteria
Symmetrical or asymmetrical edema, diffuse (limbs, trunk and abdomen) or localized (limbs), hardening and thickening of the skin and subcutaneous tissue.
Hardening of fascia with the accumulation of lymphocytes and macrophages, with or without eosinophils (full-thickness wedge biopsy of affected skin).
Minor criteria
Peripheral eosinophilia
Serum hypergammaglobulinemia
Muscle weakness and/or high serum aldolase levels
"Furrow sign" and/or skin with a peau d'orange appearance

(Box 20.2) cont.....

Box 20.2. Diagnostic criteria of EF (modified from Mazori *et al.*) [76].
Magnetic resonance imaging with hyperintense fascial signal
Exclusion criteria
Diagnosis of SSC

Box 20.3. Diagnosis criteria of EF (Jinin *et al.* 2018) [3].
Major criteria
Symmetrical plate-like sclerotic lesions that are present on the four limbs.
However, this condition lacks Raynaud's phenomenon, and SSC can be excluded.
Minor criteria 1
The histology of a skin biopsy that incorporates the fascia shows fibrosis of the subcutaneous connective tissue, with thickening of the fascia and cellular infiltration of eosinophils and monocytes.
Minor criteria 2
Thickening of the fascia is seen using imaging tests such as magnetic resonance imaging (MRI)
Note: A definitive diagnosis is made when a patient has the major criterion and one of the minor criteria, or the major criterion and two of the minor criteria.
Severity classification
Joint contracture (upper limbs): 1 point
Joint contracture (lower limbs): 1 point Limited movement (upper limbs): 1 point
Limited movement (lower limbs): 1 point
Expansion and worsening of skin rash (progression of symptoms): 1 point.
Note: A total of 2 or more points is classified as severe.

These authors also draw attention to misdiagnoses that require unnecessary laboratory tests and lead to delayed treatment and they reinforce the need for a careful history and accurate physical examination for the correct diagnosis of EF [76].

Jinnin *et al.* (2018) described, as the main criterion in the Japanese guidelines (Box **20.3**), the presence of sclerotic plaques in the four limbs, without Raynaud's phenomenon. As minor criteria, they included histopathological examination of an anatomical specimen that incorporates the muscle fascia, with fibrosis of the subcutaneous connective tissue, thickening of the fascia and presence of an infiltrate with eosinophils and monocytes. In addition, the radiological diagnosis of fascia thickening by magnetic resonance imaging (MRI) is also considered a minor criterion. Thus, a major criterion and a minor criterion give the diagnosis and EF [3].

Laboratory blood examination shows peripheral eosinophilia in 60 to 90% of the cases, which is unrelated to the prognosis [1]. Three to 72% of patients have an increase in the levels of gammaglobulinemia G or M, serum aldolase and erythrocyte sedimentation rate (ESR). Serum levels of interleukin-2 receptor, type III procollagen aminopeptide, serum immune complexes and tissue inhibitors of metalloproteinase-1 are effective markers of disease activity in EF [3].

MRI shows thickening of the fascia and can be used to monitor the response to the treatment [1]. MRI may also be used to non-invasively choose the biopsy site, showing the presence of edema and inflammation [3]. Ultrasound [77] and positron emission tomography (PET) have also been used for diagnosis [78].

Ultrasonography has been used to monitor response to treatment, correlating clinical improvement with applied therapy [76]. On ultrasound examination, thickening and abnormal echotexture of the skin, subcutaneous fat, tendons, and fascia are seen [76].

In the PET scan, impregnation of fluorinated contrast is observed in the affected fascia. Furthermore, it excludes the association with malignant disease [76].

DIFFERENTIAL DIAGNOSIS

Morphea and SSC are the two important differential diagnoses for EF (Table 20.4).

Table 20.4. Differential diagnosis of EF [73, 76].

Parameter	EF	Morphea	SSC
Age of onset	Adult 30-50 years old	Bimodal: Pediatric and adult onset.	Between 30-50 years old
Lesion morphology	Edema, local hardening, "peau d'orange" appearance, furrow sign	Erythematous to brownish indurated plaques; presence of lilac ring; at later stage may undergo softening and atrophy ensues.	Acral sclerosis, bound down skin, Raynaud's phenomenon, Vitiliginous depigmentation, with retention of peri-follicular pigmentation in a "salt and pepper" appearance, may develop flexion contracture, sclerodactyly.
Lesion distribution	Limbs and trunk	Trunk and extremities	Usually Diffuse

(Table 20.4) cont.....

Parameter	EF	Morphea	SSC
Evolution	There may be: edema; hardening and woody induration	Initially, erythema, followed by the development of induration and later atrophy.	Usually starts with Raynaud's phenomenon, followed by cutaneous sclerosis and may be accompanied or followed by internal organs system involvement.
Histo-pathology	Involves muscular fascia, with the presence of plasmacytes, lymphocytes, histiocytes and eosinophils; Thickening of the fascia	Perivascular infiltrate composed of lymphocytes and plasmacytes. Thickened collagen bundles in the papillary and reticular dermis.	Diffuse dermal sclerosis, mainly reticular dermis is composed of collagen bundles. There is a decrease in interstitial cellularity. Discrete mononuclear infiltrate around vessels.
Prognosis	Good, non-progressive	Variable	Bad prognosis depends on the affected organ.
Treatment	Steroids; hydroxychloroquine; cyclosporine; azathioprine; phototherapy	Topicals: steroids, vitamin D analogues; phototherapy: UVB-NB; PUVA. Systemic: Corticosteroids, methotrexate, cyclosporine	Immunosuppressors (cyclophosphamide, methotrexate), calcium channel blockers, angiotensin converting enzyme inhibitors, *etc.*

Morphea

Morphea has a well-defined plaque with a lilac halo in the early stages, while EF involves an area in a diffuse manner. In addition, the presence of eosinophilia in EF helps to differentiate it from morphea [73].

SSC

It is characterized by inflammation followed by fibrosis; however EF spares acral regions. Additionally, the presence of Raynaud's phenomenon is observed in SSC [73].

There have been reports of cases of EF as a paraneoplastic syndrome, most often related to hematological diseases. Aplastic anemia is the most commonly reported hematologic abnormality [79].

TREATMENT

Early diagnosis and treatment are extremely important for clinical response and complete regression of the condition [76].

Spontaneous improvement can occur; however, most cases require drug treatment (Box **20.4**), most often glucocorticoids at a dose of 0.5-1 mg/kg/day [76]. Regardless of the clinical response, eosinophilia, hypergammaglobulinemia and ESR return to normal levels [76].

There are reports of using prednisolone in pulse therapy (1,000 mg/day) for three days before starting treatment with oral prednisone at a dose of 0.5 to 1mg/kg/ body weight. This regimen showed a better therapeutic response when compared to the use of oral prednisone from the beginning [3].

The use of methotrexate in low doses (15 -25 mg per week) is the second-line treatment, mainly in patients with morphea-like skin lesions [76]. It is used as a corticosteroid-sparing agent, and there are reports of better clinical response when associated with systemic corticosteroids [76]. Methotrexate can be used with monotherapy as well as combined with the use of prednisone, having a better response rate [76].

Mycophenolate mofetil (MMF) is considered a second-line corticosteroid-sparing drug when there is a contraindication to the use of methotrexate. It is used at a dose of 1,800 mg/day [76]. MMF may also be used for weaning from steroids at the same dose [76].

Phototherapy with UV-A1 with or without psoralens can also be used as a steroid-sparing agent, with a reduction in skin thickness and improvement in elasticity [76].

Mazori *et al.* used cyclosporine as monotherapy at a dose of 3.7 to 5 mg/kg/day with a response in one month and remission of the disease in six months. There are reports of response three weeks after starting cyclosporine. The association of systemic corticosteroids with dapsone 50mg/day was effective from the second week onwards. Dapsone may be used for the gradual reduction of corticosteroids. There are reports of a return of movements after 5 months of dapsone at a dose of 50 mg/day, gradually increasing up to 150 mg/day [76].

Azathioprine at a dose of 200mg/day in a patient with a contraindication to the use of corticosteroids showed a clinical response within two months, with the improvement of the skin tightening and greater flexibility [76].

Infliximab is also used to treat EF. There are reports of use after failure of corticosteroid and methotrexate with good response [76].

The use of sirolimus in a non-reported dose and time of therapy was mentioned, promoting the resolution of the skin condition, eosinophilia, and normalization of serum IgG levels [76]. There is a report of the use of sirolimus in doses of 2 mg/day associated with systemic corticosteroids, with a response in six weeks and a total resolution of the condition in nine months [76].

The use of tocilizumab, a human monoclonal antibody against interleukin-6 (IL-6), was used in EF during weaning on steroids at a dose of 8mg/kg/month, with remission of the disease within six months [76].

The use of sirolimus, immunobiological drugs, such as infliximab, etanercept, and small molecules, such as tocilizumab had a good response in patients with contraindications to the use of corticosteroids and methotrexate [76].

D-penicillamine has been used as a corticosteroid-sparing agent, however, reports of proteinuria and bullous pemphigoid triggered by the drug have limited its use [76].

Regardless of the systemic treatment instituted, physical therapy is mandatory to prevent contractures and atrophies secondary to EF [76].

Box 20.4. Treatment of EF as monotherapy or in association [70, 76, 78].
Glucocorticoids
Methotrexate
Mycophenolate mofetil
Phototherapy with UV-A1 with or without oral psoralen
Cyclosporine
Dapsone
Azathioprine
Immunobiologicals, such as infliximab, etanercept, sirulimus and tocilizumab
D-penicillamine
Physical therapy

Factors Related to Treatment Resistance in EF

There are some factors that are associated with treatment resistance and a poor therapeutic outcome in EF [54, 74]:

• The presence of simultaneous "plaque morphea" was responsible for the decreased response to topical and systemic drugs, in addition to the need of also using immunosuppressors;

• Onset in childhood or puberty was associated with worse disease progression;

• Trunk involvement was related to a lack of response to systemic treatments; and

• The association of EF with hematological diseases or with solid tumors also results in resistance to treatment. However, the satisfactory therapeutic response of the underlying disease leads to remission of the EF

On the other hand, some factors showed no association with resistance to treatment like gender, previous physical stress, peripheral or tissue eosinophilia, hypergammaglobulinemia or high IgG level, high ESR, and positive antinuclear antibody [54, 74].

RELATIONSHIP BETWEEN EF AND MORPHEA

Morphea comprises a group of skin diseases characterized by cutaneous sclerosis. Its spectrum is much diversified, from mild presentations to severe and extensive conditions accompanied by muscle and joint contractures. In EF, the pathogenesis results from the continued formation of the extracellular matrix and immunological changes. These same processes occur in SSC [74].

In SSC, as in EF, the primary involvement of the subcutaneous tissue without superficial skin involvement is possible, but in EF, the presence of thickened dermal collagen fibers may reflect the presence of concomitant superficial morphea [74, 80].

Cutaneous and systemic manifestations of generalized morphea may overlap with eosinophilic fasciitis. The inclusion of eosinophilic fasciitis in the deep morphea group of Peterson *et al.* is still controversial [81].

However, some recent publications by prestigious authors in the dermatological literature consider eosinophilic fasciitis to be a sclerodermiform syndrome [80, 82].

Although there are some similarities between morphea and EF, we consider that EF is a distinctive entity although it is related to morphea and falls in that spectrum of disorders.

Also in EF, there is no sclerodactyly, Raynaud's phenomenon and capillary changes in the nail folds. Diagnosis of morphea is often based on characteristic clinical findings. Skin biopsies and laboratory tests are not routinely required for the diagnosis of morphea, but for EF full-thickness skin (epidermis, dermis, subcutaneous tissue, fascia and muscle tissue) specimens are essential for diagnosis [74].

PROGNOSIS

EF has a good prognosis when early physiotherapy is associated to systemic treatment, which decreases the development of flexion contracture. In most cases complete remission of the disease is observed.

Box 20.5. Learning points.
• SSC and EF both have symmetrical hardening of the limbs, however EF is characterized by the absence of sclerodactyly, Raynaud's phenomenon and capillary changes in the nail folds.
• Some authors believe that inflammation of the injured fascia stimulates an autoimmune response against antigens released into the tissue which presents clinically as EF. In EF, fibrogenesis is the result of increased levels of metalloproteinase 1 (TIMP-1) inhibitors in the tissue while there are decreased serum levels of metalloproteinase 1 (MMP-1)
• Magnetic resonance imaging (MRI) shows the thickening of the fascia and can be used to monitor the response to the treatment. MRI may also be used to non-invasively choose the biopsy site, showing the presence of edema and inflammation.
• Systemic steroids, methotrexate, mycophenolate mofetil, azathioprine, cyclosporine, biologicals, *etc.* have been used alone or in combination with good results. Regardless of the clinical response to the treatment, eosinophilia, hypergammaglobulinemia and ESR return to normal levels
• The presence of simultaneous plaque morphea, the onset of disease in childhood or puberty, trunk involvement, and association with hematological diseases or with solid tumors are the factors with poor therapeutic outcomes.

REFERENCES

[1]   Lamback EB, Resende FSS, Lenzi TCR. Eosinophilic fasciitis. An Bras Dermatol 2016; 91(5 suppl 1): 57-9.
        [http://dx.doi.org/10.1590/abd1806-4841.20164683] [PMID: 28300895]

[2]   Shulman LE. Diffuse fasciitis with eosinophilia: A new syndrome? Trans Assoc Am Physicians 1975; 88: 70-86.
        [PMID: 1224441]

[3]   Jinnin M, Yamamoto T, Asano Y, *et al.* Diagnostic criteria, severity classification and guidelines of eosinophilic fasciitis. J Dermatol 2018; 45(8): 881-90.
        [http://dx.doi.org/10.1111/1346-8138.14160] [PMID: 29235676]

[4]   Rodnan GP, DiBartolomeo AG, Medsger TA Jr. Barnes El Jr. Eosinophilic fasciitis- report of seven cases of newly recognized scleroderma like syndrome (abst). Arthritis Rheum 1975; 18: 422-234.

[5]   Barnes L, Rodnan GP, Medsger TA, Short D. Eosinophilic fasciitis. A pathologic study of twenty cases. Am J Pathol 1979; 96(2): 493-518.
        [PMID: 474708]

[6]   Yamamoto T, Ito T, Asano Y, *et al.* Characteristics of Japanese patients with eosinophilic fasciitis: A brief multicenter study. J Dermatol 2020; 47(12): 1391-4.
        [http://dx.doi.org/10.1111/1346-8138.15561] [PMID: 32860239]

[7]   Atherton DJ, Wells RS. (8)? Scleredema of Buschke? Eosinophilic fasciitis. Br J Dermatol 1976; 95 (Suppl. 14): 36-7.
        [http://dx.doi.org/10.1111/j.1365-2133.1976.tb07902.x] [PMID: 1084154]

[8] Weinstein D, Schwartz RA. Eosinophilic Fasciitis. Arch Dermatol 1978; 114(7): 1047-9.
[http://dx.doi.org/10.1001/archderm.1978.01640190035012] [PMID: 686723]

[9] Krauser RE, Tuthill RJ. Eosinophilic Fasciitis. Arch Dermatol 1977; 113(8): 1092-3.
[http://dx.doi.org/10.1001/archderm.1977.01640080094017] [PMID: 889336]

[10] Lupton GP, Goette DK. Localized eosinophilic fasciitis. Arch Dermatol 1979; 115(1): 85-7.
[http://dx.doi.org/10.1001/archderm.1979.04010010057017] [PMID: 760665]

[11] Jarratt M, Bybee JD, Ramsdell W. Eosinophilic fasciitis: An early variant of scleroderma. J Am Acad Dermatol 1979; 1(3): 221-6.
[http://dx.doi.org/10.1016/S0190-9622(79)70013-2] [PMID: 512071]

[12] Nassonova VA, Ivanova MM, Akhnazarova VD, *et al.* Eosinophilic fasciitis. Review and report of six cases. Scand J Rheumatol 1979; 8(4): 225-33.
[http://dx.doi.org/10.3109/03009747909114628] [PMID: 534317]

[13] Haim S, Friedman-Birnbaum R, Kerner H. Cutaneous sclerosis in eosinophilic fasciitis. Dermatology 1979; 159(6): 482-8.
[http://dx.doi.org/10.1159/000250661] [PMID: 510651]

[14] Abeles M, Belin DC, Zurier RB. Eosinophilic fasciitis. Arch Intern Med 1979; 139(5): 586-8.
[http://dx.doi.org/10.1001/archinte.1979.03630420072023] [PMID: 444327]

[15] Chalmers IM, Bhoola KD, Parsoo I. Eosinophilic fasciitis. A case report. S Afr Med J 1979; 55(7): 262-4.
[PMID: 441869]

[16] Robinson JK. Eosinophilic fasciitis: A problem in differential diagnosis. J Dermatol Surg Oncol 1979; 5(10): 780-3.
[http://dx.doi.org/10.1111/j.1524-4725.1979.tb00752.x] [PMID: 500924]

[17] Thivolet J, Jeune R, Faure M, Hermier C, Michel F. Shulman's syndrome: Eosinophilic fasciitis. Ann Dermatol Venereol 1979; 106(11): 859-66.
[PMID: 539697]

[18] Moore TL, Zuckner J. Eosinophilic fasciitis. Semin Arthritis Rheum 1980; 9(3): 228-35.
[http://dx.doi.org/10.1016/0049-0172(80)90009-8] [PMID: 6988969]

[19] Janin-Mercier A, Bourges M, Fonck-Cussac Y, Bussieres JL, Leblanc B, Delage J. Eosinophilic fasciitis ultrastructural study of an early biopsied case. Virchows Arch A Pathol Anat Histol 1981; 394(1-2): 177-84.
[http://dx.doi.org/10.1007/BF00431676] [PMID: 7336573]

[20] Solomon G, Barland P, Rifkin H. Eosinophilic fasciitis responsive to cimetidine. Ann Intern Med 1982; 97(4): 547-9.
[http://dx.doi.org/10.7326/0003-4819-97-4-547] [PMID: 7125411]

[21] Kennedy C, Leak A. Eosinophilic fasciitis with erosive arthritis. Clin Exp Dermatol 1982; 7(5): 469-76.
[http://dx.doi.org/10.1111/j.1365-2230.1982.tb02462.x] [PMID: 7172485]

[22] Naguwa SM, Robbins DL, Castles JJ. Eosinophilic fasciitis: A distinct clinical entity? Am J Med Sci 1983; 286(2): 32-5.
[http://dx.doi.org/10.1097/00000441-198309000-00006] [PMID: 6614045]

[23] Allen SC. Eosinophilic fasciitis in an African—possible benefit of chloroquine treatment. Postgrad Med J 1984; 60(708): 685-6.
[http://dx.doi.org/10.1136/pgmj.60.708.685] [PMID: 6494091]

[24] Silverman ED, Adornato BT, Miller JJ III. Eosinophilic fasciitis in a two-year-old child. Arthritis Rheum 1985; 28(8): 948-51.
[http://dx.doi.org/10.1002/art.1780280817] [PMID: 4026891]

[25]   Piette WW, Dorsey JK, Foucar E. Clinical and serologic expression of localized scleroderma. J Am Acad Dermatol 1985; 13(2): 342-50.
[http://dx.doi.org/10.1016/S0190-9622(85)70172-7] [PMID: 3875636]

[26]   Jones HR Jr, Beetham WP Jr, Silverman ML, Margles SW. Eosinophilic fasciitis and the carpal tunnel syndrome. J Neurol Neurosurg Psychiatry 1986; 49(3): 324-7.
[http://dx.doi.org/10.1136/jnnp.49.3.324] [PMID: 3958745]

[27]   Narayanan MN, Yin JAL, Love EM, *et al.* Eosinophilic fasciitis and aplastic anaemia. Clin Lab Haematol 1988; 10(4): 471-4.
[http://dx.doi.org/10.1111/j.1365-2257.1988.tb01197.x] [PMID: 3250793]

[28]   Valentini G, Rossiello R, Gualdieri L, Tirri G, Gerster JC, Frenck E. Morphea developing in patients previously affected with eosinophilic fasciitis. Rheumatol Int 1988; 8(5): 235-7.
[http://dx.doi.org/10.1007/BF00269201] [PMID: 3238279]

[29]   Grisanti MW, Moore TL, Osborn TG, Haber PL. Eosinophilic fasciitis in children. Semin Arthritis Rheum 1989; 19(3): 151-7.
[http://dx.doi.org/10.1016/0049-0172(89)90027-9] [PMID: 2690343]

[30]   Thomson GTD, MacDougall B, Watson PH, Chalmers IM. Eosinophilic fasciitis in a pair of siblings. Arthritis Rheum 1989; 32(1): 96-9.
[http://dx.doi.org/10.1002/anr.1780320117] [PMID: 2912468]

[31]   Cotsarelis G, Werth V. Tryptophan-induced eosinophilic fasciitis. J Am Acad Dermatol 1990; 23(5): 938-41.
[http://dx.doi.org/10.1016/S0190-9622(08)80704-9] [PMID: 2254484]

[32]   Margo M, Altomonte L, Zoli A, Mirone L, Massi G, Federico F. Eosinophilic fasciitis associated with inflammatory neutrophilic vasculitis. Rheumatology 1990; 29(2): 145-6.
[http://dx.doi.org/10.1093/rheumatology/29.2.145] [PMID: 2322770]

[33]   Hamilton ME. Eosinophilic fasciitis associated with L-tryptophan ingestion. Ann Rheum Dis 1991; 50(1): 55-6.
[http://dx.doi.org/10.1136/ard.50.1.55] [PMID: 1994870]

[34]   Ching DW, Petrie JP. Childhood eosinophilic fasciitis presenting as inflammatory polyarthritis and associated with selective IgA deficiency. Ann Rheum Dis 1991; 50(9): 647-8.
[http://dx.doi.org/10.1136/ard.50.9.647] [PMID: 1929589]

[35]   Chalker RB, Dickey BF, Rosenthal NC, Simms RW. Extrapulmonary thoracic restriction (hidebound chest) complicating eosinophilic fasciitis. Chest 1991; 100(5): 1453-5.
[http://dx.doi.org/10.1378/chest.100.5.1453] [PMID: 1935312]

[36]   Ishikawa A, Akahosi T, Okada J, Kondo H, Kasiwazaki S. A case of the eosinophilia-myalgia syndrome. Ryumachi 1992; 32(4): 327-30.
[PMID: 1411794]

[37]   Ching DWT, Leibowitz MR. Ketotifen: A therapeutic agent of eosinophilic fasciitis? J Intern Med 1992; 231(5): 555-9.
[http://dx.doi.org/10.1111/j.1365-2796.1992.tb00974.x] [PMID: 1602294]

[38]   Wong AL, Anderson-Wilms N, Mortensen SE, Colburn KK. Eosinophilic fasciitis in association with chronic vasculitic-like leg ulcerations. Clin Rheumatol 1993; 12(1): 85-8.
[http://dx.doi.org/10.1007/BF02231565] [PMID: 8467618]

[39]   Gaffney K, Kearns G, Moraes D, O'Dowd JF, Casey EB. Eosinophilic fasciitis: A good response with conservative treatment. Ir J Med Sci 1993; 162(7): 256-7.
[http://dx.doi.org/10.1007/BF02957573] [PMID: 8407264]

[40]   Juncà J, Cuxart A, Tural C, Ojanguren I, Flores A. Eosinophilic fasciitis and non-Hodgkin lymphoma. Eur J Haematol 1994; 52(5): 304-6.

[http://dx.doi.org/10.1111/j.1600-0609.1994.tb00101.x] [PMID: 8020630]

[41] O'Laughlin TJ, Klima RR, Kenney DE. Rehabilitation of eosinophilic fasciitis. A case report. Am J Phys Med Rehabil 1994; 73(4): 286-92.
[http://dx.doi.org/10.1097/00002060-199407000-00012] [PMID: 8043253]

[42] Baffoni L, Frisoni M, Maccaferri M, Ferri S. Systemic lupus erythematosus and eosinophilic fasciitis: An unusual association. Clin Rheumatol 1995; 14(5): 591-2.
[http://dx.doi.org/10.1007/BF02208164] [PMID: 8549105]

[43] Hashimoto Y, Takahashi H, Matsuo S, *et al.* Polymerase chain reaction of Borrelia burgdorferi flagellin gene in Shulman syndrome. Dermatology 1996; 192(2): 136-9.
[http://dx.doi.org/10.1159/000246339] [PMID: 8829496]

[44] Achurra AF, Mendieta MC, Llerena JM, Benitez R. Fasciitis eosinofílica. Presentación de un caso clínico y conceptos actuales para el diagnóstico y tratamiento. Rev Med Panama 1997; 22(1): 39-44. [Eosinophilic fasciitis. A report of a clinical case and the current concepts for its diagnosis and treatment].
[PMID: 9805093]

[45] Smith JD, Chang KL, Gums JG. Possible lansoprazole-induced eosinophilic syndrome. Ann Pharmacother 1998; 32(2): 196-200.
[http://dx.doi.org/10.1345/aph.17190] [PMID: 9496405]

[46] Bachmeyer C, Monge M, Dhôte R, Sanguina M, Aractingi S, Mougeot-Martin M. Eosinophilic fasciitis following idiopathic thrombocytopenic purpura, autoimmune hemolytic anemia and Hashimoto's disease. Dermatology 1999; 199(3): 282.
[http://dx.doi.org/10.1159/000018271] [PMID: 10592421]

[47] Hayashi N, Igarashi A, Matsuyama T, Harada S. Eosinophilic fasciitis following exposure to trichloroethylene: Successful treatment with cyclosporin. Br J Dermatol 2000; 142(4): 830-2.
[http://dx.doi.org/10.1046/j.1365-2133.2000.03446.x] [PMID: 10792252]

[48] Vannucci P, Gaeta P, Riccioni N. Association of Eosinophilic fasciitis and epileptic seizure. Clin Rheumatol 2001; 20(3): 223-4.
[http://dx.doi.org/10.1007/s100670170070] [PMID: 11434478]

[49] Quintero-Del-Rio AI, Punaro M, Pascual V. Faces of eosinophilic fasciitis in childhood. J Clin Rheumatol 2002; 8(2): 99-103.
[http://dx.doi.org/10.1097/00124743-200204000-00007] [PMID: 17041331]

[50] Jacob SE, Lodha R, Cohen JJ, Romanelli P, Kirsner RS. Paraneoplastic eosinophilic fasciitis: A case report. Rheumatol Int 2003; 23(5): 262-4.
[http://dx.doi.org/10.1007/s00296-003-0317-0] [PMID: 12734672]

[51] Owens WE IV, Bertorini TE, Holt HT Jr, Shadle MK. Diffuse fasciitis with eosinophilia (shulman syndrome). J Clin Neuromuscul Dis 2004; 6(2): 99-101.
[http://dx.doi.org/10.1097/00131402-200412000-00005] [PMID: 19078756]

[52] Carneiro S, Brotas A, Lamy F, *et al.* Eosinophilic fasciitis (Shulman syndrome). Cutis 2005; 75(4): 228-32.
[PMID: 15916220]

[53] Pillen S, Engelen B, Hoogen F, Fiselier T, Vossen P, Drost G. Eosinophilic fasciitis in a child mimicking a myopathy. Neuromuscul Disord 2006; 16(2): 144-8.
[http://dx.doi.org/10.1016/j.nmd.2005.12.001] [PMID: 16427783]

[54] Endo Y, Tamura A, Matsushima Y, *et al.* Eosinophilic fasciitis: report of two cases and a systematic review of the literature dealing with clinical variables that predict outcome. Clin Rheumatol 2007; 26(9): 1445-51.
[http://dx.doi.org/10.1007/s10067-006-0525-6] [PMID: 17345001]

[55] Jaimes-Hernández J, Irene Meléndez-Mercado C, Aranda-Pereira P. Fascitis eosinofílica, respuesta

favorable al tratamiento con ciclosporina A. Reumatol Clin 2008; 4(2): 55-8.
[http://dx.doi.org/10.1016/S1699-258X(08)71800-X] [PMID: 21794498]

[56] Ronneberger M, Janka R, Schett G, Manger B. Can MRI substitute for biopsy in eosinophilic fasciitis? Ann Rheum Dis 2009; 68(10): 1651-2.
[http://dx.doi.org/10.1136/ard.2008.103903] [PMID: 19748919]

[57] Servy A, Clérici T, Malines C, Le Parc JM, Côté JF. Eosinophilic fasciitis: A rare skin sclerosis. Pathol Res Int 2010; 2011: 716935.
[PMID: 21151540]

[58] Chun JH, Lee KH, Sung MS, Park CJ. Two cases of eosinophilic fasciitis. Ann Dermatol 2011; 23(1): 81-4.
[http://dx.doi.org/10.5021/ad.2011.23.1.81] [PMID: 21738370]

[59] Manzini CU, Sebastiani M, Giuggioli D, et al. D-penicillamine in the treatment of eosinophilic fasciitis: Case reports and review of the literature. Clin Rheumatol 2012; 31(1): 183-7.
[http://dx.doi.org/10.1007/s10067-011-1866-3] [PMID: 21989991]

[60] Lese AB, Dodds SD. Eosinophilic fasciitis: Case report. J Hand Surg Am 2013; 38(11): 2204-7.
[http://dx.doi.org/10.1016/j.jhsa.2013.08.106] [PMID: 24206984]

[61] Alonso-Castro L, de las Heras E, Moreno C, et al. Eosinophilic fasciitis/generalized morphea overlap successfully treated with azathioprine. Int J Dermatol 2014; 53(11): 1386-8.
[http://dx.doi.org/10.1111/j.1365-4632.2012.05741.x] [PMID: 24697582]

[62] Espinoza F, Jorgensen C, Pers YM. Efficacy of Tocilizumab in the treatment of Eosinophilic fasciitis: Report of one case. Joint Bone Spine 2015; 82(6): 460-1.
[http://dx.doi.org/10.1016/j.jbspin.2015.02.008] [PMID: 26162635]

[63] Whitlock JB, Dimberg EL, Selcen D, Rubin DI. Eosinophilic fasciitis with subjacent myositis. Muscle Nerve 2017; 56(3): 525-9.
[http://dx.doi.org/10.1002/mus.25492] [PMID: 27875630]

[64] Sato T, Goto M, Takeo N, Hatano Y. Case of generalized morphea with the manifestation of diffuse systemic cutaneous sclerosis without sclerodactyly. J Dermatol 2018; 45(5): e100-1.
[http://dx.doi.org/10.1111/1346-8138.14155] [PMID: 29215147]

[65] El-Jammal T, Gerfaud-Valentin M, Durupt F, et al. Eosinophilic fasciitis and common variable immunodeficiency: An unusual association and literature review. J Allergy Clin Immunol Pract 2019; 7(8): 2848-2849.e1.
[http://dx.doi.org/10.1016/j.jaip.2019.06.014] [PMID: 31307966]

[66] Mastrantonio S, Hinds BR, Schneider JA, Sennett R, Cotter DG. An unusual case of morphea in the setting of aplastic anemia. Cureus 2020; 12(4): e7562.
[http://dx.doi.org/10.7759/cureus.7562] [PMID: 32382464]

[67] Jiménez-García N, Aguilar-García J, Fernández-Canedo I, Blázquez-Sánchez N, Fúnez-Liébana R, Romero-Gómez C. Eosinophilic fasciitis in a pregnant woman with corticosteroid dependence and good response to infliximab. heumatol Int 2021; 41(8): 1531-9.

[68] Asaoka K, Watanabe Y, Itoh K, et al. A case of eosinophilic fasciitis without skin manifestations: A case report in a patient with lupus and literature review. Clin Rheumatol 2021; 40(6): 2477-83.
[http://dx.doi.org/10.1007/s10067-020-05416-6] [PMID: 32974835]

[69] Daniels P, Shilian R, Huq M, Hostoffer R. Eosinophilic fasciitis in common variable immunodeficiency with hypereosinophilia. Ann Allergy Asthma Immunol 2021; 126(1): 99-100.
[http://dx.doi.org/10.1016/j.anai.2020.08.395] [PMID: 32891788]

[70] Pinal-Fernandez I, Selva-O' Callaghan A, Grau JM. Diagnosis and classification of eosinophilic fasciitis. Autoimmun Rev 2014; 13(4-5): 379-82.
[http://dx.doi.org/10.1016/j.autrev.2014.01.019] [PMID: 24424187]

[71]   Ihn H. Eosinophilic fasciitis: From pathophysiology to treatment. Allergol Int 2019; 68(4): 437-9.
[http://dx.doi.org/10.1016/j.alit.2019.03.001] [PMID: 30910631]

[72]   Wollina U, Hansel G, Schönlebe J, *et al.* Eosinophilic fasciitis: Report of three cases and review of the literature. Open Access Maced J Med Sci 2019; 7(18): 2964-8.
[http://dx.doi.org/10.3889/oamjms.2019.296] [PMID: 31850100]

[73]   Falanga V, Soter NA, Kerdel FA. Increased plasma histamine level in eosinophilic fasciitis. Arch Dermatol 1989; 125(6): 805-8.
[http://dx.doi.org/10.1001/archderm.1989.01670180077010] [PMID: 2730101]

[74]   Mertens JS, Seyger MMB, Thurlings RM, Radstake TRDJ, de Jong EMGJ. Morphea and eosinophilic fasciitis: An update. Am J Clin Dermatol 2017; 18(4): 491-512.
[http://dx.doi.org/10.1007/s40257-017-0269-x] [PMID: 28303481]

[75]   Huang KW, Chen XH. Pathology of eosinophilic fasciitis and its relation to polymyositis. Can J Neurol Sci 1987; 14(4): 632-7.
[PMID: 3690437]

[76]   Mazori DR, Femia AN, Vleugels RA. Eosinophilic fasciitis: An updated review on diagnosis and treatment. Curr Rheumatol Rep 2017; 19(12): 74.
[http://dx.doi.org/10.1007/s11926-017-0700-6] [PMID: 29101481]

[77]   Mondal S, Goswami RP, Sinha D, Ghosh A. Ultrasound is a useful adjunct in diagnosis of eosinophilic fasciitis: Fig. 1. Rheumatology 2015; 54(11): 2041.
[http://dx.doi.org/10.1093/rheumatology/kev290] [PMID: 26316576]

[78]   Kim HJ, Lee SW, Kim GJ, Lee JH. Usefulness of FDG PET/CT in the diagnosis of eosinophilic fasciitis. Clin Nucl Med 2014; 39(9): 801-2.
[http://dx.doi.org/10.1097/RLU.0000000000000260] [PMID: 24152641]

[79]   Haddad H, Sundaram S, Magro C, Gergis U. Eosinophilic fasciitis as a paraneoplastic syndrome. A case report and review of the literature. Hematol Oncol Stem Cell Ther 2014; 7(2): 90-2.
[http://dx.doi.org/10.1016/j.hemonc.2013.12.003] [PMID: 24525268]

[80]   Watanabe Y, Yamamoto M, Yamamoto T. A case of eosinophilic fasciitis and generalized morphea overlap. Dermatol Online J 2020; 26(2): 13030/qt96f64417.https://escholarship.org/uc/item/96f64417
[http://dx.doi.org/10.5070/D3262047425]

[81]   Peterson LS, Nelson AM, Su WP, Mason T, O'Fallon WM, Gabriel SE. The epidemiology of morphea (localized scleroderma) in Olmsted County 1960-1993. J Rheumatol 1997; 24(1): 73-80.
[PMID: 9002014]

[82]   Bielsa Marsol I. Update on the classification and treatment of localized scleroderma. Actas Dermo-Sifiliográficas 2013; 104(8): 654-66.
[http://dx.doi.org/10.1016/j.adengl.2012.10.012] [PMID: 23948159]

SUBJECT INDEX

www.ingramcontent.com/pod-product-compliance
Lightning Source LLC
Chambersburg PA
CBHW080018240326